ANNALS OF THE NEW YORK ACADEMY OF SCIENCES

Volume 1005

EDITORIAL STAFF

Director, Publishing and New Media
SARAH GREENE

Managing Editor
JUSTINE CULLINAN

Associate Editor
STEFAN MALMOLI

The New York Academy of Sciences
2 East 63rd Street
New York, New York 10021

THE NEW YORK ACADEMY OF SCIENCES
(Founded in 1817)

BOARD OF GOVERNORS, September 2003 – September 2004

TORSTEN N. WIESEL, *Chairman of the Board*
GERALD D. FISCHBACH, *Vice Chairman*
JOHN T. MORGAN, *Treasurer*
ELLIS RUBINSTEIN, *Chief Executive Officer* [ex officio]

Honorary Life Governors
WILLIAM T. GOLDEN   JOSHUA LEDERBERG

Governors

KAREN E. BURKE	PETER B. CORR	R. BRIAN FERGUSON
RONALD L. GRAHAM	MARNIE IMHOFF	WENDY EVANS JOSEPH
JACQUELINE LEO	RODERT W. LUCKY	PAUL MARKS
BRUCE McEWEN	RONAY MENSCHEL	JOHN F. NIBLACK
SANDRA PANEM	PETER RINGROSE	DAVID D. SABATINI
	LEE G. VANCE	DEBORAH WILEY

HELENE L. KAPLAN, *Counsel* [ex officio]   LARRY R. SMITH, *Secretary* [ex officio]

IMMUNOLOGY OF DIABETES II
PATHOGENESIS FROM MOUSE TO MAN

ANNALS OF THE NEW YORK ACADEMY OF SCIENCES

Volume 1005
November 2003

IMMUNOLOGY OF DIABETES II
PATHOGENESIS FROM MOUSE TO MAN

Editors
C. B. SANJEEVI AND G. S. EISENBARTH

This volume is the result of the **Sixth International Congress of the Immunology of Diabetes Society and American Diabetes Association Research Symposium**, held October 3–6, 2002, in Copper Mountain, Colorado.

CONTENTS

Preface. *By* C. B. SANJEEVI AND G. S. EISENBARTH.....................	xiii
The Second Murine Autoantibody Workshop: Remarkable Interlaboratory Concordance for Radiobinding Assays to Identify Insulin Autoantibodies in Nonobese Diabetic Mice. *By* LIPING YU, GEORGE EISENBARTH, EZIO BONIFACIO, JAMES THOMAS, MARK ATKINSON, AND CLIVE WASSERFALL..	1

Part I. Environmental Triggers of Autoimmunity

Can Enteroviruses Cause Type 1 Diabetes? *By* SISKO TAURIAINEN, KIMMO SALMINEN, AND HEIKKI HYÖTY.................................	13
Establishing Evidence for Enterovirus Infection in Chronic Disease. *By* M. STEVEN OBERSTE AND MARK A. PALLANSCH.................	23

Part II. Beta Cell Death and Protection

Beta Cell Death and Protection. *By* THOMAS MANDRUP-POULSEN..........	32
Oxidative Stress in Type 1 Diabetes. *By* KATHRYN HASKINS, BRENDA BRADLEY, KATHERINE POWERS, VALERIE FADOK, SONIA FLORES, XIAOFENG LING, SUBBIAH PUGAZHENTHI, JANE REUSCH, AND JENNIFER KENCH..	43

Use of Microarray Analysis to Unveil Transcription Factor and Gene Networks Contributing to β Cell Dysfunction and Apoptosis. *By* DECIO L. EIZIRIK, BURAK KUTLU, JOANNE RASSCHAERT, MARTINE DARVILLE, AND ALESSANDRA K. CARDOZO 55

Part III. Immunoregulation

The T Cell Response to Glutamic Acid Decarboxylase 65 in T Cell Receptor Transgenic NOD Mice. *By* HUGH MCDEVITT 75

Detection of $CD4^+$ Autoreactive T Cells in T1D Using HLA Class II Tetramers. *By* HELENA REIJONEN, WILLIAM W. KWOK, AND GERALD T. NEPOM 82

Kinetic Evolution of a Diabetogenic CD8+ T Cell Response. *By* PERE SANTAMARIA 88

Part IV. Antigen/MHC

Multiple and High-Titer Single Autoantibodies in Schoolchildren Reflecting the Genetic Predisposition for Type 1 Diabetes. *By* MICHAEL SCHLOSSER, RALF WASSMUTH, MARTINA STREBELOW, ILONA RJASANOWSKI, AND MANFRED ZIEGLER 98

Insulin Autoimmunity: Immunogenetics/Immunopathogenesis of Type 1A Diabetes. *By* GEORGE S. EISENBARTH 109

MHC-Linked Susceptibility to Type 1 Diabetes: A Structural Perspective. *By* KAI W. WUCHERPFENNIG 119

Part V. Therapy

Using Regulatory APCs to Induce/Maintain Tolerance. *By* AMY E. JUEDES AND MATTHIAS G. VON HERRATH 128

Cell-Based Therapies for Diabetes: Progress towards a Transplantable Human β Cell Line. *By* PAMELA ITKIN-ANSARI, IFAT GERON, ERGENG HAO, CARLA DEMETERCO, BJORN TYRBERG, AND FRED LEVINE 138

Islet Cell Autoimmunity and Transplantation Tolerance: Two Distinct Mechanisms? *By* TODD PEARSON, THOMAS G. MARKEES, DAVID V. SERREZE, MELISSA A. PIERCE, LINDA S. WICKER, LAURENCE B. PETERSON, LEONARD D. SHULTZ, JOHN P. MORDES, ALDO A. ROSSINI, AND DALE L. GREINER 148

Part VI. Type 1 Diabetes in Animal Models

Characterization of Early Developments in the Splenic Leukocyte Transcriptome of NOD Mice. *By* I. C. GERLING, C. ALI, AND N. LENCHIK 157

Autoimmune Diabetes in the NOD Mouse: An Essential Role of Fas-FasL Signaling in β Cell Apoptosis. *By* DIEGO G. SILVA, LUIS SOCHA, BRETT CHARLTON, WILLIAM COWDEN, AND NIKOLAI PETROVSKY 161

Fas and Fas Ligand Immunoexpression in Pancreatic Islets of NOD Mice during Spontaneous and Cyclophosphamide-Accelerated Diabetes. *By* SHIVA REDDY AND JACQUELINE M. ROSS 166

Type 1 Diabetes in Swedish Bank Voles (*Clethrionomys glareolus*): Signs of Disease in Both Colonized and Wild Cyclic Populations at Peak Density. *By* BO NIKLASSON, BIRGER HÖRNFELDT, ERIK NYHOLM, MATTHIAS NIEDRIG, OLIVER DONOSO-MANTKE, HANS R. GELDERBLOM, AND ÅKE LERNMARK 170

Defective Activation-Induced Cell Death in NOD T Lymphocytes: 1,25-Dihydroxyvitamin D_3 Restores Defect. *By* B. DECALLONNE AND C. MATHIEU 176

The Role of Endoplasmic Reticulum Stress in Nonimmune Diabetes: NOD.k iHEL, a Novel Model of β Cell Death. *By* L. SOCHA, D. SILVA, S. LESAGE, C. GOODNOW, AND N. PETROVSKY 178

Defective Maturation of Myeloid Dendritic Cell (DC) in NOD Mice Is Controlled by IDD10/17/18. *By* RUIHUA PENG, K. BATHJAT, Y. LI, AND M. J. CLARE-SALZLER 184

Absence of the T-bet Gene Coding for the Th1-Related Transcription Factor Does Not Affect Diabetes-Associated Phenotypes in Balb/c Mice. *By* EVIE MELANITOU, EDWIN LIU, DONGMEI MIAO, LIPING YU, LAURIE H. GLIMCHER, AND GEORGE EISENBARTH 187

Immunolocalization of Caspase-3 in Pancreatic Islets of NOD Mice during Cyclophosphamide-Accelerated Diabetes. *By* SHIVA REDDY, JOSHUA BRADLEY, AND JACQUELINE M. ROSS 192

Congenic Mapping and Candidate Sequencing of Susceptibility Genes for Type 1 Diabetes in the NOD Mouse. *By* HIROSHI IKEGAMI, TOMOMI FUJISAWA, SUSUMU MAKINO, AND TOSHIO OGIHARA 196

Establishing Insulin 1 and Insulin 2 Knockout Congenic Strains on NOD Genetic Background. *By* JOHANNA PARONEN, HIROAKI MORIYAMA, NORIO ABIRU, KAMILA SIKORA, EVIE MELANITOU, SUNANDA BABU, FEI BAO, EDWIN LIU, DONGMEI MIAO, AND GEORGE S. EISENBARTH .. 205

Relationship between β Cell Mass of NOD Donors and Diabetes Development of NOD-scid Recipients in Adoptive Transfer System. *By* SATORU YAMADA, AKIRA SHIMADA, KEIICHI KODAMA, JIRO MORIMOTO, RYUJI SUZUKI, YOICHI OIKAWA, JUNICHIRO IRIE, AND TAKAO SARUTA 211

Hen Egg White Lysozyme Vaccination Induces Acute Shock in NOD Mice. *By* DUMITRU D. BRANISTEANU, LUTGART OVERBERGH, BRIGITTE DECALLONNE, AND CHANTAL MATHIEU 215

In Vivo Expression of B:9–23 Peptide/I-A^{g7} Complex May Abrogate the Inhibition of Diabetes Induced by RGD-Fiber-Mutant Adenovirus in NOD Mice. *By* NORIO ABIRU, FUYAN SUN, EIJI KAWASAKI, HIRONORI YAMASAKI, KATSUYA OSHIMA, YUJI NAGAYAMA, HIROYUKI MIZUGUCHI, TAKAO HAYAKAWA, DONGMEI MIAO, EDWIN LIU, GEORGE S. EISENBARTH, AND KATSUMI EGUCHI 218

Part VII. Type 1 Diabetes in Humans—Immunology

Abnormal Peripheral Blood Dendritic Cell Populations in Type 1 Diabetes. *By* RUIHUA PENG, Y. LI, K. BREZNER, SALLY LITHERLAND, AND M. J. CLARE-SALZLER 222

Characterization of Dendritic Cells in Humans with Type 1 Diabetes.
By KELLY L. SUMMERS, MARGARET T. BEHME, JEFFERY L. MAHON,
AND BHAGIRATH SINGH.. 226

NKT Cell Frequency in Japanese Type 1 Diabetes. *By* YOICHI OIKAWA,
AKIRA SHIMADA, SATORU YAMADA, YOSHIKO MOTOHASHI,
YOSHINORI NAKAGAWA, JUN-ICHIRO IRIE, TARO MARUYAMA,
AND TAKAO SARUTA... 230

IL-6 Modulates Hyperglycemia-Induced Changes of Na+ Channel Beta-3
Subunit Expression by Schwann Cells. *By* DUSANKA S. SKUNDRIC,
RUJUAN DAI, AND PHILIP MATAVERDE............................. 233

Glucose-Responsive Expression of the Human Insulin Promoter in HepG2
Human Hepatoma Cells. *By* BRANT R. BURKHARDT, SCOTT A. LOILER,
JO ANNE ANDERSON, MICHAEL S. KILBERG, JAMES M. CRAWFORD,
TERENCE R. FLOTTE, KEVIN S. GOUDY, TAMIR M. ELLIS,
AND MARK ATKINSON.. 237

Interleukin-6 Protects MIN6 β Cells from Cytokine-Induced Apoptosis.
By HYEWON PARK, YUHERN AHN, CHUNG-KYU PARK, HEE-YONG
CHUNG, AND YONGSOO PARK..................................... 242

Part VIII. Type 1 Diabetes in Humans—Antigens and Antibodies

A Diabetes-Related Epitope of GAD65: A Major Diabetes-Related Conformational Epitope on GAD65. *By* MARK A. MYERS, GUSTAVO FENALTI,
ROBYN GRAY, MARITA SCEALY, JONATHAN C. TONG, OSSAMA
EL-KABBANI, AND MERRILL J. ROWLEY........................... 250

SOX13 Autoantibodies Are Likely to Be a Supplementary Marker for Type 1
Diabetes in Korea. *By* YONGSOO PARK, HYEWON PARK, EUNKYUNG
YOO, AND DUKHEE KIM.. 253

Development and Validation of a Radioligand Binding Assay to Measure
Insulin Specific IgG Subclass Antibodies in Human Serum.
By D. FINCO-KENT, A. MORRONE, M. MOXNESS, V. BEDIAN,
A. KRASNER, J. FOLEY, M. STENE, AND T. KAWABATA.............. 259

Development and Validation of Radioligand Binding Assays to Measure
Total, IgA, IgE, IgG, and IgM Insulin Antibodies in Human Serum.
By MICHAEL MOXNESS, JIM FOLEY, MARK STENE, DEBORAH FINCO-
KENT, VAHE BEDIAN, ALAN KRASNER, AND THOMAS KAWABATA..... 265

Induction of Diabetes-Related Autoantibodies below Cutoff for "Positivity" in
Young Nondiabetic Children. *By* HANNA HOLMBERG, OUTI VAARALA,
KARIN FÄLTH-MAGNUSSON, AND JOHNNY LUDVIGSSON.............. 269

Cow-Milk-Free Diet during Last Trimester of Pregnancy Does Not Influence
Diabetes-Related Autoantibodies in Nondiabetic Children.
By JOHNNY LUDVIGSSON... 275

Difference in Gene Expression Profiles between Human CD4+CD25+ and
CD4+CD25− T Cells. *By* NIRUPMA PATI, SOUMITRA GHOSH,
MARTIN J. HESSNER, HUOY-JII KHOO, AND XUJING WANG........... 279

The Design of a Gene Chip for Functional Immunological Studies on a High-
Quality Control Platform. *By* JILL WAUKAU, PARTHAV JAILWALA,
YOUMIN WANG, HUOY-JII KHOO, SOUMITRA GHOSH, XUJING WANG,
AND MARTIN J. HESSNER....................................... 284

Relationship between T and B Cell Responses to Proinsulin in Human Type 1 Diabetes. *By* IVANA DURINOVIC-BELLÓ, NICOLA MAISEL, MICHAEL SCHLOSSER, HUBERT KALBACHER, MARTIN DEEG, THOMAS EIERMANN, WOLFRAM KARGES, AND BERNHARD O. BOEHM 288

Part IX. Type 1 Diabetes in Humans—Genetics

Inheritance of MHC Class II Genes in Lithuanian Families with Type 1 Diabetes. *By* VAIVA SADAUSKAITE-KUEHNE, KEN VEYS, JOHNNY LUDVIGSSON, ZILVINAS PADAIGA, AND CARANI B. SANJEEVI 295

Ethnic Differences in the Associations between the HLA-DRB1*04 Subtypes and Type 1 Diabetes. *By* AMANDA REWERS, SUNANDA BABU, TIAN BAO WANG, TEODORICA L. BUGAWAN, KATHY BARRIGA, GEORGE S. EISENBARTH, AND HENRY A. ERLICH 301

MIC-A Genotypes 4/5.1 and 9/9 Are Positively Associated with Type 1 Diabetes Mellitus in Brazilian Population. *By* VALERIA TICA, LIENE NIKITINA-ZAKE, EDUARDO DONADI, AND CARANI B. SANJEEVI 310

HLA-DRB1 and *MICA* in Autoimmunity: Common Associated Alleles in Autoimmune Disorders. *By* J. RAMÓN BILBAO, AINHOA MARTÍN-PAGOLA, GUIOMAR PÉREZ DE NANCLARES, BEGOÑA CALVO, JUAN CARLOS VITORIA, FEDERICO VÁZQUEZ, AND LUIS CASTAÑO 314

5'-Insulin Gene VNTR Polymorphism Is Specific for Type 1 Diabetes: No Association with Celiac nor Addison's Disease. *By* GUIOMAR PÉREZ DE NANCLARES, J. RAMÓN BILBAO, BEGOÑA CALVO, JUAN CARLOS VITORIA, FEDERICO VÁZQUEZ, AND LUIS CASTAÑO 319

Nicotinamide Adenine Dinucleotide Phosphate Oxidase (NADPH Oxidase) P22 Phox C242T Gene Polymorphism in Type 1 Diabetes. *By* SEIKO MATSUNAGA, TARO MARUYAMA, SATORU YAMADA, YOSHIKO MOTOHASHI, TOSHIKATSU SHIGIHARA, AKIRA SHIMADA, AND TAKAO SARUTA 324

Stromal Cell-Derived Factor-1 Chemokine Gene Polymorphism Is Not Associated with Onset Age of Japanese Type 1 Diabetes. *By* TOSHIKATSU SHIGIHARA, AKIRA SHIMADA, SATORU YAMADA, TARO MARUYAMA, HIROSHI HIROSE, AND TAKAO SARUTA 328

Mutation Scan of a Type 1 Diabetes Candidate Gene: The Human Interleukin-18 Binding Protein Gene. *By* RÚNA L. NOLSØE, FLEMMING POCIOT, DANIELA NOVICK, MENACHEM RUBINSTEIN, SOO-HYUN KIM, CHARLES A. DINARELLO, AND THOMAS MANDRUP-POULSEN 332

Caspase 7 Is a Positional Candidate Gene for IDDM 17 in a Bedouin Arab Family. *By* SUNANDA R. BABU, FEI BAO, CHRISTINE M. ROBERTS, ALLISON K. MARTIN, KATHERINE GOWAN, GEORGE S. EISENBARTH, AND PAMELA R. FAIN 340

Interleukin-10 Gene Promoter Region Polymorphisms in Patients with Type 1 Diabetes and Autoimmune Thyroid Disease. *By* AKANE IDE, EIJI KAWASAKI, NORIO ABIRU, FUYAN SUN, TETSUYA FUKUSHIMA, REIKO ISHII, RYOKO TAKAHASHI, HIRONAGA KUWAHARA, NARUHIRO FUJITA, ATSUSHI KITA, MISA IMAIZUMI, KATSUYA OSHIMA, TOSHIRO USA, SHIGEO UOTANI, ERI EJIMA, HIRONORI YAMASAKI, KIYOTO ASHIZAWA, YOSHIHIKO YAMAGUCHI, AND KATSUMI EGUCHI 344

Single Nucleotide Polymorphism Study of IDDM 17 in a Bedouin Arab Family. *By* FEI BAO, SUNANDA R. BABU, CHRISTINE M. ROBERTS, ALLISON K. MARTIN, KATHERINE GOWAN, GEORGE S. EISENBARTH, AND PAMELA R. FAIN.. 348

No Evidence for Linkage in Swedish Multiplex T1DM Families to IL12B on Chromosome 5q33–34. *By* PERNILLA HOLM, HOLGER LUTHMAN, AND INGRID KOCKUM.. 352

Part X. LADA

Frequency of Latent Autoimmune Diabetes in Adults in Asian Patients Diagnosed as Type 2 Diabetes in Birmingham, United Kingdom. *By* VALERIA TICA, M. WASIM HANIF, ANNIKA ANDERSSON, G. VALSAMAKIS, A. H. BARNETT, SUDESH KUMAR, AND C. B. SANJEEVI............... 356

Two Cases of "Fulminant" Type 1 Diabetes Suggesting Involvement of Autoimmunity. *By* YOSHINORI NAKAGAWA, AKIRA SHIMADA, YOICHI OIKAWA, JUN-ICHIRO IRIE, TOSHIKATSU SHIGIHARA, KAZUHIRO TSUMURA, SHOSAKU NARUMI, AND TAKAO SARUTA................. 359

Multicenter Prevention Trial of Slowly Progressive Type 1 Diabetes with Small Dose of Insulin (the Tokyo Study): Preliminary Report. *By* TARO MARUYAMA, AKIRA SHIMADA, AZUMA KANATSUKA, AKIRA KASUGA, IZUMI TAKEI, JUNICHI YOKOYAMA, AND TETSURO KOBAYASHI....... 362

Late-Onset Autoimmune Diabetes in Relatives of People with Type 1 Diabetes. *By* SPIROS FOURLANOS, PETER G. COLMAN, AND LEONARD C. HARRISON....................................... 370

Insulin Resistance in Latent Autoimmune Diabetes of Adulthood. *By* M. T. BEHME, J. DUPRÉ, S. B. HARRIS, I. M. HRAMIAK, AND J. L. MAHON... 374

Detection of GAD-Reactive CD4+ Cells in So-Called "Type 1B" Diabetes. *By* AKIRA SHIMADA, KEIICHI KODAMA, JIRO MORIMOTO, YOICHI OIKAWA, JUNICHIRO IRIE, YOSHINORI NAKAGAWA, KOICHI MATSUBARA, TARO MARUYAMA, AND TAKAO SARUTA............... 378

Autoantibodies to GAD65 and IA-2 Antibodies Are Increased, but Not Tissue Transglutaminase (TTG-Ab) in Type 2 Diabetes Mellitus (T2DM) Patients from South India. *By* C. B. SANJEEVI, M. BALAJI, V. BALAJI, AND V. SESHIAH... 387

IA-2 Autoantibodies Are Predominant in Latent Autoimmune Diabetes in Adults Patients from Eastern India. *By* ALOK KANUNGO AND C. B. SANJEEVI... 390

Part XI. Prediction and Prevention

Parents Want to Know if Their Child Is at High Risk of Getting Diabetes. *By* U. GUSTAFSSON STOLT, P-E. LISS, AND J. LUDVIGSSON FOR THE ABIS STUDY GROUP.. 395

Population-wide Infant Screening for HLA-Based Type 1 Diabetes Risk via Dried Blood Spots from the Public Health Infrastructure. *By* EMILY WION, MICHAEL BRANTLEY, JEFF STEVENS, SUSAN GALLINGER, HUI PENG, MICHAEL GLASS, AND WILLIAM HAGOPIAN............... 400

Vaccinations May Induce Diabetes-Related Autoantibodies in One-Year-Old Children. *By* J. WAHLBERG, J. FREDRIKSSON, O. VAARALA, AND J. LUDVIGSSON FOR THE ABIS STUDY GROUP 404

Inhibition of STAT4 Activation by Lisofylline Is Associated with the Protection of Autoimmune Diabetes. *By* ZANDONG YANG, MENG CHEN, LAWRENCE B. FIALKOW, JUSTIN D. ELLETT, RUNPEI WU, AND JERRY L. NADLER 409

Reduced Thymic Expression of Islet Antigen Contributes to Loss of Self-Tolerance. *By* C. E. MATHEWS, S. L. PIETROPAOLO, AND M. PIETROPAOLO 412

Dietary Microbial Toxins and Type 1 Diabetes. *By* M. A. MYERS, K. D. HETTIARACHCHI, J. P. LUDEMAN, A. J. WILSON, C. R. WILSON, AND P. Z. ZIMMET 418

Prevention of Autoimmune Diabetes through Immunostimulation with Q Fever Complement-Fixing Antigen. *By* D. G. SILVA, B. CHARLTON, W. COWDEN, AND N. PETROVSKY 423

AIRE-1 (Autoimmune Regulator Type 1) as a Regulator of the Thymic Induction of Negative Selection. *By* YONGSOO PARK, YOOMI MOON, AND HEE-YONG CHUNG 431

Association of Interleukin-18 Gene Promoter Polymorphisms in Type 1 Diabetes and Autoimmune Thyroid Disease. *By* AKANE IDE, EIJI KAWASAKI, NORIO ABIRU, FUYAN SUN, TETSUYA FUKUSHIMA, REIKO ISHII, RYOKO TAKAHASHI, HIRONAGA KUWAHARA, NARUHIRO FUJITA, ATSUSHI KITA, MISA IMAIZUMI, KATSUYA OSHIMA, TOSHIRO USA, SHIGEO UOTANI, ERI EJIMA, HIRONORI YAMASAKI, KIYOTO ASHIZAWA, YOSHIHIKO YAMAGUCHI, AND KATSUMI EGUCHI 436

Epitope Analysis of GAD65 Autoantibodies in Japanese Patients with Autoimmune Diabetes. *By* EIJI KAWASAKI, NORIO ABIRU, AKANE IDE, FUYAN SUN, TETSUYA FUKUSHIMA, RYOKO TAKAHASHI, HIRONAGA KUWAHARA, NARUHIRO FUJITA, ATSUSHI KITA, KATSUYA OSHIMA, SHIGEO UOTANI, HIRONORI YAMASAKI, YOSHIHIKO YAMAGUCHI, AND KATSUMI EGUCHI 440

Index of Contributors 449

Financial assistance was received from:

Conference Grants
- JUVENILE DIABETES RESEARCH FOUNDATION
- NATIONAL INSTITUTES OF HEALTH

Contributors
- AVENTIS PHARMACEUTICALS, INCORPORATED
- CENTERS FOR DISEASE CONTROL
- CHILDREN'S DIABETES FOUNDATION
- NEUROCRINE BIOSCIENCES
- NOVO NORDISK
- PFIZER, INCORPORATED
- SANKYO PHARMA RESEARCH INSTITUTE

The New York Academy of Sciences believes it has a responsibility to provide an open forum for discussion of scientific questions. The positions taken by the participants in the reported conferences are their own and not necessarily those of the Academy. The Academy has no intent to influence legislation by providing such forums.

Preface

C. B. SANJEEVI[a] AND G. S. EISENBARTH[b]

[a]Karolinska Institute, Stockholm, Sweden
[b]Barbara Davis Center for Childhood Diabetes, University of Colorado Health Sciences Center, Denver, Colorado, USA

The Immunology of Diabetes Society (IDS), which meets every 18 months in different continents to discuss the progress made by the researchers working in the field of type 1 diabetes, met at Copper Mountain in Colorado in October 2002 for their Sixth International Congress. The meeting was conducted in association with the American Diabetes Association, with chairpersons, Katie Haskins and George Eisenbarth. This volume is produced from the proceedings of the meeting and is entitled *Immunology of Diabetes II: Pathogenesis from Mouse to Man*. This volume is *Immunology of Diabetes II* because the previous IDS meeting held in Chennai, India, in February 2001 produced a volume entitled *Immunology of Diabetes: Autoimmune Mechanisms and the Prevention and Cure of Type 1 Diabetes*.

Workshops are an important component of the IDS conferences. The Sixth IDS meeting conducted autoantibody workshops for both animal models and humans, as well as a T cell workshop. Substantial progress was illustrated by the individual workshop components, plenary lectures, and meet-the-professor sessions. The meeting highlighted important areas like "Environmental Triggers of Autoimmunity", "Beta Cell Death and Protection", "Immunoregulation", "Antigen/MHC", and "Therapy", in addition to oral and poster presentations on type 1 diabetes in mouse models and humans.

Papers selected for this volume represent all these important areas. The next meeting will be held in Cambridge, United Kingdom, in March 2004 under the chairmanship of Edwin Gale.

We would like to thank Valeria Tica, a visiting scientist from Romania to the lab at Karolinska Hospital, for valuable help in putting this volume together. We also would like to thank Robin Parks, Shirley Ash, and Linda Cann for their valuable help with the Sixth IDS meeting. The fine editorial skills of Stefan Malmoli, Associate Editor at the New York Academy of Sciences, must be acknowledged as well.

Address for correspondence: Dr. C. B. Sanjeevi, M.D., M.Sc., Ph.D., Associate Professor, Karolinska Institute, Director, Center for Molecular Medicine, Head, Molecular Immunogenetics Group, Department of Molecular Medicine, Karolinska Hospital, CMM, L8:00, S-171 76 Stockholm, Sweden. Voice: +46-8-517-76254; fax: +46-8-517-76179.
sanjeevi.carani@molmed.ki.se

The Second Murine Autoantibody Workshop

Remarkable Interlaboratory Concordance for Radiobinding Assays to Identify Insulin Autoantibodies in Nonobese Diabetic Mice

LIPING YU,[a] GEORGE EISENBARTH,[a] EZIO BONIFACIO,[b] JAMES THOMAS,[c] MARK ATKINSON,[d] AND CLIVE WASSERFALL[d]

[a]*Barbara Davis Center for Childhood Diabetes, University of Colorado Health Sciences Center, Denver, Colorado, USA*

[b]*Department of Medicine, Istituto Scientifico San Raffaele, Milan, Italy, and Diabetes Research Institute, Munich, Germany*

[c]*Department of Medicine, Vanderbilt University, Nashville, Tennessee, USA*

[d]*Department of Pathology, University of Florida, Gainesville, Florida, USA*

ABSTRACT: In October 2000, the First Murine Autoantibody Workshop was held as part of an *International Workshop on Lessons from Animal Models for Human Type 1 Diabetes*. This first workshop identified insulin, but not glutamic acid decarboxylase (GAD) or IA-2, as specific autoantigens of humoral immunity in nonobese diabetic (NOD) mice. The goals of the Second Murine Autoantibody Workshop, part of the *Sixth Annual Meeting of the IDS*, were to increase the number of participating investigators, attempt standardization of insulin autoantibody (IAA) results across laboratories, identify serologic evidence of humoral immunity to other beta cell antigens, and allow for validation of ELISA assays for autoantibody detection in NOD mice. Sixty-three coded samples (26 pooled NOD sera, 23 pooled C57BL/6 sera, and 14 diluted samples of an anti-insulin monoclonal antibody) were distributed to 12 participating laboratories. This second workshop demonstrated that, for nearly all laboratories, IAA measured by radioimmunoassay (RIA) provided a sensitive and specific assay capable of distinguishing diabetes-prone from nondiabetes-prone mice. Analyses involving the serially diluted anti-insulin monoclonal antibody offered hope that a standard reference unit for reactivity could be established. Surprisingly, two ELISA assays for IAA detection proved remarkably sensitive (i.e., 65% and 92%). However, subsequent absorption studies performed after the workshop (presented at the IDS meeting) brought into question whether ELISA assays for IAA do, in reality, detect anti-insulin immunities and whether assays for GAD and IA-2 autoantibodies distinguish diabetes-prone from nondiabetes-prone mice. In sum, this workshop continued to support the notion that IAA, as determined by RIA, could provide a sensitive and specific marker of anti-beta cell immunity in NOD mice.

KEYWORDS: autoantibodies; insulin; NOD mice; type 1 diabetes

Address for correspondence: Clive Wasserfall, Department of Pathology, University of Florida, Box 100275 JHMHC, 1600 SW Archer Road, Gainesville, FL 32610. Voice: 352-392-0048.
clive@ufl.edu

Ann. N.Y. Acad. Sci. 1005: 1–12 (2003). © 2003 New York Academy of Sciences.
doi: 10.1196/annals.1288.002

INTRODUCTION

Over the past three decades, thousands of articles have been published involving assessment of autoantibodies against islet cells or their products utilizing serum from patients with type 1 diabetes. In addition to their providing an aid in the diagnosis of type 1 diabetes, autoantibodies can also serve as indicators of the prediabetic phase in this disorder.[1,2] Specifically, their presence in persons who otherwise seem healthy denotes a population having an increased risk for later development of the disease.[3] Furthermore, methods involving autoantibody detection are often utilized as the principal means for selection of persons deemed suitable for participation in clinical trials aimed at disease prevention.[1,4] These diagnostic and predictive abilities did not naturally present themselves since much of the early literature (i.e., 1970s to late 1980s) regarding autoantibodies in type 1 diabetes was subject to controversies and conflicting information, factors in large part due to variances in the methods and substrates used for autoantibody detection. Considerable advances towards overcoming these difficulties came through the voluntary performance of many investigators in over a dozen international autoantibody workshops, often organized under the auspices of the Immunology of Diabetes Workshops, an organization that later became known as the Immunology of Diabetes Society (IDS). Among their many findings, these workshops validated insulin, glutamic acid decarboxylase (GAD), and IA-2 as autoantigens associated with type 1 diabetes in humans; identified sensitive and specific methods for autoantibody measurement; and introduced reference standards for diabetes-associated autoantibodies.[5–15]

The nonobese diabetic (NOD) mouse spontaneously develops islet autoimmunity and overt hyperglycemia, and serves as a model for type 1 diabetes of humans.[16] Similar to the human disease, insulin, GAD, and IA-2 have each been implicated as target autoantigens in the NOD mouse. Also similar to studies of humans, some of these works have been conflicting in terms of the frequency of or even the mere presence of specific autoantibodies to these antigens. A recent meeting, sponsored in part by the Juvenile Diabetes Research Foundation (JDRF), was formed to review and assess the proper use of animal models (e.g., NOD mice, BB rats, streptozotocin-induced diabetes) for type 1 diabetes in humans.[17] As part of this meeting, *Lessons from Animal Models for Human Type 1 Diabetes*, an international workshop was held to establish which, if any, of the aforementioned autoantigens commonly associated as targets of autoantibodies in type 1 diabetes in humans could also be validated as being the targets of humoral immunity in the NOD mouse. This first workshop demonstrated many things. The notion that insulin autoantibodies (IAA) exist in NOD mice was largely supported by the demonstration in multiple laboratories that radioimmunoassays (RIA) for IAA distinguished diabetes-prone from nondiabetes-prone mice.[18] Disappointingly, ELISA assays for IAA were discordant with results obtained by RIA. ELISA assays did detect GADA and IA-2A and, remarkably, their frequencies varied by the source colony from which the serum was derived (i.e., 6 laboratories donated serum for analyses). Furthermore, serum with increased binding to GAD and IA-2 also demonstrated increased binding to the unrelated antigen, myelin oligodendrocyte glycoprotein (MOG), and binding to GAD could not be inhibited by excess unlabeled (irrelevant) antigen. Collectively, this workshop validated that IAA measured by sensitive RIA can serve as a marker of autoimmunity in NOD mice and drew into question the true nature of GADA and IA-2A in this animal model.

Continuing such workshops would appear important as the number of independent studies reporting autoantibodies in NOD mice are increasing.[19,20] The Second Murine Autoantibody Workshop, the subject of this report, was established to further advance the findings obtained in the first workshop involving IAA and, in addition, allow for additional questions surrounding the nature of GADA, IA-2A, and ELISA to be addressed.

WORKSHOP DESIGN AND METHODS

Workshop Design

Workshop participation was open and in large part subject to investigator registration for the *Sixth Annual Meeting of the IDS* (Copper Mountain, CO, October 2002) as well as previous utilization of assays monitoring humoral immunity in NOD mice. Participating investigators and laboratory locations are noted in TABLE 1.

The goals, priorities, and workshop design were established prior to the workshop by the workshop organizers (Liping Yu, Clive Wasserfall). As part of this process, it was agreed that participating labs would be allowed to use methods subject to current utilization within their labs rather than to employ a common method. Serum was collected from animals purchased from Taconic labs (Germantown, NY) and, in addition, a monoclonal antibody (designated 125) was provided by James Thomas (Vanderbilt University, Nashville, TN).

Assay Methods

In accordance with the workshop design, participating laboratories performed autoantibody assays as indicated in TABLE 1.

TABLE 1. Participating laboratories and investigators in the Second Murine Autoantibody Workshop

Laboratory location	Investigators
Australia	Peter Colman, Shane Gellert, Thomas Kay
Canada	Edwin Lee-Chan, Bhagirath Singh
Germany	Kersten Koczwara, Annette Ziegler
Italy	Ezio Bonifacio
Japan	Eiji Kawasaki
Korea	Yong-Soo Park
United Kingdom	
Bristol	Polly Bingley, Alistair Williams
London	Mohammed Hawa
United States	
Colorado	George Eisenbarth, Liping Yu
Florida	Mark Atkinson, Tamir Ellis, Clive Wasserfall
Massachusetts	Tihammer Orban
Tennessee	James Thomas

Statistical Analysis

Comparisons of antibody levels between control and NOD mice were performed using the rank-sum test and regression analysis for correlation between assays.

RESULTS AND DISCUSSION

Autoantibodies against Insulin in NOD versus Control Mice

All but one of the 12 participating laboratories observed increased IAA signals in serum samples obtained from NOD mice in comparison to control mice (FIG. 1). Each laboratory's reported index value divided by its own reported cutoff value was calculated for purposes of this presentation. Indeed, as reliably can be observed, only lab number 7 (utilizing an RIA method) observed low sensitivity and specificity in terms of the IAA assay. Like the situation observed in the first NOD autoantibody workshop, both RIA as well as ELISA-based methods appeared to discriminate NOD from control serum based on an IAA index. Thus, from these data, one could conclude that, for most laboratories, assays capable of distinguishing NOD from control serum based on the presence of IAA do represent a technical reality.

To address the question of whether sensitivity could be increased through alteration of specificity, the workshop organizers recalculated each laboratory's IAA assay sensitivity under conditions of 96% specificity (FIG. 2). For a majority of the labs, this action resulted in only a modest increase in terms of sensitivity (i.e., average 0–15% increase). The overall interpretation of this finding was that, for a majority of labs, IAA, in and of themselves, represent sensitive markers in NOD mice and adjustment of specificity to the 96th percentile only increased this parameter for a minority of labs.

Correlation and Concordance of IAA Results between Laboratories as a Function of Assay Methodology: RIA versus RIA and ELISA versus ELISA

A remarkably good degree of agreement in terms of reported index values was observed for the 26 NOD samples (FIG. 3). In order to examine concordance, IAA levels in NOD mice were expressed as index scores ranging from 0 to more than 25 and subject to ranking (placed in increasing order of IAA levels). IAA levels in NOD mice were highly correlated ($p < 0.01$) among 9 of the 10 RIA laboratories (lab 7 was removed from these analyses due to the aforementioned reasons of low assay specificity and sensitivity). For ELISA assay, despite the smaller number of participating laboratories, direct correlation was feasible. This comparison (FIG. 4) revealed a significant degree of correlation ($p < 0.0001$) among the 2 laboratories. Hence, while results obtained in the first workshop suggested some correlation between RIA labs for individual IAA index values, the results of this workshop suggest an improved concordance despite the increase in the number of participating laboratories. The reasons for this improvement are unclear, but may include improvements in assay methodologies or increased technical performance. In addition, unlike the situation in the first workshop wherein sera were submitted from a variety of centers (i.e., 6), samples in the second workshop were collected from a more limited number of participating centers. Results from the first NOD autoantibody workshop suggested that serum autoantibody values may vary as a function of the source colony, but the reason for this finding remains unclear. Unfortunately, as the first workshop only had one ELISA participant, such comparisons for that assay methodology over time are not possible.

Correlation of IAA Results between Laboratories as a Function of Assay Methodology: RIA versus ELISA

In order to examine concordance between the two assay formats, IAA levels in the 26 NOD mice from a representative RIA lab (lab 1) were compared to those

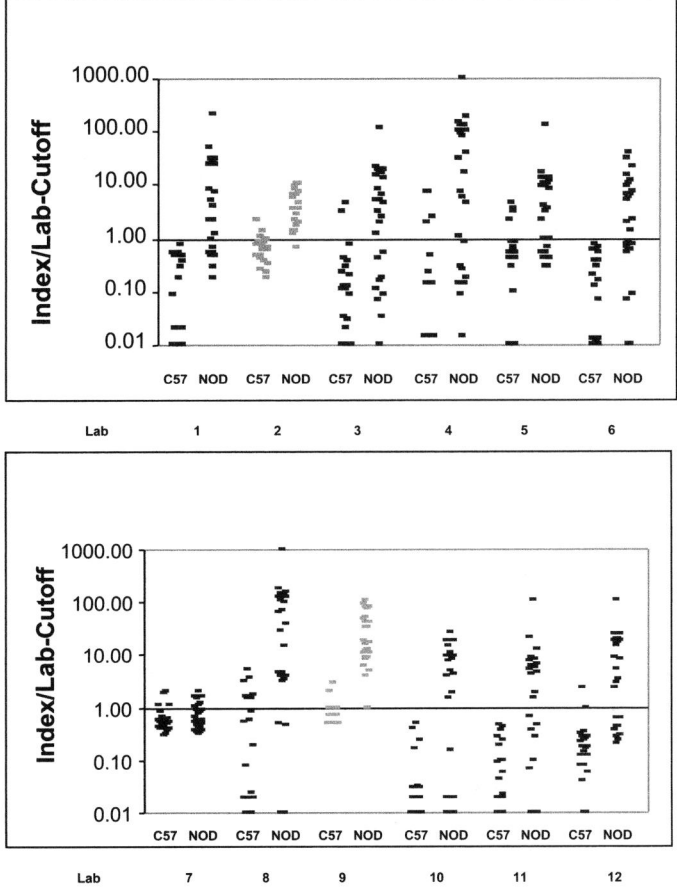

FIGURE 1. IAA levels in sera included in the Second Murine Autoantibody Workshop. Antibody levels are shown for control (C57BL/6; noted as C57) and NOD mice. Results are presented as the index units reported by each of the 12 laboratories divided by their respective laboratory cutoff.

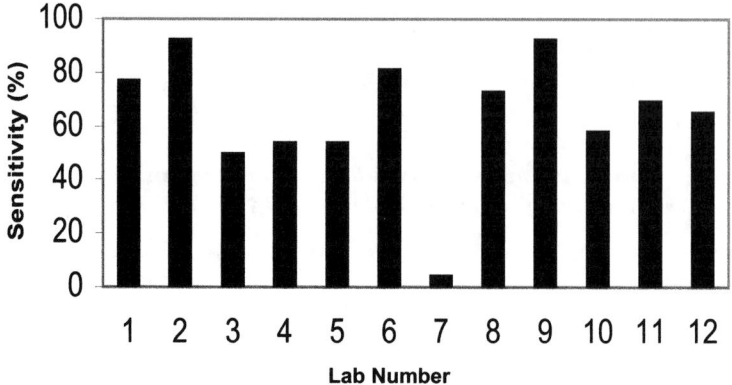

FIGURE 2. Adjusted IAA assay sensitivity with 96% specificity for the 12 laboratories participating in the Second Murine Autoantibody Workshop. An individual laboratory's sensitivity is shown on the ordinate axis as a function of the laboratory designation number (abscissa). These sensitivities were calculated by fixing the specificity for IAA detection at 96% for each laboratory. Labs 2 and 9 performed ELISA for IAA, with the remaining labs performing RIA.

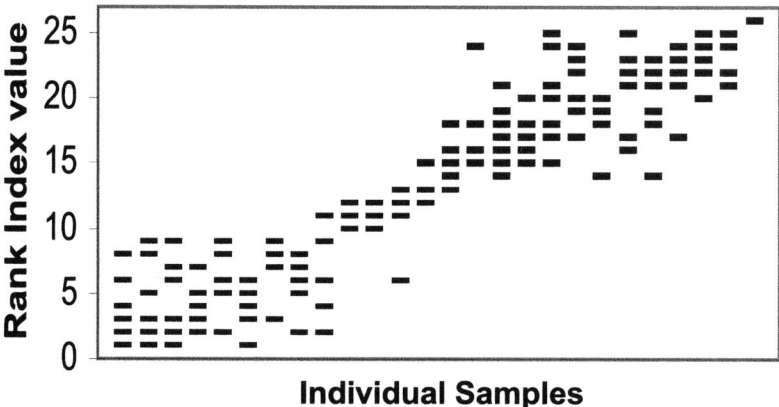

FIGURE 3. Concordance between 9 RIA laboratories for assessment of murine IAA. The index score obtained by each laboratory is shown on the ordinate axis for individual NOD mouse samples shown along the abscissa. Samples were ranked according to increasing mean index value among the 9 laboratories.

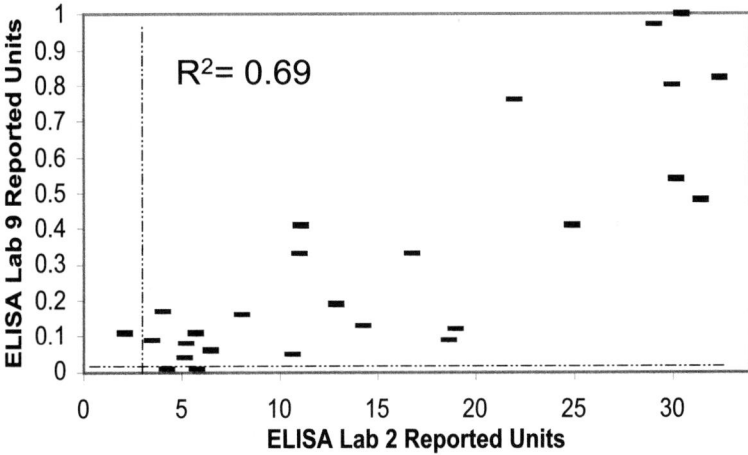

FIGURE 4. Correlation between IAA measurements from NOD mice obtained from the 2 participating laboratories performing ELISA for murine IAA. Results (each in their own distinctive reporting units) from lab 9 are shown on the ordinate axis, with those from lab 2 shown along the abscissa. The broken lines indicate the respective laboratory cutoff reported for their laboratory.

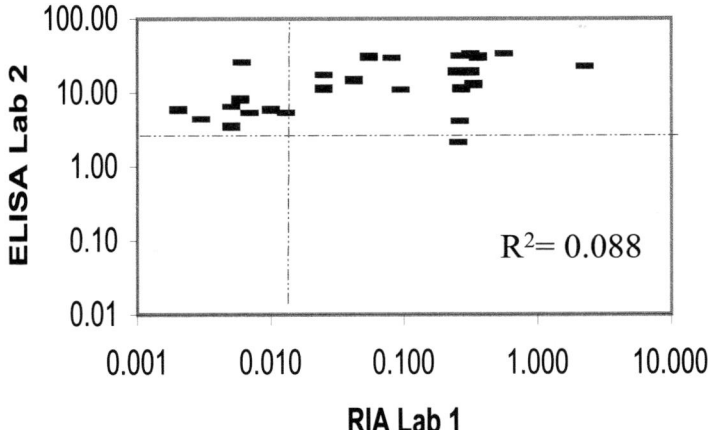

FIGURE 5. Correlation between IAA measurements from NOD mice obtained from one representative ELISA laboratory and a representative RIA laboratory. Results (each in their own distinctive reporting units) from lab 2 are shown on the ordinate axis, with those from lab 1 shown along the abscissa. The broken lines indicate the respective laboratory cutoff reported for their laboratory.

determined by a representative ELISA lab (lab 2). Values were expressed in the laboratory's own respective units. Depending on the ELISA laboratory utilized for such comparison, the degree of agreement in terms of reported index values for IAA between the two assay formats ranged from not promising (FIG. 5, $p = 0.14$) to modestly promising. Indeed, an analysis comparing RIA lab 1 with the second ELISA lab (lab 9) also revealed a limited, but somewhat more promising degree of correlation ($R^2 = 0.16$, $p = 0.04$; data not shown). Results obtained in the first workshop suggested a very limited degree of correlation between RIA and ELISA labs for individual IAA index values. Hence, results of the second workshop suggest the potential for a modest improvement in terms of assay concordance between the two formats.

Dilution Curves for the Anti-insulin mAb Utilized by the 12 Laboratories Participating in the Second Murine Autoantibody Workshop

For this second workshop, one goal was to observe whether inclusion of a standard reagent, in this case, an anti-insulin monoclonal antibody (mAb), could improve standardization. To this end, the anti-insulin mAb designated 125 was serially diluted in C57BL/6 serum and distributed in a coded fashion to each investigator for evaluation of IAA. Dilution curves were then determined by the workshop organizers (FIG. 6). As can readily be observed, most labs [the exceptions being labs 7 (RIA) and 9 (ELISA)] generated a curve from the coded samples. This suggests the ability for the various assays to quantitatively discriminate levels of anti-insulin immunity. At a dilution of 1:100, results for the IAA index were above the adjusted cutoff for 9 of the RIA labs (FIG. 7). As a result, this dilution was selected for additional analyses seeking to observe whether such a reagent could prove useful as a common standard reagent. For this determination, a unit value of 1 (as indicated on the ordinate axis) equated to 100 anti-insulin mAb units. The index score obtained by each laboratory was determined for the individual NOD mouse samples. Samples were ranked according to increasing mean index value among the 9 laboratories.

Autoantibodies to GAD and IA-2 in NOD versus Control Mice

At the first workshop, it was noted that GADA and IA-2A signals were weak, that they correlated between radiobinding assay and ELISA, that they were colony-dependent, and that positive GADA and IA-2A signals were often observed in the same samples. As such, this raised the question of whether the signals to GADA and IA-2A, as determined by ELISA, were truly representative of autoantibody binding.

To address these issues, in part, for the second workshop, 1 laboratory tested GADA by ELISA, while 2 laboratories performed GADA and IA-2A analysis by RIA, all utilizing workshop sera. As a result of this degree of participation, only

---

FIGURE 6. Dilution curves for the anti-insulin mAb utilized by the 12 laboratories participating in the Second Murine Autoantibody Workshop. The broken line indicates the lab's reported cutoff value, with the solid line representing an adjusted cutoff, determined by the workshop organizers, to represent the 99th percentile of signals obtained in all control mice included in the workshop. The adjusted sensitivity for each laboratory as a function of the adjusted cutoff is shown.

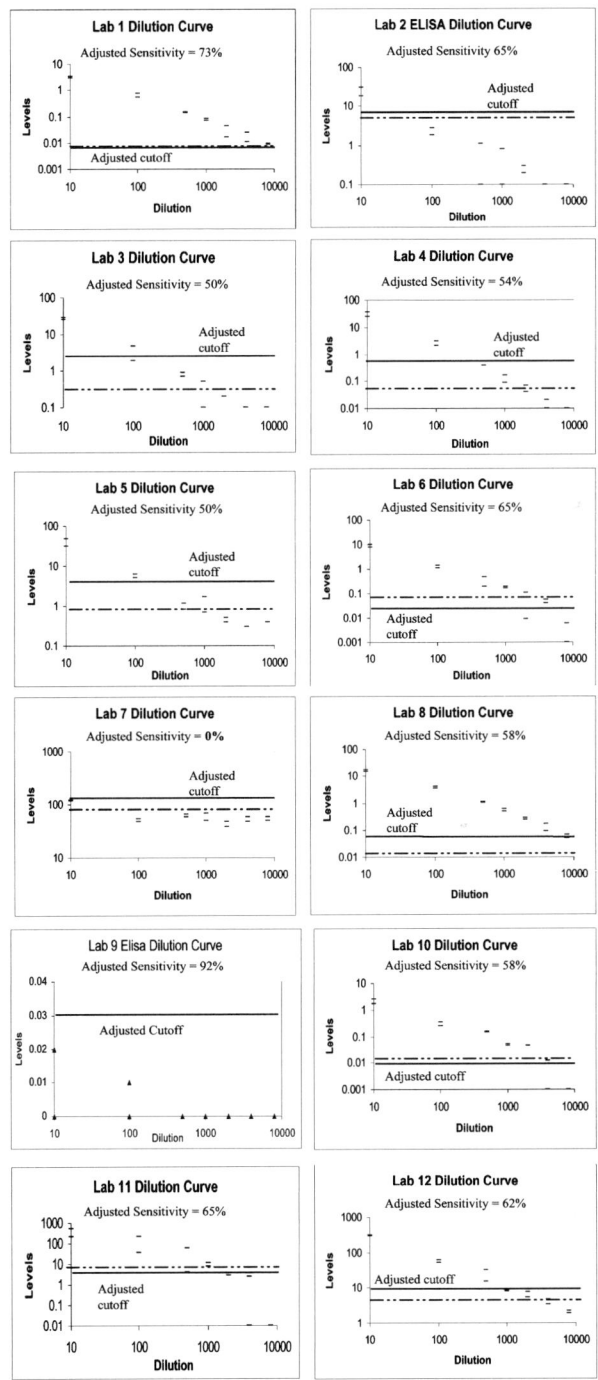

FIGURE 6. *See previous page for legend.*

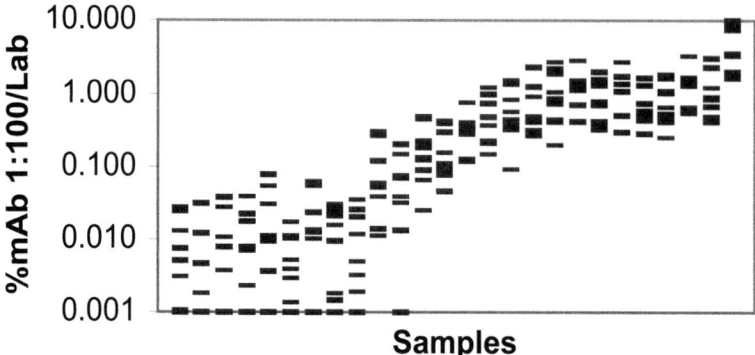

FIGURE 7. Concordance between 9 RIA laboratories in terms of assessment of NOD IAA utilizing diluted (1:100) anti-insulin mAb as a standard. For this determination, a unit value of 1 (as indicated on the ordinate axis) equated to 100 anti-insulin mAb units. The index score obtained by each laboratory is shown on the ordinate axis for individual NOD mouse samples shown along the abscissa. Samples were ranked according to increasing mean index value among the 9 laboratories.

limited notation will be discussed here. At the actual symposium, data were presented suggesting a general inability of assays for GADA and IA-2A to distinguish NOD serum from controls. Hence, debate occurred among some workshop participants as to whether increased signals in NOD mouse samples to GAD were truly observed and, in addition, whether ELISA-based assays did in fact measure true autoantibodies (including IAA). To this latter end, a limited amount of data were presented suggesting that while exogenous insulin was capable of fully displacing IAA as detected by RIA, such a technique did not show similar efficacy in terms of ELISA-based testing. Such inconsistencies and difficulties should continue to be addressed by additional workshops.

A significant portion of our knowledge regarding the pathogenesis of type 1 diabetes has been derived from studies of animal models of the disease and, in particular, the NOD mouse. However, one of the more disappointing features of studies involving NOD mice has been a relative lack of consensus in terms of investigator agreement of target antigens of beta cell autoimmunity. Indeed, while much enthusiasm has been generated towards the potential pathogenic significance of immunities to the autoantigens, insulin, GAD, and heat shock protein (HSP), in NOD mice, significant controversies remain. The outcomes of this workshop should, in part, bring partial resolution to these questions and again, in part, work to resolve existing controversies.

The data presented gave unanimous support to the concept of the autoantigenic role for insulin molecule as a target of humoral autoimmunity in NOD mice. The ability of nearly every lab (i.e., 11 out of 12) to detect such immunities, despite differences in assay format (i.e., RIA and ELISA labs), lends support to this notion, as do the facets of relative disease specificity (i.e., presence in NOD versus non-NOD strains) and good concordance in sample identity (again despite significant differences in assay formats). While subject to some degree of reader interpretation, the RIA for IAA in NOD mice did appear superior to that obtained utilizing ELISA when viewed as a function of sensitivity.

Coming out of the first workshop, a major step forward was thought to be that involving the inclusion of additional laboratories utilizing ELISA formats for IAA detection, a factor that would have allowed for improved comparisons as were performed with the RIA. In addition, increasing the number of RIA participants was also thought to allow for improved validation and scientific acceptance. While only modest success can be claimed for the first goal (increasing the number of ELISA labs), we were pleased to see the number of RIA labs increase from 4 to 10. As to the two other markers of anti-islet autoimmunity tested, GADA and IA-2A, the results of this second workshop continue (as did the first) to call their role as a target of humoral autoimmunity in NOD mice into question.

As for now, it appears safe to conclude that IAA do represent a sensitive and disease-specific marker associated with type 1 diabetes as observed in NOD mice. Further enhancements in terms of assay development are probable, as will be the increased knowledge on the pathogenesis of type 1 diabetes gained by their ascertainment.

ACKNOWLEDGMENTS

The workshop organizers acknowledge and thank all participants (indicated in TABLE 1) for their contributions to this workshop. We also wish to thank Tamir Ellis and David Serreze for their advice and recommendations for this workshop. These studies were performed, in part, with funding provided by the Barbara Davis Center for Childhood Diabetes (Denver, CO).

REFERENCES

1. GOTTLIEB, P.A. & G.S. EISENBARTH. 1998. Diagnosis and treatment of pre-insulin dependent diabetes. Annu. Rev. Med. **49:** 391–405.
2. ATKINSON, M. & G. EISENBARTH. 2001. Type 1 diabetes: new perspectives on disease pathogenesis and treatment. Lancet **358:** 221–229.
3. RABINOVICH, A. & J.S. SKYLER. 1998. Prevention of type 1 diabetes. Med. Clin. North Am. **82:** 739–755.
4. PIETROPAOLO, M. & D.J. BECKER. 2001. Type 1 diabetes intervention trials. Pediatr. Diabetes **2:** 2–11.
5. GLEICHMANN, H. & G.F. BOTTAZZO. 1987. Progress toward standardization of cytoplasmic islet cell-antibody assay. Diabetes **36:** 578–584.
6. BONIFACIO, E., Å. LERNMARK, R.L. DAWKINS et al. 1988. Serum exchange and use of dilutions have improved precision of measurement of islet cell antibodies. J. Immunol. Methods **106:** 83–88.
7. WILKIN, T., S.L. SCHOENFELD, J-L. DIAZ et al. 1989. Systemic variation accounts and differences in insulin autoantibody measurements. Diabetes **38:** 172–181.
8. PALMER, J.P., T.J. WILKIN, A.B. KURTZ et al. 1990. The Third International Workshop on the Standardisation of Insulin Autoantibody Measurement. Diabetologia **33:** 60–61.
9. BONIFACIO, E., C. BOITARD, H. GLEICHMANN et al. 1990. Report from the stage III islet cell antibody standardisation workshop: assessment of precision, concordance, specificity, and sensitivity of islet cell antibody measurement in 41 assays. Diabetologia **33:** 731–736.

10. GREENBAUM, C.J., J.P. PALMER, B. KUGLIN *et al.* 1992. Insulin autoantibodies measured by radioimmunoassay methodology are more related to insulin-dependent diabetes mellitus than those measured by enzyme-linked immunosorbent assay: results of the Fourth International Workshop on the Standardization of Insulin Autoantibody Measurement. J. Clin. Endocrinol. Metab. **74:** 1040–1044.
11. GREENBAUM, C.J., T.J. WILKIN & J.P. PALMER. 1992. Fifth International Serum Exchange Workshop for Insulin Autoantibody (IAA) Standardization: the Immunology and Diabetes Workshops and participating laboratories. Diabetologia **35:** 798–800.
12. GREENBAUM, C.J., J.P. PALMER, S. NAGATAKI *et al.* 1992. Improved specificity of ICA assays in the Fourth International Immunology of Diabetes Serum Exchange Workshop. Diabetes **41:** 1570–1574.
13. SCHMIDLI, R.S., P.G. COLMAN, E. BONIFACIO *et al.* 1994. High level of concordance between assays for glutamic acid decarboxylase antibodies (GADAb): the First International GADAb Workshop. Diabetes **43:** 1005–1009.
14. SCHMIDLI, R., P.G. COLMAN & E. BONIFACIO. 1995. Disease sensitivity and specificity of fifty-two assays for glutamic acid decarboxylase antibodies: the Second International Glutamic Acid Decarboxylase Antibody Workshop. Diabetes **44:** 636–640.
15. VERGE, C.F., D. STENGER, E. BONIFACIO *et al.* 1998. Combined use of autoantibodies (IA-2 autoantibody, GAD autoantibody, insulin autoantibody, cytoplasmic islet cell antibodies) in type 1 diabetes: Combinatorial Islet Autoantibody Workshop. Diabetes **47:** 1857–1866.
16. ATKINSON, M.A. & E.H. LEITER. 1999. The NOD mouse model of type 1 diabetes mellitus: too much of a good thing? Nat. Med. **5:** 601–604.
17. HASKINS, K. & M. ATKINSON. 2001. Predicting disease in animal models of type 1 diabetes: lessons for studies of humans? J. Autoimmun. **16:** 15–19.
18. BONIFACIO, E., M. ATKINSON, G. EISENBARTH *et al.* 2001. International Workshop on Lessons from Animal Models for Human Type 1 Diabetes: identification of insulin but not glutamic acid decarboxylase or IA-2 as specific autoantigens of humoral autoimmunity in NOD mice. Diabetes **50:** 2451–2458.
19. YU, L., D.T. ROBLES, N. ABIRU *et al.* 2000. Early expression of antiinsulin autoantibodies of humans and the NOD mouse: evidence for early determination of subsequent diabetes. Proc. Natl. Acad. Sci. USA **97:** 1701–1706.
20. GOUDY, K., S. SONG, C. WASSERFALL *et al.* 2001. Adeno-associated virus vector mediated interleukin-10 gene delivery prevents type 1 diabetes in NOD mice. Proc. Natl. Acad. Sci. USA **98:** 13913–13917.

Can Enteroviruses Cause Type 1 Diabetes?

SISKO TAURIAINEN,[a] KIMMO SALMINEN,[b] AND HEIKKI HYÖTY[a]

[a]*JDRF Center for Prevention of Type 1 Diabetes in Finland, Department of Virology, University of Tampere, and University Hospital of Tampere, Tampere, Finland*

[b]*JDRF Center for Prevention of Type 1 Diabetes in Finland, Department of Virology, University of Turku, Turku, Finland*

ABSTRACT: Enterovirus infections have long been considered as one possible environmental trigger of type 1 diabetes. These viruses have been detected from diabetic patients more often than from control subjects and they can infect beta cells in cell culture and induce diabetes in animal models. Furthermore, a same kind of seasonality has been observed in both the onset of clinical diabetes and subclinical beta cell autoimmunity (appearance of autoantibodies) as in enterovirus infections. Recently, considerable new evidence has cumulated from prospective studies indicating the risk effect of enterovirus infections long before clinical diabetes was diagnosed. In addition, several studies have reported enterovirus genome sequences in diabetic patients more often than in control subjects. Currently, the evidence for the role of enteroviruses is stronger than for most other environmental agents, but still the final proof is lacking. The ongoing studies aim to prove the risk effect in different populations and to identify the underlying mechanisms. This research field is becoming more and more important because it could open up possibilities to prevent type 1 diabetes by an enterovirus vaccine.

KEYWORDS: enterovirus; type 1 diabetes; etiology; pathogenesis

INTRODUCTION

Both genetic and environmental risk factors contribute to the risk for type 1 diabetes in humans. The most important known susceptibility genes are located in the HLA-DQ locus. Nevertheless, the genetic susceptibility is not enough to induce the disease, and environmental factors are needed to initiate and possibly also sustain, accelerate, or retard the beta cell damaging process. Suspected environmental factors include, for example, viruses, cow's milk proteins, nitrites, and lack of vitamin D. Viruses are among the most probable ones, but their role has been difficult to study, mainly due to the long time lag between their possible triggering effect and the manifestation of clinical diabetes.[1] A classical example is congenital rubella, which leads to clinical diabetes in up to 20% of infected subjects, but usually only after a very long time lag, at the age of 20–30 years.[2,3] Currently, when the effect of

Address for correspondence: Dr. Heikki Hyöty, Department of Virology, University of Tampere, Medical School, FinnMedi 3, Lenkkeilijänkatu 10, 33520 Tampere, Finland. Voice: +358-3-215-8460; fax: +358-3-215-8450.
blhehy@uta.fi

Ann. N.Y. Acad. Sci. 1005: 13–22 (2003). © 2003 New York Academy of Sciences.
doi: 10.1196/annals.1288.003

rubella infection has been attenuated by vaccinations, the most promising candidates for viral triggers are enteroviruses.[1,4] Additionally, some other viruses like mumps virus, cytomegalovirus, retrovirus, and rotavirus have occasionally been connected with type 1 diabetes, but the evidence is far less convincing.[1,5]

ENTEROVIRUSES

Enteroviruses belong to the picornavirus family. They are small nonenveloped positive-strand RNA viruses. There are over 60 different serotypes of human enteroviruses, including 3 polioviruses, 23 Coxsackie A serotypes, 6 Coxsackie B serotypes, 28 echovirus serotypes, and 4 numbered serotypes. The large number of serotypes makes their diagnosis difficult by serological assays, while several RT-PCR methods have been developed to detect all serotypes in clinical specimen. Repeated infections by different serotypes are very common throughout childhood and adolescence.[6] These infections are mostly subclinical or manifest only with mild respiratory symptoms. Still, enterovirus infections are the most common cause of aseptic meningitis and myocarditis and may cause severe systemic multiorgan infections in newborns, as well as pancreatitis and paralysis. The risk of complications is higher in males than in females and is particularly high in young infants and patients with humoral immune deficiencies.[7]

ENTEROVIRUS INFECTIONS IN DIABETIC PATIENTS

The association between enteroviruses and type 1 diabetes was reported for the first time already over 30 years ago, when coxsackievirus B antibodies were found more frequently in type 1 diabetic patients than in control subjects.[8] An additional hint was obtained from the observation that type 1 diabetes was usually diagnosed in late summer and fall, matching the seasonal pattern of enterovirus infections in northern Europe.[9] The seasonal onset of clinical diabetes has later been confirmed in several studies,[10] and seasonality has lately also been observed in the appearance of autoantibodies in high risk, but nondiabetic, children who were followed from birth.[11] This does not prove the causal link to enteroviruses, but strongly suggests that some of the triggering factors follow the same kind of seasonal pattern as enteroviruses.

Later on, enterovirus infections have been detected more frequently in diabetic patients than in healthy children in several studies.[1] However, the results are somewhat inconsistent between different research groups since all studies do not support the hypothesis.[12] Some of these studies have also been criticized because the control subjects were not matched for HLA-risk alleles, which may bias immune responsiveness to enterovirus.[13]

Enteroviruses have also been isolated from newly diagnosed type 1 diabetic patients. In one study, a coxsackievirus B4 strain was isolated from the pancreas of a child who died from diabetic ketoacidosis and this virus strain caused diabetes in a susceptible mouse strain.[14] One of the most convincing new evidence is the detection of viral RNA from the blood of diabetic patients. Seven such studies have been published from four countries indicating an increased frequency of enterovirus RNA in the peripheral blood of diabetic subjects.[15–21] The average proportion of RNA-positive patients in these studies was 33% compared to 4% of control subjects. This indicates that the virus is present in the circulation in a considerable proportion of diabetic patients as a marker of an ongoing enterovirus infection. It is not known if this reflects acute or persistent infection and if the virus replicates in the pancreas or in other organs.

Demonstration of the virus from the pancreatic islets would considerably strengthen the enterovirus hypothesis and would also help to understand the mechanisms of how the virus could induce beta cell damage. Detection of enteroviruses has been attempted from paraffin-embedded pancreatic tissues taken from diabetic patients who have died close to the onset of clinical diabetes. However, enterovirus antigens or genome sequences have not been found,[22–24] even though beta cells of diabetic patients expressed interferon-α (IFN-α),[25,26] a cytokine that is induced during virus infections, suggesting that a virus might be present in beta cells. Even if enteroviruses would infect the islets, the amount of virus might be very low, and viral proteins and genomes may also be degraded during postmortem changes and routine formalin fixation of the tissues, making these studies difficult. On the other hand, enterovirus antigens have been found in the islets in young children who have died from severe enterovirus infections, which is a clear indication that enteroviruses can infect islet cells in humans.

Other kinds of approaches have also been used to study the association between enteroviruses and diabetes. In one of theses studies, IFN-α was found in the plasma in 70% of diabetic patients, but in none of the control subjects.[18] According to the presence of IFN-α, enterovirus antibodies, and enterovirus RNA, the authors concluded that enterovirus infections, either acute or persistent, were associated with clinical diabetes in the majority of cases.[18] In some studies, increased T cell immune responses of enterovirus antigens have been found in diabetic patients as a marker of memory T cell activation, suggesting that the exposure to these viruses may have been higher in diabetic than control subjects.[27–31] One of the most important recent advances is the implementation of prospective studies, which enable detection of enterovirus infections during the early stages of the beta cell damaging process. The results from these studies are summarized below.

PROSPECTIVE STUDIES

The process leading to diabetes is slow, lasting from months to even several years. For this reason, it is difficult to identify the environmental triggers, which operate during the initiation phase of the process. These obstacles can be resolved by carrying out prospective studies, which are based on the follow-up of initially nondiabetic children until some of them will develop clinical diabetes. These studies cover the initiation phase, which can be identified by the appearance of diabetes-associated autoantibodies in circulation, such as ICA, IAA, GADA, and IA-2A. Therefore, prospective studies are much more powerful than retrospective studies in the evaluation of possible causal association.

Our research group has participated in several prospective studies. In the first such study, the Childhood Diabetes in Finland Study (DiMe), blood samples were taken every 6 months from siblings of diabetic children. Enterovirus infections were found more frequently in siblings who progressed to clinical diabetes than in control siblings, and infections were clustered to the time immediately preceding the appearance of autoantibodies.[32–35] After the DiMe study, a larger prospective study, the Finnish Diabetes Prediction and Prevention Trial (DIPP), was started. In this study, all newborns of three cities in Finland are first screened for diabetes-associated HLA-DQ alleles and those with increased genetic risk are followed starting from birth.[36] Enterovirus infections are diagnosed by antibody assays and detection of enterovirus RNA in serum and in stools (serum samples are taken every 3–6 months and stool samples every month). The frequency of infections is compared between children who turn positive for at least two autoantibodies and remain autoantibody-positive during the follow-up and control children, matched for the time of birth, gender, and HLA type. The time relationship between virus infections and the appearance of autoantibodies is evaluated by comparing the number of infections during the 6-month period preceding the appearance of autoantibodies. The time period was selected on the basis of mouse experiments where enterovirus infection induces autoantibodies within 2 months.[37,38] In addition to the DIPP trial, the role of virus infections has also been analyzed in another birth cohort study (second pilot of TRIGR trial), where the role of cow milk is primarily evaluated.

The results from all these prospective studies indicate that enterovirus infections are more frequent in children who turn autoantibody-positive than in control children, showing a clustering of infections at the time when autoantibodies first appeared.[32–36,39–41] The association holds with increasing number of subjects and with different detection methods. It was also seen when either clinical diabetes or autoantibody positivity was used as an end point. It was also specific for enteroviruses since other virus infections like rotavirus, adenovirus, cytomegalovirus, and Epstein-Barr virus infections were not associated with diabetes.

In addition to the Finnish studies, a few prospective studies have been carried out in other countries (TABLE 1). The DAISY (Diabetes Autoimmunity Study in the

TABLE 1. Summary of prospective studies evaluating the role of enteroviruses

Study	Association	Cases (n)	End point	Reference
DiMe	+ (abs)[a]	22	Diabetes	Hyöty (1995)[32]
	+ (abs)	23	Auto-abs	Hiltunen (1997)[33]
	+ (RNA)[b]	11	Diabetes	Lönnrot (1999)[57]
DIPP	+ (abs, RNA)	21	Auto-abs	Lönnrot (2000)[36]
	+ (abs, RNA)	41	Auto-abs	Salminen (2003)[41]
	+ (RNA)	25	Diabetes	Martiskainen (2002)[58]
TRIGR pilot 2	+ (abs, RNA)	19	Auto-abs	Sadeharju (2003)[39]
DAISY	– (abs, RNA)	26	Auto-abs	Graves (2003)[43]
BabyDiab				
Australia	– (abs)	24	Auto-abs	Honeyman (2000)[44]
Germany	– (abs)	28	Auto-abs	Füchtenbusch (2001)[42]

[a]Infections diagnosed by antibody assays.
[b]Infections diagnosed by detection of viral RNA by RT-PCR.

Young) in the United States and the BabyDiab in Germany failed to see any connection between enterovirus infections and diabetes.[42,43] One prospective study has also been published from Australia suggesting that rotavirus infections may be associated with diabetes, while no such effect was found in enterovirus infections.[44] The reasons for these discrepancies are not known. One possible explanation is the obvious difficulty to diagnose enterovirus infections with satisfactory sensitivity in this type of prospective series. In fact, the studies showing positive association have been based on more frequent sample intervals and a wider panel of enterovirus assays than the studies showing no association, which clearly have an effect on the sensitivity to diagnose these infections. For example, in the German BabyDiab study, only 8% of the case children had an enterovirus infection by the age of 2 years (2 infections in 25 children),[42] while over 80% of children had infection by that age in the Finnish DIPP study.[41] Another possibility is that the risk effect of enterovirus infections differs between populations. However, the detection of enterovirus RNA in diabetic patients in several countries suggests that this may not be the case.[15–20]

ROLE OF MATERNAL ENTEROVIRUS INFECTIONS DURING PREGNANCY

The possible role of *in utero* enterovirus exposures has been evaluated in a few studies. This is an interesting period of life since fetal infections can lead to viral persistence and cause congenital organ defects as seen, for example, in the case of congenital rubella. In the earliest studies, maternal enterovirus infection during pregnancy was associated with increased risk of type 1 diabetes in the offspring (TABLE 2).[32,45–47] However, these studies were based on relatively small series. A

TABLE 2. Summary of studies evaluating the role of maternal enterovirus infection during pregnancy

Country	Samples	Association	Cases (*n*)	Reference
End point clinical diabetes				
Finland	First trimester	+	96	Hyöty (1995)[32]
Sweden	At delivery	+	57	Dahlquist (1995)[46]
Sweden	At delivery	+	55	Dahlquist (1995)[45]
Sweden	First trimester	+	85	Dahlquist (1999)[47]
Finland	First trimester	–[a]	948	Viskari (2002)[48]
End point autoantibodies				
Germany	At delivery	–	16	Füchtenbusch (2001)[42]
Finland	Whole pregnancy	–	21	Sadeharju (2001)[40]
Finland	Whole pregnancy	+	19	Sadeharju (2003)[39]
Finland	Whole pregnancy	–	41	Salminen (2003)[41]

[a]No clear association, but a small trend, which was not significant after correction for multiple comparisons.

larger study was recently published on the possible role of first trimester enterovirus infection.[48] It included 948 mothers of children who developed clinical diabetes and control mothers with a nondiabetic child. A serum sample, taken at the end of the first trimester of pregnancy, was analyzed for enterovirus antibodies and enterovirus RNA. In this study, no clear risk effect was seen, suggesting that first trimester enterovirus infection is not a major risk factor for diabetes.[48] However, as this study covered only the first trimester of pregnancy, a possible role of later infections could not be analyzed. The role of these later infections has been evaluated in the context of recent prospective studies covering the whole period of pregnancy (TABLE 2).[39–41] However, these series are small and the results have varied, and larger studies are needed to confirm whether infections occurring during the last two trimesters could increase the risk of diabetes in the offspring.

DO DIABETOGENIC ENTEROVIRUS STRAINS EXIST?

Virulence of enterovirus strains varies as shown previously for polioviruses (neurovirulence) and Coxsackie B viruses (cardiovirulence). Virulent and avirulent strains differ in their genetic code, which may influence replication and translation, receptor binding, and interaction with the immune system. For example, the mutations associated with the neurovirulence of polioviruses are located in the 5′ noncoding region (5′-NCR) and in the region coding for viral structural proteins.[49–53]

The ability of a virus to induce beta cell damage could be determined by a few or even just one point mutation, which could, for example, affect virus tropism (the ability to infect certain cell types). Studies with another picornavirus, encephalomyocarditis virus, have shown that diabetogenic and nondiabetogenic strains differ for certain nucleotides, and even one amino acid change may alter the phenotype of the virus.[54,55] Only a few diabetogenic enterovirus strains have been described in the literature.[14,56] These strains originate from diabetic patients, carry certain nucleotide changes compared to reference strains, and cause diabetes in animal models. However, systematic studies aiming at isolation of enterovirus strains from diabetic subjects are lacking, and it is not known for sure if the previously described strains are truly diabetogenic. The characterization of such strains is further hampered by the fact that the mouse models for enterovirus-induced diabetes are far from optimal.

The question about the existence of diabetogenic enterovirus strains is important not only for the understanding of the mechanisms of virus-induced beta cell damage, but also for the option to develop preventive vaccines. A vaccine is already available for three enterovirus types, poliovirus types 1–3, which cause paralysis. Similarly, if diabetogenic enterovirus strains belong to certain serotypes, as expected from other enterovirus diseases, the vaccine should contain these serotypes to be effective. So far, particularly coxsackievirus B serotypes have been connected to type 1 diabetes, but there are also indications that other serotypes may be involved,[14] and systematic studies have not been carried out. In addition, previous studies may have been biased by the fact that Coxsackie B serotypes grow easily in cell culture compared to many other serotypes. Thus, direct sequencing of the viral genome from diabetic patients would be better than virus isolation in the identification of diabetogenic serotypes.

FUTURE PROSPECTS

Even though the association between enterovirus infections and type 1 diabetes has been documented in several epidemiological studies, there are also conflicting findings and causality has not been proven. It is still possible that such an association is caused by some unidentified confounding factors. To minimize the effect of such factors, cases and controls should be matched carefully or these factors have to be taken into consideration when analyzing the data. This is of course difficult because many of these factors might still be unknown. For example, the possibility that HLA-risk alleles for diabetes might have biased the comparisons between diabetic patients and control subjects has gotten much attention since HLA type may modulate immune responses against enteroviruses.[13] By now, this concern has been weakened considerably since the same kind of association has also been found in recent studies where case and control subjects were matched for HLA alleles.[28,36,41]

There is an obvious need for further studies confirming whether or not enteroviruses can cause type 1 diabetes. It would be highly important to design such studies properly to achieve satisfactory sensitivity to detect enterovirus infections and to rule out the effect of confounding factors. Prospective human studies are the most important ones in this mission, but retrospective studies as well as animal and *in vitro* models are also needed. The ongoing and planned large-scale studies, carried out in different populations by international collaboration and standardized methodologies, play a key role in this process.

ACKNOWLEDGMENTS

We wish to thank Mikael Knip, Hans Åkerblom, Olli Simell, and Jorma Ilonen for successful collaboration, and the Academy of Finland, the European Commission (Contract Nos. IC15-CT98-0316 and GLK2-CT-2001-01910), the Juvenile Diabetes Research Foundation (Grant Nos. 395019 and 197114), Tampere University Hospital, and the Sigrid Juselius Foundation for their valuable support.

REFERENCES

1. HYÖTY, H. & K.W. TAYLOR. 2002. The role of viruses in human diabetes. Diabetologia **45:** 1353–1361.
2. CLARKE, W.L. *et al.* 1984. Autoimmunity in congenital rubella syndrome. J. Pediatr. **104:** 370–373.
3. MCINTOSH, E.D. & M.A. MENSER. 1992. A fifty-year follow-up of congenital rubella. Lancet **340:** 414–415.
4. HYÖTY, H. 2002. Enterovirus infections and type 1 diabetes. Ann. Med. **34:** 138–147.
5. YOON, J.W. 1995. A new look at viruses in type 1 diabetes. Diabetes Metab. Rev. **11:** 83–107.
6. JUHELA, S. *et al.* 1998. Enterovirus infections and enterovirus specific T-cell responses in infancy. J. Med. Virol. **54:** 226–232.
7. PALLANSCH, M.A. & P. RAYMOND. 2001. Enteroviruses: polioviruses, coxsackieviruses, echoviruses, and newer enteroviruses. *In* Fields Virology, pp. 723–755. Lippincott/Williams & Wilkins. Philadelphia/Baltimore.
8. GAMBLE, D.R. *et al.* 1969. Viral antibodies in diabetes mellitus. Br. Med. J. **3:** 627–630.
9. GAMBLE, D.R. & K.W. TAYLOR. 1969. Seasonal incidence of diabetes mellitus. Br. Med. J. **3:** 631–633.

10. GREEN, A. & C.C. PATTERSON. 2001. Trends in the incidence of childhood-onset diabetes in Europe 1989–1998. Diabetologia **44:** B3–B8.
11. KIMPIMÄKI, T. *et al.* 2001. The first signs of beta-cell autoimmunity appear in infancy in genetically susceptible children from the general population: the Finnish Type 1 Diabetes Prediction and Prevention Study. J. Clin. Endocrinol. Metab. **86:** 4782–4788.
12. PALMER, J.P. *et al.* 1982. Reduced Coxsackie antibody titres in type 1 (insulin-dependent) diabetic patients presenting during an outbreak of Coxsackie B3 and B4 infection. Diabetologia **22:** 426–429.
13. BRUSERUD, O., J. JERVELL & E. THORSBY. 1985. HLA-DR3 and -DR4 control T-lymphocyte responses to mumps and Coxsackie B4 virus: studies on patients with type 1 (insulin-dependent) diabetes and healthy subjects. Diabetologia **28:** 420–426.
14. YOON, J.W. *et al.* 1979. Isolation of a virus from the pancreas of a child with diabetic ketoacidosis. N. Engl. J. Med. **300:** 1173–1179.
15. ANDREOLETTI, L. *et al.* 1997. Detection of Coxsackie B virus RNA sequences in whole blood samples from adult patients at the onset of type I diabetes mellitus. J. Med. Virol. **52:** 121–127.
16. CLEMENTS, G.B., D.N. GALBRAITH & K.W. TAYLOR. 1995. Coxsackie B virus infection and onset of childhood diabetes. Lancet **346:** 221–223.
17. NAIRN, C. *et al.* 1999. Enterovirus variants in the serum of children at the onset of type 1 diabetes mellitus. Diabetes Med. **16:** 509–513.
18. CHEHADEH, W. *et al.* 2000. Increased level of interferon-alpha in blood of patients with insulin-dependent diabetes mellitus: relationship with coxsackievirus B infection. J. Infect. Dis. **181:** 1929–1939.
19. CRAIG, M. *et al.* 2000. Genotyping of enteroviruses in children at diagnosis of type 1 diabetes. Presented at the Twenty-Sixth Annual Meeting of the International Society for Pediatric and Adolescent Diabetes (ISPAD).
20. YIN, H. *et al.* 2002. Enterovirus RNA is found in peripheral blood mononuclear cells in a majority of type 1 diabetic children at onset. Diabetes **51:** 1964–1971.
21. COUTANT, R. *et al.* 2002. Detection of enterovirus RNA sequences in serum samples from autoantibody-positive subjects at risk for diabetes. Diabetes Med. **19:** 968–969.
22. BUESA-GOMEZ, J. *et al.* 1994. Failure to detect genomic viral sequences in pancreatic tissues from two children with acute-onset diabetes mellitus. J. Med. Virol. **42:** 193–197.
23. FOULIS, A.K. *et al.* 1990. A search for the presence of the enteroviral capsid protein VP1 in pancreases of patients with type 1 (insulin-dependent) diabetes and pancreases and hearts of infants who died of coxsackieviral myocarditis. Diabetologia **33:** 290–298.
24. FOULIS, A.K. *et al.* 1997. A search for evidence of viral infection in pancreases of newly diagnosed patients with IDDM. Diabetologia **40:** 53–61.
25. HUANG, X. *et al.* 1995. Interferon expression in the pancreases of patients with type I diabetes. Diabetes **44:** 658–664.
26. FOULIS, A.K., M.A. FARQUHARSON & A. MEAGER. 1987. Immunoreactive alpha-interferon in insulin-secreting beta cells in type 1 diabetes mellitus. Lancet **2:** 1423–1427.
27. JUHELA, S. *et al.* 1999. T cell responses to enterovirus antigens and to beta-cell auto-antigens in unaffected children positive for IDDM-associated autoantibodies. J. Autoimmun. **12:** 269–278.
28. JUHELA, S. *et al.* 2000. T-cell responses to enterovirus antigens in children with type 1 diabetes. Diabetes **49:** 1308–1313.
29. KLEMETTI, P. *et al.* 1999. Relation between T-cell responses to glutamate decarboxylase and coxsackievirus B4 in patients with insulin-dependent diabetes mellitus. J. Clin. Virol. **14:** 95–105.
30. VARELA-CALVINO, R. *et al.* 2002. Characterization of the T-cell response to coxsackie-virus b4: evidence that effector memory cells predominate in patients with type 1 diabetes. Diabetes **51:** 1745–1753.
31. JONES, D.B. & I. CROSBY. 1996. Proliferative lymphocyte responses to virus antigens homologous to GAD65 in IDDM. Diabetologia **39:** 1318–1324.
32. HYÖTY, H. *et al.* 1995. A prospective study of the role of Coxsackie B and other enterovirus infections in the pathogenesis of IDDM: Childhood Diabetes in Finland (DiMe) Study Group. Diabetes **44:** 652–657.

33. HILTUNEN, M. et al. 1997. Islet cell antibody seroconversion in children is temporally associated with enterovirus infections: Childhood Diabetes in Finland (DiMe) Study Group. J. Infect. Dis. **175:** 554–560.
34. ROIVAINEN, M. et al. 1998. Several different enterovirus serotypes can be associated with prediabetic autoimmune episodes and onset of overt IDDM: Childhood Diabetes in Finland (DiMe) Study Group. J. Med. Virol. **56:** 74–78.
35. LÖNNROT, M. et al. 2000. Enterovirus RNA in serum is a risk factor for beta-cell autoimmunity and clinical type 1 diabetes: a prospective study—Childhood Diabetes in Finland (DiMe) Study Group. J. Med. Virol. **61:** 214–220.
36. LÖNNROT, M. et al. 2000. Enterovirus infection as a risk factor for beta-cell autoimmunity in a prospectively observed birth cohort: the Finnish Diabetes Prediction and Prevention Study. Diabetes **49:** 1314–1318.
37. GERLING, I., N.K. CHATTERJEE & C. NEJMAN. 1991. Coxsackievirus B4–induced development of antibodies to 64,000-Mr islet autoantigen and hyperglycemia in mice. Autoimmunity **10:** 49–56.
38. SEE, D.M. & J.G. TILLES. 1995. Pathogenesis of virus-induced diabetes in mice. J. Infect. Dis. **171:** 1131–1138.
39. SADEHARJU, K. et al. 2003. Enterovirus infections as a risk factor for type 1 diabetes—virus analyses in a dietary intervention trial. Clin. Exp. Immunol. **132:** 271–277.
40. SADEHARJU, K. et al. 2001. Enterovirus antibody levels during the first two years of life in prediabetic autoantibody-positive children. Diabetologia **44:** 818–823.
41. SALMINEN, K. et al. 2003. Enterovirus infections are associated with the induction of beta-cell autoimmunity in a prospective birth cohort study. J. Med. Virol. **69:** 91–98.
42. FÜCHTENBUSCH, M. et al. 2001. No evidence for an association of Coxsackie virus infections during pregnancy and early childhood with development of islet autoantibodies in offspring of mothers or fathers with type 1 diabetes. J. Autoimmun. **17:** 333–340.
43. GRAVES, P.M. et al. 2003. Prospective study of enteroviral infections and development of beta-cell autoimmunity: Diabetes Autoimmunity Study in the Young (DAISY). Diabetes Res. Clin. Pract. **59:** 51–61.
44. HONEYMAN, M.C. et al. 2000. Association between rotavirus infection and pancreatic islet autoimmunity in children at risk of developing type 1 diabetes. Diabetes **49:** 1319–1324.
45. DAHLQUIST, G. et al. 1995. Indications that maternal Coxsackie B virus infection during pregnancy is a risk factor for childhood-onset IDDM. Diabetologia **38:** 1371–1373.
46. DAHLQUIST, G.G. et al. 1995. Maternal enteroviral infection during pregnancy as a risk factor for childhood IDDM: a population-based case-control study. Diabetes **44:** 408–413.
47. DAHLQUIST, G.G., J.E. BOMAN & P. JUTO. 1999. Enteroviral RNA and IgM antibodies in early pregnancy and risk for childhood-onset IDDM in offspring. Diabetes Care **22:** 364–365.
48. VISKARI, H.R. et al. 2002. Maternal first-trimester enterovirus infection and future risk of type 1 diabetes in the exposed fetus. Diabetes **51:** 2568–2571.
49. REZAPKIN, G.V. et al. 1999. Reevaluation of nucleotide sequences of wild-type and attenuated polioviruses of type 3. Virus Res. **65:** 111–119.
50. TATEM, J.M. et al. 1992. A mutation present in the amino terminus of Sabin 3 poliovirus VP1 protein is attenuating. J. Virol. **66:** 3194–3197.
51. EVANS, D.M. et al. 1985. Increased neurovirulence associated with a single nucleotide change in a noncoding region of the Sabin type 3 poliovaccine genome. Nature **314:** 548–550.
52. KAWAMURA, N. et al. 1989. Determinants in the 5' noncoding region of poliovirus Sabin 1 RNA that influence the attenuation phenotype. J. Virol. **63:** 1302–1309.
53. MACADAM, A.J. et al. 1991. The 5' noncoding region of the type 2 poliovirus vaccine strain contains determinants of attenuation and temperature sensitivity. Virology **181:** 451–458.
54. NELSEN-SALZ, B. et al. 1996. Analysis of sequence and pathogenic properties of two variants of encephalomyocarditis virus differing in a single amino acid in VP1. Virus Res. **41:** 109–122.

55. BAE, Y.S. & J.W. YOON. 1993. Determination of diabetogenicity attributable to a single amino acid, Ala776, on the polyprotein of encephalomyocarditis virus. Diabetes **42:** 435–443.
56. CHAMPSAUR, H.F. *et al.* 1982. Virologic, immunologic, and genetic factors in insulin-dependent diabetes mellitus. J. Pediatr. **100:** 15–20.
57. LÖNNROT, M. *et al.* 1999. Diagnosis of enterovirus and rhinovirus infections by RT-PCR and time-resolved fluorometry with lanthanide chelate labeled probes. J. Med. Virol. **59:** 378–384.
58. MARTISKAINEN, M. *et al.* 2002. Enterovirus RNA in type 1 diabetic children. Presented at EuropicAmerica 2002 (May 13–19), Falmouth, MA.

Establishing Evidence for Enterovirus Infection in Chronic Disease

M. STEVEN OBERSTE AND MARK A. PALLANSCH

Respiratory and Enteric Viruses Branch, Division of Viral and Rickettsial Diseases, National Center for Infectious Diseases, Centers for Disease Control and Prevention, Atlanta, Georgia, USA

> ABSTRACT: Viruses have long been considered among potential environmental triggers of type 1 diabetes mellitus. Epidemiologic and seroprevalence studies have associated enterovirus infection with development of prediabetic autoimmunity and with the onset of clinical diabetes. Enterovirus infection has also been temporally correlated with disease onset by virus isolation or by detection of viral genome by reverse transcription–polymerase chain reaction (RT-PCR). For the large-scale prospective studies that are required to firmly establish a causal relationship between enterovirus infection and development of prediabetic autoimmunity or progression from autoimmunity to clinical diabetes, sensitive RT-PCR methods must be used to detect virus prior to the onset of diabetic symptoms. We have developed an RT-seminested PCR protocol to detect enteroviruses in clinical specimens. This method is approximately 10,000-fold more sensitive than conventional, single-amplification PCR. Further, we have developed molecular methods to rapidly and reliably identify enterovirus serotype, bypassing the cumbersome and often problematic neutralization test. The molecular serotyping approach will be valuable in examining the relationships between particular virus serotypes or genotypes and specific diseases.
>
> KEYWORDS: enterovirus; type 1 diabetes mellitus; RT-PCR; seminested PCR; molecular typing

While host genetic determinants have a major influence on an individual's risk of developing type 1 diabetes mellitus (T1DM), environmental factors, such as foods and infectious agents, are thought to play a role in the genesis of prediabetic autoimmunity or in the progression from persistent beta cell autoimmunity to clinical diabetes.[1,2] Immunity to one or more beta cell autoantigens, such as insulin, GAD65, or IA-2, may lead to destruction of beta cells and a loss of the capacity to produce insulin, ultimately resulting in clinical insulin-dependent diabetes mellitus. Postulated mechanisms by which infectious agents may trigger T1DM include (i) direct cytolytic infection of beta cells, resulting in destruction of beta cells and loss of capacity to synthesize insulin; (ii) a virus-induced immune response against infected beta cells, such as T cell–induced killing of virus-infected cells; (iii) nonspecific "innocent

---

Address for correspondence: M. Steven Oberste, Centers for Disease Control and Prevention, 1600 Clifton Road NE, Mailstop G-17, Atlanta, GA 30333. Voice: 404-639-5497; fax: 404-639-4011.
soberste@cdc.gov

bystander" killing of beta cells through activation of nonspecific immune mediators; and (iv) induction of an autoimmune response to islet antigens by cross-reactivity with viral antigens (molecular mimicry) or disruption or normal immune tolerance mechanisms.

Several viruses have been proposed as infectious triggers of diabetes, but the enteroviruses (family *Picornaviridae*, genus *Enterovirus*) are the subject of the most intense scrutiny at present.[3,4] Numerous studies have provided evidence for an association between enterovirus infection and prediabetic autoimmunity or clinical diabetes. Diabetes incidence has been epidemiologically linked to the incidence of enteroviral meningitis or enterovirus outbreaks.[5] Serologic studies have shown that there is a correlation between enterovirus seroprevalence in patients with prediabetic autoimmunity or diabetes compared to unaffected control individuals.[6,7] Direct enterovirus detection in pancreas, blood, serum, or stool has suggested a temporal correlation between enterovirus infection and onset of diabetes.[8–10]

Enteroviruses are among the most common of human viruses, infecting an estimated 50 million people annually in the United States and possibly a billion or more annually worldwide.[11,12] Most infections are inapparent, but enteroviruses may cause a wide spectrum of acute disease, including mild upper respiratory illness (common cold), febrile rash (hand-foot-and-mouth disease and herpangina), aseptic meningitis, pleurodynia, encephalitis, acute flaccid paralysis (paralytic poliomyelitis), and neonatal sepsis-like disease. Enterovirus infections result in 30,000 to 50,000 hospitalizations per year in the United States, with aseptic meningitis cases accounting for the vast majority of the hospitalizations.[12] In addition to these acute illnesses, enteroviruses have also been associated with severe chronic diseases such as myocarditis,[13,14] T1DM,[3,15] and neuromuscular diseases.[16] Enteroviruses are transmitted primarily by the fecal-oral route, but respiratory transmission to close contacts may also be important. The incubation period between infection and onset of symptoms is usually 4–7 days. The intestinal mucosa or upper respiratory tract is the site of primary infection, with secondary spread to the central nervous system and other tissues. Viremia is usually short-lived, often waning before the onset of symptoms, except in very young children. Virus is excreted in the stool for up to 8 weeks (average 2–4 weeks), but maximal virus shedding occurs before the onset of symptoms. The maximum virus titer in stool is ~10^4 infectious virus particles per gram.

Of the 89 recognized enterovirus serotypes, 64 are known to infect humans.[12] In addition to the human enteroviruses, human pathogenic viruses are found in 4 other picornavirus genera: *Rhinovirus* (human rhinoviruses), *Hepatovirus* (human hepatitis A virus), *Parechovirus* (human parechoviruses 1 and 2, formerly echoviruses 22 and 23, respectively), and *Kobuvirus* (aichivirus, an agent of gastroenteritis). Most of the human enterovirus serotypes were discovered and described between 1947 and 1963 as a result of the application of cell culture and suckling mouse inoculation to the investigation of cases of infantile paralysis (paralytic poliomyelitis) and other central nervous system diseases.[17,18] The human enteroviruses were originally classified on the basis of human disease (polioviruses), replication and pathogenesis in newborn mice (Coxsackie A and B viruses), and growth in cell culture without causing disease in mice (echoviruses), but they have recently been reclassified, based largely on molecular properties, into four species, A through D.[19] Sequences in various portions of the enterovirus coding region correlate with species, but only capsid sequence correlates with serotype.

The neutralization test, long the "gold standard" for enterovirus typing, is generally reliable, but it is labor-intensive and time-consuming, and may fail to identify an isolate because of aggregation of virus particles or antigenic drift (the widely used standardized typing antisera were raised against prototype strains that were isolated 40 to 50 years ago[20]). Antisera to all serotypes are not generally available and isolates that are not of a known human enterovirus serotype (new serotypes or serotypes that normally infect animals other than humans) would obviously also present difficulties in identification by antigenic means as the neutralization method requires the use of serotype-specific reagents. In addition, neutralization requires virus isolation, which may require the use of multiple cell lines and adds to the time required to make an identification.

The application of PCR has improved the speed and accuracy of general enterovirus detection[21,22] and has found wide acceptance in the clinical diagnostic laboratory. Since the enterovirus serotype is rarely relevant to clinical case management, many clinical virology laboratories are bypassing virus isolation entirely in favor of PCR detection of viral nucleic acid directly in clinical specimens such as cerebrospinal fluid, nasopharyngeal swabs, or tissue specimens.[21] This approach uses genus-specific primers targeted to the 5'-nontranslated region (FIG. 1), often coupled to probe-hybridization and detection of product in a microplate format.[21] Specimens of choice for the direct detection of enteroviruses by RT-PCR are stool or rectal swab (stool is preferred because it contains a larger amount of fecal material and, hence, virus), oro- or nasopharyngeal specimens (throat swab, nasopharyngeal swab or aspirate, saliva), cerebrospinal fluid (if there is concomitant CNS disease), fresh-frozen or formalin-fixed tissue, and serum/plasma. Serum and plasma are generally

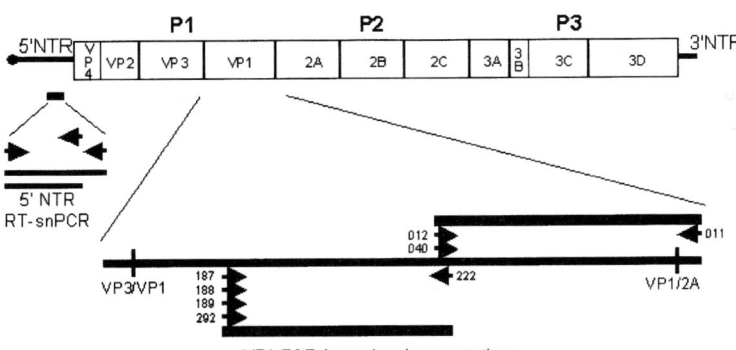

FIGURE 1. Schematic representation of the enterovirus genome, indicating regions that have been targeted for development of PCR diagnostics. The genome is a positive-stranded, polyadenylated RNA of ~7400 nucleotides, with a viral protein (3B/VPg) covalently linked to the 5'-end. The genome is divided into five functional regions: the 5'-nontranslated region (NTR) (control of viral translation initiation and initiation of positive-strand RNA synthesis); P1 (encodes the structural proteins that comprise the virus capsid); P2 and P3 (encode the nonstructural proteins involved in RNA replication, proteolytic processing of polyprotein, and host cell shutdown); and 3'-NTR (involved in initiation of negative-strand RNA synthesis).

only useful for RT-PCR in infants because viremia may still be present after onset of symptoms. If virus is detected only in a nonsterile site, such as stool or nasopharynx, a large number of patients are needed to establish the association between infection and disease.

Despite the advantages of enterovirus detection by RT-PCR, challenges remain. In the case of chronic diseases, the virus may act indirectly (e.g., through immune-mediated pathology). The virus may be cleared well before disease onset or virus may be present in the patient, but not in the diseased tissue. Even in acute illnesses, the titer is relatively low in all specimens. As a result, a "conventional" single-step RT-PCR amplification may not be sensitive enough for direct detection from the original clinical specimen. Designing a prospective study and collecting multiple specimens, at multiple time points throughout the duration of the study, may overcome some of these problems; however, the only way to solve the sensitivity problem is by increasing the sensitivity of the detection method. To address this issue, we have developed an enterovirus-specific seminested RT-PCR assay (5'-NTR RT-snPCR) that targets the conserved regions of the 5'-NTR (FIG. 1). FIGURE 2 shows the sensitivity of our standard, conventional RT-PCR[23] compared with that of the 5'-NTR RT-snPCR. Tenfold serial dilutions of a virus isolate (10^{-1} to 10^{-10}) were prepared with uninfected cell extract as diluent. RNA was extracted using the QIAamp viral RNA mini-kit (Qiagen, Inc., Valencia, CA) and reverse-transcribed using the antisense primer. PCR was performed using a single round of amplification (conventional PCR) or two rounds of amplification (seminested PCR). The second round of the seminested amplification used the same primers as the conventional

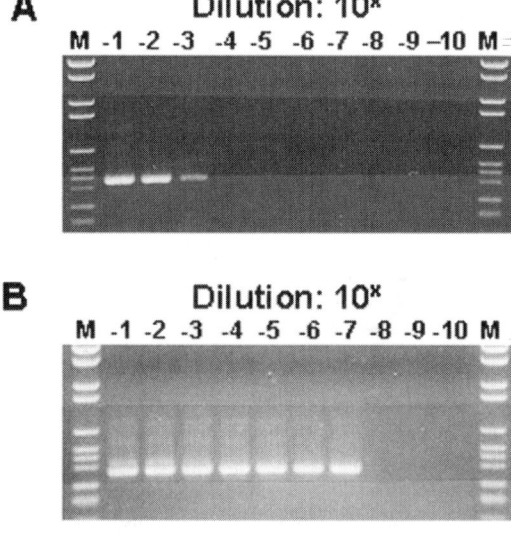

FIGURE 2. Sensitivity of pan-enterovirus RT-PCR methods; M, molecular weight marker. Virus dilutions are shown at the top of each panel. (**A**) Titration of conventional two-primer RT-PCR. (**B**) Titration of RT-seminested (three-primer) PCR.

PCR. Amplification products were visualized by polyacrylamide gel electrophoresis and staining with ethidium bromide. The RT-snPCR method (FIG. 2B) was ~10,000-fold more sensitive than the conventional RT-PCR (FIG. 2A). The 10^{-7} dilution corresponds to less than 20 infectious virus particles.

Enterovirus infection elicits a serotype-specific immune response directed against epitopes on the surface of the viral capsid. Mucosal immunity is most important. Antibody alone fully protects from disease, probably by limiting virus spread from the gut, but antibody does not necessarily protect from infection. The virus-specific T cell response, directed against epitopes on both the structural and nonstructural proteins, is probably involved in virus clearance, but it is not needed for protection. Antigenic sites are located in each of the three enterovirus structural proteins, VP1, VP2, and VP3,[24,25] but the epitopes responsible for serotype specificity have not been identified. Since the picornavirus VP1 protein contains a number of immunodominant neutralization domains, we hypothesized that VP1 sequence should correspond with neutralization properties (serotype).[26] Due to the high frequency of recombination among picornaviruses,[27–29] sequence information from noncapsid regions is of little value in characterizing new serotypes within known genera.

VP1 sequence relationships within a serotype, within a species, between species, and between human enteroviruses and other picornaviruses were analyzed by comparison of the nucleotide and deduced amino acid sequences of all possible human enterovirus VP1 sequence pairs.[26] The relationships were visualized by plotting the frequency of pairwise identity scores versus percent identity, rounded down to the nearest integer value, as a histogram (FIG. 3). For both the nucleotide (FIG. 3A) and amino acid (FIG. 3B) pairwise identity distributions, the scores fell into four categories. The highest scores (nucleotide identity of ≥75%; amino acid identity of ≥85%) depict relationships among viruses of the same serotype. Nucleotide identity scores for pairwise comparisons within a species ranged from 48.9% to 73.2% and defined a peak that was clearly delineated from the homologous pairs and from the peak of scores comparing viruses of different species (FIG. 3A). Scores among viruses in *Human Enterovirus A* (HEV-A) ranged from 58.5% to 73.2%, while those among HEV-C viruses ranged from 55.9% to 70.6%. Viruses in HEV-B appeared to be somewhat more heterogeneous, with scores ranging from 48.9% to 71.8%. Scores in the heterologous comparison peak ranged from 42.1% to 64.5% nucleotide identity and depict relationships between serotypes of different species. The final peak, containing the lowest scores, represented comparisons of viruses of different genera within the family Picornaviridae. In the amino acid identity distribution (FIG. 3B), the heterologous species peak appeared to be composed of two overlapping peaks. The peak with higher scores represented comparisons of viruses from phylogenetically related species (e.g., HEV-B and HEV-C), whereas the peak with lower scores represented comparisons among viruses of more distantly related species (e.g., HEV-A and HEV-B).

Practical criteria must be established before molecular sequence information can be applied routinely to picornavirus identification. A partial or complete VP1 nucleotide sequence identity of at least 75% (minimum 85% amino acid sequence identity) between a clinical enterovirus isolate and serotype prototype strain may be used to establish the serotype of the isolate.[26,30,31] These criteria also appear to apply to comparisons among isolates of foot-and-mouth-disease virus (family Picornaviridae, genus *Aphthovirus*),[32] but a study directly comparable to the enterovirus studies has

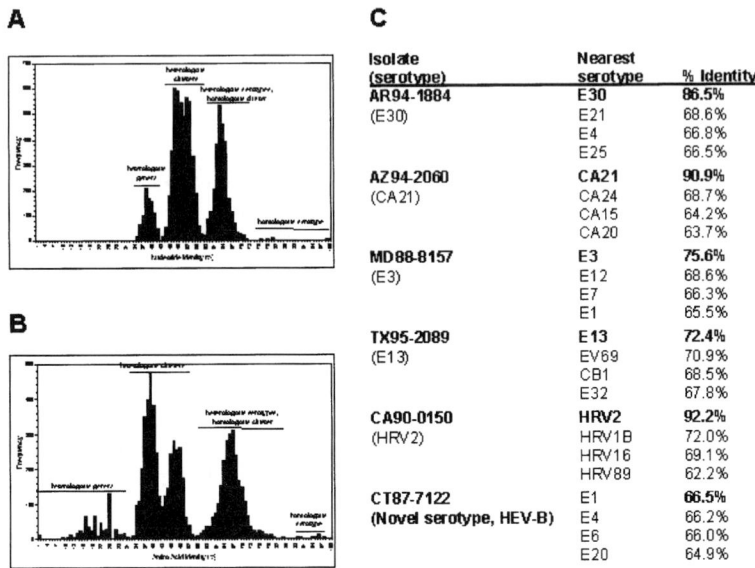

FIGURE 3. Frequency distribution of pairwise identity scores for comparison of VP1 nucleotide and deduced amino acid sequences. (**A**) Nucleotide sequence distribution. (**B**) Amino acid sequence distribution. (**C**) Example of the application of partial VP1 sequence comparisons to the identification of clinical isolates.

not yet been performed. A best-match nucleotide sequence identity of between 70% and 75% or a second-highest score of greater than 70% may provide a tentative identification, pending confirmation by other means, such as neutralization with monospecific antisera[31] or more extensive sequencing. A best-match nucleotide sequence identity below 70% (less than 85% amino acid sequence identity) may indicate that the isolate represents an unknown serotype.[31,33] Sequencing of the complete capsid coding region may be useful in confirming this result, but complete capsid sequences are available for less than half of the known enterovirus serotypes, limiting the utility of complete capsid sequence comparisons until more sequence becomes available. More extensive characterization, possibly including complete genome sequences, may be required for viruses that appear to represent previously unknown genera.[34–37]

Recognizing the technical difficulties and limitations inherent in the classic approach to enterovirus identification, we developed RT-PCR and sequencing primers that target the VP1 capsid gene and may be used to determine enterovirus serotype by sequencing of the amplicon and comparison to a database of the VP1 sequences of all enterovirus serotypes.[26,30,31] Our first set of primers amplified the prototype strains of 44 of the 64 enterovirus serotypes, as well as clinical isolates of several additional serotypes. These primers (012-040-011) amplify a product of ~450 bp corresponding to the 3′-half of VP1 (FIG. 1),[30] but they failed to amplify some of the prototype strains, primarily because of variability in the annealing site of primer 011 in 2A. The failure of primers 012-040-011 to amplify all enterovirus serotypes limited their usefulness in routine diagnostic testing.[30,31] Analysis of the complete VP1 amino acid sequences of all 64 enterovirus serotypes revealed 2 amino acid motifs that were highly conserved among all serotypes, corresponding to VP1 amino acids (NQT)A(AV)ETG and M(FIY)VPPG, respectively. A primer set targeting the sites encoding these motifs was developed for identification of isolates that were not amplified by 012-040-011.[31] Primers 187, 188, and 189 anneal to analogous sites encoding the (NQT)A(AV)ETG motif in viruses of HEV-B, HEV-C and -D, and HEV-A, respectively (FIG. 1). Primer 292 represents a consensus of 187, 188, and 189 (FIG. 1). Primer 222 anneals to the site encoding the M(FIY)VPPG motif. Primers 187-188-189-222 (and 292-222) amplify all enterovirus serotypes, producing a PCR product of about 350 nucleotides and allowing the simple and rapid identification of any enterovirus isolate. Some human rhinoviruses may also be amplified. An example of the application of this system is shown in FIGURE 3C. The highest scores for 4 of the isolates (AR94-1884, AZ94-2060, MD88-8157, and CA90-0150) were greater than 75%, ranging from 75.6% to 92.2%. These high scores were clearly resolved from the second-highest scores, which were 68.2% to 72.0%. By contrast, the high score for TX95-2089 was only 72.4% (to echovirus 13) and the second-highest score was 71.9% (to enterovirus 69). Similar scores were obtained with complete VP1 sequence. However, the isolate was fully neutralized by anti-echovirus 13 antisera, but not by antisera to any of the 3 next-highest-scoring serotypes.[30] For CT87-7122, all of the scores were less than 67% and it was not neutralized by any of the antisera,[31] strongly suggesting that it represents a new enterovirus serotype. Since 1998, over 1200 isolates of 57 different serotypes have been identified in our laboratory using the molecular serotyping approach. Only CA1, CA7, CA11, CA19, CA22, E31, and EV69 were never encountered.

These molecular detection and typing methods, when coupled with well-designed prospective studies, will be useful in addressing the potential causal relationship between enterovirus infection and development of prediabetic autoimmunity or progression from persistent autoimmunity to clinical diabetes.

REFERENCES

1. YOON, J-W. 1990. The role of viruses and environmental factors in the induction of diabetes. Curr. Top. Microbiol. Immunol. **164**: 95–123.
2. SEE, D.M. & J.G. TILLES. 1998. The pathogenesis of viral-induced diabetes. Clin. Diagn. Virol. **9**: 85–88.
3. LEINIKKI, P. 1998. Viruses and type 1 diabetes: elusive problems and elusive answers. Clin. Diagn. Virol. **9**: 65–66.
4. HYÖTY, H. et al. 1998. Enterovirus infections and insulin dependent diabetes mellitus—evidence for causality. Clin. Diagn. Virol. **9**: 77–84.
5. KARVONEN, M. et al. 1993. A review of the recent epidemiological data on the worldwide incidence of type 1 (insulin-dependent) diabetes mellitus: World Health Organisation DIAMOND Project. Diabetologia **36**: 883–892.
6. HILTUNEN, M. et al. 1997. Islet cell antibody seroconversion in children is temporally associated with enterovirus infections. J. Infect. Dis. **175**: 554–560.
7. HELFAND, R.F. et al. 1995. Serologic evidence of an association between enteroviruses and the onset of type 1 diabetes mellitus: Pittsburgh Diabetes Research Group. J. Infect. Dis. **172**: 1206–1211.
8. YOON, J-W. et al. 1979. Isolation of a virus from the pancreas of a child with diabetic ketoacidosis. N. Engl. J. Med. **300**: 1173–1179.

9. ANDREOLETTI, L. *et al.* 1997. Detection of Coxsackie B virus RNA sequences in whole blood samples from adult patients at the onset of type I diabetes mellitus. J. Med. Virol. **52:** 121–127.
10. CLEMENTS, G.B. *et al.* 1995. Coxsackie B virus infection and onset of childhood diabetes. Lancet **346:** 221–223.
11. MORENS, D.M. & M.A. PALLANSCH. 1995. Epidemiology. *In* Human Enterovirus Infections, pp. 3–23. ASM Press. Washington, D.C.
12. PALLANSCH, M.A. & R.P. ROOS. 2001. Enteroviruses: polioviruses, coxsackieviruses, echoviruses, and newer enteroviruses. *In* Fields' Virology, pp. 723–775. Lippincott/Williams & Wilkins. Philadelphia/Baltimore.
13. MARTINO, T.A. *et al.* 1995. Enteroviral myocarditis and cardiomyopathy: a review of clinical and experimental studies. *In* Human Enterovirus Infections, pp. 291–351. ASM Press. Washington, D.C.
14. KIM, K-S. *et al.* 2001. The group B coxsackieviruses and myocarditis. Rev. Med. Virol. **11:** 355–368.
15. REWERS, M. & M. ATKINSON. 1995. The possible role of enteroviruses in diabetes mellitus. *In* Human Enterovirus Infections, pp. 353–385. ASM Press. Washington, D.C.
16. DALAKAS, M.C. 1995. Enteroviruses and human neuromuscular diseases. *In* Human Enterovirus Infections, pp. 387–398. ASM Press. Washington, D.C.
17. COMMITTEE ON ENTEROVIRUSES. 1962. Classification of human enteroviruses. Virology **16:** 501–504.
18. PANEL FOR PICORNAVIRUSES. 1963. Picornaviruses: classification of nine new types. Science **141:** 153–154.
19. KING, A.M.Q. *et al.* 2000. Picornaviridae. *In* Virus Taxonomy: Seventh Report of the International Committee on Taxonomy of Viruses, pp. 657–678. Academic Press. San Diego.
20. LIM, K.A. & M. BENYESH-MELNICK. 1960. Typing of viruses by combinations of antiserum pools: application to typing of enteroviruses (Coxsackie and ECHO). J. Immunol. **84:** 309–317.
21. ROTBART, H.A. & J.R. ROMERO. 1995. Laboratory diagnosis of enteroviral infections. *In* Human Enterovirus Infections, pp. 401–418. ASM Press. Washington, D.C.
22. ROTBART, H.A. *et al.* 1997. Diagnosis of enterovirus infection by polymerase chain reaction of multiple specimen types. Ped. Infect. Dis. J. **16:** 409–411.
23. YANG, C-F. *et al.* 1992. Genotype-specific *in vitro* amplification of sequences of the wild type 3 polioviruses from Mexico and Guatemala. Virus Res. **24:** 277–296.
24. MINOR, P.D. 1990. Antigenic structure of picornaviruses. Curr. Top. Microbiol. Immunol. **161:** 121–154.
25. MATEU, M.G. 1995. Antibody recognition of picornaviruses and escape from neutralization. Virus Res. **38:** 1–24.
26. OBERSTE, M.S. *et al.* 1999. Molecular evolution of the human enteroviruses: correlation of serotype with VP1 sequence and application to picornavirus classification. J. Virol. **73:** 1941–1948.
27. KOPECKA, H. *et al.* 1995. Genotypic variation in coxsackievirus B5 isolates from three different outbreaks in the United States. Virus Res. **38:** 125–136.
28. KING, A.M.Q. 1988. Genetic recombination in positive strand RNA viruses. *In* RNA Genetics, pp. 149–165. CRC Press. Boca Raton, FL.
29. SANTTI, J. *et al.* 1999. Evidence of recombination among enteroviruses. J. Virol. **73:** 8741–8749.
30. OBERSTE, M.S. *et al.* 1999. Typing of human enteroviruses by partial sequencing of VP1. J. Clin. Microbiol. **37:** 1288–1293.
31. OBERSTE, M.S. *et al.* 2000. Comparison of classic and molecular approaches for the identification of "untypable" enteroviruses. J. Clin. Microbiol. **38:** 1170–1174.
32. VOSLOO, W. *et al.* 1992. Genetic relationships between southern African SAT-2 isolates of foot-and-mouth-disease virus. Epidemiol. Infect. **109:** 547–558.
33. OBERSTE, M.S. *et al.* 2001. Molecular identification of new picornaviruses and characterization of a proposed enterovirus 73 serotype. J. Gen. Virol. **82:** 409–416.
34. HYYPIÄ, T. *et al.* 1992. A distinct picornavirus group identified by sequence analysis. Proc. Natl. Acad. Sci. USA **89:** 8847–8851.

35. MARVIL, P. *et al.* 1999. Avian encephalomyelitis virus is a picornavirus and is most closely related to hepatitis A virus. J. Gen. Virol. **80:** 653–662.
36. NIKLASSON, B. *et al.* 1999. A new picornavirus isolated from bank voles (*Clethrionomys glareolus*). Virology **255:** 86–93.
37. YAMASHITA, T. *et al.* 1998. Complete nucleotide sequence and genetic organization of Aichi virus, a distinct member of the Picornaviridae associated with acute gastroenteritis in humans. J. Virol. **72:** 8408–8412.

Beta Cell Death and Protection

THOMAS MANDRUP-POULSEN

Steno Diabetes Center, Gentofte, Denmark, and Department of Molecular Medicine, Karolinska Institute, Stockholm, Sweden

ABSTRACT: Type 1 diabetes is an immune-mediated disease critically dependent upon the interaction between antigen-presenting cells and T cells. Clearly, both CD4+ and CD8+ T cells are required, but activated CD4+ T cells are both necessary and sufficient in causing disease. The mechanism of the Th1/Th2 immunoregulatory imbalance is unclear and needs to be further investigated. CD8+ T cells are not commonly sufficient in causing disease, but CD8 T cells are necessary in initiation (<14 weeks in the NOD mouse), but not in the later (>14 weeks) effector phase of the disease. It is still unclear whether the CD8+ T cell exerts its function as a classical effector cell or mainly as an immunomodulatory cell acting in synergy with the CD4+ T cell. The relative role of T cell effector mechanisms such as Fas/FasL, perforin/granzyme, and the TRAIL systems is unclear. Proinflammatory cytokines, reactive oxygen species, and other immune mediators seem to be involved in beta cell destruction, but much is to be learned about signaling, molecular mechanisms, and *in vivo* importance.

KEYWORDS: T cell; beta cell; type 1 diabetes; tolerance; immune; signaling

INTRODUCTION

Type 1 diabetes is a complex multifactorial disease.[1] The etiology involves multiple environmental and genetic components. Recent theories on the nongenetic components suggest that not only presence, but maybe also absence of environmental stressors (infectious agents, climatic and nutritional factors, environmental toxins) may trigger disease. Thus, notably the high incidence of spontaneous diabetes in animal models[1] can only be maintained in specific pathogen-free environments, and the incidence of type 1 diabetes has been increasing with increased standards of living and improved hygiene. Similarly, genetic susceptibility to type 1 diabetes is likely to be conferred by a combination of presence of predisposing and absence of protective genes. Genes that control responses to acute disease caused by environmental pathogens provide evolutionary advantages by ensuring survival from environmental threats, but may have the adverse effect of predisposing to autoimmunity (see Serreze *et al.* in this volume). However, our insight does not allow intervention on the etiological level at present.

The pathogenesis of type 1 diabetes shares the complexity of most autoimmune conditions.[1] There is most likely more than one driving autoantigen, and there is

Address for correspondence: Thomas Mandrup-Poulsen, Steno Diabetes Center, 2 Niels Steensensvej, DK-2820 Gentofte, Denmark. Voice: +45-44-43-91-01; fax: +45-44-43-82-32.
tmpo@steno.dk

presently no definite identification of those antigens in type 1 diabetes, although there are attractive candidates, such as insulin/proinsulin, GAD, and IA-2. The mechanisms of breaking of tolerance are elusive and involve genetically determined alterations in thymic presentation and recognition of autoantigens, and genetic as well as environmental alterations in peripheral tolerance. Despite progress in the understanding of the basics of the immunoregulatory events that allow the activation and expansion of autoreactive T cell clones, the details of this process are still incompletely understood. Accordingly, the mechanism of action explaining recent promising results of the induction of remission by usage of short-term administration of nondepleting anti-CD3 antibodies in new-onset type 1 diabetes[2] is unknown.

We still do not precisely understand the way that beta cells are destroyed. The histopathology of type 1 diabetes in human and animal models is characterized by lymphocytic infiltration and production of inflammatory mediators such as chemokines, cytokines, prostaglandins, and reactive oxygen species (ROS). The lesion can be described morphologically as a chronic atrophic lymphocytic insulitis;[3] however, in terms of phenotype and composition of infiltrating cells, expression of cytokines, and other mediators, the pathology monotonously resembles that seen in most other autoimmune diseases.

It is generally accepted that beta cell autoantigen is picked up and processed by dendritic cells or macrophages in the pancreatic islets and carried to the draining pancreatic lymph nodes.[4] Here, the processed autoantigen is presented to autoreactive T cells escaping thymic negative selection and evading peripheral tolerance, leading to T cell activation, clonal expansion, and migration to the islets of the activated T cells. Once in the islets, they are further activated by local antigen-presenting cells to produce cytokines and chemokines that attract and activate other T cells and macrophages.[5] The recruited cells build up the inflammatory infiltrate in which mutual activation and costimulation maintain and amplify the immune response. As will be detailed below, the effector mechanisms have not been clarified, but most likely involve both CD4+ and CD8+ T cells; the proinflammatory cytokines IL-1, IFNγ, and TNFα; and ROS.[6] These effectors elicit a complex of signaling pathways in the beta cells resulting in apoptosis and necrosis.[7] Eventually, with the elimination of the antigenic load and the result of generation of inhibitory cytokines, the inflammatory response is dampened and islet inflammation resolves.

It is becoming clear that the target cells in many autoimmune diseases are not passive bystanders to their own destruction. Rather, they participate in the death process by *de novo* expression of hundreds of genes and activation of constitutively expressed proteins including protein kinases and other signaling pathways, leading to programmed cell death.[7] Thus, the diverse phenotypes of immune-mediated diseases arise from a redundant inflammatory reaction, with specificity being defined by a combination of antigen-specific immune activation and the tissue-specific response of the target cells to mediators of immune destruction. For example in rheumatoid arthritis, cartilage destruction is the result of the loss of tolerance to collagen, CD4+ T cell activation, production of T cell cytokines that activate synovial cells to the synthesis of proinflammatory cytokines, and selective inducibility by cytokines, especially TNF, of chondrocyte metalloproteinases and synoviocyte collagenases.[8] In autoimmune thyroid disease, inflammation leads to induction in the thyrocyte of many proinflammatory cytokines that probably potentiate tissue damage by further recruiting and activating inflammatory cells.[9] In type 1 diabetes, the irreversible loss of insulin secretory capacity is, as mentioned, most likely the result of a combination of antigen-specific mechanisms (CD4 and CD8 T cell–mediated destruction) and antigen-nonspecific mechanisms (inflammatory mediators such as cytokines and ROS).[6] The inherent properties of the beta cell may well contribute to the susceptibility to immune attack. The beta cell expresses cytokine receptors that signal destruction by induction of the Fas receptor, selective induction of inducible NO synthase (iNOS), activation of mitogen-activated protein kinases (MAPK), PKCδ, and NFκB.[7] The signaling events operate on a background of active Ca^{2+} handling important for insulin exocytosis and a high metabolic activity. These factors may amplify proapoptotic signaling and explain why beta cells are so prone to apoptosis-inducing agents. The physiological role of these apparently inappropriate characteristics of the beta cell may be related to the importance of being able to control beta cell mass,[10] for example, in the remodeling of beta cell mass required postpartum or after severe weight loss in obese patients, situations where beta cell mass has been increased to compensate for increased demand/insulin resistance.

Disconcertingly, two recently completed large-scale intervention studies in risk individuals have failed to show therapeutic advantage. The ENDIT trial was designed to test if nicotinamide treatment provided beta cell protection against the consequences of NAD depletion caused by oxidative DNA damage and activation of the DNA repair enzyme, poly(ADP)ribose polymerase. The sc arm of the DPT-1 trial tested the hypothesis that low-dose sc insulin would protect beta cells to ongoing immune destruction either by inducing beta cell rest shown to be effective *in vitro* or by immune modulation.[11] Although it cannot be excluded that the failure of these two well-designed and well-conducted trials was due to inappropriate dosing, pharmacokinetics, or timing in relation to the pathogenic process, they raise the important question if our knowledge about the disease process is sufficient to embark on intervention studies. Therefore, clearly much more needs to be known about basic elements of the pathogenesis to be able to rationally devise evidence-based therapy in nonarbitrary doses and time windows.

The purpose of this review is to give a short oversight of our current understanding of the mechanisms underlying immune-mediated beta cell destruction to serve as a general introduction to the following few papers, dealing each in detail with central elements of beta cell destruction and defense, that is, the Fas/FasL system, cytokine effects on gene expression, the suppressors of cytokine signaling (SOCS) family, oxidative stress, and PARP.

THE ROLE OF T CELL EFFECTORS

It is unquestionable that CD4+ T cells are both necessary and sufficient to cause type 1 diabetes in animal models.[12] Thus, all measures that interfere with CD4+ T cell function have been shown to be effective in preventing disease. Further, transfer of islet reactive CD4+ T cells is sufficient to transfer disease without CD8+ T cells.[13] The role and function of CD8+ T cells as effectors have been widely debated. Although most islet reactive T cell clones are not able to transfer diabetes in the absence of CD4+ T cells, with the exception of CD8+ clones derived from special T cell receptor transgenic mice (e.g., the 8.3 clone),[14] they are required for disease initiation as disease development is prevented for up to 14 weeks of age in beta-2 microglobulin deficient and thereby class I MHC and CD8+ T cell response deficient mice.[15] It should be noted, however, that beta-2 microglobulin may have other functions than being a part of the MHC class I complex and that other cells may express low levels of CD8. Further, it remains to be shown that the requirement for CD8+ T cells is related to their function as CTLs. It is possible that CD8+ T cells act by amplifying CD4+ T cell responses and other inflammatory responses in the infiltrate. Very recent studies by Queen *et al.* (this conference) seem to indicate that CD8+ T cell determinants may be upstream to CD4 T cell determinants. Moreover, it has not been shown that the diabetogenic function of the 8.3 T cell clone can be abrogated by antisense to Fas or perforin.

Taken together with our general knowledge about the inflammatory response, it is most likely that all elements of the inflammatory response take part in destroying the islet beta cells, introducing redundancies in the ways by which beta cells can be destroyed. If this theory proves to be true, it will complicate the development of curative treatment and may explain the failure of drugs exerting their effects on single pathways of the pathogenetic process.

RELATIVE ROLE OF FAS/FASL, PERFORIN/GRANZYME, AND TRAIL IN T CELL–MEDIATED BETA CELL DESTRUCTION

As shown in TABLE 1, effector T cells can kill target cells by direct contact with surface membrane–bound ligands of apoptosis-inducing receptors such as FasL, TNF-related apoptosis-inducing ligand (TRAIL), and membrane-bound TNFα. By binding of these ligands to their respective receptors that are induced on many target cells by proinflammatory cytokines including IL-1, apoptosis is induced in the target cells via the death domains of the receptors and activation of caspases. In addition, T cells can mediate target cell killing without cell-to-cell contact by secretion of humoral substances such as perforin molecules that are inserted into the cell membrane of the target cell as tubular complexes through which the proteases granzyme A and B can pass and activate nucleases in the cell. Further, secretion of proinflammatory cytokines such as IFNγ and lymphotoxin can, together with other cytokines, signal apoptosis in target cells.

Animal studies trying to elucidate which effector mechanisms are used by T cells to kill beta cells in type 1 diabetes have been difficult to interpret because manipulation of the T cell effector system inevitably also affects T cell–mediated killing of

TABLE 1. T cell effector mechanisms

Granule-dependent
    Perforin: tubular pore complexes
    Granzyme A/B: proteases, activates nucleases

Granule-independent
    Fas/FasL: activates caspases
    TRAIL/TRAIL-RI-II: activates caspases
    IFNγ, TNFα, lymphotoxin: signals apoptosis, activates macrophages

immune cells, thereby theoretically affecting CD4, CD8, and bystander suppressor cells. Currently available evidence suggests mainly immune regulatory and not beta cell effector functions of the Fas/FasL system and of the perforin/granzyme system.[16] Very little is known regarding the role of the TRAIL/TRAIL-ligand system in beta cell destruction and clearly further studies are needed to identify the main T cell effector pathway involved in beta cell killing.

INFLAMMATORY MEDIATORS: *IN VITRO* AND ANIMAL STUDIES

In rodent islets, IL-1 alone or in synergy with IFNγ/TNFα causes nitric oxide (NO) synthesis, necrosis, and apoptosis. In human islets, a combination of the three cytokines is required to induce the same phenomena.[7] It is unknown whether intra-islet IFNγ or TNFα secretion secondary to exposure to IL-1 may deliver the triple combination needed in human islets or whether IL-1 alone is sufficient to cause beta cell destruction in rodent islets. Clearly, human beta cells exposed to cytokines die mainly in a process of apoptosis, whereas beta cell destruction in rodent islets constitutes a mixture of necrosis and apoptosis. NO synthesis is dispensable for cytokine-mediated beta cell destruction in human islets,[17] whereas NO seems to be a main mediator of rodent islet beta cell necrotic cell death. These species differences are partially related to the generation of different protective responses between the species. For example, heat shock protein 70 is an important protective factor in human islets against cytokine-mediated beta cell destruction.[18] Further comparative studies between species and insights into the protective responses of, in particular, human islets may lead to identification of clinically important targets for intervention.

In early insulitis in the NOD mouse and the BB rat, expression of IL-1, TNFα, and IFNγ can be detected.[19,20] Thus, the beta cell cytotoxic combination of pro-inflammatory cytokines has been demonstrated to be present in relevant animal models. Intraperitoneal IL-1 injections into nondiabetes-prone normal rats causes insulinopenia and hyperglycemia,[21] but whether this is due to a direct effect of IL-1 on pancreatic beta cells or to a secondary phenomenon has not been clarified. Beta cell overexpression of certain cytokines (IFNα/γ) in nondiabetes-prone mice, TNFα in NOD neonates, and IL-10 in adult NOD leads to diabetes.[7] It is unlikely that transgenic beta cell expression of the single cytokines is causing diabetes. Beta cell destruction is rather the result of massive islet infiltration and inflammatory response elicited by the beta cell secretion of these proinflammatory and chemotactic factors.

At this meeting, it was reported that the IL-1 receptor type 1 knockout mice had a reduced diabetes incidence of about 30%, emphasizing the importance of IL-1 signaling in type 1 diabetes in the NOD mouse (Kay Thomas *et al.*, this conference). The fact that protection was only partial may be due to the fact that TNFα and IFNγ signaling was not prevented, and synergy between these three cytokines has been demonstrated in terms of beta cell destruction *in vitro*. Thus, in particular, TNFα may compensate for the lack of IL-1 signaling since TNFα shares many signaling pathways with IL-1.

IL-1 converting enzyme (ICE) is responsible for processing pro-IL-1β to mature IL-1β. At this meeting, Schott *et al.*[22] reported that the ICE knockout NOD mouse was not protected against diabetes. This does not exclude involvement of IL-1 signaling because IL-1α may be the most important mouse IL-1, pro-IL-1α processing is ICE-independent and mainly requires membrane calpains and extracellular proteases, and finally membrane-bound pro-IL-1α is fully active. This study does, however, indicate that ICE may not be important as an initiator of caspase-dependent apoptosis in type 1 diabetes.[22]

Anticytokine approaches such as IL-1 receptor antagonist, soluble IL-1 receptor, anti-IL-6 antibody, anti-TNFα antibody, and anti-IFNγ antibody therapy have all individually been shown to reduce diabetes incidence in animal models.[7] It remains to be demonstrated that these effects are exerted by blocking cytokine action directly on the beta cells and not by immune modulatory effects of these cytokine antagonists, although the protective effect of soluble IL-1 receptor was not associated with alterations of T cell function. Combinations of anticytokine strategies may be needed to induce complete remission as observed for other autoimmune diseases, for example, in animal models of arthritis. A reduction in disease activity in animal models of arthritis was only partial by the employment of either anti-TNF or anti-IL-1, but was almost complete by the combination of these therapeutic principles (ACR abstract[8]). Anti-IL-1 combined with anti-TNF or anti-IFNγ therapy should be tested in animal models and perhaps even considered in clinical trials in type 1 diabetes. The potential risk of severely inhibiting the innate immune system leading to a higher propensity for severe infections should be kept in mind.

OXIDATIVE STRESS AND BETA CELL DESTRUCTION

Apart from proinflammatory cytokines, activated immune cells especially of the monocytic lineage produce reactive oxygen species (ROS), a term covering free oxygen radicals, hydroxyl radicals, and NO species, as well as derivatives such as peroxynitrite. NO species are also produced by cytokine action in beta cells because cytokines selectively induce the expression of iNOS in beta cells, but not in non-beta cells.[7,23] As mentioned, NO seems to be an important inducer of necrosis and perhaps even apoptosis especially in rodent islets, whereas NO is dispensable in terms of cytokine induction of apoptosis in human islets.[17] Due to the extremely short half-life of these species, they have been difficult to demonstrate directly. By the use of paramagnetic resonance, it has been possible to directly detect beta cell generation of NO in response to cytokines,[24] and peroxynitrite, a marker of ROS, has also been demonstrated in NOD beta cells *in vivo*.[25] Despite attempts, it has not been possible to use direct spin trapping methods to detect free oxygen radicals or hydroxyl radicals, but indirect probes as well as lipid peroxidation have lent support to the induction of these oxygen radicals, for example, by cytokines.

There is no doubt that chemical donors of ROS are beta cell cytotoxic, but also toxic to non-beta islet cells. It is therefore more likely that intracellularly produced ROS contribute to selective beta cell destruction rather than ROS produced by inflammatory cells.

Contributing also to beta cell sensitivity to ROS is the extraordinarily low level of ROS scavenging capacity in beta cells.[26] Correcting this deficiency, for example by overexpressing the mitochondrial form of superoxide dismutase (Mn-SOD), protects beta cells *in vitro* against oxidative stress and cytokines.[27,28] If beta cells have targeted overexpression of the cytosolic SOD (Cu/Zn-SOD), autoimmune and low-dose streptozotocin-induced diabetes in animal models are prevented.[29,30]

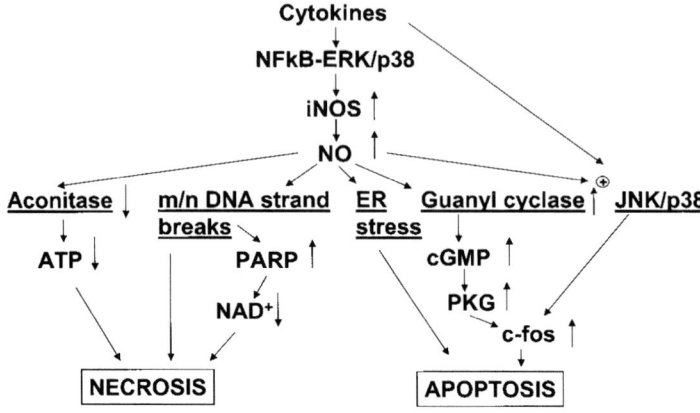

FIGURE 1. Model for NO-mediated beta cell destructive pathways. NO could elicit beta cell necrosis via the inhibition of aconitase, DNA strand breaks, and/or NAD depletion secondary to DNA repair. Beta cell apoptosis can be caused by NO-induced endoplasmic reticulum (ER) stress, NO activation of guanyl cyclase and protein kinase G, as well as potentiation of MAPK. Reproduced with permission from *Diabetologia*. Modified after reference 7.

In general, the effect of antioxidative therapy in clinical disorders such as cancer, cardiovascular disease, and other autoimmune diseases has been disappointing. The recent failure of nicotinamide, in part believed to have antioxidative capacity, might discourage the use of this approach in attempts to prevent type 1 diabetes. However, most of the antioxidants used in clinical trials have been noncatalytic substances such as vitamins E and C and the timing as well as the pharmacokinetics of antioxidants may be critical. Therefore, it is encouraging that SOD mimetics with longer half-life were recently shown to protect against diabetes induced by the islet reactive BDC-2.5 T cell clone in NOD.scid mice.[31] Further studies along this line are needed to evaluate the clinical utility of antioxidative therapy (see Haskins *et al.*, this volume). ROS can also induce cell toxicity by causing DNA strand breaks (FIG. 1). DNA strand breaks can be lethal if sufficiently extensive. Sublethal DNA strand breaks can be toxic via activation of the DNA repair enzyme, poly(ADP)ribose polymerase (PARP). This enzyme repairs DNA strand breaks, but also uses and depletes the cell of the coenzyme, nicotinamide adenosine dinucleotide (NAD), and this may lead to necrosis.[32] PARP knockout mice are resistant to low-dose streptozotocin-induced diabetes.[33] As mentioned above, failure of nicotinamide to prevent type 1 diabetes may be related to timing and dosing of this compound. Further studies on alternative PARP inhibitors (Rabinovitch, this conference) are therefore warranted with the aim of investigating this approach further.

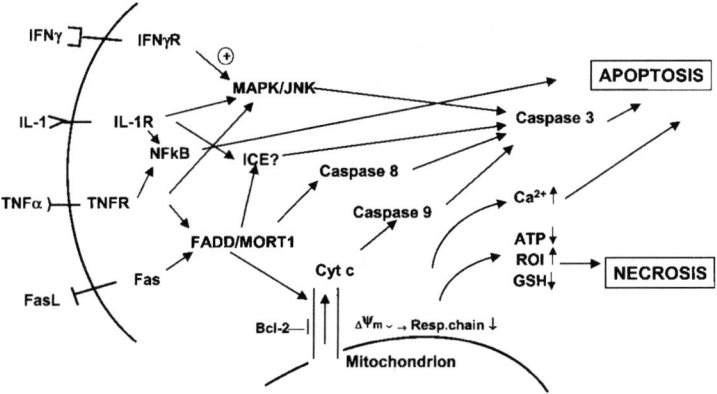

FIGURE 2. Model for NO-independent beta cell destructive pathways. IFNγ, IL-1, and TNFα signaling converges on MAP kinases, in particular JNK, which probably activates apoptosis via modification of gene expression and activation of effector caspases. IL-1 and TNF also converge for activation of the nuclear factor κB (NFκB), which by translocation to the nucleus activates many proapoptotic genes in the beta cell. The TNF receptor 1 death domain (TRADD) could also elicit apoptosis via interaction with the Fas-associated death domain protein (FADD), also known as mediator of receptor-induced toxicity 1 (MORT-1). FADD causes mitochondrial outer membrane transition pore opening leading to release of cytochrome c and caspase activation and the liberation of calcium that can also signal apoptosis. Further decreases in ATP generation, increased formation of reactive oxygen intermediates (ROI), and decrease of the reducing in potential can lead to necrosis. Reproduced by permission from *Diabetologia*. Modified after reference 7.

NO-independent intracellular pathways of beta cell destruction as shown in FIGURE 2 induced by Fas and cytokines may cause beta cell destruction.[7] The proposed pathways in FIGURE 2 are being investigated as candidate proteins and genes in the pathophysiology of type 1 diabetes by classical biochemical and cell biology techniques. There is, however, a need for screening methods to reveal novel pathways involved in immune-mediated beta cell destruction. Both the use of messenger RNA microarray and proteomic analysis have been employed to analyze protein and gene regulation in beta cells exposed to immune mediators.[34,35] More than 100 transcripts are modified by exposure to IL-1 for 24 h and this number is even higher when adding IFNγ (see Eizirik *et al.*, this volume). Further grouping and characterization of these genes may lead to interesting novel targets both in terms of proteins involved in the destruction, but perhaps more importantly in the identification of protective proteins that can be used therapeutically. Similarly, by using high-resolution 2D gel electrophoresis, more than 100 proteins were found to be altered by exposure to IL-1, of which >60 proteins have presently been identified by mass spectrometry.[35] Interestingly and in contrast to expectation, most of these proteins are not altered secondarily to NO, but seem primary or secondary to other IL-1-induced pathways.[36] Identification of the functional role of these proteins may open new avenues to therapeutic approaches.

NATURAL INHIBITORS OF CYTOKINE SIGNALING: CAN THEY BE USED AS THERAPEUTICS?

As mentioned above, inflammation leads to the expression and synthesis of proinflammatory cytokines that may participate in destruction of target cells. To avoid the adverse effect of these potent mediators, naturally occurring antagonists, soluble receptors, decoy receptors, and inhibitors of intracellular signaling of cytokines are devised by nature to dampen and downregulate the inflammatory response to avoid adverse effects and tissue destruction. An example of signaling regulators are the suppressors of cytokine signaling (SOCS) family of cytokine inducible proteins that can negatively regulate several cytokine pathways by negative feedback. Thus, SOCS proteins are induced by IFNγ signaling via the Jak-STAT pathway. These inhibitory proteins prevent IFN signaling by binding to IFN receptor components including the JAK kinases. Interestingly and unexpectedly, overexpression of SOCS-3 and clonal beta cells was found to inhibit IL-1β-induced cell death,[37] and SOCS-1 knockout islets were found to be more sensitive to TNF, but not to IL-1 actions, and this was signaled via the p38 MAPK pathway[38] (see also Kay, this conference). Studying the mechanism of action of these naturally occurring inhibitors of cytokine signaling may provide clues to how cytokine signaling can be affected. Preliminary studies have shown that SOCS-3 overexpression alters a finite number of IL-1-induced gene changes in beta cells. Interestingly, SOCS-3 did not equally inhibit all genes induced by IL-1: potentially protective genes were not inhibited, whereas potentially deleterious genes were suppressed by 40–60% (P. Heding, unpublished). These findings support the concept that inhibitors of cytokine signaling can constructively modulate the expression of many IL-1-regulated genes favoring beta cell survival. The possibilities of constructively modulating cytokine-induced changes in gene expression may lead to identification targets for prevention of type 1 diabetes.

ACKNOWLEDGMENTS

Karen Kruse is thanked for preparing this manuscript.

REFERENCES

1. POCIOT, F., A.E. KARLSEN & T. MANDRUP-POULSEN. 2002. Etiology and pathogenesis of insulin-dependent diabetes mellitus. *In* Endocrinology and Metabolism, pp. 593–606. McGraw–Hill International. London.
2. HEROLD, K.C., W. HAGOPIAN, J.A. AUGER *et al.* 2002. Anti-CD3 monoclonal antibody in new-onset type 1 diabetes mellitus. N. Engl. J. Med. **346:** 1692–1698.
3. GEPTS, W. 1965. Pathologic anatomy of the pancreas in juvenile diabetes mellitus. Diabetes **14:** 619–633.
4. HOGLUND, P., J. MINTERN, C. WALTZINGER *et al.* 1999. Initiation of autoimmune diabetes by developmentally regulated presentation of islet cell antigens in the pancreatic lymph nodes. J. Exp. Med. **189:** 331–339.
5. BERGHOLDT, R., P. HEDING, K. NIELSEN *et al.* 2002. Type 1 diabetes mellitus, an inflammatory disease of the islet. *In* Type 1 Diabetes: Molecular, Cellular and Clinical Immunology [http://www.uchsc.edu/misc/diabetes/bdc.html].
6. BENOIST, C. & D. MATHIS. 1997. Cell-death mediators in autoimmune diabetes—no shortage of suspects. Cell **89:** 1–3.

7. EIZIRIK, D.L. & T. MANDRUP-POULSEN. 2001. A choice of death—the signal-transduction of immune-mediated beta-cell apoptosis. Diabetologia **44:** 2115–2133.
8. DINARELLO, C.A. & L.L. MOLDAWER. 2002. Immunopathogenesis of rheumatoid arthritis in humans. *In* Proinflammatory and Anti-inflammatory Cytokines in Rheumatoid Arthritis, pp. 131–138. AMGEN Inc. California.
9. WEETMAN, A.P. & A.M. MCGREGOR. 1994. Autoimmune thyroid-disease—further developments in our understanding. Endocr. Rev. **15:** 788–830.
10. BONNER-WEIR, S. 2000. Perspective: postnatal pancreatic beta cell growth. Endocrinology **141:** 1926–1929.
11. RILEY, W.J., N.K. MACLAREN, J. KRISCHER *et al.* 1990. A prospective study of the development of diabetes in relatives of patients with insulin-dependent diabetes. N. Engl. J. Med. **323:** 1167–1172.
12. WONG, F.S., B.N. DITTEL & C.A. JANEWAY. 1999. Transgenes and knockout mutations in animal models of type I diabetes and multiple sclerosis. Immunol. Rev. **169:** 93–106.
13. PETERSON, J.D., B. PIKE, M. MCDUFFIE & K. HASKINS. 1994. Islet-specific T-cell clones transfer diabetes to nonobese diabetic (NOD) F1-mice. J. Immunol. **153:** 2800–2806.
14. GRASER, R.T., T.P. DILORENZO, F.M. WANG *et al.* 2000. Identification of a CD8 T cell that can independently mediate autoimmune diabetes development in the complete absence of CD4 T cell helper functions. J. Immunol. **164:** 3913–3918.
15. DILORENZO, T.P., R.T. GRASER, T. ONO *et al.* 1998. Major histocompatibility complex class I–restricted T-cells are required for all but the end stages of diabetes development in nonobese diabetic mice and use a prevalent T-cell receptor-alpha chain gene rearrangement. Proc. Natl. Acad. Sci. USA **95:** 12538–12543.
16. KIM, S., K.A. KIM, D.Y. HWANG *et al.* 2000. Inhibition of autoimmune diabetes by Fas ligand: the paradox is solved. J. Immunol. **164:** 2931–2936.
17. RABINOVITCH, A., W.L. SUAREZ-PINZON, K. STRYNADKA *et al.* 1994. Human pancreatic islet β-cell destruction by cytokines is independent of nitric oxide production. J. Clin. Endocrinol. Metab. **79:** 1058–1062.
18. WELSH, N., B. MARGULIS, L.A.H. BORG *et al.* 1995. Differences in the expression of heat-shock proteins and antioxidant enzymes between human and rodent pancreatic islets: implications for the pathogenesis of insulin-dependent diabetes mellitus. Mol. Med. **1:** 806–820.
19. JIANG, Z. & B.A. WODA. 1991. Cytokine gene expression in the islets of the diabetic BioBreeding/Worcester rat. J. Immunol. **146:** 2990–2994.
20. TOYODA, H., B. FORMBY, D. MAGALONG *et al.* 1994. *In situ* islet cytokine gene expression during development of type I diabetes in the non-obese diabetic mouse. Immunol. Lett. **39:** 283–288.
21. REIMERS, J.I., U. BJERRE, T. MANDRUP-POULSEN & J. NERUP. 1994. Interleukin 1β induces diabetes and fever in normal rats by nitric oxide via induction of different nitric oxide synthases. Cytokine **6:** 512–520.
22. SCHOTT, W., R. BAGLEY, B. HASKELL & E. LEITER. 2002. Caspase-1 is not required for diabetes in NOD mice [abstract]. Diabetes/Metabolism **18:** suppl. 4.
23. CORBETT, J.A., J.L. WANG, M.A. SWEETLAND *et al.* 1992. Interleukin 1β induces the formation of nitric oxide by β-cells purified from rodent islets of Langerhans: evidence for the β-cell as a source and site of action of nitric oxide. J. Clin. Invest. **90:** 2384–2391.
24. CORBETT, J.A., J.R. LANCASTER, JR., M.A. SWEETLAND & M.L. MCDANIEL. 1991. Interleukin-1 beta-induced formation of EPR-detectable iron-nitrosyl complexes in islets of Langerhans. J. Biol. Chem. **266:** 21351–21354.
25. SUAREZ-PINZON, W.L., C. SZABO & A. RABINOVITCH. 1997. Development of autoimmune diabetes in NOD mice is associated with the formation of peroxynitrite in pancreatic-islet beta-cells. Diabetes **46:** 907–911.
26. LENZEN, S., J. DRINKGERN & M. TIEDGE. 1996. Low antioxidant enzyme gene-expression in pancreatic-islets compared with various other mouse-tissues. Free Radical **B20:** 463–466.

27. HOHMEIER, H.E., A. THIGPEN, V.V. TRAN et al. 1998. Stable expression of manganese superoxide-dismutase (mnsod) in insulinoma cells prevents IL-1-beta-induced cytotoxicity and reduces nitric-oxide production. J. Clin. Invest. **101:** 1811–1820.
28. LORTZ, S., M. TIEDGE, T. NACHTWEY et al. 2000. Protection of insulin-producing RINm5F cells against cytokine-mediated toxicity through overexpression of antioxidant enzymes. Diabetes **49:** 1123–1130.
29. KUBISCH, H.M., J. WANG, R. LUCHE et al. 1994. Transgenic copper/zinc superoxide dismutase modulates susceptibility to type I diabetes. Proc. Natl. Acad. Sci. USA **91:** 9956–9959.
30. KUBISCH, H.M., J.Q. WANG, T.M. BRAY & J.P. PHILLIPS. 1997. Targeted overexpression of Cu/Zu superoxide-dismutase protects pancreatic beta-cells against oxidative stress. Diabetes **46:** 1563–1566.
31. PIGANELLI, J.D., S.C. FLORES, C. CRUZ et al. 2002. A metalloporphyrin-based superoxide dismutase mimic inhibits adoptive transfer of autoimmune diabetes by a diabetogenic T-cell clone. Diabetes **51:** 347–355.
32. MANDRUP-POULSEN, T., J.I. REIMERS, H.U. ANDERSEN et al. 1993. Nicotinamide treatment in the prevention of insulin-dependent diabetes mellitus. Diabetes Metab. Rev. **9:** 295–309.
33. BURKART, V., Z.Q. WANG, J. RADONS et al. 1999. Mice lacking the poly(ADP-ribose) polymerase gene are resistant to pancreatic beta-cell destruction and diabetes development induced by streptozocin. Nat. Med. **5:** 314–319.
34. CARDOZO, A.K., M. KRUHOFFER, R. LEEMAN et al. 2001. Identification of novel cytokine-induced genes in pancreatic beta-cells by high-density oligonucleotide arrays. Diabetes **50:** 909–920.
35. LARSEN, P.M., S.J. FEY, M.R. LARSEN et al. 2001. Proteome analysis of interleukin-1 beta-induced changes in protein expression in rat islets of Langerhans. Diabetes **50:** 1056–1063.
36. JOHN, N.E., H.U. ANDERSEN, S.J. FEY et al. 2000. Cytokine- or chemically derived nitric oxide alters the expression of proteins detected by two-dimensional gel electrophoresis in neonatal rat islets of Langerhans. Diabetes **49:** 1819–1829.
37. KARLSEN, A.E., S.G. RONN, K. LINDBERG et al. 2001. Suppressor of cytokine signaling 3 (SOCS-3) protects beta-cells against interleukin-1 beta- and interferon-gamma-mediated toxicity. Proc. Natl. Acad. Sci. USA **98:** 12191–12196.
38. CHONG, M.M.W., H.E. THOMAS & T.W.H. KAY. 2002. Suppressor of cytokine signaling-1 regulates the sensitivity of pancreatic beta cells to tumor necrosis factor. J. Biol. Chem. **277:** 27945–27952.

Oxidative Stress in Type 1 Diabetes

KATHRYN HASKINS,[a] BRENDA BRADLEY,[a] KATHERINE POWERS,[a]
VALERIE FADOK,[b] SONIA FLORES,[c] XIAOFENG LING,[c]
SUBBIAH PUGAZHENTHI,[d] JANE REUSCH,[d] AND JENNIFER KENCH[a]

[a]*Department of Immunology and* [b]*Department of Pediatrics, University of Colorado Health Sciences Center, and National Jewish Medical and Research Center, Denver, Colorado, USA*

[c]*Webb Waring Institute for Antioxidant Research, University of Colorado Health Sciences Center, Denver, Colorado, USA*

[d]*VA Medical Center, Denver, Colorado, USA*

ABSTRACT: We have been investigating the effects of preventing oxidative stress on pathogenesis and complications of type 1 diabetes in the NOD mouse model. Our studies have shown that damage caused by oxidative stress is higher in islets and vascular tissue of NOD mice than in nonautoimmune controls or a diabetes-resistant NOD mouse. In addition, phagocytic function and cytokine production by macrophages are aberrant in the NOD. We have demonstrated that treatment of prediabetic NOD mice for 2 weeks with a metalloporphyrin superoxide dismutase (SOD) mimetic results in marked reduction of oxidative stress in islets and vascular tissue and a reversal of macrophage defects.

KEYWORDS: oxidative stress; SOD mimetic; autoimmune diabetes

INTRODUCTION

Oxidative stress is now known to be associated with nearly all pathological states, especially those involving the inflammatory process.[1] Oxidative stress is characterized by increased production of cellular oxidants (e.g., superoxide, hydrogen peroxide, and nitric oxide) and/or decreased concentrations of antioxidants and antioxidant enzymes (e.g., glutathione, vitamin E, ascorbate, glutathione peroxidase, superoxide dismutases, and catalase). In autoimmune diabetes, a considerable body of evidence supports the concept that T cell–mediated infiltration of the pancreas leads to generation of reactive oxygen species (ROS), in addition to the proinflammatory cytokines, TNFα, IL-1β, and IFNγ.[2–5] Locally produced ROS are involved in the effector mechanisms of β cell destruction *in vitro*,[2–4,6–8] and T cell and macrophage cytokines such as IFNγ, IL-1β, and TNFα induce the production of ROS by β cells. The β cell destruction by ROS, whether induced by oxidants given exogenously or elicited by cytokines, is a process that occurs through both apoptotic and necrotic

Address for correspondence: Kathryn Haskins, Department of Immunology, University of Colorado Health Sciences Center, and National Jewish Medical and Research Center, 1400 Jackson Street, K823, Denver, CO 80206. Voice: 303-270-2093; fax: 303-270-2325.
katie.haskins@uchsc.edu

mechanisms.[9–13] There appears to be an intrinsic sensitivity of islet β cells to oxidative stress in the NOD mouse, a property that may extend to human patients.

There are also indications that oxidative stress is involved in other aspects of autoimmune diabetes including macrophage-mediated clearance of apoptotic cells and complications that develop in the vasculature of diabetic patients. Our question is whether inhibition of oxidative stress will affect not only islet β cells in the NOD mouse, but also macrophage function and damage to the vascular endothelium. We are investigating the effects of oxidative stress at the molecular level as well as in tissues and cells. For example, an important player in cell function and regulation is the transcription factor, CREB (cAMP-response element), which binds to a specific target sequence in the promoter regions of many genes and activates transcription when phosphorylated.[14–16] CREB is a key survival factor[17,18] and is important for cellular differentiation.[19] CREB also regulates the expression of MnSOD[20] and its function is impaired by oxidative stress.[21] It may be that an important mechanism of autoimmune-mediated oxidant generation is decreased CREB function in both islet β cells and in vascular endothelium, thereby increasing susceptibility to apoptosis.

Reduction of oxidative stress can protect cells from oxidant-induced damage. The enzyme, superoxide dismutase (SOD), an abundant and ubiquitous free radical scavenger, provides the body's principal defense against the highly destructive superoxide radical and is thereby a major protective mechanism against damage induced by oxidative stress. The overexpression of SOD in cells in culture or in whole animals has provided protection against the deleterious effects of a wide range of conditions involving oxidative stress.[22,23] For example, β cells engineered to overexpress antioxidant proteins have been shown to be resistant to damage from ROS and nitric oxide,[24–30] and the stable expression of manganese superoxide dismutase (MnSOD) in insulinoma cells prevented IL-1β-induced cytotoxicity and reduced

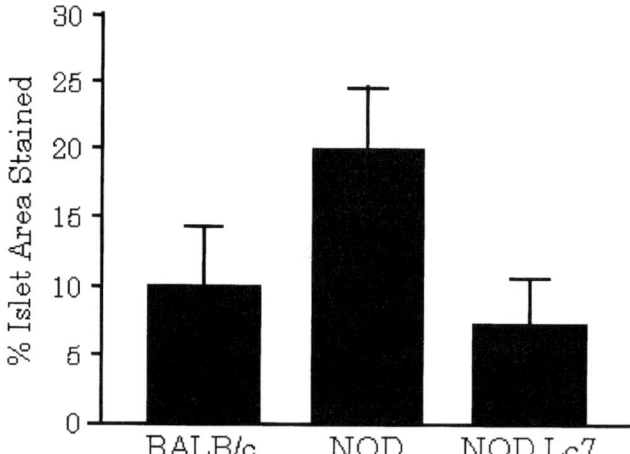

FIGURE 1. Antinitrotyrosine staining of NOD islets. Pancreatic sections were obtained from BALB/c, NOD, and diabetes-resistant NOD.Lc7 mice, 8–10 weeks of age. Sections were stained with an antibody to nitrotyrosine, and staining (3–5 islets from 2 or 3 mice from each mouse strain) was quantified using Image-Pro analysis.

nitric oxide production.[31] It has also been demonstrated that transgenic mice with β cell targeted overexpression of either Cu/ZnSOD or MnSOD[31–34] are resistant to autoimmune and streptozotocin-induced diabetes. Because there has been mixed success with the use of enzymes as therapeutic agents,[35–38] we have been investigating as an alternative approach the use of a low-molecular-weight SOD mimetic. We have previously described experiments with a metalloporphyrin SOD mimetic that could inhibit the T cell–mediated generation of ROS and proinflammatory cytokines in an adoptive transfer system with a diabetogenic T cell clone, BDC-2.5, ultimately preserving pancreatic β cell function.[39] We further determined that the SOD mimetic has an immunomodulatory effect since it directly inhibited APC effector function, APC-dependent T cell proliferation, and IFNγ production. We report here on continued studies in the NOD mouse and our new findings of how the SOD mimetic can alter the effects of oxidative stress in islets, in vascular tissue, and on macrophage function. The questions we are currently trying to address are directed at gaining a better understanding of how oxidative stress contributes to the pathogenesis of autoimmune diabetes and how treatment to prevent oxidative stress may protect against disease.

RESULTS AND DISCUSSION

Islet β Cells in the Autoimmune NOD Mouse Are Inherently More Susceptible to Damage Mediated by Oxidative Stress

Our first goal in these studies was to determine whether markers of oxidative stress in NOD islets are increased over those in nonautoimmune or diabetes-resistant mice. The graph in FIGURE 1 represents the levels of nitrotyrosine in islets from NOD and two other strains of mice at 8–10 weeks of age. Nitrotyrosine is one of the major indicators of oxidative stress in cells and increases as tyrosine groups on proteins are nitrosylated by a major cellular oxidant, peroxynitrite, which accumulates when superoxide reacts with NO. Pancreatic sections were stained with an antibody to nitrotyrosine and tissue from NOD mice was compared to islets from BALB/c and a diabetes-resistant NOD congenic mouse, NOD.Lc7. Although the NOD.Lc7 congenic mouse is autoimmune and develops insulitis like the NOD, the onset of hyperglycemia is delayed and diabetes incidence is much lower than in NOD.[40] This resistance to disease may be due to the fact that, in most of these mice, islets appear to be healthy and intact, suggesting that they are protected against β cell damage.[40] As illustrated in FIGURE 1, the staining of NOD islets with antinitrotyrosine antibody was considerably greater than that observed with BALB/c or NOD.Lc7 islets. This result suggests that oxidative damage reaches high levels in NOD islets during the prediabetic stage.

The higher levels of nitrotyrosine in NOD islets suggest that the β cells in NOD are more susceptible to oxidative stress and these findings are complemented by the results from another experiment in which we investigated apoptosis in NOD islets compared to that in islets from a diabetes-resistant mouse. In this experiment, islets were isolated from NOD and from diabetes-resistant NOD.Lc7 mice and were examined for apoptosis using an antibody against a neo-epitope on caspase 3 that appears following its cleavage and activation, providing a marker of early apoptosis

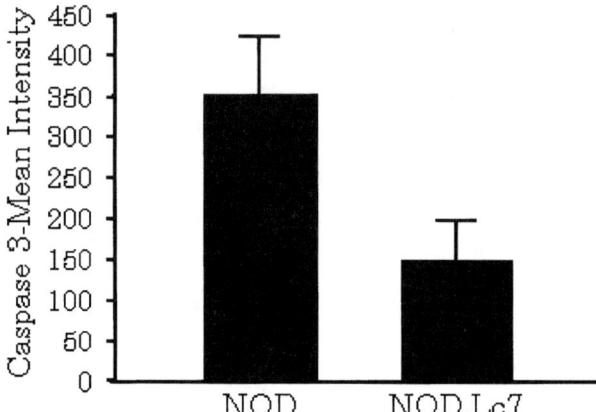

FIGURE 2. Apoptosis in islet β cells from diabetes-resistant NOD.Lc7 mice is less than in NOD islets. Islets isolated from NOD and diabetes-resistant NOD.Lc7 mice were fixed in 4% paraformaldehyde and permeabilized prior to incubation with anticaspase-3. The secondary antibody linked to cy3 (red) was used to visualize active caspase-3 and FITC (green) was used to stain for insulin. Fluorescence intensity was quantified using the Slide Book Application software. *$p < 0.01$ when compared to NOD.

in cells. As shown in FIGURE 2, the amount of apoptosis in NOD islets was profoundly elevated compared to that in NOD.Lc7. These data suggest that NOD islets are also more susceptible to apoptosis and that preservation of islets seen in NOD.Lc7 islets may in part be due to decreased cell death.

Inhibition of Oxidative Stress in Islet β Cells of the NOD Mouse by SOD Mimetic

To determine whether oxidative stress in islets, as represented by higher levels of nitrotyrosine, could be decreased or prevented by treatment of NOD mice with the SOD mimetic, we treated 6- to 8-week-old NOD mice with daily ip injections of the mimetic, 10 mg/kg, for 10 days. The mice were sacrificed, and pancreatic sections were stained with antinitrotyrosine and compared to sections from untreated NOD controls. As illustrated in the photos in FIGURE 3, a marked difference could be seen in pancreatic sections from some of the mimetic-treated NOD mice when compared to controls. In these mice, islets showed much reduced staining with antinitrotyrosine, indicating that, in at least some animals, the mimetic may be protective. However, in other mimetic-treated animals (2/6), islets were not very different from untreated NOD controls, perhaps reflecting a more advanced stage of disease in these mice (data not shown). Variation in histological results among NOD mice of the same age is common and it might be expected in some animals that the disease process is further along. These results are preliminary and it may be that, in order to get consistent results in the treatment of prediabetic NOD mice with the SOD mimetic, the animals will have to be treated at an earlier time point before insulitis is under way.

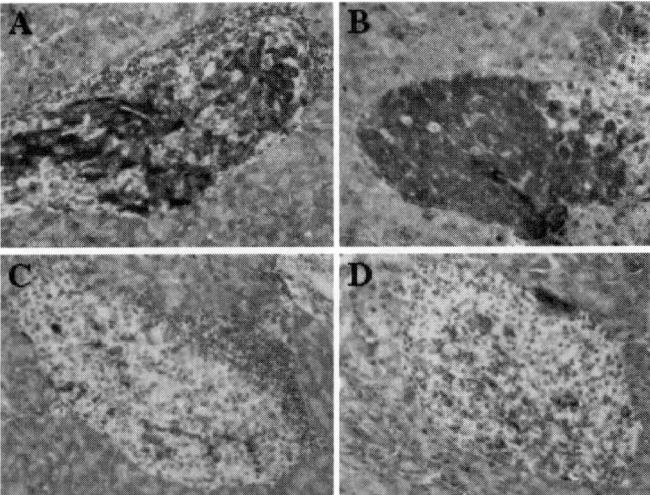

FIGURE 3. Islets from 8- to 10-week-old female NOD mice treated with the SOD mimetic and stained with antinitrotyrosine antibody: **(A, B)** untreated NOD controls; **(C, D)** islets from two different mimetic-treated mice.

Impaired Clearance of Apoptotic β Cells in the NOD Mouse Is Reversed by SOD Mimetic

ROS are known to participate in oxidative stress–mediated programmed cell death or apoptosis, and many studies now suggest that these molecules also have important signaling roles that regulate the induction of apoptosis.[41] Because clearance of dying cells is critical to the control of inflammation,[42–49] phagocytic recognition and engulfment of cells dying by apoptosis must occur prior to cell lysis in order to prevent the release of proinflammatory intracellular contents and possibly the generation of new antigens. It has recently been reported that clearance of apoptotic cells in both the BB rat and the NOD mouse is defective.[50] Engulfment of apoptotic cells by macrophages is a process critical to efficient clearance and we have been investigating whether macrophage engulfment function is normal in the NOD mouse. Results of an experiment to test engulfment function of macrophages are shown in FIGURE 4. Macrophages were elicited with thioglycollate in 8- to 10-week-old NOD and BALB/c mice at 3 days prior to harvest of peritoneal exudate cells (PEC), which were then assayed for engulfment function. The graph in FIGURE 4 shows that there is a profound engulfment defect exhibited by NOD macrophages. Also shown is the result of treating macrophages *in vitro* with SOD mimetic, in which instance it appeared that the engulfment defect was restored.

Functional Defects Observed in Circulating Macrophages of the Autoimmune NOD Mouse Are Corrected by SOD Mimetic

In normal mice (BALB/c), high levels of inflammatory mediators are observed only upon induction, with LPS for example, and are returned to low levels upon

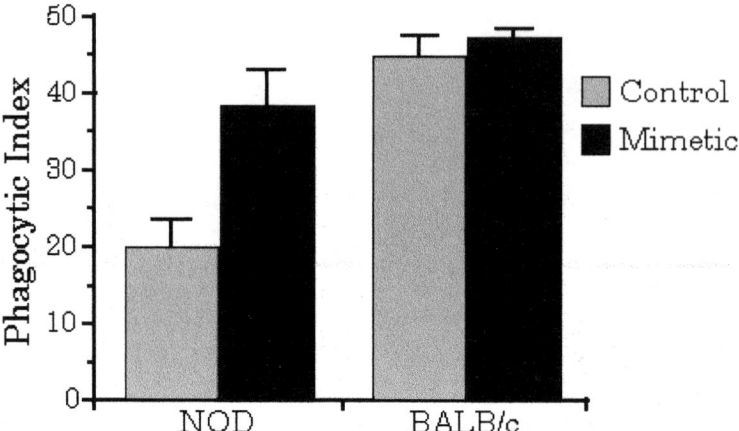

FIGURE 4. Defective engulfment of apoptotic cells in NOD mice is corrected by SOD mimetic. Peritoneal macrophages were harvested from the abdominal cavities of mice injected 72 h earlier with thioglycollate, the cells were resuspended in HBSS + 2% FCS at 1×10^6/mL, and slides were prepared by cytocentrifugation. The cytospins were stained using Wright's Giemsa and the number of free apoptotic bodies counted per HPF (400×); 10 fields per slide were counted. The data represent the mean and SEM for 10 individual female mice in each group. Black bars represent results from macrophages treated *in vitro* for 18 h with mimetic at 34 µM concentration; $N = 10 \pm$ SEM.

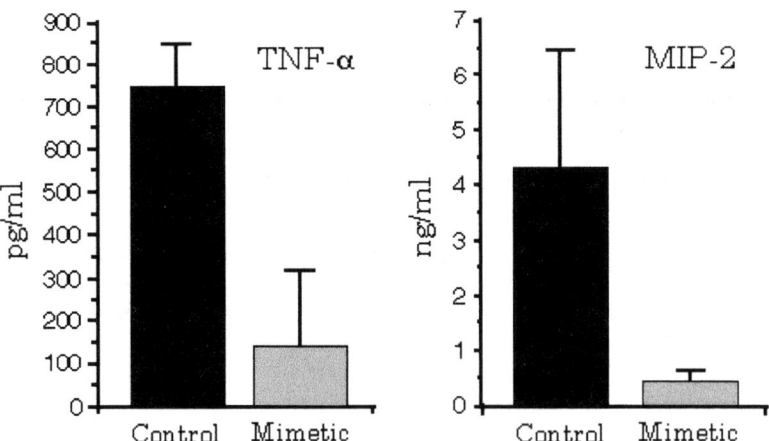

FIGURE 5. Defective cytokine responses of NOD macrophages are corrected by treatment with SOD mimetic. Macrophages were cultured in *ex vivo* medium in the absence of serum for 24 h and supernatants were collected for evaluation of cytokine production by ELISA.

exposure to apoptotic cells.[51-54] In contrast, in NOD macrophages, there is high spontaneous production of proinflammatory cytokines and chemokines as indicated in FIGURE 5. The high level of proinflammatory mediators in NOD macrophages is unaffected by either LPS or exposure to apoptotic cells (data not shown). However, if NOD mice were first treated with the SOD mimetic, the TNFα and MIP-2 levels were restored to normal (FIG. 5). These data suggest that the abnormally high production of proinflammatory cytokines and chemokines in NOD macrophages can be corrected by inhibitors of oxidative stress.

Inhibition of Oxidative Stress Can Prevent or Moderate Diabetic Complications in Vascular Tissue of NOD Mice

We have begun studies to determine whether markers of oxidative stress are higher in aortic tissue from NOD mice than in normal BALB/c animals by investigating levels of carbonyl and nitrotyrosylated proteins in aortic tissue. Carbonyl protein content, an index of increased protein oxidation from lipid hydroperoxides, was measured by immunoblots with a DNPH antibody. FIGURE 6A shows that aortae from 8- to 10-week-old NOD mice have increased oxidation of several proteins when compared with the age-matched BALB/c controls. Interestingly, since these mice were prediabetic, the results suggest that there is an intrinsic abnormality in the radical detoxifying capacity of vascular tissues of NOD mice, and that this abnormality is not a result of increased plasma glucose concentration. We then tested whether prediabetic NOD have increased reactive nitrogen species generation by

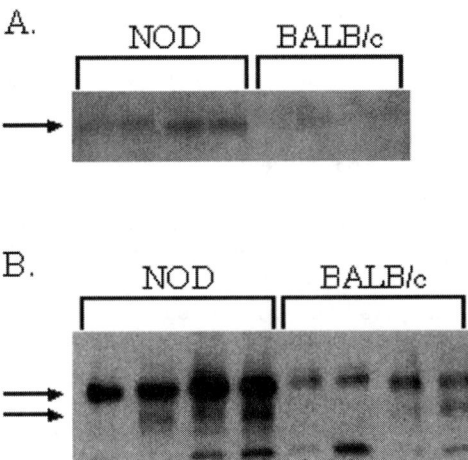

FIGURE 6. (**A**) Nitrotyrosine staining in mouse aortae. Aortic protein lysates from 10-week-old BALB/c or NOD mice were immunoblotted with an antinitrotyrosine antibody. A nitrated protein of molecular weight of approximately 24,000 was detected in the NOD lysates, but not in the BALB/c lysates. (**B**) Carbonyl protein content in aortae. Aortae from 4 separate 10-week-old NOD and BALB/c mice were homogenized and total protein lysates derivatized with DNPH. DNPH-protein adducts were detected via immunoblot analyses.

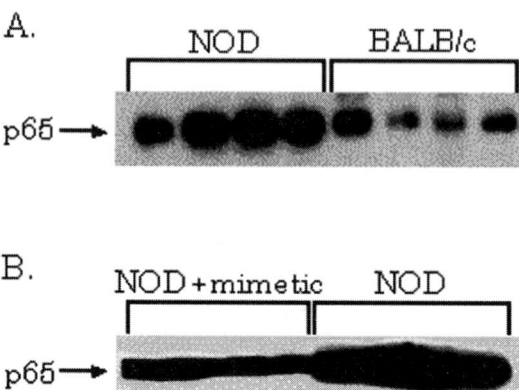

FIGURE 7. NF-κB in aortic tissue. **(A)** Immunoblot analysis of NF-κB p65 protein in lysates from aortae of 4 separate 10-week-old BALB/c and NOD mice. **(B)** NF-κB p65 levels in prediabetic aortae are decreased by mimetic treatment for 2 weeks.

measuring nitrotyrosine levels. FIGURE 6B shows that levels of nitrotyrosine were also elevated in NOD aortae and, although this technique does not provide exact identification of the nitrated proteins, we were able to identify a band of molecular weight of approximately 24,000 nitrated only in the aortae from the NOD mice (arrow in FIG. 6B). Since the molecular weight of mouse MnSOD is in this range, the possibility exists that MnSOD is nitrated in the aortae of prediabetic NOD and its activity is consequently decreased. The fact that generation of reactive nitrogen and/or oxygen species is already higher in prediabetic aortae of young (10-week) NOD mice suggests that oxidative stress leads to downstream functional abnormalities even if overt inflammatory infiltration or plaque formation is not evident.

We have also investigated NF-κB levels in aortic tissue of NOD mice. In the family of NF-κB transcriptional factors, which includes c-Rel, RelB, p52, p50, and p65, constitutive p65 levels are a good reflection of whether a particular tissue will be hyperresponsive to an inflammatory stimulus. For example, there are high levels of p65 in vasculature with a high probability of developing arteriosclerotic plaques,[55] and aortae from diabetic gerbils have increased NF-κB.[56] The results shown in FIGURE 7A demonstrate that levels of p65 were consistently higher in aortae from NOD mice, suggesting the possibility that this tissue is already primed for inflammation. However, if NOD mice were first treated with the SOD mimetic, the levels of p65 were decreased (FIG. 7B). These results provide further evidence that the NOD mouse has a global defect in oxidant/antioxidant balance.

Regulation of CREB May Provide a Mechanism for Damage Mediated by Oxidative Stress in the Autoimmune NOD Mouse

Bcl-2 is a critical regulator of survival in numerous cell types, including cells, and it has been shown that CREB plays a positive role in inducing this antiapoptotic gene.[57] We have observed a decrease in CREB-dependent bcl-2 protein expression

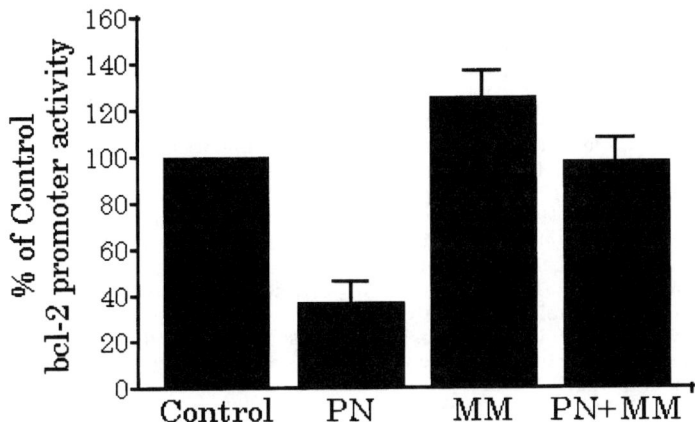

FIGURE 8. SOD mimetic restores peroxynitrite-induced downregulation of bcl-2 promoter in NIT-1 cells. NIT-1 β tumor cells were transfected with bcl-2 promoter linked to luciferase reporter gene. The transfected cells were exposed to peroxynitrite (250 μM) and/or SOD mimetic (30 μM) for 36 h. Peroxynitrite-induced inhibition of bcl-2 promoter activity was significantly blocked by the mimetic.

in islets isolated from prediabetic NOD mice when compared to normal or diabetes-resistant NOD.Lc7 mice, an observation suggesting that autoimmunity interferes with CREB-dependent gene expression in NOD islets. To determine whether loss of CREB-dependent gene expression can be restored by treating animals with the SOD mimetic, we have carried out studies in cell lines in which we showed that bcl-2 promoter activity was decreased by >50% in the presence of the potent oxidant, peroxynitrite. Treatment of control cells with the mimetic enhanced bcl-2 promoter activity, and concomitant treatment with the oxidant and the mimetic blocked oxidant-mediated downregulation of bcl-2 gene expression (FIG. 8). These studies demonstrate that antioxidant treatment of oxidant-stressed β cells can restore CREB-dependent gene expression.

CONCLUDING REMARKS

New studies in NOD mice with a novel antioxidant, a metalloporphyrin SOD mimetic, have shown that damage mediated by oxidative stress may be a primary contributor to the pathogenesis and complications of type 1 diabetes. Treatment of prediabetic NOD mice with this mimetic lowered levels of nitrotyrosylated proteins in islets, reversed defective cytokine production in peritoneal macrophages, lowered oxidant and NF-κB levels in vascular tissue, and restored CREB-dependent gene expression in a β cell tumor line. These results suggest that treatment with a highly efficient antioxidant may hold considerable promise for therapy in humans.

REFERENCES

1. MCCORD, J.M. 1995. Superoxide radical: controversies, contradictions, and paradoxes. Proc. Soc. Exp. Biol. Med. **209:** 112–117.
2. RABINOVITCH, A. et al. 1996. Inducible nitric oxide synthase (iNOS) in pancreatic islets of nonobese diabetic mice: identification of iNOS-expressing cells and relationships to cytokines expressed in the islets. Endocrinology **137:** 2093–2099.
3. MANDRUP-POULSEN, T. 1996. The role of interleukin-1 in the pathogenesis of IDDM. Diabetologia **39:** 1005–1029.
4. EIZIRIK, D.L. et al. 1996. The harmony of the spheres: inducible nitric oxide synthase and related genes in pancreatic beta cells. Diabetologia **39:** 875–890.
5. MANDRUP-POULSEN, T. et al. 1996. Cytokines and the endocrine system: II. Roles in substrate metabolism, modulation of thyroidal and pancreatic endocrine cell functions, and autoimmune endocrine diseases. Eur. J. Endocrinol. **134:** 21–30.
6. GRANKVIST, K. et al. 1979. Superoxide dismutase, catalase, and scavengers of hydroxyl radical protect against the toxic action of alloxan on pancreatic islet cells in vitro. Biochem. J. **182:** 17–25.
7. KRONCKE, K.D. et al. 1991. Activated macrophages kill pancreatic syngeneic islet cells via arginine-dependent nitric oxide generation. Biochem. Biophys. Res. Commun. **175:** 752–758.
8. CORBETT, J.A. et al. 1992. Interleukin 1 beta induces the formation of nitric oxide by beta-cells purified from rodent islets of Langerhans: evidence for the beta-cell as a source and site of action of nitric oxide. J. Clin. Invest. **90:** 2384–2391.
9. KANETO, H. et al. 1995. Apoptotic cell death triggered by nitric oxide in pancreatic beta-cells. Diabetes **44:** 733–738.
10. KURRER, M.O. et al. 1997. Beta cell apoptosis in T cell–mediated autoimmune diabetes. Proc. Natl. Acad. Sci. USA **94:** 213–218.
11. O'BRIEN, B.A. et al. 1997. Apoptosis is the mode of beta-cell death responsible for the development of IDDM in the nonobese diabetic (NOD) mouse. Diabetes **46:** 750–757.
12. CHERVONSKY, A.V. et al. 1997. The role of Fas in autoimmune diabetes. Cell **89:** 17–24.
13. ITOH, N. et al. . 1997. Requirement of Fas for the development of autoimmune diabetes in nonobese diabetic mice. J. Exp. Med. **186:** 613–618.
14. GONZALEZ, G.A. & M.R. MONTMINTY. 1989. Cyclic AMP stimulates somatostatin gene transcription by phosphorylation of CREB at serine 133. Cell **59:** 675–680.
15. WHEAT, W.H., W.J. ROESLER & D.J. KLEMM. 1994. Simian virus 40 small tumor antigen inhibits dephosphorylation of protein kinase A–phosphorylated CREB and regulates transcriptional stimulation. Mol. Cell. Biol. **14:** 5881–5890.
16. FOLCO, E.J. & G. KOREN. 1997. Degradation of the inducible cAMP early repressor (ICER) by the ubiquitin-proteasome pathway. Biochem. J. **328:** 37–43.
17. FINKBEINER, S. 2000. CREB couples neurotrophin signals to survival messages. Neuron **25:** 11–14.
18. PUGAZHENTHI, S., E. MILLER, C. SABLE et al. 1999. Insulin-like growth factor-I induces bcl-2 promoter through the transcription factor cAMP-response element binding protein. J. Biol. Chem. **274:** 27529–27535.
19. RUDOLPH, D., A. TAFURI, P. GASS et al. 1998. Impaired fetal T cell development and perinatal lethality in mice lacking the cAMP response element binding protein. Proc. Natl. Acad. Sci. USA **95:** 4481–4486.
20. KIM, H.P., J.H. ROE, P.B. CHOCK & M.B. YIM. 1999. Transcriptional activation of the human manganese superoxide dismutase gene mediated by tetradecanoylphorbol acetate. J. Biol. Chem. **274:** 37455–37460.
21. ZHANG, L. & R. JOPE. 1999. Oxidative stress differentially modulates phosphorylation of ERK, p38, and CREB induced by NGF or EGF in PC12 cells. Neurobiol. Aging **20:** 271–278.
22. LI, G. et al. 1997. Catalase-overexpressing transgenic mouse heart is resistant to ischemia-reperfusion injury. Am. J. Physiol. **273:** H1090–H1095.
23. THIBEAULT, D.W. et al. 1991. Prevention of chronic pulmonary oxygen toxicity in young rats with liposome-encapsulated catalase administered intratracheally. Pediatr. Pulmonol. **11:** 318–327.

24. GRANKVIST, K., S.L. MARKLUND & I.B. TALJEDAL. 1981. CuZn-superoxide dismutase, Mn-superoxide dismutase, catalase, and glutathione peroxidase in pancreatic islets and other tissues in the mouse. Biochem. J. **199:** 393–398.
25. MALAISSE, W.J. *et al.* 1982. Determinants of the selective toxicity of alloxan to the pancreatic B cell. Proc. Natl. Acad. Sci. USA **79:** 927–930.
26. LENZEN, S., J. DRINKGERN & M. TIEDGE. 1996. Low antioxidant enzyme gene expression in pancreatic islets compared with various other mouse tissues. Free Radical Biol. Med. **20:** 463–466.
27. TIEDGE, M. *et al.* 1997. Relation between antioxidant enzyme gene expression and antioxidative defense status of insulin-producing cells. Diabetes **46:** 1733–1742.
28. BENHAMOU, P.Y. *et al.* 1998. Adenovirus-mediated catalase gene transfer reduces oxidant stress in human, porcine, and rat pancreatic islets. Diabetologia **41:** 1093–1100.
29. TIEDGE, M. *et al.* 1998. Complementary action of antioxidant enzymes in the protection of bioengineered insulin-producing RINm5F cells against the toxicity of reactive oxygen species. Diabetes **47:** 1578–1585.
30. TIEDGE, M. *et al.* 1999. Protection against the co-operative toxicity of nitric oxide and oxygen free radicals by overexpression of antioxidant enzymes in bioengineered insulin-producing RINm5F cells. Diabetologia **42:** 849–855.
31. HOHMEIER, H.E. *et al.* 1998. Stable expression of manganese superoxide dismutase (MnSOD) in insulinoma cells prevents IL-1beta-induced cytotoxicity and reduces nitric oxide production. J. Clin. Invest. **101:** 1811–1820.
32. KUBISCH, H.M. *et al.* 1994. Transgenic copper/zinc superoxide dismutase modulates susceptibility to type I diabetes. Proc. Natl. Acad. Sci. USA **91:** 9956–9959.
33. KUBISCH, H.M. *et al.* 1997. Targeted overexpression of Cu/Zn superoxide dismutase protects pancreatic beta-cells against oxidative stress. Diabetes **46:** 1563–1566.
34. LORTZ, S. *et al.* 2000. Protection of insulin-producing RINm5F cells against cytokine-mediated toxicity through overexpression of antioxidant enzymes. Diabetes **49:** 1123–1130.
35. WISPE, J.R. *et al.* 1992. Human Mn-superoxide dismutase in pulmonary epithelial cells of transgenic mice confers protection from oxygen injury. J. Biol. Chem. **267:** 23937–23941.
36. LARDOT, C. *et al.* 1996. Exogenous catalase may potentiate oxidant-mediated lung injury in the female Sprague-Dawley rat. J. Toxicol. Environ. Health **47:** 509–522.
37. SIMONSON, S.G. *et al.* 1997. Aerosolized manganese SOD decreases hyperoxic pulmonary injury in primates: I. Physiology and biochemistry. J. Appl. Physiol. **83:** 550–558.
38. PATEL, M. & B.J. DAY. 1999. Metalloporphyrin class of therapeutic catalytic antioxidants. Trends Pharmacol. Sci. **20:** 359–364.
39. PIGANELLI, J.D. *et al.* 2002. A metalloporphyrin-based superoxide dismutase mimic inhibits adoptive transfer of autoimmune diabetes by a diabetogenic T-cell clone. Diabetes **51:** 347–355.
40. MCDUFFIE, M. 2000. Derivation of diabetes-resistant congenic lines from the nonobese diabetic mouse. Clin. Immunol. **96:** 119–130.
41. WYLLIE, A.H., J.F. KERR & A.R. CURRIE. 1980. Cell death: the significance of apoptosis. Int. Rev. Cytol. **68:** 251–306.
42. HASLETT, C. *et al.* 1994. Granulocyte apoptosis and the control of inflammation. Philos. Trans. R. Soc. Lond. B Biol. Sci. **345:** 327–333.
43. SAVILL, J. 1994. Apoptosis in disease. Eur. J. Clin. Invest. **24:** 715–723.
44. SAVILL, J. 1997. Apoptosis in resolution of inflammation. J. Leukocyte Biol. **61:** 375–380.
45. FADOK, V.A. & P.M. HENSON. 1998. Apoptosis: getting rid of the bodies. Curr. Biol. **8:** R693–R695.
46. REN, Y. & J. SAVILL. 1998. Apoptosis: the importance of being eaten. Cell Death Differ. **5:** 563–568.
47. SAVILL, J. & V. FADOK. 2000. Corpse clearance defines the meaning of cell death. Nature **407:** 784–788.
48. FADOK, V.A. & G. CHIMINI. 2001. The phagocytosis of apoptotic cells. Semin. Immunol. **13:** 365–372.
49. MEAGHER, L.C. *et al.* 1992. Phagocytosis of apoptotic neutrophils does not induce macrophage release of thromboxane $B2$. J. Leukocyte Biol. **52:** 269–273.

50. O'BRIEN, B.A., Y. HUANG, X. GENG *et al.* 2002. Phagocytosis of apoptotic cells by macrophages from NOD mice is reduced. Diabetes **51:** 2481–2488.
51. VOLL, R.E. *et al.* 1997. Immunosuppressive effects of apoptotic cells. Nature **390:** 350–351.
52. FADOK, V.A. *et al.* 1998. Macrophages that have ingested apoptotic cells *in vitro* inhibit proinflammatory cytokine production through autocrine/paracrine mechanisms involving TGF-beta, PGE2, and PAF. J. Clin. Invest. **101:** 890–898.
53. MCDONALD, P.P. *et al.* 1999. Transcriptional and translational regulation of inflammatory mediator production by endogenous TGF-beta in macrophages that have ingested apoptotic cells. J. Immunol. **163:** 6164–6172.
54. HUYNH, M.L., V.A. FADOK & P.M. HENSON. 2002. Phosphatidylserine-dependent ingestion of apoptotic cells promotes TGF-beta1 secretion and the resolution of inflammation. J. Clin. Invest. **109:** 41–50.
55. HAJRA, L., A.I. EVANS, M. CHEN *et al.* 2000. The NF-kappaB signal transduction pathway in aortic endothelial cells is primed for activation in regions predisposed to atherosclerotic lesion formation. Proc. Natl. Acad. Sci. USA **97:** 9052–9057.
56. NISHIGAKI, R., F. GUO, M. ONDA *et al.* 1999. Ultrastructural changes and immunohistochemical localization of nitric oxide synthase, advanced glycation end products, and NF-kappa B in aorta of streptozotocin treated Mongolian gerbils. Nippon Ika Daigaku Zasshi **66:** 166–175.
57. PUGAZHENTHI S., A. NESTEROVA, C. SABLE *et al.* 2000. Akt/protein kinase B up-regulates Bcl-2 expression through cAMP-response element-binding protein. J. Biol. Chem. **275:** 10761–10766.

Use of Microarray Analysis to Unveil Transcription Factor and Gene Networks Contributing to β Cell Dysfunction and Apoptosis

DECIO L. EIZIRIK, BURAK KUTLU, JOANNE RASSCHAERT, MARTINE DARVILLE, AND ALESSANDRA K. CARDOZO

Laboratory of Experimental Medicine, Université Libre de Bruxelles, B-1070 Brussels, Belgium

ABSTRACT: The β cell fate following immune-mediated damage depends on an intricate pattern of dozens of genes up- or downregulated in parallel and/or sequentially. We are utilizing microarray analysis to clarify the pattern of gene expression in primary rat β cells exposed to the proapoptotic cytokines, IL-1β and/or IFN-γ. The picture emerging from these experiments is that β cells are not passive bystanders of their own destruction. On the contrary, β cells respond to damage by activating diverse networks of transcription factors and genes that may either lead to apoptosis or preserve viability. Of note, cytokine-exposed β cells produce and release chemokines that may contribute to the homing and activation of T cells and macrophages during insulitis. Several of the effects of cytokines depend on the activation of the transcription factor, NF-κB. NF-κB blocking prevents cytokine-induced β cell death, and characterization of NF-κB-dependent genes by microarray analysis indicated that this transcription factor controls diverse networks of transcription factors and effector genes that are relevant for maintenance of β cell differentiated status, cytosolic and ER calcium homeostasis, attraction of mononuclear cells, and apoptosis. Identification of this and additional "transcription factor networks" is being pursued by cluster analysis of gene expression in insulin-producing cells exposed to cytokines for different time periods. Identification of complex gene patterns poses a formidable challenge, but is now technically feasible. These accumulating evidences may finally unveil the molecular mechanisms regulating the β cell "decision" to undergo or not apoptosis in early T1DM.

KEYWORDS: pancreatic beta cells; diabetes mellitus; microarray analysis; interleukin-1; interferon-γ; nitric oxide; chemokines; MCP-1; apoptosis; ER stress

Address for correspondence: D. L. Eizirik, Laboratory of Experimental Medicine, ULB, 808 Route de Lennik, B-1070 Brussels, Belgium. Voice: +32-2-555-62-42; fax: +32-2-555-62-39.
deizirik@ulb.ac.be

INTRODUCTION

The immune system utilizes diverse mediators to kill pancreatic β cells during the course of insulitis. Among them are soluble mediators, such as cytokines and free radicals, the ligand of the Fas receptor (FasL), and the perforin-granzyme system. Accumulating evidence suggests that apoptosis is the main form of β cell death in spontaneous models of autoimmune diabetes, and that the cytokines, interleukin-1β (IL-1β), interferon-γ (IFN-γ), and tumor necrosis factor-α (TNF-α), are key contributors in triggering the cell death program in β cells. Against this background, several groups have been searching for many years for the signals delivered by cytokines that "convince" the β cells to initiate the apoptotic program.[1]

In vitro studies in which whole pancreatic islets or FACS-purified rodent or human β cells were exposed to cytokines indicated that *de novo* gene and protein expression is required for triggering apoptosis. A long search for the gene(s) responsible for this phenomenon, using both the "candidate gene approach" and differential display by RT-PCR, failed to identify individual genes or proteins that could explain the phenomenon.[2] This raised the possibility that cytokine-induced apoptosis was a much more complex phenomenon than initially assumed, and that we and other scientists in the field were trying to oversimplify the problem, thus failing to understand it. This trend was well described by Tolstoy in *War and Peace* (1869), when analyzing the reasons for the Napoleonic wars in Russia: "… and the human intellect with no inkling of the immense variety and complexity of circumstances conditioning a phenomenon, any one of which may be separately conceived as the cause of it, snatches at the first and the most easily understood approximation, and says, 'Oh, here is the cause!'". How, then, to analyze as a whole "the immense variety and complexity of circumstances" leading to cytokine-induced β cell apoptosis? This question is the main focus of the present review. For more extensive reviews on immune-mediated β cell apoptosis, the reader is referred to references 1 and 3–5.

HIGH-DENSITY OLIGONUCLEOTIDE ARRAY ANALYSIS OF CYTOKINE-MODIFIED GENES IN PANCREATIC β CELLS

High-density arrays of oligonucleotides or complementary cDNAs are a novel and powerful technique for the quantitative and parallel measurements of the expression of thousands of genes.[6] Nucleic acid arrays work by hybridization of fluorescent-labeled RNA or DNA in solution to DNA molecules attached at specific locations at a surface. The arrayed DNA fragments could be cDNA or oligonucleotides attached to a glass substrate.[6] The GeneChip™ technology developed by Affymetrix (http://www.affymetrix.com) and utilized in our work[7,8] uses photolithography and solid phase chemistry to produce arrays containing oligonucleotide probes packed at extremely high densities: around 400,000 probes can be synthesized in 1.28×1.28 cm arrays. Each gene or expressed sequence tag (EST) is represented in the array by 16–20 pairs of perfect match (PM) and mismatch (MM) probes of 25-mer. The MM probe is identical to the PM probe, except for a single base mismatch in its center. The probe pairs (PM and MM) allow the quantification and subtraction of signals caused by nonspecific cross-hybridization. The difference in hybridization signals between partners (i.e., PM − MM), as well as their intensity ratios, serve as indicators of specific target abundance. Different labeled cRNA populations to be compared are hybridized in separate arrays. Image analysis is obtained by confocal scanning, arrays are normalized, and data are analyzed by specific software.[9] Two features of expression profiles make it presently the most rewarding approach to study complex biological systems. First, the efficiency to obtain global and quantitative information with DNA arrays surpasses that of proteomic techniques with the presently available technology. Second, RNA expression profiles provide a precise and reproducible signature of the state of a cell, reflecting, albeit indirectly, the functional state of most cell proteins.[10]

β cell exposure to IL-1β induces functional impairment, whereas β cell culture for 3–9 days in the presence of IL-1β + IFN-γ leads to cell death mostly by apoptosis.[1] As mentioned above, the prolonged time required for eliciting apoptosis in β cells suggests that *de novo* gene expression is involved in this process. In order to identify early and late genes involved in cytokine-induced β cell dysfunction/death or recovery/repair, we have already analyzed by high-density oligonucleotide arrays the expression profile of FACS-purified rat β cells exposed for 6 and 24 h to IL-1β (50 U/mL), IFN-γ (1000 U/mL), or IL-1β + IFN-γ[7,8] (Rasschaert, Liu, Kutlu, Cardozo, and Eizirik, manuscript in preparation). We have also performed a detailed time-course analysis of INS-1E cells exposed for 1, 2, 4, 8, 12, and 24 h to IL-1β + IFN-γ, with or without the presence of the iNOS inhibitor, L-methyl-arginine (Kutlu, Cardozo, and Eizirik, manuscript in preparation). In these experiments cytokine-treated cells are compared to their respective controls, that is, FACS-purified β cells or INS-1E cells cultured under the same conditions and for the same period of time, but without the presence of cytokines.

The choice of cytokine concentrations was based on previous data from our group[1] and aimed to identify genes that are directly induced by cytokine(s) and/or result from β cell responses to cellular stress. After 24-h exposure to IL-1β + IFN-γ, most β cells are still viable (no significant difference vs. controls), but 10% of the β cell population is already committed to undergo cell death (FIG. 1). By 48 h of

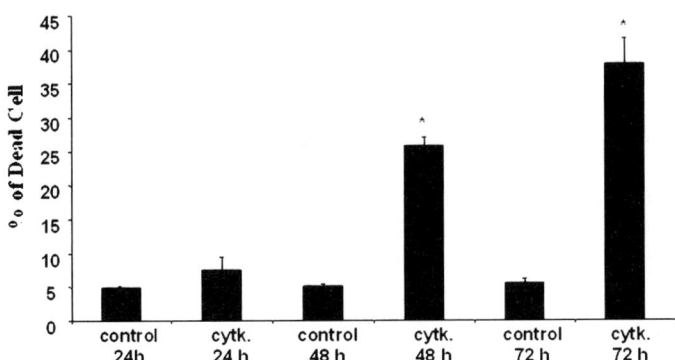

FIGURE 1. Viability of FACS-purified and reaggregated β cells exposed for different time points to IL-1β (50 U/mL) + IFN-γ (1000 U/mL). The percentage of dead cells was determined by the DNA-binding dyes, HO and PI, as previously described.[11] Data are the means ± SEM of four experiments; *$p < 0.01$ vs. respective control (paired *t* test).

cytokine exposure, 20% of the β cells show evidence of early apoptosis as evaluated by nuclear dyes ($p < 0.05$ vs. controls; FIG. 1). Degradation of cellular mRNA is a general early apoptosis-induced event,[12] suggesting that determination of β cell mRNA after 36–48 h of exposure to cytokines is of little value to understand the mechanisms leading to cell death. Against this background, our initial experiments were performed in FACS-purified and reaggregated β cells (preparations containing >90% β cells; same conditions as in FIG. 1) exposed for 6 or 24 h to cytokines.

For our different microarray analysis, FACS-purified β cells from 4–6 separate experiments were pooled for mRNA extraction, and the resulting biotinylated cRNAs hybridized in duplicate to the Affymetrix U-34A oligonucleotide array. From the 8740 probes present on the array, β cells or INS-1E cells consistently express around 3000 genes or ESTs. Based on this information, we are presently building a "β Cell Gene Bank", which will serve as a useful resource for future studies on β cell physiological and pathological phenotypes. Six hours of exposure to IL-1β + IFN-γ led to modification (i.e., >2.5-fold increased or decreased expression compared to control cells) in the expression of nearly 100 known genes in rat β cells. A prolonged exposure to these cytokines (24 h) almost doubled the number of modified genes, while 24-h exposure to IL-1β alone induced differential expression of 105 known genes.[7,8] IFN-γ alone modified expression of 89 and 51 genes after respectively 6 and 24 h of exposure (Rasschaert, Liu, Kutlu, Cardozo, and Eizirik, manuscript in preparation). Of note, the number of cytokine-modified genes increased to 700 when a more detailed time-course analysis (1, 2, 4, 8, 12, and 24 h) was performed in well-differentiated insulin-producing INS-1E cells exposed to IL-1β + IFN-γ (Kutlu, Cardozo, and Eizirik, manuscript in preparation).

Validation of our initial microarray results was achieved by two approaches: (i) by comparing the data obtained in the array with previously described cytokine-induced gene/protein expression in β cells or islets cells (for a review on previously described genes, see ref. 2); from 25 genes represented in the array, and previously described as induced or inhibited by cytokines, 22 (88%) were detected as "changed" in the array analysis; (ii) by performing RT-PCR analysis for 27 "novel" (not described before) cytokine-induced genes in independent samples, that is, samples different from the ones used in the array; we could confirm by RT-PCR 24 (89%) of the mRNAs as cytokine-modified.[7,8] These observations, together with the good agreement between duplicates, and the fact that genes observed as changed by cytokines in one array were confirmed as changed in >80% of the cases in subsequent arrays (in analysis performed months or even years later), suggest that microarray analysis is a reliable approach to study massive variations in β cell gene expression.

Genes that were modified by cytokines were clustered according to the putative biological function of their encoded proteins[7,8] (Rasschaert, Liu, Kutlu, Cardozo, and Eizirik, manuscript in preparation). Our present view of the broad effects of cytokines on pancreatic β cells is provided in FIGURE 2. This model is based on the diverse microarray analysis already performed by our group[7,8] (Rasschaert, Liu, Kutlu, Cardozo, and Eizirik, manuscript in preparation; Kutlu, Cardozo, and Eizirik, manuscript in preparation). Discussion of individual genes can be found in these publications; only some of the genes depicted in FIGURE 2, deemed of particular relevance, will be discussed here.

One of the biggest cytokine-modified cluster represents the genes related to β cell metabolism, with an initial increase at 1–2 h (Kutlu, Cardozo, and Eizirik, manu-

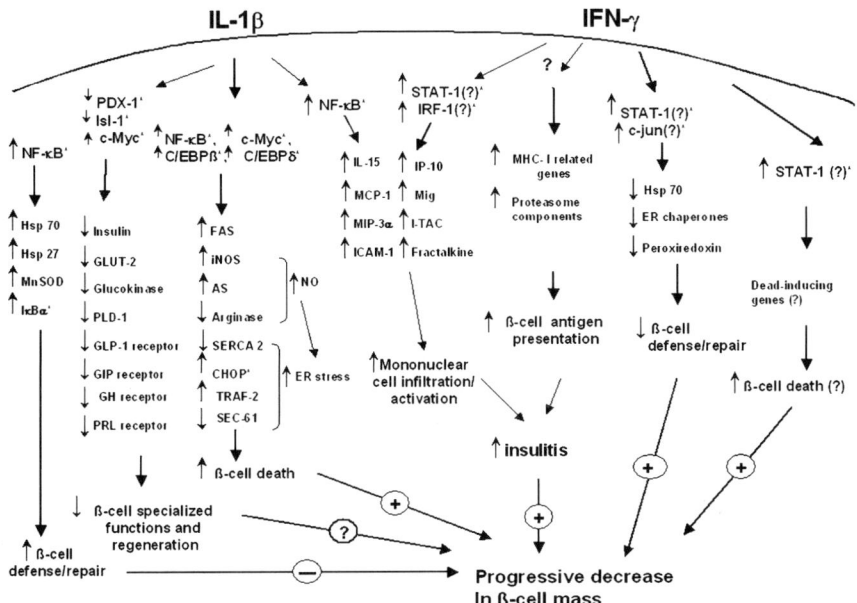

FIGURE 2. Proposed model, based on our diverse microarray analysis, of the different transcription factors (indicated with an asterisk) and "effector" genes involved in cytokine-induced β cell dysfunction/death. The figure is adapted from refs. 7 and 8. Definitions of all abbreviations and detailed discussion of the figure are provided in the text and in refs. 7 and 8.

script in preparation) followed by a progressive decrease (12–24 h) in the expression of key genes regulating glucose metabolism and the process of insulin biosynthesis and release[7,8] (Kutlu, Cardozo, and Eizirik, manuscript in preparation). This pattern of gene expression correlates well with the functional effects of IL-1β, which induces an early (1–2 h) increase in β cell glucose oxidation and insulin release, followed by a late (after 8–12 h) inhibition of substrate metabolism, insulin mRNA expression, and insulin release.[13,14] The late "inhibitory phase" is, to a significant extent, secondary to IL-1β-induced activation of the transcription factor NF-κB, causing increased expression of the inducible form of nitric oxide synthase (iNOS) and synthesis of the radical nitric oxide (NO).[15] Increased NO levels contribute to the decreased expression of the transcription factor PDX-1.[7,16] PDX-1 is an essential regulator of pancreatic cell development and islet adult β cell function,[17] transactivating the promoter regions of insulin, GLUT-2, glucokinase, PC-1, and GAD67.[18–20] Note that all these PDX-1-dependent genes were detected as inhibited by cytokines in the array analysis.[7,8] Decreased PDX-1 expression *in vivo* results in decreased GLUT-2 expression and glucose intolerance.[21,22] Thus, it is conceivable that the observed inhibition of PDX-1 expression, coupled to posttranscriptional effects of NO, such as blocking the Krebs enzyme aconitase,[23] contributes to the loss of specialized β cell functions during *in vitro* rat β cell exposure to cytokines, and perhaps also during the early stages of T1DM in humans and in rodent models of the disease.[24]

Besides PDX-1 and PDX-1-dependent genes, other transcription factors and "effector" genes probably contribute to cytokine-induced β cell dysfunction. Thus, the array analysis detected an NF-κB-dependent decrease and increase in respectively Isl-1 and c-myc expression.[7,8] Isl-1 is crucial for islet development,[25] and a recent study has shown that Isl-1 expression, together with PDX-1, is necessary for expression of insulin in immature intestinal stem cells.[26] It remains to be clarified whether Isl-1 plays a relevant role in the maintenance of a differentiated phenotype in adult β cells. Increased expression of c-myc mRNA is also observed in β cells exposed to high glucose concentrations, and c-myc overexpression suppresses both insulin gene transcription and glucose-stimulated insulin release.[27] Furthermore, transgenic c-myc overexpression under the control of the rat insulin II promoter suppresses insulin and GLUT-2 mRNA expression, and leads to diabetes due to increased rates of β cell apoptosis.[28] It is thus conceivable that IL-1β-induced c-myc expression contributes to two of the deleterious effects of the cytokine: namely, decreased insulin mRNA expression and increased susceptibility to apoptosis. The observed cytokine-induced downregulation of the incretin receptors, cholecystokinin-A (CCK), gastric inhibitory peptide (GIP), and glucagon-like peptide 1 receptor (GLP-1), in concert with downregulation of receptors for prolactin (PRL) and growth hormone (GH)[7,8] (FIG. 2), may further hamper β cell function *in vivo* and decrease the ability of these cells to compensate for the progressive loss of β cells in early T1DM.

It is noteworthy that major modifications in the expression of metabolism-related genes have also been observed by microarray analysis of FACS-purified rat β cells exposed for 24 h to low glucose,[29] or of insulin-secreting MIN6 cells exposed for 24 or 48 h to respectively high glucose[30] or elevated concentration of free fatty acids (FFA).[31] These three conditions cause β cell dysfunction and, under some experimental conditions, lead to β cell death.[32–35] β cells serve as "fuel sensors", responding to changes in the circulating pool of nutrients with appropriate insulin secretion. Substrate metabolism and the consequent production of ATP are the main signals for insulin secretion.[36] It thus seems logical that metabolism-related genes are affected early, and to a major extent, when β cells are exposed to stressful conditions. It remains to be determined whether change in the expression of these genes is only related to modifications in insulin expression and release, or whether it also contributes to cell death. For instance, NO-mediated impairment in mitochondrial metabolism probably plays an important role for the necrotic component of rodent β cell death,[2] but it has a less relevant role in cytokine-induced apoptosis in rodent and human β cells.[2,11,37,38]

Two other important gene clusters regulated by IL-1β and IFN-γ are (i) the group of genes potentially involved in the execution of β cell death and (ii) the genes involved in β cell defense and repair (FIG. 2). It is noteworthy that the transcription factor NF-κB plays a regulatory role in both the "pro"- and "anti"-apoptotic gene clusters[7] (FIG. 2). This regulation can be effected directly as indicated by studies of the molecular regulation of MnSOD,[39] iNOS,[15] Fas,[40] and MCP-1[41] expression in insulin-producing cells using reporter constructs and gel shift assays. We have recently confirmed, by chromatin immunoprecipitation (ChIP) assay, that NF-κB binds *in vivo* to the promoter region of at least two of these genes, namely MCP-1[41] and Fas (FIG. 3). For other genes, such as hsp27, hsp70, SERCA2, and CHOP, the effect of NF-κB is mediated via iNOS expression and NO production.[7,11] Moreover, as discussed below, increased NO production is probably responsible for changes in

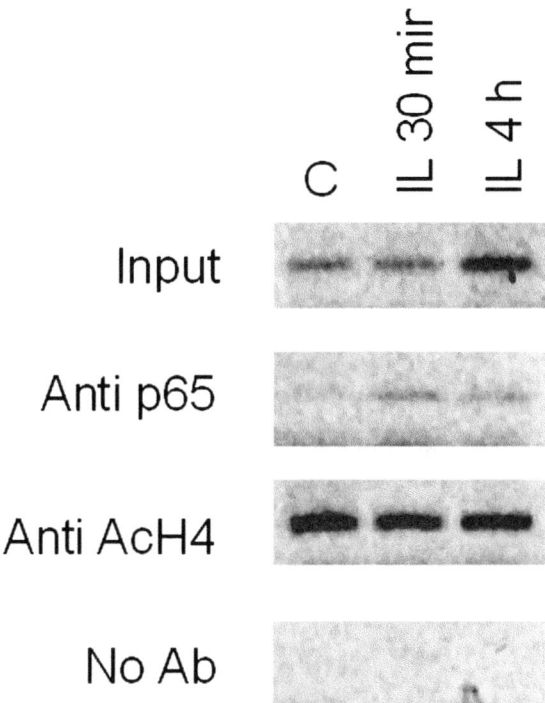

FIGURE 3. Chromatin immunoprecipitation (ChIP) analysis of the Fas promoter in insulin-producing RINm5F cells. RINm5F cells were exposed to control medium (C) or to IL-1β for 30 min or 4 h, and then fixed in 1% formaldehyde and lysed for ChIP analysis as previously described.[41] The nuclear fraction was sonicated to shear the chromatin to 0.5-kb to 1.5-kb fragments and immunoprecipitated with either an anti-p65 antibody or an anti-acetylated histone H4 antibody (used as positive control). Chromatin not exposed to antibody (no Ab) was used as negative control. Immunoprecipitated DNA was analyzed by PCR using primers specific for the Fas promoter, followed by electrophoresis on agarose gel. DNA purified before immunoprecipitation (input) was assayed in parallel as a control for amplification.

the expression of a large proportion of cytokine-induced/inhibited genes after 12–24 h of cytokine exposure (Kutlu, Cardozo, and Eizirik, manuscript in preparation).

IL-1β alone suppresses, but does not kill, FACS-purified β cells, while a combination of IL-1β + IFN-γ leads to β cell death after several days of exposure. This indicates that IFN-γ-regulated transcription factors and genes are crucial for triggering β cell death. Unfortunately, much less is known regarding the key transcription factors and genes induced by IFN-γ in β cells as compared to the knowledge already obtained for IL-1β signaling.[1] We have previously shown that IRF-1, a well-characterized IFN-γ-induced transcription factor, does not mediate the proapoptotic effects of the cytokine *in vitro* and *in vivo*,[42,43] and we are presently examining whether such effects are mediated via activation of STAT-1. Of note, IFN-γ induces an early decrease in the expression of genes related to β cell defense/repair, including hsp70, peroxiredoxin, and chaperones located in the endoplasmic reticulum (ER) (Rasschaert, Liu, Kutlu, Cardozo, and Eizirik, manuscript in preparation). Thus, conceivably, while IL-1β induces several proapoptotic genes, IFN-γ contributes to cell death by both potentiating the expression of some IL-1β-induced "pro-death" genes (as, for instance, iNOS) and decreasing β cell defenses (FIG. 2).

A good example of the synergism between IL-1β and IFN-γ is the induction of β cell ER stress. ER stress is an adaptive cellular response to the accumulation of misfolded or aggregated proteins in the ER lumen and/or to loss of the normal Ca^{2+} homeostasis in the organelle. The ER stress response can lead to resolution of the problem, via translation attenuation, increase in the expression of ER chaperones, and ER-associated degradation, or, if excessive, lead to apoptosis via increased expression of CHOP/Gadd 153 and activation of JNK and caspase 12.[44,45] β cells have a heavy engagement in insulin biosynthesis (which may reach >50% of the total protein biosynthesis) and release, making it particularly sensitive to ER stress. ER stress–related proteins, such as Ire1α and Perk, are highly expressed in β cells.[46,47] Perk is the kinase responsible for phosphorylating eIF2 during ER stress,[48] leading to decreased mRNA translation and thus diminishing the "protein overload" on the stressed organelle. Perk knockout mice have progressive loss of β cells and diabetes mellitus, suggesting that the loss of this line of defense is sufficient to trigger ER stress in β cells, which seem to work near the limit of their capacity for protein synthesis and sorting at physiological conditions.[47]

Depletion of ER Ca^{2+} by thapsigargin [a blocker of the sarcoplasmic-endoplasmic-reticulum pump Ca^{2+}-ATPase (SERCA)2b, which brings Ca^{2+} into the ER] or NO triggers the ER stress pathway in insulin-producing MIN6 cells, leading to Gadd153/CHOP expression and apoptosis.[46,49] We observed that IL-1β-induced iNOS expression and NO production in β cells (a phenomenon potentiated by IFN-γ) can decrease SERCA2b mRNA expression,[7] depleting ER Ca^{2+} (Cardozo, Herschuelz, and Eizirik, manuscript in preparation) and, as a probable consequence, triggering Gadd153/CHOP expression.[7,8] Gadd153/CHOP participates in the "execution phase" of ER stress–induced apoptosis, suggesting that ER stress is one of the mechanisms by which cytokines trigger β cell apoptosis. Cytokines also modify the expression of other genes involved in the ER stress response, including upregulation of TRAF-2 (an effect of IL-1[7]), c-jun (an effect of IFN-γ that may increase the action of JNK; Rasschaert, Liu, Kutlu, Cardozo, and Eizirik, manuscript in preparation), and c-myc (an effect of IL-1β) and downregulation of several ER chaperones (an effect of IFN-γ, which probably reduces the capacity of β cells to deal with accumulating misfolded proteins in the ER)[7,8] (Rasschaert, Liu, Kutlu, Cardozo, and Eizirik, manuscript in preparation). Thus, the accumulating information generated by several microarray analyses starts to unveil the mechanisms by which IL-1β and IFN-γ cooperate for the induction of β cell death.

Of note, it has been described that some transgenic mice with foreign proteins placed under the control of the insulin promoter present β cell dysfunction and, in some cases, death of unknown cause.[50] Taking into account the issues discussed above, it is conceivable that the extra load imposed by the synthesis and sorting of the transgenic protein may be sufficient to induce β cell ER stress. This could either directly trigger apoptosis or render the β cells more sensitive to additional pro-apoptotic stimuli. To exclude this possibility, phenotypic evaluation of β cells in transgenic models based on the insulin promoter should search for the presence of "basal" ER stress, for instance by measuring mRNA expression of ER stress–related genes such as CHOP and Bip.

A surprising finding from our microarray data was that IL-1β and IFN-γ induced expression of several chemokines by pancreatic β cells.[7,8,51] These chemokines were expressed in parallel with induction of cytokines, such as IL-15 and IL-6, and adhesion molecules, such as ICAM. In addition, IFN-γ upregulated several mRNA encoding components of the "machinery" for MHC presentation, including MHC class I, the peptide transporters MTP-1 and MTP-2, and several subunits of the proteasome.[7,8] Increased expression of β cell autoantigens, in cooperation with local chemokine production, will probably increase homing, adhesion, and activation of mononuclear cells, thus aggravating insulitis and β cell destruction (FIG. 2).

The results discussed above raise the possibility that an important part of the "autoimmune triggered battle" that will culminate, or not, in β cell destruction and clinical diabetes mellitus is fought inside the β cell, more precisely at the level of β cell gene expression. Considering the microarray-based model proposed in FIGURE 2, the next question is how to design adequate experiments to clarify a phenomenon putatively regulated by the parallel and/or sequential up- and/or downregulation of dozens of genes. For this purpose, we are taking two main approaches: (i) to select and examine in detail particular groups of genes using *in vitro* and *in vivo* models of β cell dysfunction/death; this is illustrated by our ongoing work on chemokines (see below); (ii) to modify expression of transcription factors, instead of individual genes, thus modulating expression of a large number of coregulated mRNAs (see below).

HOMING OF MONONUCLEAR CELLS TO THE ISLETS IN EARLY INSULITIS: A CHEMOKINE-MEDIATED DIALOGUE BETWEEN INVADING CELLS AND PANCREATIC β CELLS?

Chemokines are chemotatic cytokines that direct normal leukocyte migration and activation, and regulate hematopoiesis, selectin/integrin upregulation, angiogenesis, and adaptative immunity.[52] More then 50 chemokine proteins have been already identified and they are divided in 4 families on the basis of the relative position of their initial cysteine (C) residues.[52,53] Chemokines act through chemokine receptors (XCR1, CCR1–11, CXCR1–5, and CX_3CR1) that are present in different types of leukocytes. The specificity and complexity of the chemokine system are derived from both the release of specific chemokines in distinct inflammatory reactions and the regulated expression of their receptors, which also vary in diverse immune responses [reviewed in refs. 52–54].

Expression of chemokines and their receptors is altered in autoimmune diseases such as multiple sclerosis and rheumatoid arthritis.[55,56] This also seems to be the case for T1DM. Thus, elevated levels of the Th1-associated chemokines, MIP-1α, MIP-1β, and IP-10 are present in the serum of newly diagnosed type 1 diabetic patients.[57–60] CXCR3 and CCR5 receptors are expressed in activated CD4+ Th1 cells, whereas expression of CCR3, CCR4, and CCR8 is observed in Th2 cells.[61–64] Patients with early-onset T1DM have reduced numbers of peripheral cells expressing the chemokine receptors CCR5 and CXCR3, suggesting homing of these Th1 cells to the inflammated islets.[60] CD4+ Th1 cells that are able to promote diabetes in NOD mice express CCR5 receptor and diverse chemokines, such as the CCR5

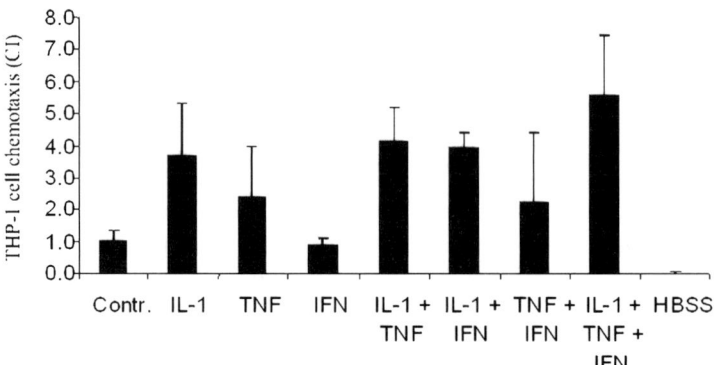

FIGURE 4. Chemotactic activity from supernatant of human pancreatic islets exposed to cytokines. Human pancreatic islets were isolated and treated with the cytokines, IL-1β (50 U/mL), IFN-γ (1000 U/mL), and/or TNF-α (1000 U/mL), as previously described.[70] Supernatants from each condition were used as chemoattractants for the human monocytic cell line THP-1. Chemotactic assay was performed as described.[72] CI, chemotactic index.

ligands RANTES and MIP-1α, the CXCR3 ligand IP-10, as well as lymphotactin, MCP-1, MCP-3, and MCP-5.[65,66] MIP-1α NOD knockout mice have reduced insulitis and are protected from diabetes,[65] while deletion of the CCR5 receptor leads to a switch from a Th1 to a Th2 response, delaying islet allograft destruction in mice.[67] Finally, transgenic expression of MCP-1 in β cells leads to insulitis,[68] and high basal MCP-1 production by human islets correlates with a poor clinical outcome following islet transplantation in patients with T1DM.[69]

FACS-purified rat β cells exposed to IL-1β + IFN-γ, or to double-stranded RNA, have increased expression of mRNAs encoding for several cytokines and chemokines, including MCP-1, IP-10, MIP-3α, fractalkine, and IL-15.[8,51,70,71] Furthermore, human islets exposed to IL-1β and IFN-γ have increased mRNA expression of IL-15, IP-10, MCP-1, MIP-3α, and fractalkine and secrete IL-15, MCP-1, IP-10, Mig, I-TAC, and MIP-3α into the culture medium.[51,70] These chemokines, or at least part of them, are functional, as suggested by the observation that supernatants from human islets exposed to cytokines have chemotactic activity for human THP-1 cells (FIG. 4).

To evaluate whether these chemokines and cytokines are expressed in pancreatic islets during early insulitis, we examined their mRNA expression in islets isolated from diabetes-prone NOD mice during the prediabetic period. Increased levels of IP-10 and MCP-1 mRNA were observed already at 4–6 weeks of age,[51,70] before major insulitis is present.[70] In line with these observations, high levels of IP-10 protein were also observed in islet cells from NOD mice at 8 weeks of age.[55] Macrophages are among the first cells to infiltrate the islets of NOD mice and BB rats,[1,73] and depletion or inactivation of macrophages prevents diabetes in these experimental models.[74,75] IP-10 and MCP-1 attract macrophages, and the early expression of IP-10 and MCP-1 in NOD islet cells[51,70] probably contributes to the recruitment of macrophages during the early stages of insulitis.

Induction of IL-15 mRNA in NOD islets was observed at 6 weeks and paralleled the increased IFN-γ expression, while MIP-3α induction was detected later (10 weeks), coinciding with the peak of IL-1β expression.[51] Induction of IL-15 mRNA was also observed during cyclophosphamide-induced insulitis in NOD mice.[76] The expression of MCP-1, IL-15, IP-10, and MIP-3α in NOD islets[51,70] occurs in parallel with the increased infiltration by macrophages, dendritic cells, T helper and cytotoxic lymphocytes, and NK cells in NOD islets (observed around 4–10 weeks[77]), suggesting a causal role for chemokines. Note that T cells are required for development of diabetes in both NOD mice and BB rats,[77,78] and the increased expression of IP-10, IL-15, and MIP-3α by the islet cells may contribute to T cell and dendritic cell recruitment.

Diabetic NOD mice transplanted with syngeneic islets show histological evidence of an early and severe graft infiltration, leading to β cell destruction and recurrence of diabetes at 6–10 days after transplantation.[79] Both CD4+ and CD8+ T cells producing Th1-type cytokines (principally IFN-γ) participate in the destruction of transplanted β cells.[80] A state of inflammation, characterized by high levels of IL-1 expression, is present soon (8 h) after islet transplantation in NOD mice.[51,81] This high local cytokine production leads to an early production of chemokines such as MCP-1 and IP-10 by the transplanted islets, possibly contributing to the attraction of immune-competent cells and eventual graft destruction.[51]

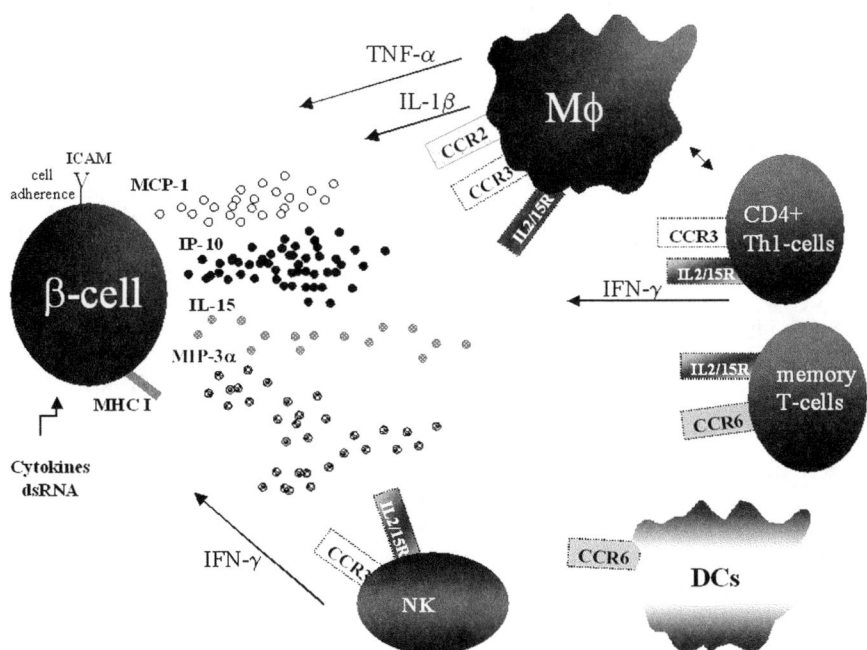

FIGURE 5. Proposed model for the chemokine-mediated "dialogue" between infiltrating mononuclear cells and the target β cells during the course of insulitis. Chemokines are represented as spheres.

The findings described above suggest that chemokines are involved in the pathogenesis of T1DM. Moreover, they raise the possibility of a "dialogue" between the invading monocytes, dendritic cells, and Th1 cells and the target β cells during the course of insulitis (FIG. 5). Thus, activated Th1 cells and macrophages homing into the islets produce cytokines such as IFN-γ and IL-1, inducing the β cells to release chemokines such as MCP-1, IP-10, and MIP-3α. These positively charged chemokines will possibly adhere to negatively charged proteoglycan proteins in the extracellular space around the islets, as described for other tissues, creating a chemokine gradient that will attract additional mononuclear cells. If this vicious circle is not interrupted, it will evolve to massive accumulation of macrophages and T cells around and inside the islets. In case the model proposed in FIGURE 5 proves to be correct, chemoattractant proteins and their receptors may be good candidates for therapeutic interventions to prevent T1DM.

TRANSCRIPTION FACTOR NETWORKS AND THE REGULATION OF β CELL APOPTOSIS

As discussed above, several of the cytokine-induced genes in pancreatic β cells are potentially regulated by the transcription factor NF-κB (FIG. 2). Resting β cells have negligible binding of NF-κB to the nucleus, but following 15–30 min of exposure to IL-1β the transcription factor is detected in the nucleus by both gel shift analysis[82] and chromatin immunoprecipitation (FIG. 3). It is noteworthy that NF-κB remains bound for at least 4 h to the promoter region of some cytokine-induced genes in β cells, such as Fas (FIG. 3) and MCP-1.[41] NF-κB is a transcription factor formed by dimers of proteins from the rel family, which includes p65, c-rel, relB, p50/p105, and p52/p100. Although most of these dimers are transcriptionally active (i.e., p50/p65, p50/c-rel, p65/p65, and p65/c-rel), some combinations act as inactive or repressive complexes (p50/p50 and p52/p52).[83] NF-κB is sequestered as an inactive protein in the cytoplasm of nonstimulated cells due to interaction with IκB proteins, which mask NF-κB localization signal and thus prevent its nuclear migration.[83] The best characterized IκB is IκBα. Following stimulation by different agonists, such as cytokines, bacterial products, or viruses, IκBα is phosphorylated at two NH_2-terminal serine residues (S32 and S36) by an IκB kinase complex, leading to its degradation in the proteasome. IκB degradation releases NF-κB, which rapidly translocates to the nucleus where it binds specific decanucleotide sequences in the promoter region of NF-κB-responsive genes, activating or inhibiting gene transcription. Mutation of serines 32 and 36 in the IκBα protein prevents its degradation and consequent NF-κB activation.[84]

NF-κB-regulated genes have been shown to inhibit the apoptotic program in diverse cell types. In a few cell types, however, the transcription factor also acts as an apoptosis inducer.[85,86] To test whether cytokine-induced activation of NF-κB in pancreatic β cells was mostly pro- or antiapoptotic, we infected β cells with an adenovirus containing a mutant form of IκBα, where S32 and S36 were substituted by alanine residues [AdIκB$^{(S/A)2}$], creating an IκB "superrepressor" protein. As described for other cell types,[87,88] AdIκB$^{(S/A)2}$ specifically blocked cytokine-induced NF-κB activation in FACS-purified rat β cells, preventing expression of the known NF-κB-dependent genes, iNOS, Fas, and MnSOD.[89] Moreover, the AdIκB$^{(S/A)2}$

prevented cytokine-induced β cell death via both apoptosis and necrosis.[89] In agreement with these findings, blocking of NF-κB activation by an IκB superrepressor prevented double-stranded RNA (dsRNA; a common by-product of viral infections) plus IFN-γ-induced apoptosis in rat β cells,[71] and also inhibited IL-1β-induced NO formation and Fas-mediated cell death in human islet cells.[90] Moreover, stable overexpression of mutant IκBα in insulin-producing MIN6 cells inhibited cytokine-induced NO production and cell death.[91] NF-κB regulates the expression of both genes involved in β cell death and defense/repair (FIG. 2), but the findings described above suggest that NF-κB activation has mostly a proapoptotic role in β cells, at least under conditions where β cells are exposed for prolonged periods of time to cytokines or dsRNA + cytokines. However, when β cells are exposed for a limited period (24 h) to low concentrations of IL-1β, the "protective" effects of NF-κB-regulated genes seem to preponderate, increasing β cell resistance to a subsequent assault by alloxan, streptozotocin, or chemical NO donors.[16] Three important questions remain to be answered in the context of the findings discussed above: (1) does blocking of NF-κB prevent β cell death *in vivo* in animal models of autoimmune diabetes or islet transplantation?; (2) why is NF-κB activation mostly proapoptotic in β cells and some neuronal cells, as contrasted to its antiapoptotic role in most other cell types?; (3) what are the cytokine-induced and NF-κB-dependent genes in pancreatic β cells?

To answer the third question (and perhaps to contribute to solve the second question), we combined two experimental approaches to identify the cytokine-induced and NF-κB-regulated genes in β cells. This was achieved by blocking NF-κB activation with IκB$^{(S/A)2}$ and studying the broad pattern of gene expression by microarray analysis.[7] Nearly 70 cytokine-modified and NF-κB-regulated genes were identified in primary β cells. Of special interest, NF-κB controls directly or indirectly (mostly via NO production) the expression of several other key transcription factors, such as PDX-1, Isl-1, c-myc, Gadd153/CHOP, C/EBPβ, and C/EBPδ[7] (FIG. 6). Based on these observations, we proposed that NF-κB functions as a "master switch", controlling distinct networks of transcription factors and effector genes of relevance for maintaining the β cell differentiated state, cytosolic and ER calcium homeostasis, attraction and activation of immune cells, and β cell apoptosis.[7] Moreover, and in line with evidence obtained in animal models of type 2 diabetes mellitus,[92,93] it seems that the process of β cell dysfunction and death in T1DM is, at least in part, a "transcription factor malaise".[7] These transcription factor and gene networks are probably not unidirectional, as depicted in FIGURE 2 (see also refs. 7 and 8), but should include positive and negative feedbacks, and cross-talk between the different pathways (FIG. 6). For instance, β cells probably utilize several mechanisms to downregulate NF-κB action following the initial wave of activation (FIG. 6). These negative feedback components include upregulation of IκBα,[7,8] MnSOD,[94] and NO production.[95] IκBα expression is regulated by NF-κB in β cells[7] and, as suggested for other cell types, increased IκBα expression will both prevent additional NF-κB translocation to the nucleus and remove NF-κB from its nuclear binding sites.[83,96,97] MnSOD expression is also regulated by NF-κB in β cells,[39] and increased expression of this mitochondrial free radical scavenging enzyme has been recently shown to decrease cytokine-induced NF-κB activation in insulin-producing cells.[94] iNOS is another NF-κB-dependent gene in β cells, and NO, the product of the iNOS reaction, both inhibits NF-κB activation and iNOS expression.[95] Considering the potential lethal effects of prolonged NF-κB activation in β cells, it seems

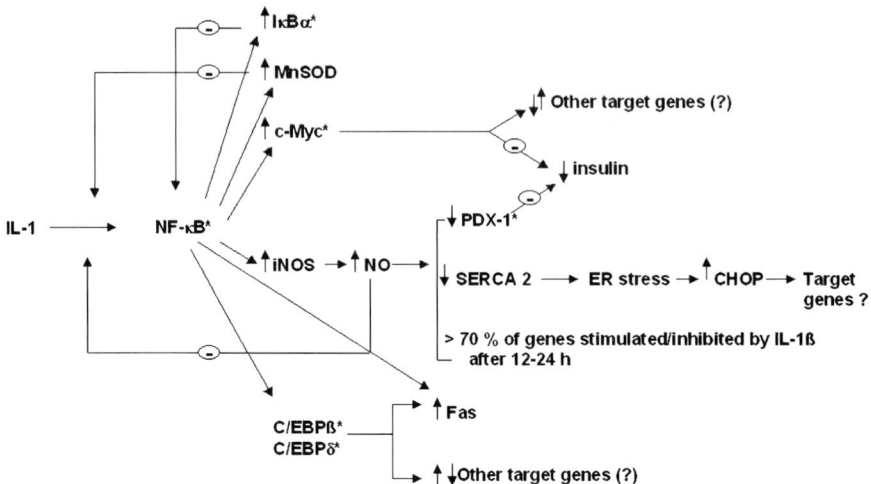

FIGURE 6. The role of NF-κB as a "master switch" for the transcription factor and gene networks contributing to cytokine-induced β cell dysfunction and death. Transcription factors are indicated with an asterisk.

logical that this cell utilizes different mechanisms to downregulate NF-κB activity. It is noteworthy that NO has a major effect on the late (>12 h) effect of cytokines on β cells. Indeed, >70% of the genes stimulated/inhibited in insulin-producing INS-1 cells after 12–24 h of exposure to IL-1β, including key genes such as PDX-1, SERCA-2, and CHOP, are regulated by NO generation (Kutlu, Cardozo, and Eizirik, manuscript in preparation). On the other hand, the fact that iNOS blocking, or genetic absence of iNOS expression, decreases necrosis, but does not prevent cytokine-induced apoptosis in INS-1E cells, rodent β cells, or human islet cells[11,37,38] (Kutlu, Cardozo, and Eizirik, manuscript in preparation) suggests that NO-independent genes are crucial for β cell fate. These genes may comprise early induced genes, preceding iNOS upregulation, and/or the 30% "late" induced, but NO-unrelated genes. Our ongoing microarray analysis of INS-1E cells exposed to cytokines in the presence of iNOS blockers will hopefully identify these genes (Kutlu, Cardozo, and Eizirik, manuscript in preparation).

CONCLUSIONS AND FUTURE PERSPECTIVES

The development of microarray analysis allows, for the first time, the study of the global responses of β cells to immune-mediated damage. The data generated are complex, but provide a more realistic view of the problem than the previous "gene-by-gene" approach. There are, however, important caveats that must be considered when analyzing the microarray data. Among them are the following: (1) The available arrays do not contain all genes expressed in β cells, and the global pattern of β cell gene expression will need to be reevaluated once complete arrays, that is, containing all genes expressed in human, mouse, and rat cells, become available. (2) The annotation of the genes included in the arrays is not always complete or correct. Gene functions are often assigned based on available data from other tissues, and a gene first described in neutrophils or platelets may have a completely different function in β cells. Moreover, >50% of the putative 30,000–35,000 genes present in the human genome do not have an identified function;[98,99] the situation is worse regarding the rat and mouse genome. These unknown genes, or pieces of these genes, are included in the arrays as ESTs, posing a formidable task to identify their physiological role. (3) mRNA expression does not necessarily lead to protein synthesis, and phenomena such as alternative splicing or posttranslational protein modification can cause important discrepancies between the mRNA data and the final protein product. Thus, as the methods for proteomic analysis improve, it will be crucial to compare the available microarray data with proteomic analysis. (4) Once a pattern of gene expression is detected, and associated with a biological phenomenon based on the temporal pattern of gene expression, the question then becomes how to prove this association. When dealing with single genes, there are well-defined methods to inhibit or induce gene expression *in vitro* or to develop transgenic and KO mice. How can we, however, down- or upregulate gene clusters that may include hundreds of genes? The approach described here, namely to target specific transcription factors regulating a group of genes of special biological interest, is clearly useful, but it lacks specificity and it may be difficult to use in situations where multiple transcription factors regulate the phenomenon under study.

The decision of the β cell to undergo or not apoptosis seems to be an extremely complex phenomenon, regulated at least in part at the level of gene expression. If we wish to understand this phenomenon, it is imperative that we address it at its real level of complexity. The analysis of complex patterns of gene expression, and their biological meaning, is a very difficult task, requiring large amounts of time and resources, and deep reflection. Instead of discouraging us, these difficulties should stimulate additional research and the development of better global approaches to understand the process of β cell death. We believe that this knowledge is a basic requirement for the development of rational approaches to prevent β cell loss in type 1 diabetes mellitus.

[NOTE ADDED IN PROOF: Two new microarray papers from our group, referred to in the text as "manuscript in preparation", are now "in press": KUTLU, B., A.K. CARDOZO, M.I. DARVILLE *et al.* 2003. Discovery of gene networks regulating cytokine-induced dysfunction and apoptosis in insulin-producing INS-1 cells. *Diabetes*. In press; RASSCHAERT, J., D. LIU, A.K. CARDOZO *et al.* 2003. Global profiling of double stranded RNA- and IFN-γ-induced genes in rat pancreatic beta cells. *Diabetologia*. In press.]

ACKNOWLEDGMENTS

We are grateful to P. Proost, Laboratory of Medical Immunology, Rega Institute for Medical Research, Katholieke Universiteit Leuven, for help and advice in the performance of the chemotactic analysis shown in FIGURE 4. We also acknowledge the rewarding collaboration with C. Mathieu and C. Gysemans and with T. Ortonft and M. Kruhoffer on, respectively, *in vivo* chemokine studies and microarray analysis. Research activities by the authors described in the present review were supported by grants from the Juvenile Diabetes Foundation International (JDRF), the Fonds National de la Recherche Scientifique (FNRS), and the Funds voor Wetenschappelijk Onderzoek (FWO), Belgium. Ongoing research by the authors on β cell apoptosis is conducted in collaboration with and supported by the JDRF Center for Prevention of β Cell Destruction in Europe under Grant No. 4-2002-457.

REFERENCES

1. EIZIRIK, D.L. & T. MANDRUP-POULSEN. 2001. A choice of death—the signal-transduction of immune-mediated β-cell apoptosis. Diabetologia **44:** 2115–2133.
2. EIZIRIK, D.L. & M.I. DARVILLE. 2001. β-Cell apoptosis and defense mechanisms: lessons from type 1 diabetes. Diabetes **50**(suppl. 1)**:** S64–S69.
3. MAURICIO, D. & T. MANDRUP-POULSEN. 1998. Apoptosis and the pathogenesis of IDDM: a question of life and death. Diabetes **47:** 1537–1543.
4. THOMAS, H.E. & T.W. KAY. 2001. How beta cells die in type 1 diabetes. Curr. Dir. Autoimmun. **4:** 144–170.
5. MATHIS, D., L. VENCE & C. BENOIST. 2001. β-Cell death during progression to diabetes. Nature **414:** 792–798.
6. LIPSHUTZ, R.J., S.P. FODOR, T.R. GINGERAS et al. 1999. High density synthetic oligonucleotide arrays. Nat. Genet. **21:** 20–24.
7. CARDOZO, A.K., H. HEIMBERG, Y. HEREMANS et al. 2001. A comprehensive analysis of cytokine-induced and nuclear factor-κB-dependent genes in primary rat pancreatic β-cells. J. Biol. Chem. **276:** 48879–48886.
8. CARDOZO, A.K., M. KRUHOFFER, R. LEEMAN et al. 2001. Identification of novel cytokine-induced genes in pancreatic β-cells by high-density oligonucleotide arrays. Diabetes **50:** 909–920.
9. LOCKHART, D.J. & E.A. WINZELER. 2000. Genomics, gene expression, and DNA arrays. Nature **405:** 827–836.
10. YOUNG, R.A. 2000. Biomedical discovery with DNA arrays. Cell **102:** 9–15.
11. LIU, D., D. PAVLOVIC, M.C. CHEN et al. 2000. Cytokines induce apoptosis in β-cells isolated from mice lacking the inducible isoform of nitric oxide synthase (iNOS–/–). Diabetes **49:** 1116–1122.
12. DEL PRETE, M.J., M.S. ROBLES, A. GUAO et al. 2002. Degradation of cellular mRNA is a general early apoptosis-induced event. FASEB J. **16:** 2003–2006.
13. BORG, L.A. & D.L. EIZIRIK. 1990. Short-term exposure of rat pancreatic islets to human interleukin-1β increases cellular uptake of calcium. Immunol. Lett. **26:** 253–258.
14. EIZIRIK, D.L. 1991. Interleukin-1β induces an early decrease in insulin release, (pro)insulin biosynthesis, and insulin mRNA in mouse pancreatic islets by a mechanism dependent on gene transcription and protein synthesis. Autoimmunity **10:** 107–113.
15. DARVILLE, M.I. & D.L. EIZIRIK. 1998. Regulation by cytokines of the inducible nitric oxide synthase promoter in insulin-producing cells. Diabetologia **41:** 1101–1108.
16. LING, Z., M. VAN DE CASTEELE, D.L. EIZIRIK et al. 2000. Interleukin-1β-induced alteration in a β-cell phenotype can reduce cellular sensitivity to conditions that cause necrosis, but not to cytokine-induced apoptosis. Diabetes **49:** 340–345.
17. MCKINNON, C.M. & K. DOCHERTY. 2001. Pancreatic duodenal homeobox-1, PDX-1, a major regulator of beta cell identity and function. Diabetologia **44:** 1203–1214.
18. PEDERSEN, A.A., H.V. PETERSEN, N. VIDEBAEK et al. 2002. PDX-1 mediates glucose responsiveness of GAD(67), but not GAD(65), gene transcription in islets of Langerhans. Biochem. Biophys. Res. Commun. **295:** 243–248.
19. WAEBER, G., N. THOMPSON, P. NICOD et al. 1996. Transcriptional activation of the GLUT2 gene by the IPF-1/STF-1/IDX-1 homeobox factor. Mol. Endocrinol. **10:** 1327–1334.
20. BAEZA, N., A. HART, U. AHLGREN et al. 2001. Insulin promoter factor-1 controls several aspects of β-cell identity. Diabetes **50**(suppl. 1)**:** S36.

21. THOMAS, M.K., O.N. DEVON, J.H. LEE et al. 2001. Development of diabetes mellitus in aging transgenic mice following suppression of pancreatic homeoprotein IDX-1. J. Clin. Invest. **108:** 319–329.
22. LOTTMANN, H., J. VANSELOW, B. HESSABI et al. 2001. The Tet-On system in transgenic mice: inhibition of the mouse pdx-1 gene activity by antisense RNA expression in pancreatic β-cells. J. Mol. Med. **79:** 321–328.
23. WELSH, N., D.L. EIZIRIK, K. BENDTZEN et al. 1991. Interleukin-1β-induced nitric oxide production in isolated rat pancreatic islets requires gene transcription and may lead to inhibition of the Krebs cycle enzyme aconitase. Endocrinology **129:** 3167–3173.
24. EIZIRIK, D.L., S. SANDLER & J.P. PALMER. 1993. Repair of pancreatic β-cells: a relevant phenomenon in early IDDM? Diabetes **42:** 1383–1391.
25. AHLGREN, U., S.L. PFAFF, T.M. JESSELL et al. 1997. Independent requirement for ISL1 in formation of pancreatic mesenchyme and islet cells. Nature **385:** 257–260.
26. KOJIMA, H., T. NAKAMURA, Y. FUJITA et al. 2002. Combined expression of pancreatic duodenal homeobox 1 and islet factor 1 induces immature enterocytes to produce insulin. Diabetes **51:** 1398–1408.
27. KANETO, H., A. SHARMA, K. SUZUMA et al. 2002. Induction of c-Myc expression suppresses insulin gene transcription by inhibiting NeuroD/BETA2-mediated transcriptional activation. J. Biol. Chem. **277:** 12998–13006.
28. LAYBUTT, D.R., G.C. WEIR, H. KANETO et al. 2002. Overexpression of c-Myc in β-cells of transgenic mice causes proliferation and apoptosis, downregulation of insulin gene expression, and diabetes. Diabetes **51:** 1793–1804.
29. FLAMEZ, D., V. BERGER, M. KRUHOFFER et al. 2002. Critical role for cataplerosis via citrate in glucose-regulated insulin release. Diabetes **51:** 2018–2024.
30. WEBB, G.C., M.S. AKBAR, C. ZHAO et al. 2000. Expression profiling of pancreatic β cells: glucose regulation of secretory and metabolic pathway genes. Proc. Natl. Acad. Sci. USA **97:** 5773–5778.
31. BUSCH, A.K., D. CORDERY, G.S. DENYER et al. 2002. Expression profiling of palmitate- and oleate-regulated genes provides novel insights into the effects of chronic lipid exposure on pancreatic β-cell function. Diabetes **51:** 977–987.
32. LEIBOWITZ, G., M. YULI, M.Y. DONATH et al. 2001. β-Cell glucotoxicity in the *Psammomys obesus* model of type 2 diabetes. Diabetes **50**(suppl. 1)**:** S113–S117.
33. HOORENS, A., M. VAN DE CASTEELE, G. KLOPPEL et al. 1996. Glucose promotes survival of rat pancreatic β cells by activating synthesis of proteins which suppress a constitutive apoptotic program. J. Clin. Invest. **98:** 1568–1574.
34. CNOP, M., J.C. HANNAERT, A. HOORENS et al. 2001. Inverse relationship between cytotoxicity of free fatty acids in pancreatic islet cells and cellular triglyceride accumulation. Diabetes **50:** 1771–1777.
35. UNGER, R.H. 1995. Lipotoxicity in the pathogenesis of obesity-dependent NIDDM: genetic and clinical implications. Diabetes **44:** 863–870.
36. MAECHLER, P. & C.B. WOLLHEIM. 2001. Mitochondrial function in normal and diabetic β-cells. Nature **414:** 807–812.
37. DELANEY, C.A., D. PAVLOVIC, A. HOORENS et al. 1997. Cytokines induce deoxyribonucleic acid strand breaks and apoptosis in human pancreatic islet cells. Endocrinology **138:** 2610–2614.
38. ZUMSTEG, U., S. FRIGERIO & G.A. HOLLANDER. 2000. Nitric oxide production and Fas surface expression mediate two independent pathways of cytokine-induced murine β-cell damage. Diabetes **49:** 39–47.
39. DARVILLE, M.I., Y.S. HO & D.L. EIZIRIK. 2000. NF-κB is required for cytokine-induced manganese superoxide dismutase expression in insulin-producing cells. Endocrinology **141:** 153–162.
40. DARVILLE, M.I. & D.L. EIZIRIK. 2001. Cytokine induction of Fas gene expression in insulin-producing cells requires the transcription factors NF-κB and C/EBP. Diabetes **50:** 1741–1748.
41. KUTLU, B., M. DARVILLE, A.K. CARDOZO et al. 2003. Molecular regulation of monocyte chemoattractant protein-1 (MCP-1) expression in pancreatic β-cells. Diabetes **52:** 348–355.

42. PAVLOVIC, D., M.C. CHEN, C.A. GYSEMANS et al. 1999. The role of interferon regulatory factor-1 in cytokine-induced mRNA expression and cell death in murine pancreatic β-cells. Eur. Cytokine Netw. **10:** 403–412.
43. GYSEMANS, C.A., D. PAVLOVIC, R. BOUILLON et al. 2001. Dual role of interferon-gamma signalling pathway in sensitivity of pancreatic beta cells to immune destruction. Diabetologia **44:** 567–574.
44. OYADOMARI, S., E. ARAKI & M. MORI. 2002. Endoplasmic reticulum stress-mediated apoptosis in pancreatic β-cells. Apoptosis **7:** 335–345.
45. VERKHRATSKY, A. & O.H. PETERSEN. 2002. The endoplasmic reticulum as an integrating signalling organelle: from neuronal signalling to neuronal death. Eur. J. Pharmacol. **447:** 141–154.
46. OYADOMARI, S., K. TAKEDA, M. TAKIGUCHI et al. 2001. Nitric oxide–induced apoptosis in pancreatic β cells is mediated by the endoplasmic reticulum stress pathway. Proc. Natl. Acad. Sci. USA **98:** 10845–10850.
47. HARDING, H.P., H. ZENG, Y. ZHANG et al. 2001. Diabetes mellitus and exocrine pancreatic dysfunction in perk−/− mice reveals a role for translational control in secretory cell survival. Mol. Cell **7:** 1153–1163.
48. HARDING, H.P., Y. ZHANG & D. RON. 1999. Protein translation and folding are coupled by an endoplasmic-reticulum-resident kinase. Nature **397:** 271–274.
49. ZHOU, Y.P., D. TENG, F. DRALYUK et al. 1998. Apoptosis in insulin-secreting cells: evidence for the role of intracellular Ca2+ stores and arachidonic acid metabolism. J. Clin. Invest. **101:** 1623–1632.
50. LEITER, E.H. 2002. Mice with targeted gene disruptions or gene insertions for diabetes research: problems, pitfalls, and potential solutions. Diabetologia **45:** 296–308.
51. CARDOZO, A.K., P. PROOST, C. GYSEMANS et al. 2003. IL-1β and IFN-γ induce the expression of diverse chemokines and IL-15 in human and rat pancreatic islet cells, and in islets from pre-diabetic NOD mice. Diabetologia **46:** 255–266.
52. COLVIN, B.L. & A.W. THOMSON. 2002. Chemokines, their receptors, and transplant outcome. Transplantation **74:** 149–155.
53. LUSTER, A.D. 1998. Chemokines—chemotactic cytokines that mediate inflammation. N. Engl. J. Med. **338:** 436–445.
54. CHRISTOPHERSON, K., II & R. HROMAS. 2001. Chemokine regulation of normal and pathologic immune responses. Stem Cells **19:** 388–396.
55. ARIMILLI, S., W. FERLIN, N. SOLVASON et al. 2000. Chemokines in autoimmune diseases. Immunol. Rev. **177:** 43–51.
56. GODESSART, N. & S.L. KUNKEL. 2001. Chemokines in autoimmune disease. Curr. Opin. Immunol. **13:** 670–675.
57. SHIMADA, A., J. MORIMOTO, K. KODAMA et al. 2001. Elevated serum IP-10 levels observed in type 1 diabetes. Diabetes Care **24:** 510–515.
58. HANIFI-MOGHADDAM, P., S. KAPPLER, A. ZWINDERMANN et al. 2002. Distinct cytokine and chemokine serum levels are associated with different stages of disease in diabetes mellitus type 1. Diabetes Metab. Res. Rev. **18**(suppl. 4): S8.
59. NICOLETTI, F., I. CONGET, M. DI MAURO et al. 2002. Serum concentrations of the interferon-γ-inducible chemokine IP-10/CXCL10 are augmented in both newly diagnosed type I diabetes mellitus patients and subjects at risk of developing the disease. Diabetologia **45:** 1107–1110.
60. LOHMANN, T., S. LAUE, U. NIETZSCHMANN et al. 2002. Reduced expression of Th1-associated chemokine receptors on peripheral blood lymphocytes at diagnosis of type 1 diabetes. Diabetes **51:** 2474–2480.
61. SALLUSTO, F., C.R. MACKAY & A. LANZAVECCHIA. 1997. Selective expression of the eotaxin receptor CCR3 by human T helper 2 cells. Science **277:** 2005–2007.
62. SALLUSTO, F., D. LENIG, C.R. MACKAY et al. 1998. Flexible programs of chemokine receptor expression on human polarized T helper 1 and 2 lymphocytes. J. Exp. Med. **187:** 875–883.
63. LOETSCHER, P., M. UGUCCIONI, L. BORDOLI et al. 1998. CCR5 is characteristic of Th1 lymphocytes. Nature **391:** 344–345.

64. BONECCHI, R., G. BIANCHI, P.P. BORDIGNON et al. 1998. Differential expression of chemokine receptors and chemotactic responsiveness of type 1 T helper cells (Th1s) and Th2s. J. Exp. Med. **187:** 129–134.
65. CAMERON, M.J., G.A. ARREAZA, M. GRATTAN et al. 2000. Differential expression of CC chemokines and the CCR5 receptor in the pancreas is associated with progression to type I diabetes. J. Immunol. **165:** 1102–1110.
66. BRADLEY, L.M., V.C. ASENSIO, L.K. SCHIOETZ et al. 1999. Islet-specific Th1, but not Th2, cells secrete multiple chemokines and promote rapid induction of autoimmune diabetes. J. Immunol. **162:** 2511–2520.
67. ABDI, R., R.N. SMITH, L. MAKHLOUF et al. 2002. The role of CC chemokine receptor 5 (CCR5) in islet allograft rejection. Diabetes **51:** 2489–2495.
68. GREWAL, I.S., B.J. RUTLEDGE, J.A. FIORILLO et al. 1997. Transgenic monocyte chemoattractant protein-1 (MCP-1) in pancreatic islets produces monocyte-rich insulitis without diabetes: abrogation by a second transgene expressing systemic MCP-1. J. Immunol. **159:** 401–408.
69. PIEMONTI, L., B.E. LEONE, R. NANO et al. 2002. Human pancreatic islets produce and secrete MCP-1/CCL2: relevance in human islet transplantation. Diabetes **51:** 55–65.
70. CHEN, M.C., P. PROOST, C. GYSEMANS et al. 2001. Monocyte chemoattractant protein-1 is expressed in pancreatic islets from prediabetic NOD mice and in interleukin-1β-exposed human and rat islet cells. Diabetologia **44:** 325–332.
71. LIU, D., A.K. CARDOZO, M.I. DARVILLE et al. 2002. Double-stranded RNA cooperates with interferon-γ and IL-1β to induce both chemokine expression and nuclear factor-κB-dependent apoptosis in pancreatic β-cells: potential mechanisms for viral-induced insulitis and β-cell death in type 1 diabetes mellitus. Endocrinology **143:** 1225–1234.
72. SCHUTYSER, E., S. STRUYF, P. MENTEN et al. 2000. Regulated production and molecular diversity of human liver and activation-regulated chemokine/macrophage inflammatory protein-3α from normal and transformed cells. J. Immunol. **165:** 4470–4477.
73. HANENBERG, H., V. KOLB-BACHOFEN, G. KANTWERK-FUNKE et al. 1989. Macrophage infiltration precedes and is a prerequisite for lymphocytic insulitis in pancreatic islets of pre-diabetic BB rats. Diabetologia **32:** 126–134.
74. JUN, H.S., P. SANTAMARIA, H.W. LIM et al. 1999. Absolute requirement of macrophages for the development and activation of β-cell cytotoxic CD8+ T-cells in T-cell receptor transgenic NOD mice. Diabetes **48:** 34–42.
75. OSCHILEWSKI, U., U. KIESEL & H. KOLB. 1985. Administration of silica prevents diabetes in BB-rats. Diabetes **34:** 197–199.
76. ROTHE, H., A. HAUSMANN & H. KOLB. 2002. Immunoregulation during disease progression in prediabetic NOD mice: inverse expression of arginase and prostaglandin H synthase 2 vs. interleukin-15. Horm. Metab. Res. **34:** 7–12.
77. YOON, J.W., H.S. JUN & P. SANTAMARIA. 1998. Cellular and molecular mechanisms for the initiation and progression of β cell destruction resulting from the collaboration between macrophages and T cells. Autoimmunity **27:** 109–122.
78. THOMAS, H.E. & T.W. KAY. 2000. β cell destruction in the development of autoimmune diabetes in the non-obese diabetic (NOD) mouse. Diabetes Metab. Res. Rev. **16:** 251–261.
79. CASTEELS, K., M. WAER, J. LAUREYS et al. 1998. Prevention of autoimmune destruction of syngeneic islet grafts in spontaneously diabetic nonobese diabetic mice by a combination of a vitamin D3 analog and cyclosporine. Transplantation **65:** 1225–1232.
80. SUAREZ-PINZON, W., R.V. RAJOTTE, T.R. MOSMANN et al. 1996. Both CD4+ and CD8+ T-cells in syngeneic islet grafts in NOD mice produce interferon-γ during β-cell destruction. Diabetes **45:** 1350–1357.
81. GYSEMANS, C.A., M. WAER, D. VALCKX et al. 2000. Early graft failure of xenogeneic islets in NOD mice is accompanied by high levels of interleukin-1 and low levels of transforming growth factor-β mRNA in the grafts. Diabetes **49:** 1992–1997.
82. EIZIRIK, D.L., M. FLODSTROM, A.E. KARLSEN et al. 1996. The harmony of the spheres: inducible nitric oxide synthase and related genes in pancreatic β cells. Diabetologia **39:** 875–890.

83. GHOSH, S., M.J. MAY & E.B. KOPP. 1998. NF-κB and Rel proteins: evolutionarily conserved mediators of immune responses. Annu. Rev. Immunol. **16:** 225–260.
84. BROWN, K., S. GERSTBERGER, L. CARLSON *et al.* 1995. Control of IκB-alpha proteolysis by site-specific, signal-induced phosphorylation. Science **267:** 1485–1488.
85. CHEN, L. & X. GAO. 2002. Neuronal apoptosis induced by endoplasmic reticulum stress. Neurochem. Res. **27:** 891–899.
86. BARKETT, M. & T.D. GILMORE. 1999. Control of apoptosis by Rel/NF-κB transcription factors. Oncogene **18:** 6910–6924.
87. JOBIN, C., A. PANJA, C. HELLERBRAND *et al.* 1998. Inhibition of proinflammatory molecule production by adenovirus-mediated expression of a nuclear factor κB super-repressor in human intestinal epithelial cells. J. Immunol. **160:** 410–418.
88. HELLERBRAND, C., C. JOBIN, Y. IIMURO *et al.* 1998. Inhibition of NFκB in activated rat hepatic stellate cells by proteasome inhibitors and an IκB super-repressor. Hepatology **27:** 1285–1295.
89. HEIMBERG, H., Y. HEREMANS, C. JOBIN *et al.* 2001. Inhibition of cytokine-induced NF-κB activation by adenovirus-mediated expression of a NF-κB super-repressor prevents β-cell apoptosis. Diabetes **50:** 2219–2224.
90. GIANNOUKAKIS, N., W.A. RUDERT, M. TRUCCO *et al.* 2000. Protection of human islets from the effects of interleukin-1β by adenoviral gene transfer of an IκB repressor. J. Biol. Chem. **275:** 36509–36513.
91. BAKER, M.S., X. CHEN, X.C. CAO *et al.* 2001. Expression of a dominant negative inhibitor of NF-κB protects MIN6 β-cells from cytokine-induced apoptosis. J. Surg. Res. **97:** 117–122.
92. EDLUND, H. 2001. Factors controlling pancreatic cell differentiation and function. Diabetologia **44:** 1071–1079.
93. FERRER, J. 2002. A genetic switch in pancreatic β-cells: implications for differentiation and haploinsufficiency. Diabetes **51:** 2355–2362.
94. AZEVEDO-MARTINS, A.K., S. LORTZ, S. LENZEN *et al.* 2003. Improvement of the mitochondrial antioxidant defense status prevents cytokine-induced NF-κB activation in insulin-producing cells. Diabetes **52:** 93–101.
95. NIEMANN, A., A. BJORKLUND & D.L. EIZIRIK. 1994. Studies on the molecular regulation of the inducible form of nitric oxide synthase (iNOS) in insulin-producing cells. Mol. Cell. Endocrinol. **106:** 151–155.
96. MAY, M.J. & S. GHOSH. 1998. Signal transduction through NF-κB. Immunol. Today **19:** 80–88.
97. TAK, P.P. & G.S. FIRESTEIN. 2001. NF-κB: a key role in inflammatory diseases. J. Clin. Invest. **107:** 7–11.
98. LANDER, E.S., L.M. LINTON, B. BIRREN *et al.* 2001. Initial sequencing and analysis of the human genome. Nature **409:** 860–921.
99. VENTER, J.C., M.D. ADAMS, E.W. MYERS *et al.* 2001. The sequence of the human genome. Science **291:** 1304–1351.

The T Cell Response to Glutamic Acid Decarboxylase 65 in T Cell Receptor Transgenic NOD Mice

HUGH McDEVITT

Departments of Microbiology and Immunology, and Medicine, Stanford University School of Medicine, Stanford, California, USA

ABSTRACT: Using BW 5147 T cell hybridomas isolated by fusion with spleen and lymph node cells from NOD female mice, two T cell receptor transgenic NOD mouse lines were produced. Both TCR transgenics respond to their cognate peptide/MHC (GAD65 206–220 and 286–300) and produce IL-2, IFN-γ, and small amounts of IL-10. Unexpectedly, the transgenic mice do not develop diabetes and have no insulitis. Analysis with a GAD65 286–300/I-A^{g7} tetramer reveals that transgenic T cells are negatively selected in the thymus and further negatively selected in the periphery. When crossed to the C$_\alpha^{-/-}$ NOD line, CD4 T cells were reduced by 90% in the thymus and periphery. Further, the tetramer positive GAD65 286–300 specific T cells were capable of delaying the onset of diabetes in a standard transfer system. Thus, GAD65 specific TCR transgenic T cells (1) must express a second α chain to survive negative selection, (2) produce IL-2 and IFN-γ, and (3) have a mildly protective effect on transfer of diabetes with diabetogenic spleen cells.

KEYWORDS: NOD mice; GAD65; TCR transgenes; diabetes

INTRODUCTION

The studies described below grew out of an analysis of the response of the T cell receptor repertoire to glutamic acid decarboxylase 65 (GAD65) in 12-week-old female NOD mice, either unimmunized or immunized with recombinant, baculovirus-produced GAD65 in incomplete Freund's adjuvant, injected in the hind foot pads. The draining lymph nodes were removed and their T cells used for fusion with the BW 5147 T cell tumor. Screening the resulting T cell hybridomas, first with GAD65 and then with a peptide library of 120 15-mers overlapping by 10 residues, identified three immunodominant epitopes—residues 206–220, 221–235, and 286–300. T cell hybridomas recognizing three other minor, less frequent, epitopes of GAD65 were not included in the studies described below. It should be pointed out that one experiment screened a large number of T cell hybridomas from a fusion of spleen CD4 T cells isolated from an unimmunized 12-week-old female NOD mouse with BW 5147.[1] Of

Address for correspondence: Hugh McDevitt, Departments of Microbiology and Immunology, and Medicine, Stanford University School of Medicine, 299 Campus Drive, Fairchild Science Building, Room D345, Stanford, CA 94305-5124. Voice: 650-723-5893; fax: 650-723-9180.
hughmcd@stanford.edu

the three hybridomas responding to GAD65 protein, two T cell hybridomas were specific for GAD65 286–300 and one was specific for peptide 206–220.

Two GAD65 specific TCR transgenic founders on the NOD background have been analyzed sufficiently well to characterize their immune response to GAD65 and the phenotype of the transgenic T cells.[2] PCR-amplified sequences of the variable region sequences of the α and β chains from a spontaneously occurring GAD65 206–220 T cell hybridoma and a postimmune GAD65 286–300 T cell hybridoma were used to produce TCR transgenic mice by the methods described.[2] The analyses of these mice are described below.

CHARACTERIZATION OF THE GAD65 SPECIFIC T CELL RECEPTOR TRANSGENIC NOD MICE

Since almost all of the characteristics of the two TCR transgenic lines specific for the two dominant epitopes were very similar, this discussion will present the data primarily found in the G286 TCR transgenic line, expressing a T cell receptor specific for the GAD65 286–300 epitope.[2] Both transgenic lines failed to develop diabetes, and had almost no insulitis, as shown for the G286 transgenic line in FIGURES 1A and 1B. *In vitro* stimulation with the cognate peptide/MHC presented by irradiated NOD splenocytes showed that the CD4$^+$ transgenic T cells responded well to GAD65 286–300 (FIGS. 2A and 2B). The cytokine pattern in the supernates following this *in vitro* stimulation revealed that these T cells produced moderate amounts of IL-2, IFN-γ, IL-10, and TNFα (data not shown), and no detectable IL-5.[2]

About 10–20% of CD4$^+$ T cells from the G286 TCR transgenic line and 40–50% of the CD8$^+$ T cells were tetramer positive with a streptavidin-I-A^{g7}/286–300 peptide (covalently linked). This relatively small number of tetramer positive T cells suggested that many of the T cells were expressing a second α chain. This was confirmed by crossing the TCR transgene onto the NOD.C$_\alpha^{-/-}$ background. On the C$_\alpha^{-/-}$ background, the number of CD4$^+$ T cells dropped from 40% in peripheral blood to 6%, indicating that almost all of the T cells in these transgenic animals were

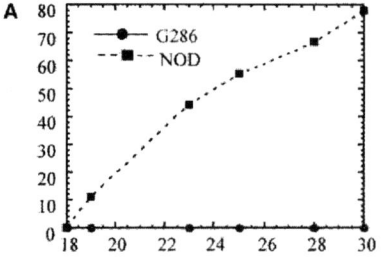
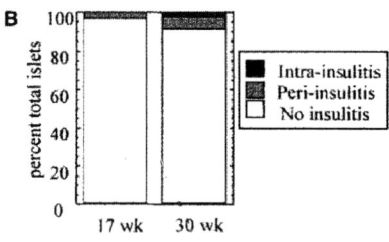

FIGURE 1. Incidence of diabetes and insulitis in G286 mice. (**A**) Diabetes incidence in female G286 (*circles*, n = 6) or NOD littermates (*squares*, n = 9). (**B**) Insulitis in 17-week-old (*left*) or 30-week-old (*right*) female G286 mice. Islets were scored as no insulitis, peri-insulitis, or intra-insulitis. Totals of 42 and 160 islets were scored in the 17-week-old and 30-week-old mice, respectively. Reproduced with permission from ref. 2.

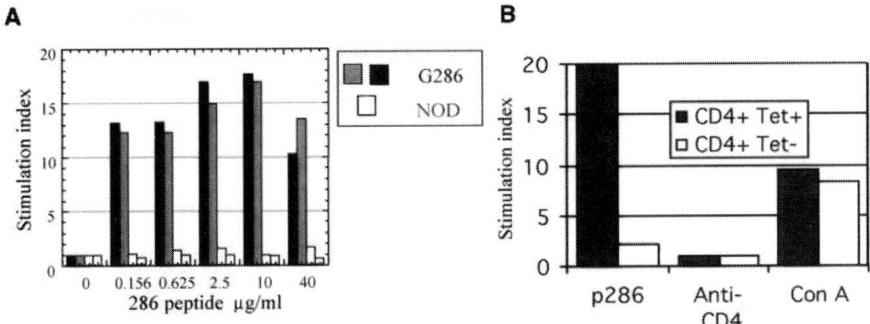

FIGURE 2. Activation and cytokine production by lymphocytes from G286 mice. Lymph node cells from G286 or NOD mice were activated *in vitro* with the indicated concentration of p286. Proliferation for total LN cells (**A**) or purified population (**B**) was determined by ^{3}[H]thymidine incorporation. In B, CD4$^+$ p286 tetramer positive and CD4$^+$ p286 tetramer negative cells were sorted and activated with 20 µg/mL p286 and irradiated NOD spleen cells; ^{3}[H]thymidine was added for the last 16 h of a 96-h incubation. Results are expressed as average stimulation index. The average background counts for the no-antigen controls were 1396 cpm (A) and 58 cpm (B). Reproduced with permission from ref. 2.

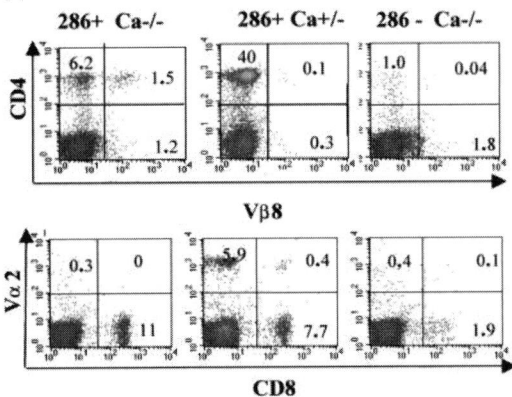

FIGURE 3. Evidence for expression of multiple TCRs in G286 mice. Peripheral blood lymphocytes from G286 $C_\alpha^{-/-}$ (*left*), G286 $C_\alpha^{+/-}$ (*middle*), and NOD $C_\alpha^{-/-}$ (*right*) mice were stained with antibodies for CD4 and Vβ8 (*top*) or CD8 and Vα2 (*bottom*). The percentages of cells in each quadrant are indicated in each corner of the plots. Reproduced with permission from ref. 2.

deleted in the thymus (FIG. 3). A plot of T cell receptor expression (detected by CD3 expression) versus tetramer positivity showed that the majority of T cells in the thymus fell on the expected diagonal line for both the CD4 and CD8 T cell populations, although in the CD4 population a large number of CD3$^+$ T cells were tetramer negative, as seen in the bottom panel of FIGURE 4. A similar analysis in the periphery (lymph nodes) revealed that the CD4 T cells that were tetramer positive fell off of the expected diagonal line, indicating that these T cells expressed a second T cell receptor that was not tetramer positive, despite the fact that the CD4 T cells were CD3$^+$. These results are shown in FIGURE 4 for both thymus and lymph node.

The inescapable conclusion from the results shown in FIGURES 3 and 4 is that transgenic T cells expressing the T cell receptor specific for GAD65 286–300 survive

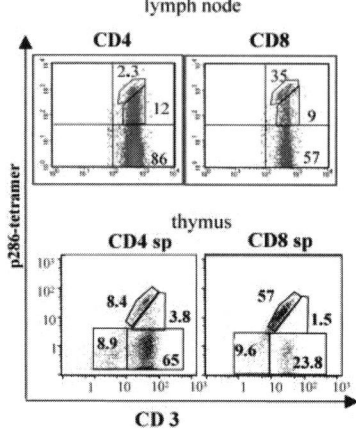

FIGURE 4. Cells from lymph node of a G286 mouse or thymus of a G286 $C_\alpha^{+/-}$ mouse were stained with antibodies for CD4, CD8, and CD3. Cells were gated on CD4$^+$ or CD8$^+$. Expression of CD3 versus I-A^{g7}-286 tetramer is shown. Cells in the diagonal gate represent cells for which the p286 specific TCR is the predominant TCR expressed. Percentages of cells in the gates drawn are indicated on the plots. Reproduced with permission from ref. 2.

negative selection in the thymus only if they are able to express a second α chain. Further, when these T cells arrive in the periphery, they are subjected to additional negative selection as indicated by the very small percentage of T cells falling on the diagonal line in the tetramer versus CD3 plot. Clearly, transgenic T cells in these mice are negatively selected in the thymus and undergo further negative selection in the periphery. Similar results were obtained with the GAD65 206–220 TCR transgenic mouse line. It should be pointed out that the 206–220 specific T cells used to produce this latter transgenic T cell receptor were isolated from an unimmunized, unmanipulated 12-week-old female NOD mouse. Since the transgenes were introduced directly into inbred NOD embryos, these results cannot be due to the introduction of alleles from other strains.

GAD65 SPECIFIC TCR TRANSGENIC T CELLS ARE NOT DIABETOGENIC AND CAN DELAY DIABETES TRANSFER

As noted above, the cytokine profiles of these T cells show the production of low levels of IFN-γ, moderate levels of TNF and IL-2, low levels of IL-10, and no production of IL-5 (data not shown). Since the transgenic animals do not develop diabetes, it was felt important to test their ability to suppress the transfer of diabetes by using transgenic T cells mixed with spleen T cells from a recently diabetic wild-type NOD female mouse. A large number of these T cell transfer experiments were carried out and are described in detail in reference 2. None of these transfer experiments showed a diabetogenic effect of the transgenic T cells. In many of these experiments, the addition of transgenic T cells in a ratio of 10 wild-type NOD spleen T cells to 1 TCR transgenic T cell resulted in a delay of the onset of diabetes and a decrease in incidence, which was variable and in some cases quite marked (FIG. 5). Similar results were obtained with transgenic T cells isolated from the GAD65 206–220 TCR transgenic mouse line.

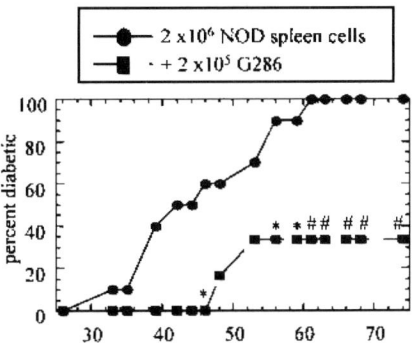

FIGURE 5. Lymphocytes from G286 mice delay transfer of diabetes. Transfer of lymphocytes from recently diabetic NOD females and from G286 mice into NOD.*scid* females: 2×10^6 diabetic spleen cells (*circles*); 2×10^6 diabetic spleen cells plus 2×10^5 peptide activated CD4$^+$ G286 cells (*squares*). Reproduced with permission from ref. 2.

TABLE 1. β islet cell target antigens

T cell target	Modifies T1DM	T cells cause diabetes or insulitis	Transgenic T cells cause diabetes
Insulin	+	+	Not done
GAD65	+	−	This study
HSP60	+	?	Not done
"BDC2.5"	Unknown	+	+
"4.1"	Unknown	+	+
"9.3"	Unknown	+	+

DISCUSSION

Although the finding that GAD65 specific TCR transgenic NOD mice develop T cells that are weakly or partially protective against transfer of type 1 diabetes at first seems anomalous, a review of the literature reveals that, with one exception,[3] most T cell clones, T cell lines, and TCR transgenic T cells specific for GAD65 either fail to cause diabetes or insulitis or in some cases are protective.[4,5] This is in contrast to two T cell receptor transgenics specific for unknown islet cell proteins that are capable of inducing both insulitis and diabetes.[6,7] In addition, T cell clones specific for insulin can also transfer both insulitis and diabetes into newborn or young NOD.*scid* mice.[8] These results are summarized in TABLE 1, which highlights the fact that two transgenic TCRs specific for unknown islet cell proteins readily transfer diabetes, while T cell clones and transgenic T cells specific for GAD65 fail to do so.

A partial and by no means complete list of possible mechanisms explaining the protective phenotype of GAD65 TCR transgenic T cells is presented in TABLE 2. The first postulated mechanism—very low level of expression of GAD65 and GAD67 in

TABLE 2. Mechanisms

(1) Low level expression of GAD65 and GAD67 in mice

(2) Activation of CTLA-4 and/or IL-10

(3) GAD protein in thymic APCs

(4) $CD4^+CD25^+$ T cells

---

mice compared to rats and humans—has been at least partly excluded by recent experiments that are still unpublished. In these experiments, G286 and 206–220 TCR transgenic mice were crossed with two lines expressing increased levels of human GAD65 in the pancreatic islets. Despite documented expression of hGAD65 in the islets in these NOD TCR transgenic mice, there was still no diabetes or insulitis in these mice. The second postulated mechanism—activation of CTLA-4 and/or IL-10—is currently being tested by crossing the 286 and 206 TCR transgenic lines to the NOD.CTLA-4 null allele and to the IL-10 null allele, both on the NOD background. The third possibility, namely that GAD protein may be expressed in thymic APCs, resulting in negative selection of GAD65 specific T cells, has been given considerable support by the recent findings of Kyewski et al.[9] that mRNA for GAD65 and GAD67 is present in thymic medullary epithelial cells, and by the more recent demonstration by Mathis and Benoist[10] that the *AIRE* gene determines expression of a large number of self-proteins, particularly endocrine organ proteins, in medullary epithelial cells in the thymus. While this would explain the negative selection that these T cells appear to undergo as noted above, it does not explain the protective phenotype of those T cells that do survive negative selection in the thymus and in the periphery. A recent publication has put forth evidence that low levels of IFN-γ can actually be anti-inflammatory in several experimental situations[11] and this possibility is currently being pursued.

Finally, the hypothesis that the protective phenotype seen in these transgenic mice is due to the production of $CD4^+CD25^+$ T cells has been partially excluded by the demonstration that the numbers of $CD4^+CD25^+$ T cells in the thymus and spleen in transgenic mice are essentially similar to those seen in wild-type littermates.[2] Further, removal of $CD4^+CD25^+$ T cells from G286 $CD4^+$ spleen T cells did not block their protective effect.[2]

The phenomenon of expression of a second α chain to escape negative selection has been observed in a number of transgenic animal lines (see citations in ref. 2). At the present time, the 286 and 206 TCR transgenic lines are being crossed to NOD mice carrying the CTLA-4 null allele, the IL-10 null allele, and the TGFβ null allele. The first of these crosses will be bred for homozygous CTLA-4 deletion in the presence of the G286 or 206 TCR transgene to determine whether this induces diabetes. (In transgenic mice, the CTLA-4 null phenotype is not fatal in the early weeks of life as it is in mice expressing a wild-type T cell receptor repertoire.) The possibility that IFN-γ is acting in a regulatory manner in these transgenic T cells[11] will be explored by treating TCR transgenic mice with moderate doses of antibody to murine IFN-γ.

If all of these studies fail to develop a pathogenic phenotype, with induction of at least insulitis and/or diabetes, the possibility needs to be entertained that the immune response to GAD65 in NOD mice, and possibly in patients with type 1 diabetes, may be a protective response and may play a role in the long prediabetic phase that is seen in many patients who ultimately develop overt diabetes. This possibility has important implications for the design of antigen-specific immunotherapies. Ideally, if the response to GAD65 is protective, it would be counterproductive to attempt to delete GAD65 specific T cells in these individuals.

ACKNOWLEDGMENTS

This work was supported by NIDDK Grant No. 51667 and JDRF Grant No. 1-2000-162.

REFERENCES

1. CHAO, C.C., H.K. SYTWU, E.L. CHEN et al. 1999. The role of MHC class II molecules in susceptibility to type I diabetes: identification of peptide epitopes and characterization of the T cell repertoire. Proc. Natl. Acad. Sci. USA **96**(16): 9299–9304.
2. TARBELL, K.V., M. LEE, E. RANHEIM et al. 2002. CD4(+) T cells from glutamic acid decarboxylase (GAD)65–specific T cell receptor transgenic mice are not diabetogenic and can delay diabetes transfer. J. Exp. Med. **196**(4): 481–492.
3. ZEKZER, D., F.S. WONG, O. AYALON et al. 1998. GAD-reactive CD4+ Th1 cells induce diabetes in NOD/SCID mice. J. Clin. Invest. **101**(1): 68–73.
4. WEGMANN, D.R., N. SHEHADEH, K.J. LAFFERTY et al. 1993. Establishment of islet-specific T-cell lines and clones from islet isografts placed in spontaneously diabetic NOD mice. J. Autoimmun. **6**(5): 517–527.
5. TISCH, R., B. WANG, M.A. ATKINSON et al. 2001. A glutamic acid decarboxylase 65–specific Th2 cell clone immunoregulates autoimmune diabetes in nonobese diabetic mice. J. Immunol. **166**(11): 6925–6936.
6. KATZ, J.D., B. WANG, K. HASKINS et al. 1993. Following a diabetogenic T cell from genesis through pathogenesis. Cell **74**(6): 1089–1100.
7. SCHMIDT, D., J. VERDAGUER, N. AVERILL & P. SANTAMARIA. 1997. A mechanism for the major histocompatibility complex–linked resistance to autoimmunity. J. Exp. Med. **186**(7): 1059–1075.
8. HASKINS, K. & D. WEGMANN. 1996. Diabetogenic T-cell clones. Diabetes **45**(10): 1299–1305.
9. DERBINSKI, J., A. SCHULTE, B. KYEWSKI & L. KLEIN. 2001. Promiscuous gene expression in medullary thymic epithelial cells mirrors the peripheral self. Nat. Immunol. **2**(11): 1032–1039.
10. ANDERSON, M.S., E.S. VENANZI, L. KLEIN et al. 2002. Projection of an immunological self shadow within the thymus by the AIRE protein. Science **298**(5597): 1395–1401.
11. FLAISHON, L., I. TOPILSKI, D. SHOSEYOV et al. 2002. Anti-inflammatory properties of low levels of IFN-γ. J. Immunol. **168**: 3707–3711.

Detection of CD4+ Autoreactive T Cells in T1D Using HLA Class II Tetramers

HELENA REIJONEN,[a] WILLIAM W. KWOK,[a] AND GERALD T. NEPOM[a,b]

[a]*Benaroya Research Institute at Virginia Mason, Seattle, Washington, USA*
[b]*University of Washington School of Medicine, Seattle, Washington, USA*

ABSTRACT: The use of soluble class II MHC tetramers has enabled the identification of autoantigen-specific T cells in the peripheral blood of type 1 diabetes patients. Our approach takes advantage of the appearance of highly activated T cells expressing a CD25+/CD4^{high+} phenotype induced by immobilized class II MHC monomer containing the GAD65 peptide. Almost all T cells that stain with the specific tetramer reside in this population and, since this activation profile is not present in normal subjects, it may provide a useful tool for analysis of the T cell response in autoimmune diabetes. The utilization of tetramer techniques in the detection of autoreactive T cells is a powerful tool to gain insight into mechanisms of the molecular basis of autoimmunity. The phenotyping of T cells should provide useful markers for progression of immune-mediated β cell reactivity and can be utilized in clinical trials to evaluate the efficacy of the immunomodulatory therapies targeting intervention/prevention of autoimmune diseases.

KEYWORDS: HLA molecules; autoimmune diabetes; T cells; flow cytometry; autoantigens

The antigen-specific T cell–mediated response to autoantigens involves recognition of selected peptide epitopes presented in the context of MHC molecules. A promising method has been developed recently, using multimeric peptide-MHC complexes ("tetramers") to detect and analyze responding CD8+ and CD4+ T cells specific for viral antigens,[1–5] which has been extended to the identification of CD4+ T cells in type 1 diabetes.[6] In this latter study, *in vitro* amplification of autoreactive cells was crucial for detection of tetramer-positive cells since a major problem in detecting and quantitating autoreactive T cells from type 1 diabetes patients is their extremely low precursor frequency in the peripheral blood. This amplification is accompanied by the upregulation of the CD4 and CD25 as activation markers, which can be used to guide the tetramer analysis. Our approach to detect tetramer-responsive peripheral blood mononuclear cells (PBMCs) in newly diagnosed type 1 diabetes patients using tetramers containing an immunodominant peptide derived from a major islet autoantigen, GAD65, is briefly described below.

Address for correspondence: Helena Reijonen, Ph.D., Benaroya Research Institute at Virginia Mason, 1201 Ninth Avenue, Seattle, WA 98101. Voice: 206-223-8813; fax: 206-223-7543.
reijonen@benaroyaresearch.org

Susceptibility to type 1 diabetes is strongly associated with HLA DRB1*0401 and 0404. The construction of the expression vectors for generation of class II tetramers containing the DRA*0101/DRB1*0401-encoded molecule has been described previously.[4] Briefly, a target biotinylation sequence was added to the 3'-end of a DRB1*0401 or DR404 cDNA spliced to a zipper cassette, which was then incorporated into a Cu-inducible *Drosophila* expression vector. Vectors containing DR-A and DR-B constructs were cotransfected into Schneider S-2 cells, and the expressed class II molecules were then purified, concentrated, and biotinylated. Specific peptide was loaded by a detergent-facilitated exchange procedure, and tetramers were formed by incubation with PE-labeled streptavidin.

An immunodominant epitope 555–567 from GAD65 is contained within a naturally processed peptide, identified by using a combination of chromatography and mass spectrometry of peptides bound to surface DR401 of GAD65 transfected cells.[7] We used a modified version of the wild-type 555–567 peptide, NFIRMVIS-NPAAT, with an F → I substitution at position 557. This change has been shown to enhance agonist activity for proliferation and cytokine release from DR4-restricted T cells.[8] This peptide binds well to both DR401 and 404, and it induces activation of T cells specific for GAD65.

FIGURE 1 illustrates the approach used to analyze PBMCs from type 1 diabetes patients and normal controls. PBMCs are resuspended in culture media at a density of 5×10^6/mL and cultured in the presence of 10 µg/mL of GAD65 555–567 (557I). On day 10, the cells are transferred onto microtiter wells coated with DR401 or DR404 monomer that contains the same peptide as used in the primary culture, in the presence of 1 µg/mL anti-CD28 antibody to provide costimulation. At 72 h later, the cells are stained with 10 µg/mL of PE-labeled HLA-DR401 or 404 tetramer, with fluorochrome-labeled anti-CD25 and anti-CD4, and analyzed by flow cytometry.

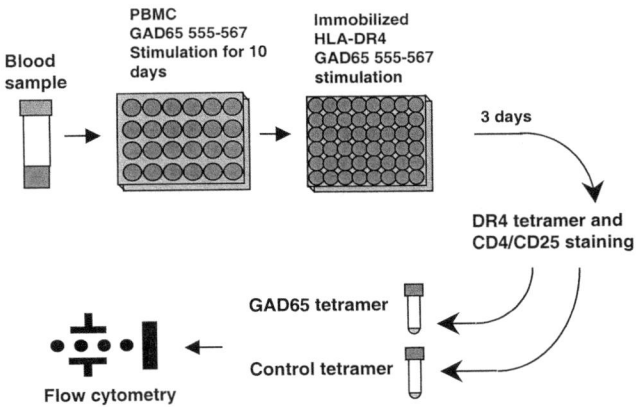

FIGURE 1. Schematic outline of the T1D tetramer assay. *In vitro* amplification of the rare autoreactive CD4+ T cells in peripheral blood is necessary for detection by fluorescence-based flow cytometry.

FIGURE 2 shows an example of cells from a type 1 diabetes patient who displayed a highly activated T cell subset expressing a $CD25^+/CD4^{high+}$ phenotype. This activation phenotype was not present in normal subjects. FIGURE 3 shows an example of tetramer binding analysis of these activated cells using HLA-DR401 GAD65 tetramers to stain cells gated on $CD25^+/CD4^{high+}$ markers. Almost a third of the cells expressing $CD25^+/CD4^{high+}$ phenotype present in a type 1 diabetes patient stained with the specific GAD65 tetramer (FIG. 3A). Binding to HSVp61-control tetramer was 1%. In some subjects, the tetramer staining was lower; for example, in FIGURES 3B and 3C, the tetramer staining was 6.5% and 2.5% of the activated population.

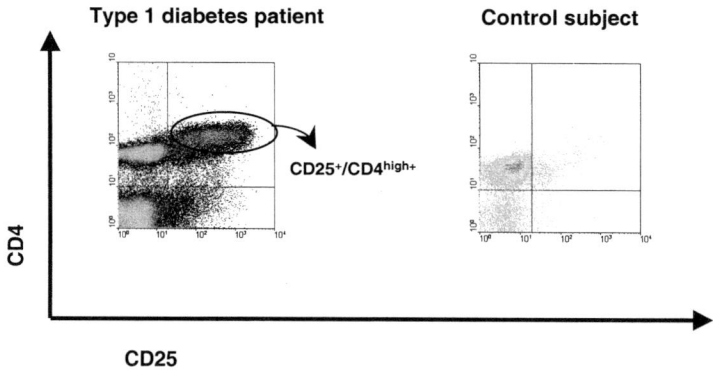

FIGURE 2. GAD65-responsive cells display $CD25^+/CD4^{high+}$ phenotype. Flow cytometry analysis of PBMCs restimulated with a GAD65 557I peptide HLA-DR401 monomer.

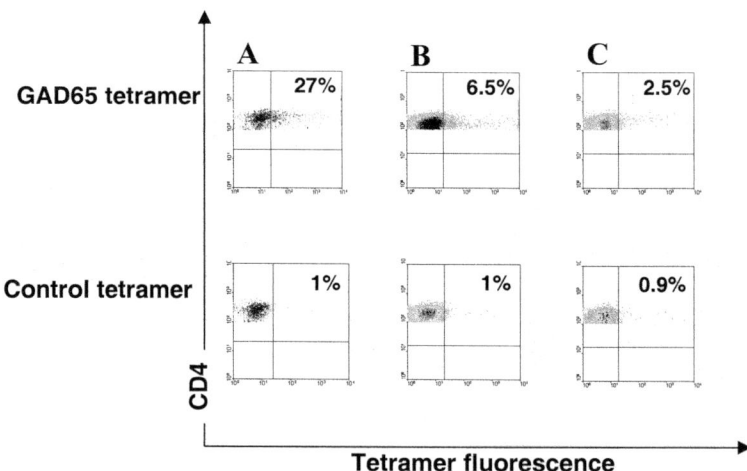

FIGURE 3. Tetramer-binding GAD65-specific cells reside in the $CD25^+/CD4^{high+}$ population. Examples of the detection of tetramer-positive cells by flow cytometry of the $CD25^+/CD4^{high+}$ cell population from type 1 diabetes patients are shown. The percentage of tetramer$^+$/$CD4^{high+}$ cells is shown in the upper right quadrant.

Specificity of the T cell activation profile was examined in a more detailed fashion using single-cell sorting of the activated $CD25^+/CD4^{high+}$ cells. T cell clones were obtained that proliferated in the presence of either the 557I superagonist or the wild-type peptide GAD65 555–567 (FIG. 4). These clones also responded to native GAD65 protein processed and presented by human antigen-presenting cells. In the preliminary study, approximately 40–60% of the HLA-DR4 patients recently diagnosed with type 1 diabetes display this type of T cell response detected by the

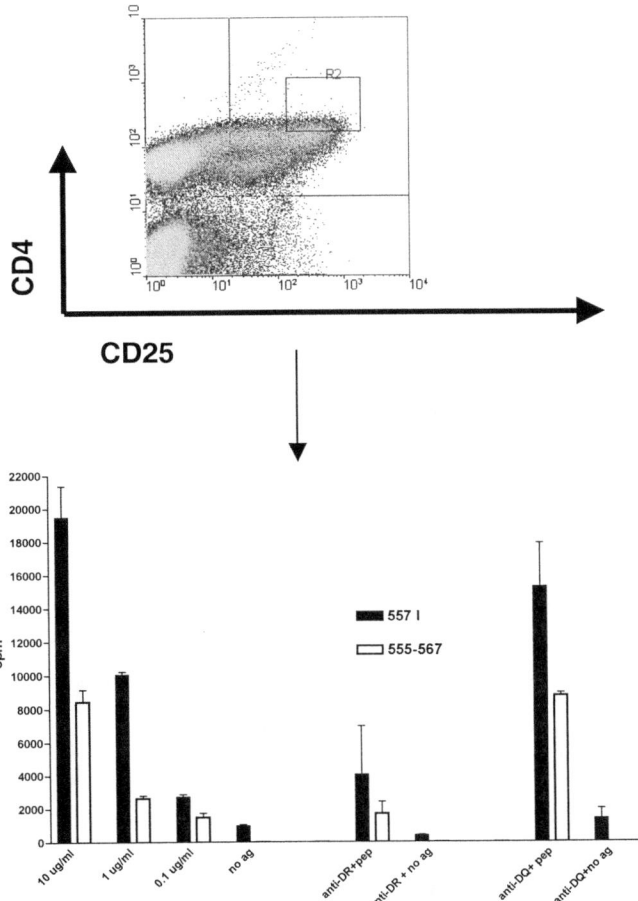

FIGURE 4. Single-cell sorted $CD25^+/CD4^{high+}$ cells are GAD65-specific. PBMCs from the $DR401^+$ T1D patient were stimulated as described above. Single-cell sorting was performed on the top 1% of the $CD25^+/CD4^{high+}$ cell population. The T cell clones (one example shown) were tested for proliferation in the presence of GAD65 557I and 555–567 (wild-type) peptides at concentrations of 0.1–10 µg/mL and in the absence of the peptide antigen. Restriction of T cell clones was confirmed by blocking the proliferation by anti-DR antibody. Error bars represent SE.

HLA-DR4-GAD tetramers. The use of tetramers in the search of autoreactive T cells is based on the presumption that the peptide on the tetramer corresponds to an immunodominant epitope of interest that is prevalent in the disease process. In type 1 diabetes, T responses to several other epitopes occur and it is likely that epitope spreading often occurs during the progression of the disease, including the GAD555–567 epitope. It is still unknown how the natural history of the disease correlates with the appearance of different epitopes and how persistent the T cell reactivity to one particular epitope is, thus making interpretation of negative tetramer staining or a low activation profile challenging. Furthermore, there may be differences in the processing of epitopes between individuals and different APCs.[9,10] All these variables could create differences in the selection of autoreactive T cells and potentially limit the utility of the approach described here.

Our studies indicate that CD4$^+$ T cells that are able to bind GAD tetramers reside in the highly activated antigen-specific cell population characterized by the simultaneous high level of expression of CD25 and CD4.[11,12] Because of the need to amplify these autoreactive cells for detection, however, problems associated with *in vitro* culture may arise, including potential changes in the phenotype of the CD4$^+$ antigen-specific T cells, preferential proliferation of high-affinity T cells, and activation-induced cell death. For these reasons, future improvements in tetramer-based assays will seek to focus on more sensitive detection and characterization of the rare autoreactive cells circulating in peripheral blood.

REFERENCES

1. ALTMAN, J.D., P.A.H. MOSS, P.J.R. GOULDER *et al.* 1996. Phenotypic analysis of antigen-specific T lymphocytes. Science **274:** 94–96.
2. CWYNARSKI, K., J. AINSWORTH, M. COBBOLD *et al.* 2001. Direct visualization of cytomegalovirus-specific T-cell reconstitution after allergenic stem cell transplantation. Blood **97:** 1232–1240.
3. PREZZI, C., M.A. CASCIARO, V. FRANCAVILLA *et al.* 2001. Virus-specific CD8$^+$ T cells with type 1 or type 2 cytokine profile are related to different disease activity in chronic hepatitis C virus infection. Eur. J. Immunol. **31:** 894–906.
4. NOVAK, E.J., A.W. LIU, G.T. NEPOM & W.W. KWOK. 1999. MHC class II tetramers identify peptide-specific human CD4(+) T cells proliferating in response to influenza A antigen. J. Clin. Invest. **104:** R63–R67.
5. KWOK, W.W., A.W. LIU, E.J. NOVAK *et al.* 2000. HLA-DQ tetramers identify epitope-specific T cells in peripheral blood of herpes simplex virus type 2–infected individuals: direct detection of immunodominant antigen-responsive cells. J. Immunol. **164:** 4244–4249.
6. REIJONEN, H., E.J. NOVAK, S. KOCHIK *et al.* 2002. Detection of GAD65-specific T-cells by major histocompatibility complex class II tetramers in type 1 diabetic patients and at-risk subjects. Diabetes **51(5):** 1375–1382.
7. NEPOM, G.T., J.D. LIPPOLIS, F.M. WHITE *et al.* 2001. Identification and modulation of a naturally processed T cell epitope from the diabetes-associated autoantigen human glutamic acid decarboxylase 65 (hGAD65). Proc. Natl. Acad. Sci. USA **98:** 1763–1768.
8. MASEWICZ, S.A., G.K. PAPADOPOULOS, E. SWANSON *et al.* 2002. Modulation of T cell response to hGAD65 peptide epitopes. Tissue Antigens **59:** 101–112.
9. MICHAELSSON, E., M. HOLMDAHL, A. ENGSTROM *et al.* 1995. Macrophages, but not dendritic cells, present collagen to T cells. Eur. J. Immunol. **25:** 2234–2241.
10. REIJONEN, H., J.F. ELLIOTT, P. VAN ENDERT & G. NEPOM. 1999. Differential presentation of glutamic acid decarboxylase (GAD65) T-cell epitopes among HLA-DRB1*0401 positive individuals. J. Immunol. **163:** 1674–1681.

11. RIDGWAY, W., M. FASSO & C.G. FATHMAN. 1998. Following antigen challenge, T cells up-regulate cell surface expression of CD4 *in vitro* and *in vivo*. J. Immunol. **161:** 714–720.
12. NOVAK, E.J., S.A. MASEWICZ, A.W. LIU *et al.* 2001. Activated human epitope-specific T cells identified by class II tetramers reside within a $CD4^{high}$, proliferating subset. Int. Immunol. **13:** 799–806.

Kinetic Evolution of a Diabetogenic CD8+ T Cell Response

PERE SANTAMARIA

Julia McFarlane Diabetes Research Center and Department of Microbiology and Infectious Disease, University of Calgary Faculty of Medicine, Calgary, Alberta, Canada T2N 4N1

ABSTRACT: Nonobese diabetic (NOD) mice develop overt diabetes following prolonged periods of pancreatic islet inflammation involving both CD4+ and CD8+ T cells. The initiation and progression of autoimmune diabetes require the recruitment of beta cell–reactive CD8+ T cells to the pancreatic lymph nodes, their activation by antigen, and their subsequent migration into pancreatic islets. We and others have shown that a significant fraction of NOD islet-associated CD8+ T cells express highly homologous TCRα chains (Vα17 and Jα42 joined by the same N-region sequence) and that they recognize the peptide NRP-A7 in the context of the MHC class I molecule $H-2K^d$. We have also shown that this T cell subpopulation undergoes a process of "avidity maturation" that is associated with progression of benign insulitis to overt diabetes. This paper will summarize our current understanding of the mechanisms that drive the recruitment and activation of this CD8+ T cell subpopulation.

KEYWORDS: antigen-presenting cell (APC); cytotoxic T lymphocyte (CTL); dendritic cell (DC); nonobese diabetic (NOD); major histocompatibility complex (MHC); pancreatic lymph node (PLN); recombination-activating gene (RAG); type 1 diabetes (T1D); T cell receptor (TCR)

ROLE OF CD4+ AND CD8+ T CELLS IN THE INITIATION OF T1D

Type 1 diabetes (T1D) in both humans and NOD mice is the result of a T cell–mediated autoimmune process directed against the pancreatic beta cells. T cell transfer studies have shown that T1D requires both CD4+ and CD8+ T cells.[1–11] Since beta cells do not express MHC class II molecules,[12] it has been proposed that autoreactive CD4+ cells differentiate into effectors by engaging beta cell antigens (shed by a prior insult) on local antigen-presenting cells (APCs).[13,14] Studies of CD8+ T cell–deficient NOD mice[15–18] have suggested that this initial insult is mediated by CD8+ cytotoxic T cells (CTLs), which are consistently present in NOD islets.[14,19–25] This view is compatible with two other findings: that restoring MHC class I expression on beta cells of β2-microglobulin (β2m)–deficient NOD mice restores insulitis susceptibility[26] and that NOD splenocytes cannot transfer insulitis into β2m-

Address for correspondence: Dr. Pere Santamaria, Department of Microbiology and Infectious Diseases, University of Calgary Faculty of Medicine, 3330 Hospital Drive N.W., Calgary, Alberta, Canada T2N 4N1. Voice: 403-220-8735; fax: 403-270-8520.
psantama@ucalgary.ca

deficient NOD.*scid* mice.[27] This hypothesis, however, is in apparent conflict with observations suggesting that T1D is "initiated" by CD4+ T cells. For example, NOD splenic CD4+ T cells can transfer insulitis into NOD.scid mice, but splenic CD8+ T cells cannot.[1,5] Furthermore, susceptibility to insulitis and T1D are profoundly affected by polymorphisms of MHC class II genes,[28,29] which specifically control the development of CD4+ cells. Whatever their role, there is evidence for the involvement of CD8+ T cells in human T1D. Thus, human T1D is associated with certain MHC class I alleles,[30–34] and CD8+ T cells are abundant among the mononuclear cells that infiltrate the pancreas (or pancreas isografts) at disease onset.[35–41]

REPERTOIRE OF DIABETOGENIC CD8+ T CELLS

Little is known about the antigenic repertoire of the CD8+ T cells that are involved in the initiation and/or progression of T1D in NOD mice. Wong *et al.* have reported the existence, in islets of 3- to 4-week-old NOD mice, of a CD8+ subpopulation that recognizes an insulin-derived peptide.[42] This subpopulation wanes with age[42,43] and is replaced, in part, by another subpopulation of diabetogenic CD8+ T cells that use highly homologous TCRα chains (Vα17-Jα42).[24,25,44,45] In fact, the majority of the islet-associated CD8+ T cells of transgenic NOD mice expressing the TCRβ chain of a representative CD8+ clone (NY8.3, which uses this particular TCRα rearrangement) express an endogenously derived TCRα chain that is identical to the one employed by the clonotype donating the TCRβ transgene.[25] In addition, a significant percentage of the CD8+ T cells that can be propagated from the earliest insulitic lesions of NOD mice use TCRα chains that are very similar (or even identical) to those used by 8.3-CD8+ T cells (Vα17 and Jα42 elements joined by the N-region sequence MRD/E).[45]

There is now ample evidence indicating that these and other CD8+ CTL specificities function as major effectors of beta cell lysis in T1D, along with CD4+ T cells. CD8+ CTLs are consistently present in islets of NOD mice,[19,20–23] can transfer diabetes into NOD.*scid* mice,[19,20] and can kill beta cells of T1D-resistant mice *in vivo*.[46] Our study of NOD mice expressing the 8.3-TCRβ transgene provided *in vivo* evidence for a contribution of CD8+ CTLs to beta cell loss in spontaneous T1D: these mice have a minor (but selective) increase in the frequency of beta cell–reactive CD8+ T cells and develop accelerated T1D, owing to an accelerated recruitment of CD8+ T cells.[25] Furthermore, transgenic NOD mice expressing the 8.3-TCRαβ heterodimer develop T1D shortly after the onset of insulitis.[44] Although 8.3-CD8+ CTLs kill beta cells via Fas exclusively,[47] studies of perforin-deficient NOD mice have shown that CD8+ CTL clonotypes recruited to islets later on kill beta cells via perforin.[48]

ROLE OF AUTOREACTIVE CD8+ T CELLS IN THE PROGRESSION OF ISLET INFLAMMATION TO OVERT DIABETES: AVIDITY MATURATION

By screening combinatorial peptide libraries, we originally identified two major peptide ligands for CD8+ T cells expressing the prevalent Vα17-MRD-Jα42 TCRα chain: NRP and NRP-A7.[49] Although clearly not the only antigenic specificity, the NRP/NRP-A7-reactive, Vα17-Jα42+ subset in T1D is large in size[43] and thus allows the study of mechanisms underlying the recruitment of CD8+ T cells in T1D.

NOD mice begin to develop insulitis at 3 weeks, but do not develop T1D until at least 9 weeks later. Since many of the CTL clones derived from islets of diabetic NOD mice express Vα17-MRD/E-Jα42 rearrangements and recognize NRP-A7, we hypothesized that progression of insulitis to diabetes might be driven by the accumulation of NRP/NRP-A7-reactive CTLs in islets. Studies of the fate of the NRP/NRP-A7-reactive T cell subpopulation in wild-type NOD mice using peptide/ MHC tetramers revealed that progression of islet inflammation to overt diabetes in the NOD mouse is driven, at least in part, by the "avidity maturation" of CD8+ T cells, including NRP/NRP-A7-reactive CTLs.[43] As prediabetic NOD mice age, their islet-associated CD8+ T cells contain increasing numbers of NRP-A7-reactive cells, and these cells bind NRP-A7/K^d tetramers with increasing avidity. Repeated treatment of prediabetic NOD mice with soluble NRP-A7 peptide blunted the avidity maturation of the NRP-A7-reactive CD8+ T cell population by deleting those clonotypes expressing TCRs with the highest affinity and lowest dissociation rates for peptide/MHC binding, and by expanding clonotypes expressing low-affinity TCRs. This inhibited the production of CTLs and halted the progression of insulitis to diabetes. These observations led to the conclusion that avidity maturation of pathogenic T cell populations is a key event in the progression of benign inflammation to overt disease in autoimmunity.

To investigate the molecular basis of this "avidity maturation" process, we recently examined the TCR repertoire of pancreatic islet-derived NRP-A7-reactive CD8+ T cells. Pancreatic islet-associated T cells from nondiabetic NOD mice were stained with NRP-A7 tetramer and anti-CD8 mAb, and the NRP-A7 tetramer-positive and tetramer-negative CD8+ cells sorted by flow cytometry. The TCR repertoires of each subpopulation were determined by generating TCRα- and TCRβ-specific cDNA libraries by anchor-PCR, and by sequencing multiple recombinants from each library. As this strategy does not employ TCR-V family-specific primers and as recombinants derived from different cDNAs have unique lengths and characteristic oligodGTP tails, comparison of multiple sequences within libraries provides information about the clonality of the donor cell populations. NRP-A7 tetramer-negative CD8+ T cells expressed highly heterogeneous TCRα and TCRβ sequences. In contrast, 96 of 121 different TCRα cDNAs from NRP-A7 tetramer-positive CD8+ T cells used Vα17 elements rearranged to a Jα42 element via an identical complementarity determining region-3 (CDR3). This T cell population was also polyclonal, however, as it expressed a heterogeneous TCRβ repertoire. As T cells can express TCRα rearrangements from both *tcra* loci, these results indicated that virtually all NRP-A7 tetramer-binding CD8+ T cells expressed the same TCRα chains, but diverse TCRβ rearrangements.

To determine the molecular basis of this T cell avidity maturation process, we subsequently sequenced TCRα and TCRβ rearrangements expressed by NRP-A7-reactive CD8+ cells from 9- and 20-week-old NOD mice (binding tetramer with low and high avidity, respectively[43]). Islet-associated T cells were sorted by flow cytometry into tetramer-positive and tetramer-negative CD8+ T cells. The TCRα and TCRβ repertoires of each population were determined by sequencing recombinants from TCR-specific cDNA libraries generated by anchor-PCR. Most TCRα

cDNAs from NRP-A7+ CD8+ cells of 9- and 20-week-old mice used Vα17 and Jα42 elements joined by the MRD CDR3 sequence. The tetramer-negative cells from both age groups expressed heterogeneous TCRα rearrangements, and both the tetramer-positive and -negative cells from 9- and 20-week-old NOD mice used heterogeneous TCRβ rearrangements. Detailed analyses of the Vα17 and Vβ elements used by cells from 9- and 20-week-old NOD mice suggested that the avidity maturation of the NRP-A7-reactive population was associated with changes in Vα and/or Vβ gene usage. Interestingly, the CD8+ T cells isolated from 9-week-old mice use the three different Vα17 elements expressed by the NOD mouse (unpublished data). In contrast, the CD8+ T cells isolated from 20-week-old mice only use two of these elements, owing to a substantial increase in the usage of one of these elements at the expense of another, compatible with clonal competition for stimuli. Experiments with TCR transfectants confirmed that 8.3-like TCRs employing the Vα17 element predominantly expressed by islet-associated CD8+ T cells in 20-week-old NOD mice recognize peptide/MHC with significantly higher avidity than those employing the Vα17 element predominantly expressed by cells derived from 9-week-old NOD mice (unpublished data).

CHANGES IN THE FINE SPECIFICITY OF THE NRP-REACTIVE CD8+ T CELL POPULATION WITH DISEASE PROGRESSION

With the goal of ascertaining the degree of antigenic promiscuity of NRP-reactive TCRs, we set out to determine which amino acid substitutions could be introduced at each position of NRP without inducing a major loss of functional activity (as defined using 8.3-CD8+ T cells). We then searched on-line protein databases using a supertope that included all the tolerated residues. This analysis resulted in the identification of 92 potential mimics of NRP.[50] Thirty-eight of these peptides were able to restore expression of H-2K^d molecules on RMA-SK^d cells, and 24 were able to elicit the cytokine secretion, proliferation, and/or cytotoxicity of 8.3-CD8+ T cells.[50]

We next tested the ability of 18 of these mimics to elicit the IFN-γ secretion by islet-derived CD8+ T cells from 9- and 20-week-old NOD mice (low and high avidity, respectively). Interestingly, cells from 20-week-old mice recognized more NRP mimics than cells from 9-week-old mice, suggesting that "high avidity" T cells can respond to a greater number of mimics of the target peptide than "low avidity" T cells. Studies on nonautoreactive TCRs have suggested that the TCR's antigen-binding site is flexible, that the low affinity and slow kinetics of TCR-peptide/MHC-binding are a consequence of this flexibility, and that this flexibility accounts for the cross-reactivity of TCRs for different peptide/MHC complexes.[51–53] It will thus be interesting to determine whether the increased peptide promiscuity of TCRs on "high" versus "low avidity" NRP-A7-reactive CD8+ T cells is associated with increased flexibility of the peptide/MHC-binding site, as determined by thermodynamic measurements. If true, this would be in contrast to what has been described in antibody responses, where increases in affinity are associated with reductions in both the conformational flexibility of antibodies and their antigenic promiscuity.[54]

DETECTION OF NRP-REACTIVE CD8+ T CELLS IN PERIPHERAL BLOOD WITH HIGH-AFFINITY TETRAMERS CAN BE USED TO PREDICT THE ONSET OF DIABETES IN NOD MICE

The above studies resulted in the identification of a particular mimic of NRP (NRP-V7) that is a much more powerful agonist of 8.3-CD8+ T cells than NRP-A7. 8.3-CD8+ T cells bind NRP-V7/K^d tetramers with significantly higher avidity than NRP or NRP-A7/K^d tetramers. Importantly, recent studies of peripheral and islet-associated CD8+ T cells in wild-type NOD mice using the NRP-V7 tetramer have shown that ~18% of all CD8+ T cells contained in freshly isolated islets (without prior *in vitro* culture) are 8.3-like.[55] Most importantly, this tetramer allows the detection of 8.3-like CD8+ T cells in the circulation (~0.5–1% of circulating CD8+ T cells). Interestingly, enumeration of changes in the size of the circulating 8.3-like CD8+ T cell pool can predict, with high degrees of specificity and sensitivity, which mice within the NOD colony will progress to overt disease and which ones will remain diabetes-free. This is an important observation because it suggests that enumeration of CD8+ T cell responses against dominant beta cell autoantigens in humans might one day allow the "quantitation" of diabetes risk in genetically predisposed individuals.

MECHANISMS DRIVING THE RECRUITMENT AND ACTIVATION OF NRP-REACTIVE CD8+ T CELLS

Role of CD154 in the Priming of 8.3-CD8+ T Cells

Although CD4+ T cells are not an absolute requirement for the development of 8.3-CD8+ T cell–induced diabetes, naïve 8.3-CD8+ T cells require CD4+ T cell help to reach their maximum pathogenic potential.[44] Productive collaboration between CD4+ T helper cells and precytotoxic CD8+ T cells requires the presentation of different epitopes by the same APCs, usually a dendritic cell (DC), in a CD40/CD154-dependent manner.[56–63] CD40 ligation on APCs induces the upregulation of T cell costimulatory molecules, elicits the production of proinflammatory cytokines, and endows APCs with the ability to differentiate CD8+ T cells.

To determine whether diabetogenic CD8+ T cells need to express CD154 to undergo activation in the pancreatic lymph nodes (PLNs), we compared the ability of CD154$^+$ and CD154$^{-/-}$, carboxyfluorescein diacetate succinidimyl ester (CFSE)– labeled 8.3-CD8+ T cells to proliferate in the lymphoid organs of nondiabetic NOD hosts. CD154$^+$ 8.3-CD8+ T cells and CD154$^{-/-}$ 8.3-CD8+ T cells underwent several rounds of cell division exclusively in the PLNs, confirming that 8.3-CD8+ T cells need not express CD154 to undergo antigen-driven activation in the PLNs. To confirm that 8.3-CD8+ T cells do not require CD154 to differentiate into CTLs *in vivo*, we compared the fate of 8.3-CD8+ cells in CD154$^+$ versus CD154$^{-/-}$ 8.3-TCR-transgenic NOD.RAG-2$^{-/-}$ mice. 8.3-NOD.RAG-2$^{-/-}$ and 8.3-NOD.RAG-2$^{-/-}$/CD154$^{-/-}$ mice developed diabetes with the same incidence and kinetics as 8.3-NOD.RAG-2$^{-/-}$/CD154$^+$ mice.[64] Thus, NRP-reactive CD8+ T cells do not require CD154 on their own surface to undergo activation *in vivo*.

The CD4+ T Cell–Assisted Diabetogenic Activity of 8.3-CD8+ T Cells Is CD154-Dependent, but Can Be Bypassed by Transfer of Antigen-Pulsed DCs

To investigate whether the T helper–dependent diabetogenic potential of CD8+ CTLs requires the engagement of CD40 on APCs by CD154 on CD4+ T cells, we transfused CD4+ NOD splenocytes into NOD.RAG-2$^{-/-}$/CD154$^+$ and 8.3-NOD.RAG-2$^{-/-}$/CD154$^{-/-}$ mice. CD4+ splenocytes did not induce insulitis in NOD.RAG-2$^{-/-}$/CD154$^+$ mice, but increased the incidence of T1D in 8.3-NOD.RAG-2$^{-/-}$/CD154$^{+/-}$ mice.[64] This effect was CD154-dependent as it did not occur in 8.3-NOD.RAG-2$^{-/-}$/CD154$^{-/-}$ hosts transfused with CD4+ T cells from NOD.CD154$^{-/-}$ donors.[64] These results therefore suggest that the T helper–assisted activation of NRP-reactive CD8+ T cells *in vivo* is mediated via DCs.

DC Activation in the Priming of 8.3-CD8+ T Cells

To determine whether ligation of CD40 on APCs could in fact enhance the diabetogenic activity of CD154$^{-/-}$ 8.3-CD8+ T cells, we treated 8.3-NOD.RAG-2$^{-/-}$/CD154$^{-/-}$ mice with the agonistic anti-CD40 mAb FGK45. FGK45 treatment significantly increased the incidence of T1D in 8.3-NOD.RAG-2$^{-/-}$/CD154$^{-/-}$ mice versus untreated or anti-B220 mAb–treated controls.[64] CpG oligodeoxynucleotides bind to the Toll-Like Receptor 9 on DCs, B cells, and macrophages, inducing their activation.[65] To determine whether systemic activation of DCs and/or macrophages with CpG DNA could uncouple 8.3-CD8+ T cell activation from CD4+ help, we compared the effects of CpG and non-CpG DNA on the history of T1D in 8.3-NOD.RAG-2$^{-/-}$/CD154$^{-/-}$ mice. Unlike non-CpG DNA, CpG DNA clearly enhanced the diabetogenic potential of CD154$^{-/-}$ 8.3-CD8+ T cells.[64]

Spontaneous Priming of 8.3-CD8+ T Cells in the PLNs Occurs Shortly after a Neonatal Wave of Beta Cell Apoptosis and Increases with the Extent of Beta Cell Apoptosis

Experiments with CFSE-labeled 8.3-CD8+ T cells have shown that priming of naïve 8.3-CD8+ T cells in the PLNs is undetectable before 3 weeks and that it progressively increases with age.[66] An increased incidence of beta cell apoptosis following the administration of low doses of the β cell toxin streptozotocin (STZ) augmented 8.3-CD8+ T cell priming and allowed it to occur at 2 weeks of age, when it is not observed to occur spontaneously. These results strongly implicate *in situ* beta cell-cell death in the facilitation of autoantigen-specific CD8+ T cell priming in T1D. Interestingly, the timing of 8.3-CD8+ T cell priming in NOD mice is preceded by a period of remodeling and physiologic apoptosis of the pancreatic islets that peaks at 2 weeks of age.[67] Regardless of whether this wave of apoptosis is a key event in T1D, these results demonstrate that *in situ* beta cell-cell death induced by CTLs can perpetuate the priming of their naïve precursors in the PLNs.

Constitutive Expression of Transgenic B7.1 Molecules in Beta Cells Promotes the Accumulation of 8.3-CD8+ T Cells in Islets, Even in Mice That Do Not Normally Develop Insulitis

The above studies deal with events taking place away from islets. It has been proposed that CD8+ CTLs effect some of the earliest beta cell insults in T1D. However, this hypothesis is at odds with the idea that CD8+ T cells must be primed in the PLNs prior to entering islets, presumably by antigens derived from beta cells that have apoptosed in response to other events. Alternatively, these T cells circulate through islets without the need to engage antigen in the PLNs. We have shown that most of the 8.3-NOD.RAG-$2^{-/-}$ mice that do not develop diabetes are also insulitis-free[44] and that 8.3-NOD.RAG-2^{+}/CD154$^{-/-}$ mice develop neither diabetes nor insulitis.[64] To ascertain whether naïve T cells patrol islet tissue in the absence of histologically detectable islet inflammation, we tested the ability of costimulatory B7.1 molecules on beta cells to promote the accumulation of 8.3-CD8+ T cells in insulitis-resistant mice. Whereas non-TCR-transgenic RIP-B7.1-NOD.RAG-$2^{-/-}$/CD154$^{-/-}$ mice did not develop diabetes, expression of RIP-B7.1 molecules on beta cells of both 8.3-NOD.RAG-$2^{-/-}$/CD154^{+} and 8.3-NOD.RAG-2^{+}/CD154$^{-/-}$ mice triggered insulitis and diabetes in 100% of the mice.[64] Thus, naïve 8.3-like CD8+ T cells may normally patrol islets in the absence of insulitis.

SUMMARY

In summary, this paper provides an overview of our current understanding of the mechanisms that govern the kinetic evolution of a prevalent CD8+ T cell response in murine spontaneous autoimmune diabetes. We have shown that this T cell response initiates well before the onset of pathological (insulitis) and clinical signs (hyperglycemia) of diabetes and can be used to predict diabetes development. We have also shown that this T cell response initially involves clonotypes that recognize target peptide/MHC complexes with low avidity, and that it undergoes a process of avidity maturation characterized by interclonal competition for stimulatory resources. This initial activation of low/intermediate-avidity clonotypes requires a collaboration with DCs and CD4+ T cells in a CD40-CD154-dependent manner. Elucidation of the molecular nature of the self-antigen that drives this T cell response[68] will certainly open new avenues of inquiry into how spontaneous autoimmune responses are initiated and evolve. Ultimately, we hope that the new paradigms brought forth by this research will help us and others unravel the enormous complexity of spontaneous, organ-specific autoimmunity.

ACKNOWLEDGMENTS

I thank all the past and present members of my laboratory for their many contributions to the evolution of this work. I also thank Connie Courts for excellent editorial and secretarial assistance. The work was funded by grants from the Canadian Institutes of Health Research, the Natural Sciences and Engineering Research Council of Canada, the Juvenile Diabetes Research Foundation, the Canadian Diabetes

Association, and the Alberta Heritage Foundation for Medical Research (AHFMR). The author is a Senior Scholar of the AHFMR.

REFERENCES

1. CHRISTIANSON, S., L. SHULTZ & E. LEITER. 1993. Adoptive transfer of diabetes into immunodeficient NOD-scid/scid mice: relative contributions of CD4+ and CD8+ T-cells from diabetic versus prediabetic NOD.NON-thy-1a donors. Diabetes **42:** 44.
2. BENDELAC, A. et al. 1987. Syngeneic transfer of autoimmune diabetes from diabetic NOD mice to healthy neonates. J. Exp. Med. **166:** 823.
3. MILLER, B.J. et al. 1988. Both the Lyt-2+ and L3T4+ T cell subsets are required for the transfer of diabetes in non-obese diabetic mice. J. Immunol. **140:** 52.
4. YAGI, H. et al. 1992. Analysis of the roles of CD4+ and CD8+ T cells in autoimmune diabetes of NOD mice using transfer to NOD athymic nude mice. Eur. J. Immunol. **22:** 2387.
5. THIVOLET, C. et al. 1991. CD8+ T cell homing to the pancreas in the nonobese diabetic mouse is CD4+ T cell–dependent. J. Immunol. **146:** 85.
6. HASKINS, K. & M. MCDUFFIE. 1990. Acceleration of diabetes in young NOD mice with a CD4+ islet-specific T cell clone. Science **249:** 1433.
7. NAKANO, N. et al. 1991. T cell receptor V gene usage of islet beta cell-reactive T cells is not restricted in non-obese diabetic mice. J. Exp. Med. **173:** 1091.
8. BRADLEY, B. et al. 1992. CD8 T cells are not required for islet destruction induced by a CD4+ islet-specific T-cell clone. Diabetes **41:** 1603.
9. DANIEL, D. et al. 1995. Epitope specificity, cytokine production profile, and diabetogenic activity of insulin-specific T cell clones isolated from NOD mice. Eur. J. Immunol. **25:** 1056.
10. KATZ, J., C. BENOIST & D. MATHIS. 1995. T helper cell subsets in insulin-dependent diabetes. Science **268:** 1185.
11. PETERSON, J. & K. HASKINS. 1996. Transfer of diabetes in the NOD-scid mouse by CD4 T cell clones: differential requirement for CD8 T cells. Diabetes **45:** 328.
12. MCINERNEY, M., S. RATH & C. JANEWAY. 1991. Exclusive expression of MHC class II proteins on CD45+ cells in pancreatic islets of NOD mice. Diabetes **40:** 648.
13. SERREZE, D. & E. LEITER. 1994. Genetic and pathogenic basis of autoimmune diabetes in NOD mice. Curr. Opin. Immunol. **6:** 900.
14. WONG, F. et al. 1996. CD8 T cell clones from young NOD islets can transfer rapid onset of diabetes in NOD mice in the absence of CD4 T cells. J. Exp. Med. **183:** 67.
15. KATZ, J., C. BENOIST & D. MATHIS. 1993. Major histocompatibility complex class I molecules are required for the generation of insulitis in non-obese diabetic mice. Eur. J. Immunol. **23:** 3358.
16. WICKER, L. et al. 1994. β2-microglobulin-deficient NOD mice do not develop insulitis or diabetes. Diabetes **43:** 500.
17. SERREZE, D. et al. 1994. Major histocompatibility complex class I–deficient NOD.b1m^{null} mice are diabetes and insulitis resistant. Diabetes **43:** 505.
18. WANG, B. et al. 1996. The role of CD8+ T-cells in initiation of insulin-dependent diabetes mellitus. Eur. J. Immunol. **26:** 1762.
19. GRASER, R.T. et al. 2000. Identification of a CD8 T cell that can independently mediate autoimmune diabetes development in the complete absence of CD4 T cell helper functions. J. Immunol. **164:** 3913.
20. NAGATA, M. et al. 1994. Evidence for the role of CD8+ cytotoxic T cells in the destruction of pancreatic beta cells in NOD mice. J. Immunol. **152:** 2042.
21. HAYAKAWA, M. et al. 1991. Morphological analysis of selective destruction of pancreatic beta cells by cytotoxic T lymphocytes in NOD mice. Diabetes **40:** 1210.
22. NAGATA, M. & J-W. YOON. 1992. Studies on autoimmunity for T cell–mediated beta cell destruction: distinct difference in the destruction of beta cells between CD4+ and CD8+ T cell clones derived from lymphocytes infiltrating the islets of NOD mice. Diabetes **41:** 998.

23. SHIMIZU, J., O. KANAGAWA & E. UNANUE. 1993. Presentation of beta cell antigens to CD4+ and CD8+ T cells of non-obese diabetic mice. J. Immunol. **151:** 1723.
24. SANTAMARIA, P. *et al.* 1995. Beta cell cytotoxic CD8+ T cells from non-obese diabetic mice use highly homologous T cell receptor alpha chain CDR3 sequences. J. Immunol. **154:** 2494.
25. VERDAGUER, J. *et al.* 1996. Acceleration of spontaneous diabetes in TCRβ-transgenic nonobese diabetic mice by beta cell–cytotoxic CD8+ T cells expressing identical endogenous TCRα chains. J. Immunol. **157:** 4726.
26. KAY, T. *et al.* 1996. RIP-β2-microglobulin transgene expression restores insulitis, but not diabetes, in β2-microglobulin^{null} nonobese diabetic mice. J. Immunol. **157:** 3688.
27. SERREZE, D. *et al.* 1997. Initiation of autoimmune diabetes in NOD/Lt mice is MHC class I–dependent. J. Immunol. **157:** 3978.
28. TISCH, R. & H. MCDEVITT. 1996. Insulin-dependent diabetes mellitus. Cell **85:** 291.
29. VYSE, T. & J. TODD. 1996. Genetic analysis of autoimmune disease. Cell **85:** 311.
30. FENNESSY, M. *et al.* 1994. A gene in the HLA class I region contributes to susceptibility to IDDM in the Finnish population: Childhood Diabetes in Finland (DiMe) Study Group. Diabetologia **37:** 937–944.
31. HONEYMAN, M. *et al.* 1995. Analysis of families at risk for insulin-dependent diabetes mellitus reveals that HLA antigens influence progression to clinical disease. Mol. Med. **1:** 576–582.
32. TAIT, B. *et al.* 1995. HLA antigens and age at diagnosis of insulin-dependent diabetes mellitus. Hum. Immunol. **42:** 116–122.
33. NEJENTSEV, S. *et al.* 1997. The effect of HLA-B allele on the IDDM risk defined by DRB1*04 subtypes and DQB1*0302. Diabetes **46:** 1888–1892.
34. NAKANISHI, K. *et al.* 1999. HLA-A24 and -DQA1*0301 in Japanese insulin-dependent diabetes mellitus: independent contributions to susceptibility to the disease and additive contributions to acceleration of beta cell destruction. J. Clin. Endocrinol. Metab. **84:** 3721–3725.
35. BOTTAZZO, G.F. *et al.* 1985. *In situ* characterization of autoimmune phenomenon: an expression of HLA molecules in the pancreas of diabetic insulinitis. N. Engl. J. Med. **313:** 353–360.
36. HANNINEN, A. *et al.* 1992. Macrophages, T cell receptor usage, and endothelial cell activation in the pancreas at the onset of insulin-dependent diabetes mellitus. J. Clin. Invest. **90:** 1901.
37. ITOH, N. *et al.* 1993. Mononuclear cell infiltration and its relation to the expression of major histocompatibility complex antigens and adhesion molecules in pancreas biopsy specimens from newly diagnosed insulin-dependent diabetes mellitus patients. J. Clin. Invest. **153:** 1360–1377.
38. SOMOZA, N. *et al.* 1994. Pancreas in recent onset insulin-dependent diabetes mellitus. J. Immunol. **153:** 1360–1377.
39. SIBLEY, R.K. *et al.* 1985. Recurrent diabetes mellitus in the pancreas iso- and allograft. Lab. Invest. **53:** 132–144.
40. SANTAMARIA, P. *et al.* 1992. CD8+ T cells from isletitis of graft-recurrent type I diabetes are oligoclonal and show restricted TcR usage. Diabetes **41**(suppl. 1): 97A.
41. SANTAMARIA, P. *et al.* 1992. Isolation and characterization of T lymphocytes infiltrating a human pancreas allograft affected by isletitis and recurrent diabetes. Diabetes **41:** 53–61.
42. WONG, F. *et al.* 1999. Identification of an MHC class I–restricted autoantigen in type 1 diabetes by screening an organ-specific cDNA library. Nat. Med. **9:** 1026–1031.
43. AMRANI, A. *et al.* 2000. Progression of autoimmune diabetes driven by avidity maturation of a T-cell population. Nature **406:** 739–742.
44. VERDAGUER, J. *et al.* 1997. Spontaneous autoimmune diabetes in monoclonal T cell nonobese diabetic mice. J. Exp. Med. **186:** 1663–1676.
45. DILORENZO, T. *et al.* 1998. Major histocompatibility complex class I–restricted T cells are required for all but the end stages of diabetes development in nonobese diabetic mice and use prevalent T cell receptor α chain gene rearrangement. Proc. Natl. Acad. Sci. USA **95:** 12538–12543.

46. UTSUGI, T. *et al.* 1996. MHC class I–restricted infiltration and destruction of pancreatic islets by NOD mouse–derived beta cell–cytotoxic CD8+ T-cell clones *in vivo*. Diabetes **45:** 1121.
47. AMRANI, A. *et al.* 1999. Perforin-independent beta cell destruction by diabetogenic CD8+ T lymphocytes in transgenic nonobese diabetic mice. J. Clin. Invest. **103:** 1201.
48. KAGI, D. *et al.* 1997. Reduced incidence and delayed onset of diabetes in perforin-deficient nonobese diabetic mice. J. Exp. Med. **186:** 989.
49. ANDERSON, B. *et al.* 1999. Dominant CD8+ T-cell response against a single peptide/MHC complex in autoimmune diabetes. Proc. Natl. Acad. Sci. USA **96:** 9311.
50. AMRANI, A. *et al.* 2001. Expansion of the antigenic repertoire of a single T cell receptor upon T-cell activation. J. Immunol. **167:** 655.
51. WILLCOX, B.E. & G.F. GAO. 1999. T cell receptor binding to peptide-MHC stabilizes a flexible recognition interface. Immunity **10:** 357.
52. GARBOCZI, D. *et al.* 1996. Structure of the complex between human T-cell receptor, viral peptide, and HLA-A2. Nature **384:** 134.
53. GARCIA, K. *et al.* 1998. Structural basis of plasticity in T cell receptor recognition of a self peptide-MHC antigen. Science **279:** 1166.
54. WEDEMAYER, G. *et al.* 1997. Structural insights into the evolution of an antibody combining site. Science **276:** 1665.
55. TRUDEAU, J.D. *et al.* 2002. Autoreactive T cells in peripheral blood predict development of type 1 diabetes. J. Clin. Invest. In press.
56. STUHLER, G. & P. WALDEN. 1993. Collaboration of helper and cytotoxic T lymphocytes. Eur. J. Immunol. **23:** 2279.
57. GREWAL, I., J. XU & R. FLAVELL. 1995. Impairment of antigen-specific T-cell priming in mice lacking CD40 ligand. Nature **378:** 617.
58. ESSEN, D.V., H. KIKUTANI & D. GRAY. 1995. CD40 ligand–transduced co-stimulation of T-cells in the development of helper function. Nature **378:** 620.
59. YANG, Y. & J. WILSON. 1996. CD40 ligand–dependent T-cell activation: requirement of B7-CD28 signalling through CD40. Science **273:** 1862.
60. GREWAL, I., F.D. ROSA & P. MATZINGER. 1996. Requirement for CD40 ligand in costimulation induction, T-cell activation, and experimental allergic encephalomyelitis. Science **273:** 1864.
61. RIDGE, J., F.D. ROSA & P. MATZINGER. 1998. A conditioned dendritic cell can be a temporal bridge between a CD4+ T-helper and a T-killer cell. Nature **393:** 474.
62. BENNETT, S. *et al.* 1998. Help for cytotoxic T-cell responses is mediated by CD40 signalling. Nature **393:** 478.
63. SCHOENBERGER, S. *et al.* 1998. T-cell help for cytotoxic T lymphocytes is mediated by CD40-CD40L interactions. Nature **393:** 480.
64. AMRANI, A. *et al.* 2002. CD154-dependent activation of diabetogenic CD4[+] T-cells dissociated from APC activation. Immunity **16:** 719.
65. HEMMI, H. *et al.* 2000. A Toll-like receptor recognizes bacterial DNA. Nature **408:** 740.
66. ZHANG, Y. *et al.* 2002. *In situ* beta cell death promotes the priming of diabetogenic cytotoxic T-lymphocytes. J. Immunol. **168:** 1466.
67. TRUDEAU, J.D. *et al.* 2000. Neonatal beta-cell apoptosis: a trigger for autoimmune diabetes? Diabetes **49:** 1–7.
68. LIEBERMAN, S. *et al.* 2003. Identification of the beta cell autoantigen targeted by a prevalent population of CD8[+] T cells in autoimmune diabetes. Proc. Natl. Acad. Sci. USA **100:** 8384–8388.

Multiple and High-Titer Single Autoantibodies in Schoolchildren Reflecting the Genetic Predisposition for Type 1 Diabetes

MICHAEL SCHLOSSER,[a] RALF WASSMUTH,[b] MARTINA STREBELOW,[c] ILONA RJASANOWSKI,[d] AND MANFRED ZIEGLER[e]

[a]*Institute of Pathophysiology, Ernst Moritz Arndt University of Greifswald, Greifswald, Germany*

[b]*Institute for Clinical Immunology, Friedrich Alexander University of Erlangen-Nürnberg, Erlangen-Nürnberg, Germany*

[c]*Laboratory of Autoimmune Diagnostic-GmbH, Hennigsdorf, Branch Karlsburg, Germany*

[d]*Center of Diabetes and Metabolic Disorders, Karlsburg, Germany*

[e]*Institute of Diabetes e.V., Karlsburg, Germany*

ABSTRACT: The study aimed to compare the HLA specificities of AAb-positive healthy schoolchildren with those of patients with type 1 diabetes (T1D). HLA-DRB1 and DQB1 alleles were determined in 178 AAb-positive and 339 AAb-negative schoolchildren aged 6–17 years without first-degree relatives with T1D and in 274 patients with T1D. AAbs against glutamic acid decarboxylase (GADA), protein tyrosine phosphatase (IA-2A), and insulin (IAA) were determined by ^{125}I-antigen binding, and islet cell cytoplasmic antibodies (ICAs) immunohistochemically. Here, 82.6% (147/178) of AAb-positive schoolchildren had single AAbs and 17.4% (31/178) had multiple AAbs. In both groups, GADA occurred with highest and IAA with lowest frequency. In children with single AAbs at levels between the 99th and 99.9th percentile, frequencies of the diabetes-associated DRB1 (*03, *04) and DQB1 (*02, *0302) alleles and the protective DRB1 (*15) and DQB1 (*0602) alleles did not differ from those of controls. In patients, the positive associations were confirmed for DRB1*04 (OR = 5.39) and DQB1*0302 (OR = 9.05), whereas DRB1*15 (OR = 0.05) and DQB1*0602 (OR = 0.06) were negative-associated ($p < 0.001$). The same association was found in schoolchildren with multiple AAbs for DRB1*04 (OR = 3.84), DQB1*0302 (OR = 4.95), and DRB1*15 (OR = 0.1; $p < 0.001$–0.014), and with high-titer single AAbs (≥99.9th percentile), but none of them had DQB1*0602. The highest risk genotype DQB1*02/*0302 occurred in 36.5% of patients (OR = 21.07) and in 19.3% of children with multiple AAbs (OR = 8.8; $p < 0.001$). It is concluded that probands with multiple and high-titer single AAbs in the general population have the same genetic predisposition for T1D as patients and are therefore at highest risk for the disease.

Address for correspondence: Dr. Michael Schlosser, Institute of Pathophysiology, Ernst Moritz Arndt University of Greifswald, Greifswald, Germany. Voice: +49-3834-8619178; fax: +49-3834-8680118.
schlosse@uni-greifswald.de

KEYWORDS: type 1 diabetes risk; autoantibodies; HLA marker; screening; general population

INTRODUCTION

In type 1 diabetes (T1D), insulin deficiency occurs as the end point of an autoimmune-mediated specific destruction of insulin-producing islet beta cells in genetically predisposed subjects.[1] There has been a rapid increase in the incidence of T1D in many countries, however, with a wide range of incidence rates as shown within Europe.[2] T1D is most often associated with autoantibodies (AAbs) against beta cell antigens[3] as glutamic acid decarboxylase (GADA), protein tyrosine phosphatase (IA-2A), and insulin (IAA), as well as with the heterogeneous islet cell cytoplasmic antibodies (ICAs), including GADA, IA-2A, and others.[1] They are at present the most useful markers of beta cell destruction and precede the onset of the disease up to 10 years prior.[4]

At onset of T1D, more than 95% of patients have one or more beta cell AAbs.[5,6] Therefore, AAbs are highly predictive diagnostic markers for developing the disease in first-degree relatives of diabetic patients[5,7] and obviously also within the normal population, which actually makes up to 90% of patients with T1D.[6,8–10]

Although the complex association and linkage of HLA class II antigens with T1D are not yet fully understood, HLA-DRB1 and -DQA1/-DQB1 alleles provide for approximately 50% of the genetic risk in T1D,[11] but they are of low-positive predictive value when used alone in the general population.[12] In Caucasians, DQB1*0302 and DQB1*02 and their linked DR specificities DR4 and DR3 provide disease susceptibility, particularly in heterozygous combination,[13] whereas dominant protection is conveyed by DQB1*0602, linked to DRB1*15.[14] The relationship between HLA markers and the occurrence of AAbs has been previously examined in recent-onset patients as well as in siblings of patients with T1D, indicating positive correlations between the occurrence of diabetes-associated AAbs and high-risk HLA markers.[15] It remains, however, to be shown whether these findings from patients and their AAb-positive relatives can be correlated to AAb-positive individuals lacking a family history of T1D coming from the general population.

The purpose of this study was to compare the HLA-DRB1 and DQB1 specificities of AAb-positive and -negative healthy schoolchildren from the Karlsburg Type 1 Diabetes Risk Study of a Normal Schoolchild Population[6,10] with those of patients with T1D.

MATERIALS AND METHODS

Study Cohorts

AAb-positive and AAb-negative probands were recruited from the Karlsburg Type 1 Diabetes Risk Study of a Normal Schoolchild Population, previously published in detail.[6,10] In reexamination after primary screening,[6] 178 (98 f/80 m) probands, representing a general population of 6337 healthy schoolchildren without diabetes heredity, were found to be AAb-positive for GADA, IA-2A, and/or IAA at or above the 99th percentile and/or for ICA at or above 20 JDF units.[10] For comparison, 339 children were selected at random from the AAb-negative children as detected in the primary screening. The study protocol was authorized by the Ministry of Culture and Education of Mecklenburg-Vorpommern and approved by the ethics committee of the Ernst Moritz Arndt University of Greifswald. Informed consent was obtained from the parents or legal guardians.

For comparison, 274 geographically matched patients with longstanding T1D were involved after obtaining informed consent, followed at the Center of Diabetes and Metabolic Disorders, Karlsburg, Germany.

Autoantibody Assays

The autoantibody assays used have been previously described in detail.[6,10] Briefly, GADA and IA-2A were measured by fluid-phase ^{125}I-antigen binding assays by the use of recombinant human GAD65 (Diamyd Diagnostics AB, Stockholm, Sweden) and recombinant human IA-2ic (kindly provided by J. F. Elliot, University of Alberta, Edmonton, Canada). The assays were evaluated in the first and second Diabetes Antibody Standardization Program (DASP-1 and -2) proficiency evaluation. The anti-GAD assay had a diagnostic sensitivity and specificity of 88% and 96% (DASP-1) and 88% and 98% (DASP-2), respectively. The anti-IA-2 assay achieved a diagnostic sensitivity and specificity of 58% and 100% (DASP-1) and 50% and 100% (DASP-2), respectively, using a cutoff at or above the 98th percentile of a control group of 6877 schoolchildren without family history of diabetes or autoimmune thyroid diseases and not positive for more than one AAb.[6]

IAAs were determined by a competitive fluid-phase antigen binding microassay with and without the addition of unlabeled insulin. In DASP-2, this assay achieved a diagnostic sensitivity and specificity of 35% and 98%, respectively, at or above the 97.5th percentile calculated from 991 (537 m/454 f) healthy schoolchildren.

ICAs were measured by indirect immunofluorescence on cryosections of human pancreas. The assay achieved an analytical sensitivity and specificity of 100% for both in the Thirteenth ICA Workshop (1998). To distinguish single or multiple AAb positivity in sera with GADA + ICA and IA-2A + ICA, sera were preincubated with human recombinant GAD65 and IA-2ic, respectively, followed by testing for non-GAD ICA or non-IA-2 ICA on cryosections and for ^{125}I-antigen binding.[10]

HLA-DQB1 Typing

Genomic DNA was extracted from whole peripheral blood by standard procedures employing a salting-out technique. HLA-DRB1 and -DQB1 genotyping was performed by nonradioactive (digoxigenin-ddUTP) oligonucleotide hybridization of enzymatically amplified DNA as described previously.[10]

Statistical Analysis

For the immunogenetic analyses, odds ratios (OR) were calculated according to Woolf's method as cross-product ratios with Haldane's correction. The level of significance between groups was assessed by explorative two-sided chi-squared (χ^2) statistics with Yates' correction or Fisher's exact test where appropriate. Correction of p values was carried out according to the Bonferroni inequality method. In addition to the χ^2, the upper and lower 95% confidence intervals are indicated. All statistical

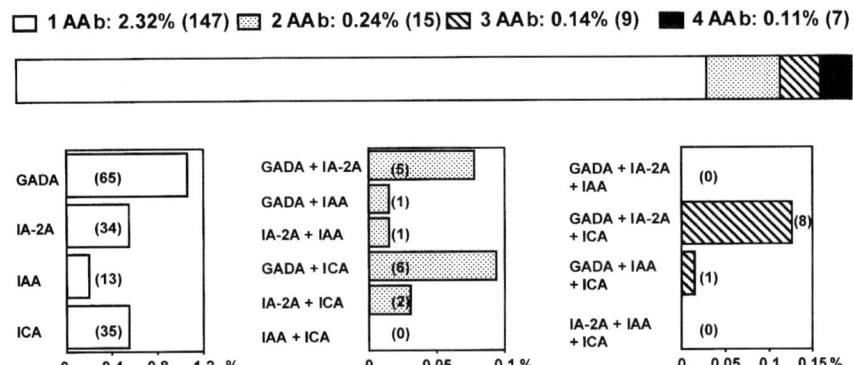

FIGURE 1. AAb-positive children: Prevalence and distribution of AAb specificities and their combinations in 178 AAb-positive schoolchildren representing 6337 probands of a normal cross-population. GADA occurred significantly enhanced compared to IAA, IA-2A, and ICA ($p < 0.001$–0.002) in children with single AAbs. In children with multiple AAbs, GADA, IA-2A, and ICA were significantly more frequent compared to IAA ($p = 0.006$–0.036).

analyses and calculations of percentiles were performed using the Statistical Package for Social Sciences, Version 10.0 (SPSS Inc., Chicago, IL). A two-tailed p value of 0.05 or less was considered to indicate statistical significance.

RESULTS

Frequency of Autoantibodies and Their Combinations in Schoolchildren

A total of 2.8% (178/6337) of the general schoolchild population was AAb-positive at or above the 99th percentile for GADA, IA-2A, or IAA, or for ICA at or above 20 JDF units. Among them, the majority of 2.32% (147/6337) had only one single AAb, whereas 0.49% (31/6337) tested positive for two or more AAbs (FIG. 1). In both groups, GADA occurred with highest and IAA with lowest frequency. In children with single AAbs, the frequency of GADA, IA-2A, and ICA was significantly higher compared to IAA ($p < 0.001$). In this group, GADA occurred also more frequent than IA-2A and ICA ($p < 0.01$). In children with multiple AAbs, the frequencies of GADA, IA-2A, and ICA did not differ significantly, but in comparison to IAA all three occurred significantly more frequent ($p = 0.006$–0.036). Among the 15 children (0.24%) positive for two AAbs, the combinations GADA + ICA ($n = 6$) and GADA + IA-2A ($n = 5$) occurred more frequently than GADA + IAA ($n = 1$), IA-2A + IAA ($n = 1$), or IA-2A + ICA ($n = 2$). The binding of the 6 sera with GADA + ICA and the 2 sera with IA-2A + ICA on cryosections was not inhibited by preincubation of sera with GAD65 or IA-2ic. No child has the combination IAA + ICA. In the 9 children (0.14%) positive for three AAbs, the combination GADA + IA-2A + ICA ($n = 8$) was significantly more frequent than GADA + IAA + ICA ($n = 1$; $p = 0.005$). Seven children have all four AAbs. All probands with multiple AAbs were positive for GADA and/or IA-2A.

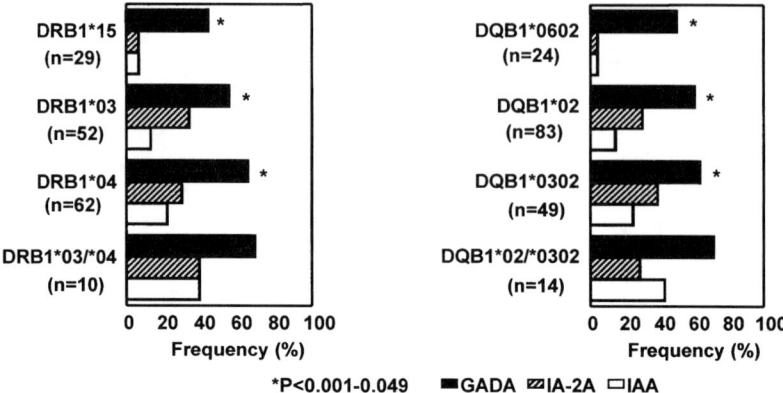

FIGURE 2. AAb-positive children: Prevalence of individual AAb specificities in HLA-defined subgroups. GADA occurred significantly more frequent in AAb-positive children with HLA markers protective and associated for T1D. Children bearing the protective DRB1 or DQB1 alleles are exclusively IA-2A- and IAA-negative.

Frequencies of Distinct HLA-DRB1 and -DQB1 Alleles in Children with GADA, IA-2A, and IAA

The probands were stratified according to occurrence of the protective alleles (HLA-DRB1*15; -DQB1*0602), the diabetes-associated alleles (HLA-DRB1*03, *04; -DQB1*02, *0302), as well as the highest risk genotype (HLA-DRB1*03/*04 and -DQB1*02/*0302). In general, among the three defined AAbs, GADAs were significantly more frequent than IA-2A or IAA in probands bearing the protective as well as the diabetes-associated DR or DQ alleles ($p < 0.001$–0.049; FIG. 2). In children bearing the dominant protective alleles, the IA-2A or IAA positivity was lowest. Among the probands with at least one diabetes-associated allele, IA-2A and IAA occurred significantly more frequent compared to those with the protective alleles. In children bearing the highest risk genotypes HLA-DRB1*03/*04 ($n = 10$) and HLA-DQB1*02/*0302 ($n = 14$), the distribution of AAb specificities did not differ significantly: again, the GADA occurred most frequently, but also IA-2A and IAA positivity was enhanced.

HLA Marker and the Relative Risk of Patients with T1D and Children with Multiple AAbs in Comparison to AAb-Negative Controls

The relative risk (OR) and the level of significance (χ^2 statistics) were calculated by cross-tabulating the frequencies of the HLA marker of patients with T1D ($n = 274$) and of healthy schoolchildren with multiple AAbs ($n = 31$) in comparison to the group of AAb-negative schoolchildren ($n = 339$; TABLE 1). In patients, the positive associations were confirmed for DRB1 haplotypes *03 and *04 ($p < 0.001$) and homozygosity for *03/*03 ($p = 0.006$) and *04/*04 ($p < 0.001$), as well as for the DQB1 haplotypes *02 and *0302 and homozygosity for *0302/*0302 ($p < 0.001$). The highest relative risk was confirmed for the DRB1*03/*04 and the DQB1*02/

TABLE 1. Frequencies of HLA marker, the relative risk (OR, odds ratio), and the level of significance (χ^2, p value) for the comparison of patients with T1D and children with multiple AAbs at or above the 99th percentile to healthy control children

	T1D ($n = 274$) [%]	OR (CI 95%)	χ^2	p	>1 AAb ($n = 31$) [%]	OR (CI 95%)	χ^2	p	Controls ($n = 339$) [%]
DRB1									
*15	1.5	0.05 (0.02–0.13)	63.0	<0.001	3.2	0.10 (0.01–0.79)	6.02	0.014	24.2
*03	52.9	3.76 (2.66–5.32)	57.3	<0.001	38.7	2.11 (0.98–4.54)	3.00	n.s.	23.0
*04	69.0	5.39 (3.81–7.62)	94.7	<0.001	61.3	3.84 (1.79–8.2)	12.03	0.001	29.2
*03/*03	4.7	5.58 (1.57–19.78)	7.4	0.006	9.7	12.00 (2.31–62.24)	8.80	0.009	0.9
*04/*04	10.6	4.34 (2.02–9.33)	15.1	<0.001	16.1	7.00 (2.2–22.58)	10.70	0.001	2.6
*03/*04	33.2	12.47 (6.78–22.92)	90.8	<0.001	16.1	4.82 (1.59–14.57)	6.81	0.009	3.8
DQB1									
*0602	1.5	0.06 (0.02–0.18)	44.9	<0.001	0	0	5.82	0.005	18.9
*02	58.4	1.97 (1.43–2.72)	16.5	<0.001	51.6	1.50 (0.72–3.13)	0.79	n.s.	41.6
*0302	66.1	9.05 (6.22–13.16)	146.5	<0.001	51.6	4.95 (2.32–10.58)	17.99	<0.001	17.7
*02/*02	8.4	1.39 (0.75–2.56)	0.8	n.s.	12.9	2.24 (0.72–7.01)	1.10	n.s.	6.2
*0302/*0302	8.8	10.75 (3.2–36.11)	20.5	<0.001	9.7	12.00 (2.31–62.24)	8.80	0.009	0.9
*02/*0302	36.5	21.07 (10.4–42.71)	116.4	<0.001	19.3	8.80 (2.9–26.71)	16.30	<0.001	2.6

*0302 genotypes ($p < 0.001$). Furthermore, the known negative association of DRB1*15 as well as DQB1*0602 ($p < 0.001$) was confirmed. In the group of healthy schoolchildren with multiple AAbs, we obtained comparable positive/negative associations for the DRB1 haplotypes *15 ($p = 0.014$) and *04 ($p = 0.001$), the genotypes *03/*03 ($p = 0.009$) and *04/*04 ($p = 0.001$), and the highest risk genotype *03/*04 ($p = 0.009$), as well as for the DQB1 haplotypes *0602 ($p = 0.005$) and *0302 ($p < 0.001$) and the genotypes *0302/*0302 ($p = 0.009$) and *02/*0302 ($p < 0.001$).

TABLE 2. Frequencies of HLA marker, the relative risk (OR, odds ratio), and the level of significance (χ^2, p value) for the comparison of children with single AAbs at or above the 99th percentile and below the 99.9th percentile and children with high-titer single AAbs at or above the 99.9th percentile to healthy controls

	1 AAb ≥99th, <99.9th (n = 138) [%]	OR (CI 95%)	χ^2	p	1 AAb ≥99.9th (n = 9) [%]	OR (CI 95%)	χ^2	p	Controls (n = 339) [%]
DRB1									
*15	20.3	0.80 (0.49–1.29)	0.63	0.426	0	0	1.66	0.123	24.2
*03	27.5	1.27 (0.81–2.0)	0.86	0.354	22.2	0.96 (0.19–4.7)	0	1.000	23.0
*04	26.8	0.89 (0.57–1.38)	0.17	0.680	66.6	4.85 (1.19–19.77)	4.20	0.024	29.2
*03/*03	3.6	4.21 (0.99–17.87)	2.95	0.086	11.1	14.00 (1.31–149.66)	1.58	0.100	0.9
*04/*04	0.7	0.27 (0.03–2.13)	0.96	0.294	22.2	10.48 (1.9–57.65)	5.50	0.029	2.6
*03/*04	2.9	0.75 (0.24–2.34)	0.05	0.788	11.1	3.13 (0.36–26.95)	0.06	0.312	3.8
DQB1									
*0602	17.4	0.90 (0.54–1.52)	0.06	0.803	0	0	1.01	0.375	18.9
*02	45.6	1.18 (0.79–1.76)	0.50	0.477	44.4	1.12 (0.3–4.26)	0	1.000	41.6
*0302	19.6	1.13 (0.68–1.87)	0.12	0.728	66.6	9.30 (2.26–38.23)	10.69	0.002	17.7
*02/*02	9.4	1.57 (0.76–3.24)	1.09	0.296	11.1	1.89 (0.23–15.85)	0	0.448	6.2
*0302/*0302	0.7	0.82 (0.08–7.93)	0	1.000	11.1	14.00 (1.31–149.66)	1.58	0.100	0.9
*02/*0302	4.3	1.67 (0.58–4.77)	0.45	0.502	22.2	10.48 (1.9–57.65)	5.50	0.029	2.6

HLA Marker and the Relative Risk of Children with Single AAbs at Different Titers in Comparison to AAb-Negative Controls

The frequencies of the HLA marker of children with single AAb positivity, differentiated according to AAb titers at or above the 99th percentile and below the 99.9th percentile (n = 138) and high AAb titers at or above the 99.9th percentile (n = 9), were compared to controls (n = 339; TABLE 2). The frequencies of the group of AAb-positive schoolchildren with AAb titers between the 99th and 99.9th percentile did not differ from those of AAb-negative control children. However, healthy children with high-titer single AAbs confirm the same positive/negative associations as shown for patients with T1D and for probands with multiple AAbs. In this group, frequencies of the HLA alleles DRB1*04 ($p = 0.024$) and DQB1*0302 ($p = 0.002$) and the genotypes DRB1*04/*04 and DQB1*02/*0302 ($p = 0.029$) are significantly different from those of AAb-negative controls. None of the children with high AAb titers bore the dominant protective haplotypes DRB1*15 or DQB1*0602.

DISCUSSION

AAbs against beta cell antigens have been shown to be useful in the assessment of diabetes risk among first-degree relatives of subjects with T1D. However, their predictive power is poorly defined in the general population, from which about 90% of newly diagnosed patients are derived. In a recent study by combined screening of GADA, IA-2A, and IAA in 4505 schoolchildren aged 14 years and recontacting 67% of them 8 years later, it has been shown that multiple AAbs prospectively identified all progressors to T1D.[9] However, several other studies have reported variable results in long-term follow-up of a general population mainly screened for ICA.[9] The Karlsburg Type 1 Diabetes Risk Study of a Normal Schoolchild Population aimed to investigate in a first primary screening, by drawing capillary blood, the occurrence of all four major AAbs—GADA, IA-2A, and IAA at or above the 98th percentile and ICA at or above 10 JDF units—in a large population of 9419 schoolchildren aged 6–17 years without family history of T1D.[6] In a second reexamination by drawing venous blood, AAbs were detected at higher specificity and lower sensitivity, for example, the 99th percentile of controls for GADA, IA-2A, and IAA and ICA ≥ 20 JDF units. Furthermore, HLA-DRB1 and -DQB1 specificities were determined.[10] The intent of the present study was first to assess the association of the immunogenetic markers with the diabetes-associated AAbs in AAb-positive children drawn from a large general population–based screening. Second, for comparison, geographically matched patients with T1D as well as AAb-negative random-selected control children were involved to assess the HLA determined risk by cross-tabulation in the AAb-defined subgroups.

A total of 178 schoolchildren, representing 2.8% of a general population of 6337 schoolchildren aged 6–17 years, were found to be AAb-positive. The majority of them, 82.6% (147/178) were positive for only one AAb specificity, whereas 17.4% (31/178) were positive for at least two AAbs. As previously demonstrated by combined analysis of GADA, IA-2A, IAA, and ICA in 86 children with T1D at time of diagnosis, the majority of them (91.87%) were positive for multiple AAbs, whereas only 7 of them (8.13%) had a single AAb only.[6] Thus, the healthy schoolchildren with multiple AAbs identified from our general population were defined as probands at increased risk for the development of the disease. It should be highlighted that, if the screening would be performed by a combination of GADA and IA-2A, none of these children would be missed. This was also true for the recently published group of children with T1D at onset; all children with multiple AAbs were identified by this AAb screening combination.[6] In both children with multiple AAbs as well as children with single AAbs, GADA occurred in highest frequency and IAA in lowest frequency in the age group investigated here. This is in accordance with results from the BABYDIAB Study demonstrating that IAA occurs most frequently in early life and often precedes other AAbs in first-degree relatives with multiple AAbs, whereas in later life a decline of IAA is seen.[16]

The clinical onset of T1D is influenced by at least three groups of factors, including genetic markers, environmental factors, and immunological events. It is currently generally accepted that the largest genetic contribution comes from genes within the MHC.[11] If the AAb-positive schoolchildren were stratified according to diabetes-associated and -protective alleles, among the three biochemically defined AAbs only GADA will occur in both groups with significantly increased frequency compared to IA-2A or IAA. In other words, GADA will occur in the probands independently if they are genetically susceptible or if "saved" by the dominant protective allele. Since only 1.5% of the patients with T1D in the present study bearing DQB1*0602 or DRB1*15 (resulting in a low relative risk of OR 0.06 or OR 0.05, respectively), but 44.8% of children with DRB1*15 and 50% of those with DQB1*0602 have GADA, the disease specificity of GADA for T1D seems to be questioned, at least if occurring as single AAb at titers below the 99.9th percentile. This was also obtained for the ICA; 41.7% of children bearing DQB1*0602 were found to be ICA-positive (data not shown). In contrast, AAb-positive children with a genetic predisposition for T1D are closely related to IA-2A positivity compared to those bearing the protective alleles. This could also be demonstrated for probands bearing the highest risk genotypes DRB1*03/*04 or DQB1*02/*0302, which are significantly more frequently positive for IA-2A and IAA compared to those bearing the protective allele. Thus, it is suggested that IA-2A and IAA are of higher specificity for T1D than GADA or ICA, especially if they occur as single AAb in the general population.

The comparison of the frequency of diabetes-associated and -protective alleles and genotypes of the patients with T1D and the AAb-negative controls clearly confirms the well-known positive associations of DRB1*03 and *04, as well as DQB1*02 and *0302, and the dominant protective effect of DRB1*15 and DQB1*0602. This was also true for the AAb-positive children at increased risk, that is, with multiple AAbs. In this group as in patients, the positive and negative associations were significantly confirmed. Furthermore, in both groups, a higher contribution of the DRB1*04–DQB1*0302 haplotype to the disease has been shown compared to the DRB1*03–DQB1*02 haplotype. The strongest associations in probands with multiple AAbs were seen for the DQB1*0302 allele and for the highest risk genotype DQB1*02/*0302. Moreover, multiple AAbs seem to imply the absence of protection since no child has the DQB1*0602 allele. In contrast, children with single AAbs between the 99th and the 99.9th percentile are not genetically susceptible to T1D because their allele frequencies did not differ significantly from those of controls. However, children with single AAbs at very high titers at or above the 99.9th percentile reflected the same genetic predisposition as patients or children with multiple AAbs, although caused by the limited number of probands in this group ($n = 9$) the differences compared to the controls were not always statistically different. None of the children with high-titer single AAbs had the protective allele. Therefore, it is assumed that the risk to develop the disease is also increased in children with single AAbs at very high concentrations. As shown by our study, HLA genotyping gives no additional information in estimating and differentiating diabetes risk in children from the general population having tested positive for high-titer single or multiple AAbs. In children with single AAbs at moderate levels, however, HLA genotyping is helpful to differentiate probands bearing the dominant protective or the "neutral" alleles and having a very low risk from those with the diabetes-associated alleles or genotypes. This is of importance for efficiently estimating risk while minimizing family anxiety because the observed AAb prevalence of 2.8% in the general population investigated here greatly exceeds the disease prevalence. However, if we look only at the children with multiple and high-titer single AAbs, a total of 0.63% ($n = 40$) in a population of 6337 children are at increased risk to develop the disease.

We conclude from the study that AAb screening performed in the general population without T1D heredity identifies also those probands with an HLA determined genetic predisposition as was shown for patients and their first-degree relatives. Probands with multiple AAbs or single AAbs at very high concentrations have the same genetic predisposition as patients and are therefore at risk for the development of the disease. The follow-up of this study will enable us to evaluate the risk of T1D more precisely based on the combined AAb screening and genotyping performed in the general population.

ACKNOWLEDGMENTS

We are grateful to Sonja Tietz, Heidi Kenk, Rosemarie Jung, and Christiane Lenth for their excellent technical assistance in AAb determinations, and to Marie-Luise Arnold and Isabel Breunig for HLA typing. This study was supported by BMFT Project 07NBL02/D4, the Ministry of Culture and Education of Mecklenburg-Vorpommern EMAU 16/1995, ABM Project 4576/98, the Community Medicine Project of the Ernst Moritz Arndt University of Greifswald, Aventis Pharma Deutschland GmbH, and BRAHMS Diagnostica GmbH. Additional support was obtained from the BMFT-funded Center for Interdisciplinary Clinical Research at the Friedrich Alexander University of Erlangen-Nürnberg (IZKF Erlangen, No. 01KS9601), the SFB 263 of the DFG, and the Association for Support of Diabetes Research (Karlsburg, Greifswald e.V.).

REFERENCES

1. CASTANO, L. & G.S. EISENBARTH. 1990. Type-I diabetes: a chronic autoimmune disease of human, mouse, and rat. Annu. Rev. Immunol. **8:** 647–679.
2. EURODIAB ACE STUDY GROUP. 2000. Variation and trends in incidence of childhood diabetes in Europe. Lancet **355:** 873–876.
3. BINGLEY, P.J., E. BONIFACIO & E.A.M. GALE. 1993. Can we really predict IDDM? Diabetes **42:** 213–220.
4. LÜHDER, F., M. SCHLOSSER, L. MAUCH et al. 1994. Autoantibodies against GAD65 rather than GAD67 precede the onset of type 1 diabetes. Autoimmunity **19:** 71–80.
5. GORUS, F.K., P. GOUBERT, C. SEMAKULA et al. 1997. IA-2-autoantibodies complement GAD65-autoantibodies in new-onset IDDM patients and help predict impending diabetes in their siblings. Diabetologia **40:** 95–99.
6. STREBELOW, M., M. SCHLOSSER, B. ZIEGLER et al. 1999. Karlsburg Type I Diabetes Risk Study of a General Population: frequencies and interactions of the four major type I diabetes associated autoantibodies studied in 9,419 schoolchildren. Diabetologia **42:** 661–670.
7. VERGE, C.F., R. GIANANI, E. KAWASAKI et al. 1996. Prediction of type I diabetes in first-degree relatives using a combination of insulin, GAD, and ICA512bdc/IA-2 autoantibodies. Diabetes **45:** 926–933.

8. BINGLEY, P.J., E. BONIFACIO, A.J.K. WILLIAMS et al. 1997. Prediction of IDDM in the general population: strategies based on combinations of autoantibody markers. Diabetes **46:** 1701–1710.
9. LaGASSE, J.M., M.S. BRANTLEY, M.J. LEECH et al. 2002. Successful prospective prediction of type 1 diabetes in schoolchildren through multiple defined autoantibodies: an 8-year follow-up of the Washington State Diabetes Prediction Study. Diabetes Care **25:** 505–511.
10. SCHLOSSER, M., M. STREBELOW, R. WASSMUTH et al. 2002. The Karlsburg Type 1 Diabetes Risk Study of a Normal Schoolchild Population: association of β-cell autoantibodies and human leukocyte antigen–DQB1 alleles in autoantibody-positive individuals. J. Clin. Endocrinol. Metab. **87:** 2254–2261.
11. TODD, J.A. & M. FARRAL. 1996. Panning for gold: genome-wide scanning for linkage in type 1 diabetes. Hum. Mol. Genet. **5:** 1443–1448.
12. HAGOPIAN, W.A., C.B. SANJEEVI, I. KOCKUM et al. 1995. Glutamate decarboxylase, insulin, and islet cell antibodies and HLA typing to detect diabetes in a general population-based study of Swedish children. J. Clin. Invest. **95:** 1505–1511.
13. MICHELSEN, B., R. WASSMUTH, J. LUDVIGSSON et al. 1990. HLA heterozygosity in insulin-dependent diabetes is most frequent at the DQ locus. Scand. J. Immunol. **31:** 405–413.
14. PUGLIESE, A., R. GIANANI, R. MOROMISATO et al. 1995. HLA-DQB1 *0602 is associated with dominant protection from diabetes even among islet cell antibody-positive first-degree relatives of patients with IDDM. Diabetes **44:** 608–613.
15. VANDEWALLE, C.L., A. FALORNI et al. 1997. Association of GAD65- and IA-2-autoantibodies with genetic risk markers in new-onset IDDM patients and their siblings: The Belgian Diabetes Registry. Diabetes Care **20:** 1547–1552.
16. ZIEGLER, A.G., M. HUMMEL, M. SCHENKER et al. 1999. Autoantibody appearance and risk for development of childhood diabetes in offspring of parents with type 1 diabetes: the 2-year analysis of the German BABYDIAB Study. Diabetes **48:** 460–468.

Insulin Autoimmunity

Immunogenetics/Immunopathogenesis of Type 1A Diabetes

GEORGE S. EISENBARTH

Barbara Davis Center for Childhood Diabetes, University of Colorado Health Sciences Center, Denver, Colorado, USA

ABSTRACT: We can now predict the development of type 1A diabetes in humans and prevent the disorder in animal models, but we cannot at present safely prevent type 1A diabetes in humans, although a series of clinical trials are under way and planned. A major lack in our current trial design is the inability to measure T lymphocytes directly responsible for beta cell destruction. Given the immunogenetics of type 1A diabetes and increasing knowledge of pathogenesis in the NOD mouse, we believe the disorder results from immune reactivity to a limited set of islet peptides, with reactivity to insulin a major determinant of disease. Insulin autoantibodies precede the development of diabetes in both humans and the NOD mouse. T lymphocytes isolated from the islets of the NOD mouse that recognize insulin peptide B:9–23 can transfer diabetes. Insulin expression within the thymus is correlated with genetic susceptibility, and insulin peptides can be used to induce diabetes and as an immunologic vaccine to prevent the disorder. Nevertheless, at present, routine measurement of anti-insulin T lymphocytes is not standardized. Better assays to monitor such autoreactivity are likely to be essential for the development and evaluation of preventive therapies.

KEYWORDS: type 1A diabetes; T cell; autoantibodies; susceptibility; insulin; islet peptide; assay; immune

INTRODUCTION

Type 1A diabetes (immune-mediated diabetes) is rapidly becoming one of the most extensively studied autoimmune disorders. There are multiple spontaneous animal models and induced animal models. Large-scale prospective natural history studies and prevention trials are under way. Recently developed trial networks (e.g., Immune Tolerance Network, Trialnet) are inviting trial proposals. We will review our current concepts of the immunogenetics and immunopathogenesis of type 1A diabetes, concentrating on anti-insulin autoimmunity, within a scaffold that divides disease pathogenesis into a series of stages beginning with genetic susceptibility and

---

Address for correspondence: George S. Eisenbarth, Barbara Davis Center for Childhood Diabetes, University of Colorado Health Sciences Center, Denver, CO 80262. Voice: 303-315-4891; fax: 303-315-4892.

george.eisenbarth@uchsc.edu

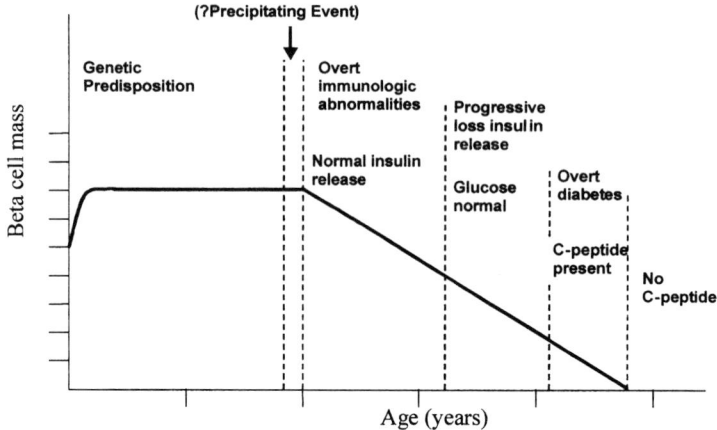

FIGURE 1. Hypothetical islet beta cell mass and stages in the development of type 1A diabetes (from: EISENBARTH, G.S. 1986. *N. Engl. J. Med.* **314**: 1360–1368).

ending with complete beta cell destruction (FIG. 1).[1] Much of the progress in understanding human type 1A diabetes over the past two decades can be encapsulated within improved ability to identify individuals at risk and predict who and at what rate individuals progress to overt diabetes. For example, we can now identify at birth individuals with risks of activating anti-islet autoimmunity that range from 1/2 (e.g., sibling of patient with type 1A diabetes with DR3/4, DQB1*0302) to <1/10,000 (e.g., DQB1*0602-positive individuals). Individuals with specific patterns of autoantibody expression have risks of progression to diabetes ranging from 20% to >90% (e.g., single autoantibody expression versus ≥2 anti-islet autoantibodies).

STAGE 1: GENETIC SUSCEPTIBILITY

The major defined determinants of type 1A diabetes are genes within the major histocompatibility complex (MHC, termed HLA for humans). Linkage studies indicate that this locus accounts for approximately 50% of the familial aggregation of type 1A diabetes.[2] Alleles of multiple genes are important with immune response genes (e.g., DQ and DR) of central relevance. For the NOD mouse model, the MHC has similar importance, with absence of I-E (homologue of DR) and specific sequences of I-A (e.g., I-A^{g7}) determining susceptibility. In addition, the normal Balb/c mouse [which has an identical I-Aα sequence to the NOD, but a different I-Aβ sequence (with aspartic acid at position 57), and expresses I-E] can be induced to express anti-insulin autoantibodies or progress to diabetes.[3] Balb/c mice, but not C57bl/6 mice, produce anti-insulin autoantibodies following immunization with the insulin B chain 9–23 peptide (congenics map the response to the MHC and not background genes of the strains). Of note, these autoantibodies react with intact insulin and cannot be absorbed by the immunizing peptide.[4] This suggests that normal Balb/c mice are sensitized to insulin and thus rapidly respond to peptide administration

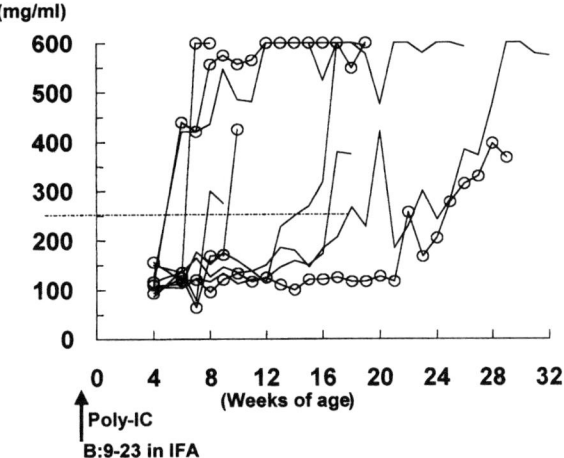

FIGURE 2. Induction of diabetes (blood glucose level) in Balb/c-derived mice (H-2^d) with islet expression of the costimulatory molecule B7.1 transgene following immunization with insulin peptide B:9–23 and the double-stranded RNA viral mimic, polyinosinic-cytidylic acid. Modified from ref. 3.

even in the absence of added adjuvant (e.g., peptide in saline). Although insulin autoantibodies can be induced, insulitis and diabetes do not occur. If the peptide is administered with poly-IC (a mimic of double-stranded viral RNA and toll receptor ligand), Balb/c mice develop insulitis, with predominant CD4 T cells.[3] Balb/c mice with islet B7.1 expression progress to diabetes following immunization with the B:9–23 peptide, with a large influx of CD8 lymphocytes (FIG. 2). It is likely that both class II alleles (e.g., I-A^d or I-A^{g7}) and class I alleles (e.g., K^d) are important for diabetes induction in both the spontaneous NOD and induced Balb/c mouse models. Autoimmune diabetes occurs spontaneously in the BB rat and the LETL (Long-Evans Tokushima Lean) rat and can be induced in a series of rat strains following neonatal thymectomy/radiation or poly-IC administration.[5] A common feature of these rat strains is RT1-U class II MHC alleles.

It is likely that, in humans, mice, and rats, class II alleles are essential for diabetes development in terms of directing the immune response to specific islet peptides and thus directing immune destruction to islet beta cells. To date, the only beta cell "specific" autoantigen (not expressed by non-beta islet cells) is insulin. In addition, recent workshops indicate that insulin autoantibodies are the only islet disease-specific autoantibodies (high-affinity autoantibodies produced by NOD and not C57bl/6 mice) of NOD mice.[6] These autoantibodies usually develop between 4 and 12 weeks of age, and early expression of insulin autoantibodies correlates with greater progression to diabetes, but probably primarily reflects insulitis.[7] MHC class II alleles can enhance or decrease disease risk, with transgenic introduction of human and mouse class II alleles directly demonstrating their importance. In humans, there is a hierarchy of disease risk with DQ2 and DQ8 alleles of very high risk, and the DQB1*0602 allele is protective (e.g., present in 20% of the general population, but

1% of children with type 1A diabetes). DR alleles can also decrease diabetes risk, such as DRB1*0403 even when present with DQB1*0302, and the allele DRB1*1401 appears to be as potent as DQB1*0602 in disease prevention (although much less common). At present, the specific mechanisms underlying disease susceptibility and protection are not completely defined, but the most likely hypothesis is that these alleles both shape the T cell repertoire (negative and positive selection) and present important islet peptides to autoreactive T cells.[8] The association of specific HLA genotypes across populations appears invariant, that is, specific DR and DQ haplotypes in studies of transmission in families have the same influence on diabetes risk throughout the world, despite dramatic differences in frequencies.[9] Unfortunately, one cannot encapsulate such disease risk with simple amino acid rules, such as aspartic acid at position 57 of the DQB chain being protective (e.g., high-risk alleles in Japan, the United States, and Norway include DQB1*0303 and DQB1*0401/0402). This worldwide uniformity of risk suggests that a single islet peptide may be an essential target. At present, one can only speculate whether such a peptide derives from one of the antigens already identified or is a completely unknown peptide. Structural data are available for human DQ for one peptide, namely, the insulin B:9–23 peptide bound in the groove of DQ8.[10] Although this peptide has been most studied in the NOD mouse, it weakly binds to I-A^{g7}, but is tightly bound by human DQ8.

Given targeting of islets related to specific MHC alleles (both class II and class I), multiple genes that influence immune function act as "diabetogenes". The search for "autoimmune" genes associated with diabetes susceptibility has been most successful in rat models. Mutation of the Ian4/5 (Immune Associated Nucleotide) gene underlies a severe T cell lymphopenia of the BB rat.[11] Inherited as an autosomal recessive trait for spontaneously diabetic BB rats, two copies of mutated Ian genes are essential for diabetes to develop. The penetrance of the lymphopenia phenotype is 100%, but progression to diabetes depends upon MHC RT1-U alleles as well as additional loci. The Cblb gene mutation was already known to influence immune function prior to its discovery as the major autosomal recessive locus essential for diabetes of LETL rats.[12] Mutations of the human homologue of the mouse Scurfy gene (a transcription factor) result in the XPID syndrome (X-Linked Polyendocrinopathy Immune Dysfunction and Diarrhea).[13] Neonates with the syndrome die of overwhelming autoimmunity (can be treated with bone marrow transplant) and develop autoimmune diabetes in the first days of life. Approximately 18% of patients with the APS-I syndrome (Autoimmune Polyendocrine Syndrome Type I) develop type 1A diabetes.[14] This syndrome results from mutations of the AIRE gene (Autoimmune Regulator Gene) that is hypothesized to contribute to autoimmunity by decreasing expression of antigens such as insulin within the thymus.[15]

Although there has been gratifying progress in identifying the above autoimmune genes, non-MHC-encoded genetic susceptibility of humans and the NOD mouse remains poorly understood, with predominantly loci rather than specific genes implicated. Polymorphisms of a VNTR (variable nucleotide tandem repeat) 5′ of the insulin gene accounts for approximately 10% of the familial aggregation of type 1 diabetes. The long form of this VNTR is associated with protection from diabetes and increased insulin message expression within the thymus. Studies by Hanahan and coworkers implicating tolerance induction by such low levels of thymic message and direct demonstration of insulin expression in mouse thymus controlled by the

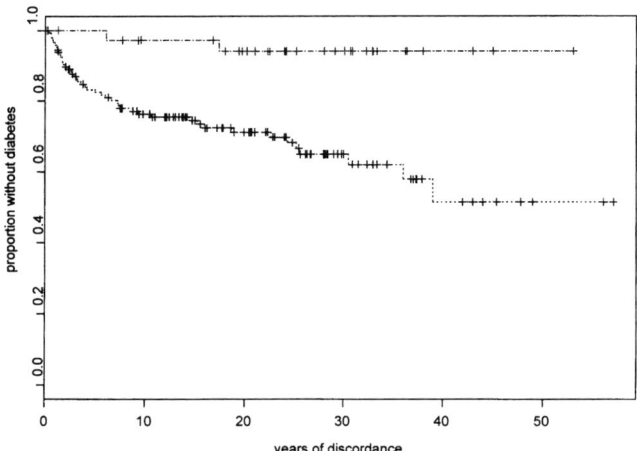

FIGURE 3. Life table analysis of progression to diabetes of monozygotic twins subdivided by whether the twin developed diabetes after age 25 (*upper line*) or before age 25 (*lower curve*). Modified from ref. 19.

insulin-2 gene have led to the hypothesis that this insulin polymorphism, by regulating thymic insulin, protects from type 1 diabetes.[16,17] Although, in the NOD mouse model, no polymorphisms of the insulin-1 and -2 gene are identified IDDM loci, we have recently discovered that knockouts of either of these genes, when bred onto the NOD mouse, dramatically influence disease.

There are two major contrasting hypotheses to account for genetic susceptibility to type 1 diabetes of humans: (i) a polygenic hypothesis (namely, multiple normal alleles combine to create above-average diabetes liability) versus (ii) an oligogenic hypothesis where there are multiple different non-MHC "mutations" plus MHC-encoded susceptibility (e.g., IDDM17 locus on chromosome 10 identified by the study of a single Bedouin Arab family).[18] It is likely that both hypotheses will be "right" for different individuals and, at present, we cannot ascertain the relative contribution of either model to human diabetes. Even groups of identical twins of patients with type 1A diabetes differ markedly in their risk of diabetes. If the first twin developed diabetes after age 25, risk for the next twin to progress to either diabetes or expression of anti-islet autoantibodies is less than 5%.[19] In contrast, if the first twin developed diabetes before age 5, the risk is 50% (FIG. 3).

STAGE 2: TRIGGERING OF ANTI-ISLET AUTOIMMUNITY

It is clear that concordance among identical twins is not 100%, that the incidence of type 1A diabetes is increasing worldwide, that congenital rubella infection increases the development of type 1A diabetes, and that multiple factors can enhance or suppress the development of diabetes of mice, all suggesting the importance of environmental factors. There is little agreement concerning the relevance of specific additional environmental factors. For example, we only have contradictory prospective studies of introduction of milk to infants or enterovirus infections.[20,21] A general paradigm, however, is developing where infants will be followed from birth (and potentially prenatally) for the development of anti-islet autoantibodies with careful environmental monitoring. With our ability to identify infants at birth with a risk approaching 50% for expressing anti-islet autoantibodies within the first 3 years of life and then progressing to diabetes, such studies are now feasible (see below). Studies of the induction of insulin autoantibodies and diabetes in Balb/c animal models suggest that immunization with an insulin peptide can be followed by insulin autoantibodies within 2 weeks (autoantibodies reacting with intact insulin and not absorbed by the peptide).[4] In addition, "nonspecific" stimulation of the innate immune system (e.g., poly-IC) enhances disease induction.[3] Thus, it is possible that multiple environmental factors (e.g., multiple RNA viruses) might contribute to disease induction and that the temporal relationship between autoimmunity and an environmental factor may be short.

STAGE 3: ACTIVATION OF AUTOIMMUNITY

At present, our best indicator of active anti-islet autoimmunity is the presence of anti-islet autoantibodies [insulin autoantibodies for the NOD mouse and insulin, GAD65, or ICA512 (IA-2) autoantibodies of humans]. Insulin autoantibodies can even precede (e.g., 3 weeks) obvious insulitis of the NOD mouse. In humans, for the youngest infants, insulin autoantibodies are usually (although not invariably) the first to appear.[7,22] Multiple international workshops indicate that these autoantibodies are best measured with highly sensitive and specific fluid-phase radioassays. There is now good standardization of assays for GAD65 and ICA512 autoantibodies and most laboratories participating in the last DASP workshop produced concordant results. In contrast, the measurement of insulin autoantibodies is more challenging, with most laboratories having low sensitivity. Nevertheless, multiple laboratories can now measure insulin autoantibodies with excellent sensitivity and specificity using what are termed microinsulin autoantibody assays.[7,23] Our laboratory in the last IDS (DASP) workshop had a sensitivity of 60% and a specificity of 98% using a convenient 96-well filtration plate assay that allows the processing by a single technician of tens of thousands of samples per year.

With completion of the DPT-1 parenteral insulin trial and the ENDIT nicotinamide trial, there is no doubt that large populations can be screened (e.g., >100,000 relatives) and relatives with high diabetes risk are identifiable with the expression of multiple anti-islet autoantibodies.[24] Of note for both trials with their long-term follow-up, there was between 40% and 60% diabetes risk at 5 years of follow-up and no indication of a plateau of risk for those with multiple autoantibodies and no influence of the studied therapy. For relatives only expressing cytoplasmic ICA or a single "biochemical" autoantibody, risk was much lower (e.g., <2% in the ENDIT trial). Studies such as DAISY indicate that screening of the general population and diabetes prediction are also possible.[25] In the DAISY study, more than 25,000 newborns from the general population of Denver have been screened and all those with the highest risk HLA genotype (DR3/4, DQB1*0302) are offered follow-up, as well as a subset of other risk genotypes. Expression of multiple biochemical anti-islet autoantibodies is associated with high diabetes risk, but quality control (e.g., analysis of blinded duplicates/triplicates) of the assays is essential and autoantibody assays are set for specificity above the 99th percentile of controls (e.g., assays of insulin, GAD65, and ICA512 autoantibodies). Almost one-half of very low positive samples are not confirmed on blinded assay of the same sample, a factor that can create considerable noise in population studies.

Measurement of T cell autoreactivity is much more difficult. This is likely due to the low frequency of autoreactive T lymphocytes in the peripheral blood, but is probably also related to available assay techniques and potentially to our lack of knowledge of appropriate disease-related peptide epitopes. A fundamental question is whether, similar to studies of T cell reactivity to infections or vaccines, robust assays for autoreactive T cells are feasible. Assays for CD8-reactive T cells using class I tetramers are well standardized, with high responses following infections. Assays for CD4 class II–restricted T cells are more difficult. Encouraging data are provided by the Nepom group studying GAD peptides and a DRB1*0401 tetramer. These studies that rely upon *in vitro* expansion of T cell subsets indicate that autoreactive T cells are usually below 1/30,000 cells and thus will be difficult to directly quantitate without *in vitro* expansion.[26] For a class I–restricted CD8 T cell, Santamaria and coworkers have presented data indicating that not only their NRP tetramer can directly identify autoreactive cells from peripheral blood of NOD mice, but those female NOD mice with a higher level of reactive cells are those that progress to diabetes.[27] This suggests that monitoring T cells in the peripheral blood, at least for NOD mice, can provide prognostic information.

It is a challenge in humans with a T cell assay to distinguish patients developing or with new onset diabetes from control.[28] Variants of ELISPOT and proliferation assays (e.g., costimulation dependence, cytokine staining) have been assessed. There is also considerable debate as to whether global changes in lymphocytes that distinguish disease from control in humans can be defined. For example, two reports indicated that NKT cells are deficient in patients with type 1 diabetes (as they are in NOD mice). Studies by Bendalac and colleagues utilizing a CD1 tetramer indicate, however, that even normal individuals stably differ by more than 100-fold in their percentage of NKT cells, but there is no difference between prediabetic, new onset diabetic, and control individuals.[29] In addition, with potent stimulation, there is no difference of NKT cell ability to secrete IL-4 when comparing control individuals and patients with diabetes.[29]

STAGE 4: PROGRESSIVE LOSS OF INSULIN SECRETION

At present, the most sensitive indicator of islet damage consists of progressive loss of first-phase insulin secretion following intravenous glucose, and the sum of the 1- plus 3-min insulin following glucose administration is the parameter most frequently utilized to ascertain diabetes risk.[30] Studies in baboons with streptozotocin-induced islet beta cell death indicate that, with destruction of approximately 40–50% of islet mass, intravenous glucose–stimulated insulin secretion approaches zero,[31] consistent with profound abnormalities of first-phase insulin secretion prior to diabetes onset. The utility of the intravenous glucose tolerance test in identifying high-risk individuals has been assessed in the largest trials of progression to diabetes such as DPT-1[32] and the nicotinamide ENDIT trial. Drawbacks to the test include a coefficient of variation in studying the same individual over time of approximately 20%, lower first-phase secretion in children particularly below the age of 8, an increase in first-phase secretion through puberty, and a large range of values for normal individuals. Thus, the test is primarily used with cutoffs of the tenth to first percentile of normal controls and is age-adjusted.

STAGE 5: OVERT DIABETES

Overt diabetes most likely occurs when there is still significant islet beta cell mass remaining. This is probably reflected by the common observation of a "honeymoon" phase for many new onset patients with type 1A diabetes. We believe it is unlikely that this honeymoon phase reflects an "immunologic" change versus metabolic improvement resulting from the reversal of hyperglycemia with insulin therapy. Anti-islet autoantibodies continue unabated through the honeymoon phase, and first-phase insulin secretion remains absent even though some patients are able to discontinue insulin therapy and maintain normal blood glucose for a matter of months. It is likely that both insulin secretion improves and insulin resistance decreases during this transient remission phase. The best determinant of beta cell function during this stage is the presence of serum C-peptide secretion, the connecting peptide cleaved from the proinsulin molecule. Maintenance of significant C-peptide secretion is associated with much improved metabolic control and there are benefits in terms of diabetes complications for those maintaining C-peptide secretion even at very low levels.[33]

For most patients developing type 1 diabetes, the time of onset of hyperglycemia is unknown, but is likely to have preceded diagnosis by months to years in that HbA1c is almost always elevated at the time of diagnosis. An acute fulminant form of diabetes recognized in Japan illustrates parameters associated with acute onset diabetes. These patients are characterized by severe hyperglycemia, but a normal HbA1c; have a characteristic HLA genotype; and have pancreatic histology with relatively little insulitis and no anti-islet autoantibodies.[34] This might be an example of a type 1B diabetes (nonimmune-mediated), but is more likely a fulminant autoimmune diabetes.[35,36]

CONCLUSIONS

Improving assays for anti-islet autoantibodies have important implications for our current understanding of the pathogenesis of type 1A diabetes and provide tools that should allow a much more refined search for environmental factors triggering the disease. They also provide us with tools to design trials for diabetes prevention. Nevertheless, most investigators believe that anti-islet autoantibodies are the smoke rather than the fire, and assays for pathogenic T cells and measures of islet beta cell mass will be essential for rapid progress toward diabetes prevention. We believe that T cells reacting with insulin peptides are central to the disease process of both humans and NOD mice, and the counting and characterizing of such cells will foster the next generation of studies.

ACKNOWLEDGMENTS

This work was supported by NIH Grant Nos. DK32083, DK32493, AI39213, 5-M01-RR00069, and M01-RR00051 (Clinical Research Centers Program); the Diabetes Endocrine Research Center (P30 DK57516) from the NIH; JDF Grant No. 1-1999-679; the Children's Diabetes Foundation; the Autoimmunity Center for Excellence (U19 AI46374); and the Autoimmunity Prevention Center (U19 AI50864).

REFERENCES

1. Buse, J.B. & G.S. Eisenbarth. 1986. Autoimmune endocrine disease. Vitam. Horm. **42:** 253–314.
2. Field, L.L. 2002. Genetic linkage and association studies of type I diabetes: challenges and rewards. Diabetologia **45:** 21–35.
3. Moriyama, H., L. Wen, N. Abiru et al. 2002. Induction and acceleration of insulitis/diabetes in mice with a viral mimic (polyinosinic-polycytidylic acid) and an insulin self-peptide. Proc. Natl. Acad. Sci. USA **99:** 5539–5544.
4. Abiru, N., A.K. Maniatis, L. Yu et al. 2001. Peptide and major histocompatibility complex–specific breaking of humoral tolerance to native insulin with the B9–23 peptide in diabetes-prone and normal mice. Diabetes **50:** 1274–1281.
5. Ellerman, K.E. & A.A. Like. 2000. Susceptibility to diabetes is widely distributed in normal class IIu haplotype rats. Diabetologia **43:** 890–898.
6. Bonifacio, E., M. Atkinson, G. Eisenbarth et al. 2001. International Workshop on Lessons from Animal Models for Human Type 1 Diabetes: identification of insulin, but not glutamic acid decarboxylase or IA-2 as specific autoantigens of humoral autoimmunity in nonobese diabetic mice. Diabetes **50:** 2451–2458.
7. Yu, L., D.T. Robles, N. Abiru et al. 2000. Early expression of antiinsulin autoantibodies of humans and the NOD mouse: evidence for early determination of subsequent diabetes. Proc. Natl. Acad. Sci. USA **97:** 1701–1706.
8. Wucherpfennig, K.W. & G.S. Eisenbarth. 2001. Type 1 diabetes. Nat. Immunol. **2:** 1–3.
9. Park, Y., J-X. She, C-Y. Wang et al. 2000. Common susceptibility and transmission pattern of HLA DRB1-DQB1 haplotypes to Korean and Caucasian patients with type 1 diabetes. J. Clin. Endocrinol. Metab. **85:** 4538–4542.
10. Lee, K.H., K.W. Wucherpfennig & D.C. Wiley. 2001. Structure of a human insulin peptide/HLA-DQ8 complex and susceptibility to type 1 diabetes. Nat. Immunol. **2:** 501–507.
11. Hornum, L., J. Romer & H. Markholst. 2002. The diabetes-prone BB rat carries a frameshift mutation in Ian4, a positional candidate of Iddm1. Diabetes **51:** 1972–1979.
12. Yokoi, N., K. Komeda, H.Y. Wang et al. 2002. Cblb is a major susceptibility gene for rat type 1 diabetes mellitus. Nat. Genet. **31:** 391–394.
13. Patel, D.D. 2001. Escape from tolerance in the human X-linked autoimmunity-allergic disregulation syndrome and the Scurfy mouse. J. Clin. Invest. **107:** 155–157.
14. Perheentupa, J. & A. Miettinen. 1999. Autoimmune polyendocrinopathy–candidiasis–ectodermal dystrophy. In Molecular Mechanisms of Endocrine and Organ Specific Autoimmunity, pp. 19–40. Landes. Austin.
15. Anderson, M.S., E.S. Venanzi, L. Klein et al. 2002. Projection of an immunological self-shadow within the thymus by the AIRE protein. Science **298:** 1395–1401.
16. Hanahan, D. 1998. Peripheral-antigen-expressing cells in thymic medulla: factors in self-tolerance and autoimmunity. Curr. Opin. Immunol. **10:** 656–662.
17. Chentoufi, A.A. & C. Polychronakos. 2002. Insulin expression levels in the thymus modulate insulin-specific autoreactive T-cell tolerance: the mechanism by which the IDDM2 locus may predispose to diabetes. Diabetes **51:** 1383–1390.
18. Verge, C.F., P. Vardi, S. Babu et al. 1998. Evidence for oligogenic inheritance of type 1A diabetes in a large Bedouin Arab family. J. Clin. Invest. **102:** 1569–1575.
19. Redondo, M.J., L. Yu, M. Hawa et al. 2001. Heterogenity of type 1 diabetes: analysis of monozygotic twins in Great Britain and the United States. Diabetologia **44:** 354–362.

20. HYÖTY, H., M. HILTUNEN & M. LONNROT. 1998. Enterovirus infections and insulin dependent diabetes mellitus—evidence for causality. Clin. Diagn. Virol. **9:** 77–84.
21. GRAVES, P.M., H.A. ROTBART, W.A. NIX et al. 2003. Prospective study of enteroviral infections and development of beta-cell autoimmunity: Diabetes Autoimmunity Study in the Young (DAISY). Diabetes Res. Clin. Pract. **59:** 51–61.
22. NASERKE, H.E., E. BONIFACIO & A-G. ZIEGLER. 1999. Immunoglobulin G insulin autoantibodies in BABYDIAB offspring appear postnatally: sensitive early detection using a protein A/G–based radiobinding assay. J. Clin. Endocrinol. Metab. **84:** 1239–1243.
23. NASERKE, H.E., N. DOZIO, A-G. ZIEGLER & E. BONIFACIO. 1998. Comparison of a novel micro-assay for insulin autoantibodies with the conventional radiobinding assay. Diabetologia **41:** 681–683.
24. SCHATZ, D.A. & P.J. BINGLEY. 2001. Update on major trials for the prevention of type 1 diabetes mellitus: the American Diabetes Prevention Trial (DPT-1) and the European Nicotinamide Diabetes Intervention Trial (ENDIT). J. Pediatr. Endocrinol. Metab. **14**(suppl. 1): 619–622.
25. REWERS, M., T.L. BUGAWAN, J.M. NORRIS et al. 1996. Newborn screening for HLA markers associated with IDDM: Diabetes Autoimmunity Study in the Young (DAISY). Diabetologia **39:** 807–812.
26. REIJONEN, H., E.J. NOVAK, S. KOCHIK et al. 2002. Detection of GAD65-specific T-cells by major histocompatibility complex class II tetramers in type 1 diabetic patients and at-risk subjects. Diabetes **51:** 1375–1382.
27. AMRANI, A., J. VERDAGUER, P. SERRA et al. 2000. Progression of autoimmune diabetes driven by avidity maturation of a T-cell population. Nature **406:** 739–742.
28. ROEP, B.O., M.A. ATKINSON, P.M. VAN ENDERT et al. 1999. Autoreactive T cell responses in insulin-dependent (type 1) diabetes mellitus: report of the First International Workshop for Standardization of T Cell Assays. J. Autoimmun. **13:** 267–282.
29. LEE, P.T., A. PUTNAM, K. BENLAGHA et al. 2002. Testing the NKT cell hypothesis of human IDDM pathogenesis. J. Clin. Invest. **110:** 793–800.
30. SRIKANTA, S., O.P. GANDA, G.S. EISENBARTH & J.S. SOELDNER. 1983. Islet cell antibodies and beta cell function in monozygotic triplets and twins initially discordant for type I diabetes mellitus. N. Engl. J. Med. **308:** 322–325.
31. MCCULLOCH, D.K., P.K. RAGHU, C. JOHNSTON et al. 1988. Defects in beta-cell function and insulin sensitivity in normoglycemic streptozotocin-treated baboons: a model of preclinical insulin-dependent diabetes. J. Clin. Endocrinol. Metab. **67:** 785–792.
32. CHASE, H.P., D.D. CUTHBERTSON, L.M. DOLAN et al. 2001. First-phase insulin release during the intravenous glucose tolerance test as a risk factor for type 1 diabetes. J. Pediatr. **138:** 244–249.
33. THE DCCT RESEARCH GROUP. 1987. Effects of age, duration, and treatment of insulin-dependent diabetes mellitus on residual beta-cell function: observations during eligibility testing for the Diabetes Control and Complications Trial (DCCT). J. Clin. Endocrinol. Metab. **65:** 30–36.
34. IMAGAWA, A., T. HANAFUSA, J. MIYAGAWA & Y. MATSUZAWA. 2000. A proposal of three distinct subtypes of type 1 diabetes mellitus based on clinical and pathological evidence. Ann. Med. **32:** 539–543.
35. SHIMADA, A., J. MORIMOTO, K. KODAMA et al. 2002. T-cell-mediated autoimmunity may be involved in fulminant type 1 diabetes. Diabetes Care **25:** 635–636.
36. RABINOWE, S.L., F.M. BROWN, M. WATTS et al. 1989. Anti-sympathetic ganglia antibodies and postural blood pressure in IDDM subjects of varying duration and patients at high risk of developing IDDM. Diabetes Care **12:** 1–6.

MHC-Linked Susceptibility to Type 1 Diabetes
A Structural Perspective

KAI W. WUCHERPFENNIG

Department of Cancer Immunology and AIDS, Dana-Farber Cancer Institute and Harvard Medical School, Boston, Massachusetts 02115, USA

ABSTRACT: The MHC represents the most important susceptibility locus for type 1 diabetes, and the MHC class II alleles that encode DQ8 and DQ2 in humans and I-A^{g7} in NOD mice represent critical elements. Even though these genetic facts have been known for a number of years, the biochemical and structural features of these MHC class II molecules have only been elucidated recently. We expressed DQ8 and I-A^{g7} as soluble proteins and observed significant structural and functional similarities between these human and murine MHC molecules. It had been postulated that I-A^{g7} and DQ8 are poor peptide binders, based on the observation that the subunits dissociate in the presence of SDS, a denaturing detergent. We observed that both DQ8 and I-A^{g7} form stable, long-lived complexes with a number of different peptides, indicating that they are not unstable in the absence of detergent. DQ8 and I-A^{g7} were found to bind similar sets of peptides, which included peptides that had been identified as immunodominant T cell epitopes of insulin and GAD 65 in NOD mice. The insulin B (9–23) peptide formed long-lived complexes with DQ8 and was thus chosen for crystallization of the complex. No defect in the peptide binding groove was evident in the crystal structure and the insulin peptide was deeply anchored in the binding site. The structure demonstrated significant similarities between DQ8 and I-A^{g7}, indicating that similar antigen presentation events are relevant in the NOD mouse model and the human disease.

KEYWORDS: type 1 diabetes; susceptibility; MHC class II; humans; NOD mice; pathogenesis; SDS; DQ8; I-A^{g7}

GENETIC SUSCEPTIBILITY TO TYPE 1 DIABETES

Role of MHC Genes in Susceptibility to the Human Disease

Genome-wide studies in humans have demonstrated that type 1 diabetes is a polygenic disease and that the MHC is the most important susceptibility locus (*IDDM1*), accounting for an estimated 42% to the familial clustering of the disease. By comparison, the contribution of other loci to familial clustering is relatively small, with an estimated 10% for *IDDM2* (insulin gene) and an even smaller fraction for other candidate loci.[1] The MHC covers a large region on the short arm of human chromosome 6, and studies in families have identified extended haplotypes that span from the class I to the class II region. Susceptibility is most closely associated with the DQB gene in the MHC class II region, based on linkage studies in families and association studies in patient and control groups.[2,3] The two alleles of the DQB gene that confer the highest risk for type 1 diabetes—DQB1*0201 and DQB1*0302— encode the β chains of the DQ2 (DQA1*0501, DQB1*0201) and DQ8 (DQB1*0301, DQB1*0302) heterodimers. The risk for type 1 diabetes is greatly increased in individuals who are homozygous for these DQB genes and thus express DQ8/DQ8 or DQ2/DQ2, and is even higher in subjects who are heterozygous and coexpress DQ8 and DQ2. Analysis of MHC genes in different populations has demonstrated that these alleles of the DQB gene confer susceptibility in a number of ethnic groups, including Caucasians, blacks, and Chinese, providing further support for the hypothesis that the DQB gene rather than a closely linked gene is critical. A notable exception is Japan, where the frequency of type 1 diabetes and these particular DQB alleles is relatively low and where a different allele of DQB (DQB1*0401) confers susceptibility to the disease. These disease associations are highly specific since DQB alleles that encode proteins that differ by only one or a few amino acids do not confer an increased susceptibility to type 1 diabetes. Among these, the DQB1*0303 allele has received the greatest attention since it differs from DQB1*0302 only at position 57 of the DQβ chain (aspartic acid versus alanine).[2–5]

MHC-Linked Protection from Type 1 Diabetes in Humans

A remarkable aspect in the genetics of type 1 diabetes is that other MHC class II haplotypes confer dominant protection from the disease. The highest level of protection is induced by the DR2/DQ6 haplotype (DRB1*1501, DQB1*0602), which is common in the general population, but rare in patients with type 1 diabetes.[2–5] Analysis of DR/DQ haplotypes in 180 Caucasian multiplex families demonstrated this haplotype in 15.5% of control subjects, but only 0.3% of patients. Dominant protection is associated with DQ rather than DR genes since a reduced diabetes incidence is observed in individuals with the DRB1*1501/DQB1*0602, but not the DRB1*1501/DQB1*0402 haplotype.[3] The protective effect of the DQB1*0602 allele has also been demonstrated in other ethnic groups, including Japanese, Mexican-Americans, and blacks. In addition, several other DR/DQ haplotypes confer protection, but to a lesser extent than the DR2/DQ6 haplotype.[3–5] These data demonstrate that coexpressed DQ molecules modulate disease susceptibility conferred by DQ8 and DQ2.

Genetic Evidence for a Role of Thymic T Cell Repertoire Development in the Pathogenesis of Type 1 Diabetes in Humans

Genetic data support the hypothesis that thymic repertoire selection represents a significant aspect in the pathogenesis of type 1 diabetes. The human *IDDM2* susceptibility gene has been mapped to the 5' region of the insulin gene, and neighboring genes (tyrosine hydroxylase and insulin-like growth factor II) have been excluded as candidates. The 5' region of the insulin gene carries a variable number of tandem repeats (VNTR) of 14–15 bp; homozygosity for the shorter VNTR (class I, average of 570 bp) is associated with an increased risk for type 1 diabetes, while the longer

VNTR (class III, average of 2200 bp) has a dominant protective effect. The class III VNTR is associated with 2- to 3-fold higher levels of insulin mRNA than class I VNTR in human fetal thymus. Higher levels of proinsulin in the thymus may promote negative selection of T cells that are relevant in the disease process.[6,7]

Strong evidence for an important role of the thymus in the pathogenesis of type 1 diabetes comes from a rare monogenic disease in which multiple endocrine organs are affected (autoimmune-polyendocrinopathy-candidiasis-ectodermal dystrophy, APECED). The disease is caused by mutations in the *AIRE* (autoimmune regulator) gene, which has sequence features of a transcriptional regulator.[8] The *AIRE* gene is primarily expressed in a distinct subpopulation of thymic medullary epithelial cells, and the nuclear localization of the protein strongly suggests that it acts as a transcription factor. This gene is therefore expressed at the anatomical site associated with negative selection and could be involved in thymic tolerance induction.[9]

MHC-Linked Susceptibility in NOD Mice

Analysis of the NOD mouse model has demonstrated a number of interesting similarities to the human disease. The MHC is a critical susceptibility locus (*Idd1*) in NOD mice, and many other loci contribute to the disease process. NOD mice that are congenic for the MHC locus are resistant to the development of type 1 diabetes, as shown by the analysis of six NOD strains congenic for different MHC haplotypes ($H2^b$, $H2^{i7}$, $H2^{i5}$, $H2^{h4}$, $H2^{h2}$, and $H2^k$). In these MHC congenic NOD strains, insulitis was only observed in a small fraction of mice from two of the six strains and disease could not even be induced by cyclophosphamide administration.[10,11] Two features of the MHC class II region of NOD mice are particularly relevant. Only I-A (but not I-E) molecules are expressed due to a deletion in the Eα promoter, and the expressed I-A molecule (I-A^{g7}) has a unique sequence at positions 56 and 57 of the I-Aβ chain (histidine–serine rather than proline–aspartic acid).[10,12] This aspect is remarkable since the relevant human alleles are also characterized by the absence of a negative charge at position 57 of the β chain (serine in I-A^{g7} and alanine in DQ8/DQ2).[2,12] The contribution of the MHC to susceptibility to diabetes in NOD mice is, however, not solely due to the *I-A*β gene since analysis of congenic mice demonstrated the presence of at least one other gene (*Idd16*) in the MHC class I region.[13]

Protection from Coexpressed MHC Class II Molecules in the NOD Mouse

Coexpressed I-E or non-NOD I-A molecules, the murine DR and DQ homologues, respectively, can provide partial or complete protection from type 1 diabetes in NOD mice.[14,15] As mentioned above, NOD mice do not express I-E molecules due a deletion in the Eα promoter. Expression of the *Eα^d* gene as a transgene results in protection from type 1 diabetes, indicating that the deficiency in I-E expression is an important feature of the *H2^{g7}* haplotype. Particularly interesting is the observation that introduction of a mutant I-A^{g7} β chain with a single amino acid substitution also results in protection from diabetes—this single amino acid change is located at position 56 (histidine to proline) in the P9 pocket of the binding site.[14] Protection has also been assessed using nontransgenic experimental approaches, an aspect that is important for ruling out that the observations discussed above reflect artifacts generated by introduction of transgenes. A striking level of protection was observed when NOD mice were crossed with six different lines of MHC-congenic NOD mice. Only a small fraction of these F_1 mice (one copy of NOD and non-NOD MHC on a NOD background) developed diabetes, and the incidence and severity of insulitis were greatly reduced.[11] Two major hypotheses have been proposed for the mechanism of MHC-linked protection: (1) protective MHC molecules act in the thymus and alter the T cell repertoire; (2) coexpressed MHC molecules affect antigen presentation in the peripheral immune system and modulate the immune response to islet antigens.[10]

FUNCTIONAL PROPERTIES OF DQ8 AND I-A^{g7}

The genetic data indicate that MHC class II molecules play a critical role in determining susceptibility and resistance to type 1 diabetes and suggest important parallels between the disease process in humans and the NOD mouse model. Understanding these MHC class II molecules at the biochemical and structural level is therefore critical for defining their role in the disease process. Purification of these MHC molecules from cell lines would have required the use of detergents, which could interfere with their function and would have provided only limited quantities. We thus expressed soluble DQ8 and I-A^{g7} in insect cells by replacing the transmembrane and cytoplasmic domains with leucine zippers from the transcription factors Fos and Jun.[16,17] These dimerization domains served as a functional replacement for the transmembrane regions that participate in the assembly of MHC class II heterodimers, and transient transfection experiments demonstrated that soluble DQ8 was only secreted when the leucine zippers were attached to the ectodomains. This approach yielded soluble heterodimers suitable for structural and functional studies. The leucine zippers were required for efficient assembly, but not for stabilization of the assembled dimer. For the crystallization of DQ8/insulin peptide complex, the leucine zippers were removed, and the heterodimers did not dissociate into individual chains.[17,18]

DQ8 and I-A^{g7} Form Long-Lived Complexes with Naturally Processed Peptides

It has recently been proposed that I-A^{g7} molecules are poor peptide binders. This hypothesis was based on the observation that I-A^{g7} heterodimers dissociate in the presence of SDS, a denaturing detergent. This assay has been used to monitor peptide occupancy of other MHC class II molecules by SDS-PAGE. This observation suggested that the interaction of I-A^{g7} with peptides is impaired, which could be relevant for thymic tolerance induction. Also, binding experiments with affinity-purified, detergent-solubilized I-A^{g7} molecules demonstrated little or no binding of peptides in that study.[19] However, an alternative explanation of these results is that the interface of the I-A^{g7} heterodimer is sensitive to SDS regardless of peptide content.

Binding experiments with soluble I-A^{g7} molecules in the absence of detergent demonstrated peptide binding properties similar to other MHC class II molecules. These soluble molecules formed long-lived complexes with naturally processed peptides that had been eluted from I-A^{g7} molecules,[20] with a half-life of greater than 72 h at an acidic pH. The stability of these complexes was further enhanced by a neutral pH, conditions that are relevant for surface display of peptides by antigen-presenting cells. These I-A^{g7}/peptide complexes dissociated in the presence of SDS, demonstrating that the SDS stability assay is not suitable for examining peptide occupancy by this MHC class II molecule.[16] Very similar observations were made for DQ8 since soluble DQ8/peptide complexes did not form SDS-resistant dimers, even though they formed long-lived complexes with certain peptides in the absence of detergent.[17] Importantly, the insulin B chain (9–23) peptide formed stable complexes with DQ8, which indicated that this peptide was suitable for crystallization experiments.[18]

Islet Peptides Cover a Wide Range of Affinities for DQ8 and I-A^{g7}

Peptide binding experiments led to the identification of islet peptides that bind with high affinity and form long-lived complexes, as well as other peptides whose interaction with these MHC molecules is relatively weak. It is important to note that low-affinity peptides can be identified for all MHC class II molecules and that low-affinity binding by some peptides does not indicate that the respective MHC class II molecule is defective. Four of nine peptides tested for binding to DQ8 formed long-lived complexes with a $t_{1/2}$ of greater than 72 h. This group included peptides from insulin (B chain, res. 9–23), heat shock protein 60 (HSP 60, res. 166–185 and 441–460) and GAD 65 (res. 121–140). The second group of peptides had an intermediate half-life, ranging from 16 to 65 h. These peptides included three GAD 65 peptides (res. 201–220, 247–266, and 571–585), a viral T cell epitope from HSV-2 VP 16 (res. 430–444), and an FcεR (105–120) peptide. These data demonstrate that DQ8 forms long-lived complexes with peptides from several islet antigens.[17]

Similar findings were made with I-A^{g7}, and two of six I-A^{g7}/peptide complexes had a long half-life ($t_{1/2}$ of >72 h). These peptides were derived from GAD 65 (res. 471–490) and mouse serum albumin (res. 560–574). Two other peptides (HSP 60, res. 441–460; and GAD 65, res. 206–220) had an intermediate half-life of 12–20 h, while the insulin (9–23) and GAD 65 (221–235) peptides had a short half-life ($t_{1/2}$ of <2 h).[16,17] These two peptides represent major T cell epitopes of insulin and GAD 65 in NOD mice, indicating that there is no strict correlation between the dissociation rate and immunodominance of a peptide *in vivo*.[21,22] In other animal models of autoimmunity, disease can be mediated by T cells specific for low- or high-affinity self-peptides. Classical examples are the N-terminal peptide of MBP (Ac1–11), which has a very low affinity, and the high-affinity PLP (139–151) peptide, both of which are highly encephalitogenic in mouse strains that express the appropriate MHC class II molecules.[23,24]

I-A^{g7} AND DQ8 SHARE SIGNIFICANT STRUCTURAL AND FUNCTIONAL SIMILARITIES

Crystal Structure of DQ8 with the Insulin B (9–23) Peptide

The insulin peptide was chosen for crystallization of a DQ8/peptide complex based on these biochemical data, as well as the large body of work on this peptide in NOD mice. DQ8 was expressed with the insulin peptide covalently linked to the N-terminus of the β chain through a flexible linker; this protein preparation could be crystallized and yielded a structure with a resolution of 2.4 Å.[18] The insulin peptide was of particular interest because it represents a prominent T cell epitope for islet-infiltrating CD4 T cells in NOD mice.[21] In addition, an epitope for CD8 T cells from NOD mice is contained within the same segment of the insulin B chain (res. 15–23), indicating that this region represents the major target for both MHC class I– and class II–restricted T cells in NOD mice.[25] A T cell response to the insulin B (9–23) peptide has also been detected in patients with recent onset of type 1 diabetes and in prediabetics, indicating that this epitope may also be relevant in the human disease.[26]

The crystal structure demonstrates that the peptide is deeply buried in the peptide binding groove and that there is no structural defect in the binding site.[18] Even though stability is difficult to assess based on a crystal structure, these results are in agreement with the functional data, which indicate a stable, long-lived interaction. An unusual feature of the structure is that two acidic residues of the insulin peptide—glutamic acid 13 and glutamic acid 21—serve as anchor residues in the P1 and P9 pockets of the binding site. This feature is unusual since many MHC molecules favor hydrophobic amino acid side chains in the major pockets.[27] A tyrosine residue of the insulin peptide is bound in the P4 pocket, which is very deep and hydrophobic.

The β57 Polymorphism and Its Effect on the Charge of the P9 Pocket

Particularly relevant are the structural features of the P9 pocket of DQ8, which is shaped by the critical β57 residue. Both DQ8 and DQ2 carry an alanine at β57, while alleles that are not associated with susceptibility to type 1 diabetes encode an aspartic acid.[2] The structure demonstrates that this polymorphism has a striking effect on the charge of the P9 pocket. In MHC class II molecules with aspartic acid at this position, the P9 pocket is electrostatically neutral since β57 aspartic acid forms a salt bridge with α76 arginine.[18,27] In contrast, the P9 pocket of DQ8 has a positive charge since α76 arginine cannot form a salt bridge with the alanine at β57. The positively charged side chain of the arginine is instead available for interaction with the peptide, and a salt bridge between glutamic acid 21 of the insulin peptide and α76 of DQ8 is observed in the structure.[18] The formation of a salt bridge between the peptide and α76 accounts for the observed preference of the P9 pocket of DQ8 for negatively charged amino acids, and this salt bridge may also contribute to the long half-life of the DQ8/insulin peptide complex.[17,28] However, it is important to note that other residues can also be accommodated in the P9 pocket of DQ8, albeit with a reduced affinity. In contrast, negatively charged peptide residues are strongly disfavored in the P9 pocket of MHC class II molecules with an aspartic acid at β57. The β57 polymorphism therefore has a dramatic effect on the peptide binding specificity of DQ8 and may profoundly alter the repertoire of peptides displayed in the thymus and secondary lymphoid structures.

The crystal structure of I-A^{g7} has also been determined, permitting a direct structural comparison of these diabetes-associated MHC molecules.[29,30] An important similarity between these structures is that the P9 pocket of both DQ8 and I-A^{g7} is basic. Peptide binding studies demonstrated that the P9 pocket of I-A^{g7} also has a preference for negatively charged residues.[16,31] In the I-A^{g7}/GAD peptide complex, a glutamic acid side chain occupies the P9 pocket and forms hydrogen bonds with α76 arginine and β57 serine.[30]

Particularly interesting is a comparison of the β chain residues of DQ8 and I-A^{g7} that shape the critical P9 pocket. Four of the six β chain residues differ between DQ8 and I-A^{g7}, including residues β55–57 (Pro-Pro-Ala in DQ8 and Arg-His-Ser in I-A^{g7}). The difference in the residues that shape the P9 pocket indicates that the alleles of DQB and *I-A*β that confer susceptibility to type 1 diabetes evolved independently from each other. The presence of a non-aspartic-acid residue at β57 and the resulting basic charge of the P9 pocket may confer an advantage in the CD4 T cell response to a particular infectious agent(s), and the increased risk for the development of type 1 diabetes may represent an unfortunate side effect.[18]

Functional Similarities between DQ8 and I-A^{g7}

Comparison of the DQ8 and I-A^{g7} structures also demonstrates significant similarities in other aspects of the peptide binding groove. As discussed above, the P9 pocket of DQ8 and I-A^{g7} has a preference for negatively charged residues and, in addition, the P4 pocket of both molecules is large and hydrophobic. Differences are observed in the detailed architecture of the P1 pocket, but this pocket can accommodate a number of different amino acid side chains in both DQ8 and I-A^{g7}.[18,29,30] These structural data clearly demonstrate why DQ8 and I-A^{g7} bind similar sets of peptides. The GAD 65 (206–220) peptide that is immunodominant in NOD mice binds with high affinity to both I-A^{g7} and DQ8.[17,31] The crystal structure of I-A^{g7} was determined with this GAD 65 peptide, and available motif data indicate that the same residues (P1 isoleucine, P4 valine, and P9 glutamic acid) are likely to also represent anchors for binding to DQ8.[30]

The structural and functional similarities between DQ8 and I-A^{g7} suggest that similar antigen presentation events are involved in the development of type 1 diabetes in humans and NOD mice.

ACKNOWLEDGMENTS

I would like to thank my colleagues and collaborators for their important contributions to work discussed here, particularly Laurent Gauthier, Bei Yu, Dorothee Hausmann, Kon Ho Lee, and Don C. Wiley. This work was supported by grants from the NIH (Nos. PO1 AI45757 and RO1 AI42316) and the Juvenile Diabetes Research Foundation International, as well as a Career Development Award from the American Diabetes Association (ADA).

REFERENCES

1. DAVIES, J.L., Y. KAWAGUCHI, S.T. BENNETT *et al.* 1994. A genome-wide search for human type 1 diabetes susceptibility genes. Nature **371:** 130–136.
2. TODD, J.A., J.I. BELL & H.O. MCDEVITT. 1987. HLA-DQ beta gene contributes to susceptibility and resistance to insulin-dependent diabetes mellitus. Nature **329:** 599–604.
3. NOBLE, J.A., A.M. VALDES, M. COOK *et al.* 1996. The role of HLA class II genes in insulin-dependent diabetes mellitus: molecular analysis of 180 Caucasian, multiplex families. Am. J. Hum. Genet. **59:** 1134–1148.
4. NEPOM, G.T. & H. ERLICH. 1991. MHC class-II molecules and autoimmunity. Annu. Rev. Immunol. **9:** 493–525.

5. ERLICH, H.A., A. ZEIDLER, J. CHANG et al. 1993. HLA class II alleles and susceptibility and resistance to insulin dependent diabetes mellitus in Mexican-American families. Nat. Genet. **3:** 358–364.
6. VAFIADIS, P., S.T. BENNETT, J. TODD et al. 1997. Insulin expression in human thymus is modulated by INS VNTR alleles at the IDDM2 locus. Nat. Genet. **15:** 289–292.
7. PUGLIESE, A., M. ZELLER, A. FERNANDEZ et al. 1997. The insulin gene is transcribed in the human thymus and transcription levels correlated with allelic variation at the INS VNTR-IDDM2 susceptibility locus for type 1 diabetes. Nat. Genet. **15:** 293–297.
8. THE FINNISH-GERMAN APECED CONSORTIUM. 1997. An autoimmune disease, APECED, caused by mutations in a novel gene featuring two PHD-type zinc-finger domains. Nat. Genet. **17:** 399–403.
9. HEINO, M., P. PETERSON, N. SILLANPAA et al. 2000. RNA and protein expression of the murine autoimmune regulator gene (AIRE) in normal, RelB-deficient and in NOD mouse. Eur. J. Immunol. **30:** 1884–1893.
10. WICKER, L.S., J.A. TODD & L.B. PETERSON. 1995. Genetic control of autoimmune diabetes in the NOD mouse. Annu. Rev. Immunol. **13:** 179–200.
11. PODOLIN, P.L., A. PRESSEY, N.H. DELARATO et al. 1993. I-E+ nonobese diabetic mice develop insulitis and diabetes. J. Exp. Med. **178:** 793–803.
12. ACHA-ORBEA, H. & H.O. MCDEVITT. 1987. The first external domain of the nonobese diabetic mouse class II I-A beta chain is unique. Proc. Natl. Acad. Sci. USA **84:** 2435–2439.
13. HATTORI, M., E. YAMATO, N. ITOH et al. 1999. Homologous recombination of the MHC class I K region defines new MHC-linked diabetogenic susceptibility gene(s) in nonobese diabetic mice. J. Immunol. **163:** 1721–1724.
14. LUND, T., L. O'REILLY, P. HUTCHINGS et al. 1990. Prevention of insulin-dependent diabetes mellitus in non-obese diabetic mice by transgenes encoding modified I-A beta-chain or normal I-E alpha-chain. Nature **345:** 727–729.
15. MIYAZAKI, T., M. UNO, M. UEHIRA et al. 1990. Direct evidence for the contribution of the unique I-A^{NOD} to the development of insulitis in non-obese diabetic mice. Nature **345:** 722–724.
16. HAUSMANN, D.H., B. YU, S. HAUSMANN et al. 1999. pH-dependent peptide binding properties of the type I diabetes-associated I-A^{g7} molecule: rapid release of CLIP at an endosomal pH. J. Exp. Med. **189:** 1723–1734.
17. YU, B., L. GAUTHIER, D.H. HAUSMANN et al. 2000. Binding of conserved islet peptides by human and murine MHC class II molecules associated with susceptibility to type I diabetes. Eur. J. Immunol. **30:** 2497–2506.
18. LEE, K.H., K.W. WUCHERPFENNIG & D.C. WILEY. 2001. Structure of a human insulin peptide-HLA-DQ8 complex and susceptibility to type 1 diabetes. Nat. Immunol. **2:** 501–507.
19. CARRASCO-MARIN, E., J. SHIMIZU, O. KANAGAWA et al. 1996. The class II MHC I-A^{g7} molecules from non-obese diabetic mice are poor peptide binders. J. Immunol. **156:** 450–458.
20. REICH, E.P., H. VON GRAFENSTEIN, A. BARLOW et al. 1994. Self peptides isolated from MHC glycoproteins of non-obese diabetic mice. J. Immunol. **152:** 2279–2288.
21. WEGMANN, D.R., M. NORBURY-GLASER & D. DANIEL. 1994. Insulin-specific T cells are a predominant component of islet infiltrates in pre-diabetic NOD mice. Eur. J. Immunol. **24:** 1853–1857.
22. CHAO, C.C. & H.O. MCDEVITT. 1997. Identification of immunogenic epitopes of GAD 65 presented by A^{g7} in non-obese diabetic mice. Immunogenetics **46:** 29–34.
23. FAIRCHILD, P.J., R. WILDGOOSE, E. ATHERTON et al. 1993. An autoantigenic T cell epitope forms unstable complexes with class II MHC: a novel route for escape from tolerance induction. Int. Immunol. **5:** 1151–1158.
24. LAMONT, A.G., A. SETTE, R. FUJINAMI et al. 1990. Inhibition of experimental autoimmune encephalomyelitis induction in SJL/J mice by using a peptide with high affinity for IAs molecules. J. Immunol. **145:** 1687–1693.
25. WONG, F.S., J. KARTTUNEN, C. DUMONT et al. 1999. Identification of an MHC class I–restricted autoantigen in type 1 diabetes by screening an organ-specific cDNA library. Nat. Med. **5:** 1026–1031.

26. ALLEVA, D.G., P.D. CROWE, L. JIN *et al.* 2001. A disease-associated cellular immune response in type 1 diabetics to an immunodominant epitope of insulin. J. Clin. Invest. **107:** 173–180.
27. STERN, L.J., J.H. BROWN, T. JARDETZKY *et al.* 1994. Crystal structure of the human class II MHC protein HLA-DR1 complexed with an influenza virus peptide. Nature **368:** 215–221.
28. KWOK, W.W., M.E. DOMEIER, M.L. JOHNSON *et al.* 1996. HLA-DQB1 codon 57 is critical for peptide binding and recognition. J. Exp. Med. **183:** 1253–1258.
29. LATEK, R.R., A. SURI, S.J. PETZOLD *et al.* 2000. Structural basis of peptide binding and presentation by the type I diabetes-associated MHC class II molecule of NOD mice. Immunity **12:** 699–710.
30. CORPER, A.L., T. STRATMANN, V. APOSTOLOPOULOS *et al.* 2000. A structural framework for deciphering the link between I-A^{g7} and autoimmune diabetes. Science **288:** 505–511.
31. STRATMANN, T., V. APOSTOLOPOULOS, V. MALLET-DESIGNE *et al.* 2000. The I-A^{g7} MHC class II molecule linked to murine diabetes is a promiscuous peptide binder. J. Immunol. **165:** 3214–3225.

Using Regulatory APCs to Induce/Maintain Tolerance

AMY E. JUEDES AND MATTHIAS G. VON HERRATH

Division of Immune Regulation, La Jolla Institute for Allergy and Immunology, San Diego, California 92121, USA

ABSTRACT: It is well established that antigen-presenting cells (APCs) such as dendritic cells (DCs) possess potent immune-stimulatory function. They are considered to be the key driving element for most immune, autoimmune, and host-defense responses. However, recent evidence suggests that as much as APCs can turn things on, they also have the capability to turn things off. To summarize the evidence for such regulatory function of APCs is the purpose of this review article. We are just beginning to understand whether regulatory APC function can be mapped to a separate lineage of APCs or whether it is more commonly acquired under certain maturation conditions. Furthermore, it becomes apparent that it is important to consider differences between human and mouse DCs as well as splenic-, lymph node–, or blood-derived APCs. We believe that, in the upcoming years, better understanding of positive and negative roles of APCs in immune regulation will benefit both sides of APC therapy: their use in enhancing immunity, for example, in vaccine design and cancer, as well as their application for the treatment of autoimmunity.

KEYWORDS: antigen-presenting cells (APCs); dendritic cells (DCs); immune; immunoregulation; maturation; type 1 diabetes (T1D)

INTRODUCTION

Autoimmune disorders such as type 1 diabetes (T1D) are thought to be caused by autoaggressive T lymphocytes that invade the target organ (i.e., pancreas) leading to tissue or cellular injury (e.g., loss of insulin-producing beta cells). Over the past decade, accumulating evidence indicates that inflammatory autoimmune processes are composed not only of autoaggressive components, but also of (autoreactive) regulatory components. Autoimmunity may result when the balance shifts too far to the aggressive side, usually associated with the production of T_H1/T_C1 cytokines such as IFN-γ and TNF-α. In contrast, if this equilibrium contains a sufficient amount of regulatory components, for example, T cells (Tregs), that produce more T_H2- or T_H3-like cytokines such as IL-4, IL-10, and TGF-β, disease may be prevented. It is important to bear in mind that effector functions of Tregs will likely involve other mechanisms than the induction of cytokines. Many experimental strategies have

Address for correspondence: Matthias G. von Herrath, M.D., La Jolla Institute for Allergy and Immunology, 10355 Science Center Drive, San Diego, CA 92121. Voice: 858-558-3571; fax: 858-558-3579.

matthias@liai.org

been devised to shift the immune response by downregulating the autoaggressive components and enhancing the regulatory response. One method that will be discussed here involves modulating the immune response using antigen-presenting cells (APCs), particularly dendritic cells (DCs).

DCs are a specialized subset of professional APCs that play a central role in immune responses due to their unique ability to prime naïve T cells. Immature DCs, which reside in the peripheral tissues, can capture antigen and, in response to "danger" signals such as microbial stimuli, migrate to peripheral lymph nodes and undergo maturation. It is in the peripheral lymph nodes that fully mature DCs interact with naïve T cells, inducing their activation and differentiation. It is clear from studies with humans and mice that DCs are a morphologically, phenotypically, and functionally heterogeneous cell population. They can be classified according to their functional ability to stimulate T cells (immature vs. mature) or by their ability to regulate the class of the T cell response. A wide body of evidence in both humans and mice indicates that specialized subtypes of DC are able to preferentially induce a T_H1 or T_H2 response. In addition, it is becoming apparent that, although DCs are instrumental in the activation of T cells in response to pathogens, they may play an equally important role in the maintenance of peripheral tolerance. These properties make DCs ideal as tools to shape the dynamics of T cell responses and thus make them an intriguing possibility for treating autoimmune diseases.

For the purposes of this article, regulation of the immune response by DCs will be grouped into several overlapping themes. One method of immunoregulation involves the use of specialized subtypes of DCs that preferentially induce a protective or regulatory T_H2 response. A second emerging theme in DC biology is the fact that DCs with an immature phenotype are thought to possess tolerogenic properties. Finally, other studies have demonstrated that it is possible to modulate DCs in order to induce regulatory properties, for example, by treatment with cytokines or costimulatory blockade. Investigations into the tolerogenic/regulatory properties of DCs have been performed using both human and animal systems and, for the most part, similar themes have emerged. Nonetheless, there are certain differences in the phenotype and origin of DCs used in these studies, and they will therefore be discussed separately.

HUMAN DCs AND IMMUNOREGULATION

The most commonly used type of DC precursors in humans are peripheral blood monocytes, which after culture with GM-CSF and IL-4 give rise to immature myeloid DCs (iDCs). Unlike DCs generated by culture with GM-CSF in mice, additional stimuli such as proinflammatory cytokines or microbial products are necessary to induce the maturation of fully stimulatory mature DCs in humans.[1,2] Mature DCs (mDCs) derived from peripheral blood monocytes are strong T_H1 inducers and have been studied extensively as tools to elicit protective immune responses against infection or tumor antigens. However, several recent studies have demonstrated the tolerogenic potential of iDCs generated from peripheral blood monocytes. iDCs grown from human blood after culture in GM-CSF/IL-4 express lower levels of costimulatory molecules and MHC than mDCs.[1] *In vitro* evidence indicates that while mDCs support the expansion of alloreactive T cells and the development of T_H1 cells, iDCs do not.[3] The T cells stimulated by iDCs do not proliferate, but differentiate into a regulatory T cell population. The mode of action of the regulatory T cells is not clear, but they can suppress proliferation of T_H1 cells in a contact- and dose-dependent manner.[3] Evidence also exists for a role of IL-10 in maintaining iDCs with tolerogenic properties. DCs grown by culture with GM-CSF and IL-4 and then further treated with IL-10 were able to induce both CD4 and CD8 anergic/regulatory T cells *in vitro*.[4,5]

Additional experiments confirm the efficacy of iDCs in inducing tolerance *in vivo*. In a study by Dhodapkar *et al.*, iDCs coated with influenza matrix peptide (MP) and KLH were injected into human subjects.[6] They found that iDC administration led to an inhibition of MP-specific CD8 T cell effector function, as well as the appearance of MP-specific IL-10-producing regulatory T cells. Later studies confirmed that T cells induced by immunization with iDCs were potent regulators of T cell effector function, again in a cell-dose-dependent manner.[7] However, inhibition was not permanent as IFN-γ-producing effectors returned to normal by 6 months after treatment.[7]

Immune regulation by DCs has also been successful using a second type of DC precursor found in humans, the plasmacytoid DC (pDC2). Plasmacytoid DC2s are a unique subset of DC precursors found in blood or tonsils that rapidly produce IFN-α and IFN-β in response to appropriate microbial stimuli.[1] pDC2s derived from blood give rise to a distinct type of immature DCs by culture with IL-3.[8,9] Without further maturation, pDC2s are poor stimulators of T cell responses.[9] One report also suggests that pDC2s have the capacity to induce an anergic state in an antigen-specific manner in CD4 T cell lines.[10] Maturation of pDC2s *in vitro* with stimuli such as CD40 ligation demonstrates that these cells (DC2s) preferentially induce a T_H2 response.[11] In addition, a recent study demonstrates that DC2s are able to induce human CD8 T regulatory T cells that produced IL-10 and could inhibit the bystander proliferation of naïve CD8 T cells.[12]

Results obtained using human iDCs and DC2s indicate that they may be a promising avenue for the treatment of autoimmune diseases as well as transplantation. It is also notable that *in vivo* studies with human iDCs demonstrate they are effective in regulating an already established immune response to influenza and need not be present at the time of priming. However, one drawback of using iDCs, especially in the context of treating autoimmune disease, is that they may be susceptible to maturation *in vivo* due to the presence of inflammatory cytokines. This may be a partial explanation for the relative ineffectiveness of immature DCs in treating animal models of autoimmune disease such as diabetes in the NOD mouse and EAE as discussed below.

MOUSE DC SUBSETS AND IMMUNOREGULATION

While in humans functional subsets of DCs (DC1 and DC2) can be generated by growth *in vitro* from distinct precursor subtypes, most work with mouse DC subsets involves direct isolation from peripheral lymphoid organs. The majority of DCs found in the peripheral lymphoid organs in mice express the surface marker CD11c. Different subsets of mouse DCs also express the T cell coreceptors CD4 or CD8, or even the B cell surface marker B220. Despite the difficulty in comparing *ex vivo* isolated DC subsets to those generated *in vitro* from human blood, similar functionally distinct populations are also apparent in the peripheral lymphoid organs of mice. The most striking functional difference so far is the ability of CD8-positive DCs to preferentially induce a T_H1 response, while CD8-negative DCs preferentially induce a T_H2 response. This was demonstrated by the adoptive transfer of purified, antigen-loaded CD8-positive or CD8-negative DCs into naïve mice. While CD8-positive DCs primed T cells that produced IFN-γ, CD8-negative DCs primed T cells that produced IL-4, IL-5, and IL-10.[13] The efficacy of targeting antigen to particular subsets of DCs was recently demonstrated in an EAE model. These authors injected an Ig chimera carrying the MOG 35–55 peptide, which induced recovery from the acute phase of disease.[14] They demonstrated that Ig-MOG uptake was mediated by FcR binding to APCs. In FcR−/− mice, protection was abolished, but was restored upon transfer of wild-type DCs. Specifically, the $CD8^- CD4^+$ subset of splenic DCs was demonstrated to be necessary for protection from EAE, and this was correlated with the production of IL-10 by the DCs themselves.

Another type of recently described DCs with potentially regulatory properties are the mouse IFN-α-producing cells (MIPCs). These DCs have a unique surface phenotype, expressing both B220 and Ly6C. They are a specialized subset of DCs that rapidly produce IFN-α and IFN-β in response to microbial stimuli and, despite differences in surface molecule expression, seem to be analogous to the plasmocytoid DC population in humans.[15–17] A recent study demonstrated that *ex vivo* isolated MIPCs induced T cell unresponsiveness, involving the differentiation of T regulatory cells capable of suppressing antigen-specific T cell proliferation.[16]

In terms of therapy of autoimmune disease, it is an intriguing idea to be able to induce a protective T_H2-like response by targeting antigens to specialized subsets of DCs. However, it is clear that another critical factor must be considered, namely, the maturation state of the DCs. For example, even specialized types of APCs such as the MIPCs mentioned above may only be tolerogenic in their nonactivated/immature state. Activation of MIPCs resulted in an upregulation of APC capacity and strong IL-12 production.[16] It is becoming increasingly evident that under steady state conditions DCs play an important role in the maintenance of peripheral tolerance. Administration of antigen selectively to DCs via a monoclonal antibody specific to a DC-restricted endocytic receptor DEC205, without additional activation or "danger" signals, results in a partial activation of CD4 T cells that is not sustained.[18] Further, these T cells become unresponsive to systemic challenge with antigen in CFA. Tolerization could be ablated by administering antigen along with DC-activating agents such as anti-CD40 agonistic antibody.

As discussed earlier, many studies in humans have demonstrated the tolerogenic potential of iDCs. Additional animal studies have demonstrated that immature DCs can be useful in inducing tolerance and prolonging allograft survival *in vivo*.[19–21] Despite the abundant evidence in both mice and humans for a role of immature DCs in tolerance induction, relatively little success has been achieved so far using *in vitro* generated immature DCs to treat autoimmune disease. One potential difficulty is the fact that DCs in mice, unlike in humans, mature spontaneously upon *in vitro* culture and it may thus be difficult to generate truly immature DCs. Nonetheless, studies with the NOD mouse have demonstrated that, surprisingly, mature BM-DCs were more potent at preventing development of diabetes than immature DCs.[22] The mature DCs used in these studies expressed high levels of MHC and costimulatory molecules, and were strong inducers of IFN-γ compared to their immature counterparts *in vitro*. However, when transferred to prediabetic recipients, it was the mature BM-DC that was most effective in preventing diabetes. Protection correlated with an increase in the production of the T_H2 cytokines IL-4 and IL-10, presumably due to the induction of regulatory cells.[23] Another recent study examined the role of immature vs. mature DCs to treat EAE. Immature DCs were generated from the BM by continuous culture with IL-10 and expressed low levels of MHC and costimulatory molecules. Mature DCs were generated by culture with the proinflammatory cytokine TNF-α or by culture with LPS and CD40 ligation. Interestingly and against the paradigm that iDCs are usually more tolerogenic, prevention of EAE was achieved only using TNF-α-matured DCs, and not immature DCs or LPS-matured DCs.[24] Again, protection was associated with an increase in the T_H2 cytokine IL-10. In the EAE study, it was also interesting that DCs matured with LPS were ineffective in preventing autoimmunity. This could be explained by their production of high levels of the T_H1-inducing cytokine IL-12, while conversely TNF-α-matured DCs produced only low levels of IL-12.[24] Likewise, it was reported that the DCs used to successfully treat diabetes in NOD mice were defective in IL-12 production.[25] Therefore, it is possible that protective DCs in these studies represent a partially mature population, expressing high levels of MHC and costimulatory molecules, but producing little IL-12. One can conclude from these studies that there are multiple factors that set apart tolerogenic from immunogenic DCs. Not only the precise maturation state, but also the type of cytokines/chemokines produced by the DCs will play an essential role. Indeed, lack of IL-12 production and increased amounts of IL-10 might be more important than lower levels of MHC and lack of costimulatory function.

APC MODULATION

Thus, which features constitute a regulatory DC? It is clear that DCs have the potential to regulate the immune response, be it by inducing T cell tolerance or the induction of regulatory T cells. However, the situation after *in vivo* transfer is certainly complex and DCs are likely to be affected by factors present at the site of inflammation. Indeed, it is possible that factors, perhaps even cytokines produced by the T cells themselves, may result in functional changes in DCs. In this way, it is an interesting idea to modulate the functional abilities of DCs *in vitro* or *in vivo* with the goal of inducing tolerance/regulation. Several examples of such approaches already exist and will be discussed here, along with some of our recent data on APC modulation *in vitro*.

Regulatory DC Phenotype Determined by Antigen Uptake

Doug Green and his colleagues made a very intriguing observation recently.[26] They reported that the precise circumstance under which a cell dies will determine whether an APC taking the debris up will possess stimulatory or tolerogenic properties. These observations support a basic concept of Polly Matzinger's[27] danger hypothesis: apoptotic, but not necrotic cells are capable of eliciting an actively tolerogenic response. In Green's study, regulatory APCs were generated after exposing them to apoptotic cells. Intriguingly, such APCs seemed to exert their effector functions by induction of regulatory CD8 lymphocytes, supporting the concept that tolerogenic DCs might act through the induction of Tregs.

Regulatory DCs Arising after Costimulatory Blockade

It is well known that activation of APCs occurs after ligation of CD40 by CD40L-expressing T cells and that this interaction enhances the ability of APC to prime T cells. Conversely, it is an attractive approach to induce tolerance by blockade of CD40/CD40L interactions. So far, the only available blocking antibody for CD40/CD40L interactions is a blocking antibody to CD40L expressed on T cells. The potential of CD40L blockade has already been examined in a number of animal models for autoimmune disease. Protection from lupus erythematosus,[28] collagen-induced arthritis,[29] EAE,[30,31] autoimmune thyroiditis,[32] myasthenia gravis,[33] and diabetes[34,35] has been successfully achieved by treating animals with CD40L-blocking antibody. In these experiments, protection was usually associated with a decrease in autoaggressive T_H1 cytokines (e.g., IFN-γ), but not an increase in T_H2 cytokines or regulatory cells.

A recent study from our laboratory examined in detail the mechanism of protection mediated by administration of a CD40L-blocking antibody during the RIP-LCMV model of type 1 diabetes (T1D).[35] In this model, the glycoprotein of lymphocytic choriomeningitis virus (LCMV) is transgenically expressed in the beta cells of the pancreas. While spontaneous diabetes is usually not observed in transgenic mice, disease can be initiated by infection with LCMV. This model is useful in that the CD8 and CD4 epitopes for LCMV are known, and a range of tools such as tetramers and intracellular cytokine staining can be employed to examine the diabetogenic antigen-specific T cells in detail. Treatment of RIP-LCMV mice with anti-CD40L antibody completely prevents diabetes and, similar to previous results in other disease models, protection was associated with reduced IFN-γ and TNF-α production as well as a decrease in the frequency of memory CTL specific for LCMV. Interestingly, CD11c+ DCs from CD40L-treated mice could transfer protection in an antigen-specific manner when injected into prediabetic recipients.[35] This indicated that blockade of CD40L during LCMV infection generated a type of DC with regulatory properties, which could presumably downregulate aggressive T cell responses. Further examination of the phenotype of the regulatory DCs indicated that they also expressed the NK cell marker DX5. In addition to presenting antigen, these NK-DCs displayed some functional characteristics of NK cells, such as the ability to kill NK-sensitive target cells. Further investigation is needed to determine the exact mechanism employed by regulatory "NK/DCs" induced by CD40L blockade, and it will also be interesting to try to generate such regulatory DCs *in vitro*. This could be especially promising as a therapeutic approach to induce antigen-specific tolerance during transplantation or autoimmune disease.

Modulation of APCs by Cytokines

Another situation where APC modulation has been examined is the exposure of APCs to regulatory cytokines. It is well known that, during autoimmune disease, protection can be achieved by shifting the class of the immune response by the induction of type 2–like regulatory T cells. Although the mechanisms of inhibition by regulatory T cells are not known, one intriguing idea is that autoantigen-specific regulatory T cells producing T_H2 cytokines act at the level of APCs to downmodulate autoaggressive T cells. Evidence for a protective role of regulatory cytokines in

TABLE 1. Effect of IL-4 or IL-10 on ability of APCs to stimulate LCMV-specific CTL

	Spleen DC	Macrophage	B cell	IL-10 BM-DC	TNF-α BM-DC
Untreated	+++	+++	++	+++	+
IL-4	+++	+/−	++++		
IL-10	+++	+++			

modulating APCs exists in several models. In the RIP-LCMV model of diabetes, IL-4 produced by T regulatory cells inhibited the local expansion of LCMV-specific CTL, and *in vitro* could inhibit the antigen-presenting function of peritoneal macrophages.[36]

In another study by King *et al.*, transgenic expression of IL-4 in the RIP-LCMV model could suppress diabetes by reducing the acquisition of cytolytic function by LCMV-specific CTL.[37] IL-4 was found to be protective by acting at the locus of the antigen-presenting DC. Transfer of wild-type DCs abolished protection in IL-4-expressing mice, while DCs treated *in vitro* with IL-4 did not. This indicated that the protection in IL-4-expressing mice seemed to be mediated by modulation of DC function. In support of this, the authors demonstrated that DCs cultured with IL-4 had enhanced B7-2 expression and decreased B7-1 expression. In another study by the same lab, TGF-β1 transgenically expressed in the pancreas was also found to be effective in preventing diabetes, this time in the NOD mouse.[38] TGF-β1 was found to inhibit B cell APC function, but not macrophage APC function *in vitro*. Evidence indicated that this led to a shift in APC preference in transgenic mice, leading to an altered GAD T cell repertoire and a shift from IFN-γ-producing to IL-4-producing T cells.

As described above, various T_H2 cytokines have been reported to modulate different types of APCs, resulting in a switch from T_H1 to T_H2 or a downregulation in their inability to stimulate autoaggressive T cells. In light of these data, our recent studies have taken a systematic approach to determining the effect of regulatory cytokines on the ability of professional APCs to stimulate LCMV-specific T cells. We have found that culture with IL-4 has different effects depending on the type of APC used. Treatment of peritoneal macrophages with IL-4 almost completely abolished their ability to stimulate LCMV-specific CTL, while treatment of B cells with IL-4 enhanced their ability to stimulate LCMV-specific CTL (TABLE 1). Surprisingly though, spleen-derived DCs were not affected by culture with IL-4 (TABLE 1). This result seems to contrast with the fact that IL-4 transgenically expressed in the pancreas specifically modulated DCs.[37] It is possible that this has to do with the strain of mice used or that only macrophages, specific DC subsets, or maturation stages are capable of modulation by IL-4.

We have also examined the role of IL-10 in modulating APCs, but found IL-10-treated DCs or macrophages were unchanged in their ability to stimulate LCMV-specific CTL (TABLE 1). However, culture of BM cells with IL-10 has a profound effect on the GM-CSF-induced maturation of DCs. Despite the fact that BM-DCs grown with IL-10 were immature, with low levels of B7, they were potent stimulators of LCMV-specific T cells; conversely, TNF-α-treated DCs, which expressed high levels of B7, were not (TABLE 1). Further investigation will focus on defining the mechanisms of cytokine modulation of APCs, as well as determining the efficacy of treatment with cytokine-modulated APCs *in vivo* using the RIP-LCMV model of diabetes.

CONCLUSIONS

At this point, it is still unclear which features constitute a regulatory APC/DC. However, several important determinants have been identified in *in vitro* and *in vivo* studies. For example, the precise cytokine environment present during APC maturation and later on during interaction with T lymphocytes seems to play an essential role. Furthermore, levels of MHC and/or costimulatory molecules will have an impact, although it is not always true that immature DCs or lower levels of costimulators and MHC will correlate with induction of tolerance. Last, the property or circumstance of antigen presentation to the APC will play a role, and a more "natural" cell death by apoptosis might predispose to a tolerogenic response. Future studies should advance our understanding in detail and thus should enable induction or transfer of regulatory DCs as a therapeutic avenue.

ACKNOWLEDGMENTS

This is manuscript no. 525 from the La Jolla Institute for Allergy and Immunology. This work was supported by NIH Grant Nos. AI51973 and DK51091 to M. G. von Herrath and a fellowship from the JDRF to A. E. Juedes. We thank Diana Frye for assistance with the manuscript preparation.

REFERENCES

1. SHORTMAN, K. & Y.J. LIU. 2002. Mouse and human dendritic cell subtypes. Nat. Rev. Immunol. **2:** 151–161.
2. STEINMAN, R.M., S. TURLEY, I. MELLMAN & K. INABA. 2000. The induction of tolerance by dendritic cells that have captured apoptotic cells. J. Exp. Med. **191:** 411–416.
3. JONULEIT, H., E. SCHMITT, G. SCHULER *et al.* 2000. Induction of interleukin 10–producing, nonproliferating CD4(+) T cells with regulatory properties by repetitive stimulation with allogeneic immature human dendritic cells. J. Exp. Med. **192:** 1213–1222.
4. STEINBRINK, K., E. GRAULICH, S. KUBSCH *et al.* 2002. CD4(+) and CD8(+) anergic T cells induced by interleukin-10-treated human dendritic cells display antigen-specific suppressor activity. Blood **99:** 2468–2476.
5. STEINBRINK, K., M. WOLFL, H. JONULEIT *et al.* 1997. Induction of tolerance by IL-10-treated dendritic cells. J. Immunol. **159:** 4772–4780.
6. DHODAPKAR, M.V., R.M. STEINMAN, J. KRASOVSKY *et al.* 2001. Antigen-specific inhibition of effector T cell function in humans after injection of immature dendritic cells. J. Exp. Med. **193:** 233–238.
7. DHODAPKAR, M.V. & R.M. STEINMAN. 2002. Antigen-bearing immature dendritic cells induce peptide-specific CD8(+) regulatory T cells *in vivo* in humans. Blood **100:** 174–177.
8. RISSOAN, M.C., V. SOUMELIS, N. KADOWAKI *et al.* 1999. Reciprocal control of T helper cell and dendritic cell differentiation. Science **283:** 1183–1186.
9. GROUARD, G., M.C. RISSOAN, L. FILGUEIRA *et al.* 1997. The enigmatic plasmacytoid T cells develop into dendritic cells with interleukin (IL)–3 and CD40-ligand. J. Exp. Med. **185:** 1101–1111.
10. KUWANA, M., J. KABURAKI, T.M. WRIGHT *et al.* 2001. Induction of antigen-specific human CD4(+) T cell anergy by peripheral blood DC2 precursors. Eur. J. Immunol. **31:** 2547–2557.
11. MOSER, M. & K.M. MURPHY. 2000. Dendritic cell regulation of TH1-TH2 development. Nat. Immunol. **1:** 199–205.

12. GILLIET, M. & Y.J. LIU. 2002. Generation of human CD8 T regulatory cells by CD40 ligand–activated plasmacytoid dendritic cells. J. Exp. Med. **195:** 695–704.
13. MALDONADO-LOPEZ, R., T. DE SMEDT, P. MICHEL et al. 1999. CD8alpha+ and CD8alpha− subclasses of dendritic cells direct the development of distinct T helper cells in vivo. J. Exp. Med. **189:** 587–592.
14. LEGGE, K.L., R.K. GREGG, R. MALDONADO-LOPEZ et al. 2002. On the role of dendritic cells in peripheral T cell tolerance and modulation of autoimmunity. J. Exp. Med. **196:** 217–227.
15. ASSELIN-PATUREL, C., A. BOONSTRA, M. DALOD et al. 2001. Mouse type I IFN-producing cells are immature APCs with plasmacytoid morphology. Nat. Immunol. **2:** 1144–1150.
16. MARTIN, P., G.M. DEL HOYO, F. ANJUERE et al. 2002. Characterization of a new subpopulation of mouse CD8alpha+ B220+ dendritic cells endowed with type 1 interferon production capacity and tolerogenic potential. Blood **100:** 383–390.
17. NAKANO, H., M. YANAGITA & M.D. GUNN. 2001. CD11c(+)B220(+)Gr-1(+) cells in mouse lymph nodes and spleen display characteristics of plasmacytoid dendritic cells. J. Exp. Med. **194:** 1171–1178.
18. HAWIGER, D., K. INABA, Y. DORSETT et al. 2001. Dendritic cells induce peripheral T cell unresponsiveness under steady state conditions in vivo. J. Exp. Med. **194:** 769–779.
19. LUTZ, M.B., R.M. SURI, M. NIIMI et al. 2000. Immature dendritic cells generated with low doses of GM-CSF in the absence of IL-4 are maturation resistant and prolong allograft survival in vivo. Eur. J. Immunol. **30:** 1813–1822.
20. O'CONNELL, P.J., W. LI, Z. WANG et al. 2002. Immature and mature CD8alpha+ dendritic cells prolong the survival of vascularized heart allografts. J. Immunol. **168:** 143–154.
21. FU, F., Y. LI, S. QIAN et al. 1996. Costimulatory molecule-deficient dendritic cell progenitors (MHC class II+, CD80dim, CD86−) prolong cardiac allograft survival in nonimmunosuppressed recipients. Transplantation **62:** 659–665.
22. FEILI-HARIRI, M., X. DONG, S.M. ALBER et al. 1999. Immunotherapy of NOD mice with bone marrow–derived dendritic cells. Diabetes **48:** 2300–2308.
23. FEILI-HARIRI, M., D.H. FALKNER & P.A. MOREL. 2002. Regulatory Th2 response induced following adoptive transfer of dendritic cells in prediabetic NOD mice. Eur. J. Immunol. **32:** 2021–2030.
24. MENGES, M., S. ROSSNER, C. VOIGTLANDER et al. 2002. Repetitive injections of dendritic cells matured with tumor necrosis factor alpha induce antigen-specific protection of mice from autoimmunity. J. Exp. Med. **195:** 15–21.
25. FEILI-HARIRI, M. & P.A. MOREL. 2001. Phenotypic and functional characteristics of BM-derived DC from NOD and non-diabetes-prone strains. Clin. Immunol. **98:** 133–142.
26. FERGUSON, T.A., J. HERNDON, B. ELZEY et al. 2002. Uptake of apoptotic antigen-coupled cells by lymphoid dendritic cells and cross-priming of CD8(+) T cells produce active immune unresponsiveness. J. Immunol. **168:** 5589–5595.
27. MATZINGER, P. 1994. Tolerance, danger, and the extended family. Annu. Rev. Immunol. **12:** 991–1045.
28. MOHAN, C., Y. SHI, J.D. LAMAN & S.K. DATTA. 1995. Interaction between CD40 and its ligand gp39 in the development of murine lupus nephritis. J. Immunol. **154:** 1470–1480.
29. DURIE, F.H., R.A. FAVA, T.M. FOY et al. 1993. Prevention of collagen-induced arthritis with an antibody to gp39, the ligand for CD40. Science **261:** 1328–1330.
30. GERRITSE, K., J.D. LAMAN, R.J. NOELLE et al. 1996. CD40–CD40 ligand interactions in experimental allergic encephalomyelitis and multiple sclerosis. Proc. Natl. Acad. Sci. USA **93:** 2499–2504.
31. HOWARD, L.M., A.J. MIGA, C.L. VANDERLUGT et al. 1999. Mechanisms of immunotherapeutic intervention by anti-CD40L (CD154) antibody in an animal model of multiple sclerosis. J. Clin. Invest. **103:** 281–290.
32. CARAYANNIOTIS, G., S.R. MASTERS & R.J. NOELLE. 1997. Suppression of murine thyroiditis via blockade of the CD40-CD40L interaction. Immunology **90:** 421–426.
33. IM, S.H., D. BARCHAN, P.K. MAITI et al. 2001. Blockade of CD40 ligand suppresses chronic experimental myasthenia gravis by down-regulation of Th1 differentiation and up-regulation of CTLA-4. J. Immunol. **166:** 6893–6898.

34. BALASA, B., T. KRAHL, G. PATSTONE et al. 1997. CD40 ligand–CD40 interactions are necessary for the initiation of insulitis and diabetes in nonobese diabetic mice. J. Immunol. **159:** 4620–4627.
35. HOMANN, D., A. JAHREIS, T. WOLFE et al. 2002. CD40L blockade prevents autoimmune diabetes by induction of bitypic NK/DC regulatory cells. Immunity **16:** 403–415.
36. HOMANN, D., A. HOLZ, A. BOT et al. 1999. Autoreactive CD4+ T cells protect from autoimmune diabetes via bystander suppression using the IL-4/Stat6 pathway. Immunity **11:** 463–472.
37. KING, C., R. MUELLER HOENGER, M. MALO CLEARY et al. 2001. Interleukin-4 acts at the locus of the antigen-presenting dendritic cell to counter-regulate cytotoxic CD8+ T-cell responses. Nat. Med. **7:** 206–214.
38. KING, C., J. DAVIES, R. MUELLER et al. 1998. TGF-beta1 alters APC preference, polarizing islet antigen responses toward a Th2 phenotype. Immunity **8:** 601–613.

Cell-Based Therapies for Diabetes: Progress towards a Transplantable Human β Cell Line

PAMELA ITKIN-ANSARI, IFAT GERON, ERGENG HAO, CARLA DEMETERCO, BJORN TYRBERG, AND FRED LEVINE

Cancer Center, University of California, San Diego, La Jolla, California, USA

ABSTRACT: Achieving normoglycemia is the goal of diabetes therapy. Potentially, there are many ways to achieve this goal, including transplantation of cells exhibiting glucose-responsive insulin secretion. However, to be applicable to the large number of people who might benefit from β cell replacement, an unlimited supply of β cells must be found. To address this problem, we have been developing cell lines from the human endocrine pancreas. In one case, a cell line, βlox5, has been developed from human islets that can be induced under some circumstances to differentiate into functional β cells exhibiting appropriate glucose-responsive insulin secretion. Inducing differentiation is complex, requiring the activation of multiple signaling pathways, including those downstream of those involved in cell-cell contact and the glucagon-like peptide-1 receptor. In addition, transfer of the PDX-1 gene is also necessary to render the cells competent for differentiation. However, it is clear that many other genes are involved in maintaining the commitment of βlox5 cells towards the β cell lineage. Understanding the complement of genes required to establish and maintain a β cell lineage commitment would be enormously helpful in efforts to develop a cell line that can be used for β cell replacement therapies. Here, we provide further information on the characteristics of cell lines that we have developed from the human pancreas that are relevant to the development of a β cell replacement therapy for diabetes.

KEYWORDS: β cell; βlox5; diabetes; islets; pancreas; therapy; transplantation

INTRODUCTION

Approaches to β Cell Replacement

The recent explosion of interest in cell replacement therapies for diabetes has been driven primarily by the dramatic progress in allogeneic islet cell transplantation.[1] For the first time, the Edmonton group demonstrated that islet transplantation is a viable therapy for diabetes. This advance was dependent largely on progress in immunosuppressive drug therapy that allowed for a steroid-free regimen. Further advances in this area are likely to result in even better long-term results as there is evidence that even the current improved drug regimens are toxic to β cells, albeit to

Address for correspondence: Dr. Fred Levine, Cancer Center, UCSD School of Medicine-0912, La Jolla, CA 92093-0912. Voice: 858-822-2039; fax: 858-822-4181.
flevine@ucsd.edu

a lesser extent than the previous steroid-containing regimens. While the success of the Edmonton trial was an important proof of principle, it did not address the major problem with islet transplantation, that is, the grossly inadequate supply of cadaveric pancreases as a source of islets. Solving this problem has been a major focus of research in β cell biology.

Many different potential sources of cells for β cell replacement, each with its own advantages and disadvantages, are being studied.[2] Overall, three major sources of cells are being pursued: embryonal stem cells, adult stem cells, and β cell lines.

Embryonal Stem Cells

The isolation of human embryonal stem cell lines has generated enormous excitement about the possibility of producing unlimited quantities of transplantable β cells. However, there are enormous gaps in our knowledge of β cell development that make it difficult to take a focused, rather than scattershot, approach to inducing β cell differentiation from early precursors such as embryonal stem cells. Islet-like cell structures have been generated at low frequency from both murine and human ES cells.[3,4] Those cells have low insulin content and some glucose-responsiveness, but not at levels appropriate for clinical transplantation studies. In one case, insulin-positive cells generated from murine ES cells did not express the critical β cell transcription factor PDX-1, raising the question of whether they were truly β cells.[3] In addition, because the process of inducing differentiation is inefficient, with undifferentiated ES remaining in the cultures, another potential problem is teratoma formation from undifferentiated cells that retain the ability to divide following transplantation *in vivo*.

Adult Stem Cells

In part because of the ethical concerns about ES cells, many studies have been directed towards inducing β cell differentiation from adult stem cells, either from the pancreas or from other sources such as bone marrow. Although many investigators have claimed that stem cells from ectopic organs such as bone marrow can be induced to differentiate into a variety of cell types such as neurons,[5] there have been no studies as yet in which β cells have been generated from adult stem cells outside of the pancreas. Recently, questions have been raised about the plasticity of adult stem cells. The possibility that apparent differentiation may result from fusion of adult stem cells with differentiated cells has been raised.[6,7] Elegant experiments using marked stem cells have not found evidence that bone marrow–derived cells can differentiate into nonhematopoietic lineages.[8]

A great deal of effort has been directed towards identifying stem cells within the pancreas.[9] It has been known for some time that the pool of β cells can be regenerated when placed under stress by a number of manipulations, including partial pancreatectomy, drugs such as streptozotocin, and immune-mediated damage. A central question in β cell biology concerns the identity of the cells that give rise to the regenerated β cells. Pancreatic epithelial cells can differentiate *in vitro* into mature β cells.[10] Some studies have found that duct cells can give rise to endocrine cells.[11,12] Others have proposed that β cells can be generated from other endocrine cells within the islet such as δ cells.[13]

A finding that has generated considerable interest and controversy involves a population of nestin-positive cells in the pancreas that has been shown to give rise to a variety of cell types, including pancreatic endocrine cells and hepatocytes. The nestin-positive cell population contains SP (side population) cells that express a member of the MDR family of transporters that is expressed on multilineage stem cells from bone marrow. However, because the cell cultures used are not completely homogeneous, it is as yet unclear whether the SP cells are also positive for nestin. In fact, the issue of whether nestin-positive cells serve as pancreatic endocrine stem cells is controversial, with recent reports that nestin is found only in pancreatic stellate and endothelial cells.[14]

Pancreatic β Cell Lines

Because of the problems with embryonal and adult stem cells, we have focused our efforts on creating an immortalized human β cell line (FIG. 1). Towards this end, we have developed a series of cell lines from the human endocrine pancreas using the potent dominant oncogenes SV40 T antigen and H-ras^{val12}.[15–18] While the cell lines are immortal and thus can be grown in unlimited quantities, they dedifferentiate over time in culture, exhibiting loss of hormone expression. Thus, it is important to determine the genes and signaling pathways that are affected by growth stimulation. Initially, we were successful in inducing endocrine differentiation in a cell line derived from islets isolated from a 24-week-gestation human fetal pancreas. This cell line, TRM-6, expresses substantial levels of somatostatin in response to retroviral vector–mediated expression of PDX-1 and aggregation into cell clusters to promote cell-cell contact.[16] More recently, we induced β cell function *in vitro* and *in vivo* in a cell line, βlox5, derived from purified adult human β cells.[18–20] Differentiation required the activation of multiple signaling pathways, including cell-cell contact, PDX-1 expression, and activation of the glucagon-like peptide-1 receptor (GLP1R). While this represents a substantial step along the road to developing a widely available cell transplantation therapy for diabetes, induction of differentiation in βlox5 is difficult and variable. To better control the process of endocrine differentiation from human pancreatic cell lines, we have been studying the expression of genes that are important in that process. The major finding is that βlox5, but not TRM-6,

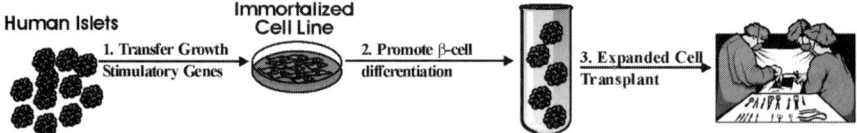

FIGURE 1. Strategy for developing human β cell lines. (1) Retroviral vectors are used to transfer growth stimulatory genes into β cells to create immortalized cell lines. (2) Immortalized cells are stimulated to differentiate into β cells, for example, by GLP1R activation, PDX-1 gene transfer, and aggregation into 3-D clusters. (3) Induced cells are transplanted into a patient to achieve glucose-responsive insulin secretion and normoglycemia. The autoimmune and allograft response to transplanted cells must be dealt with, by encapsulation, use of genetically modified cells, or systemic immunosuppression.

TABLE 1. RT-PCR

Gene	Primers	Comments
MafA	Forward: CTTCAGCAAGGAGGAGGTCA Reverse: TTGTACAGGTCCCGCTCTTT	7.5% DMSO, 57.5° annealing temp.; identity confirmed by sequencing
Nkx6.1	Forward: TACCCCTCATCAAGGATCCATT Reverse: TGTGCTTCTTCAACAGCTGCGT	60° annealing temp.; identity confirmed by sequencing[23]
Foxa2	Forward: CCGACTGGAGCAGCTACTATG Reverse: CTCAGGCTGGGACTCAAGTG	5% DMSO, 60° annealing temp.
Ngn3	Forward: TGAACTTGGCGACCAGAAG Reverse: TCAGTGCCAACTCGCTCTTA	60° annealing temp.
GLP1R	Forward: CAGCTCCTGTTCCTCTACAT Reverse: AGCAGTGTGTACAGGTACAC	60° annealing temp.

expresses the β cell–specific transcription factor Nkx6.1, consistent with it having an origin from a primary β cell.

MATERIALS AND METHODS

RT-PCR

RNA and cDNA preparation as well as PCR conditions for PDX-1 were as previously described.[21] PCR for the housekeeping gene, porphobilinogen deaminase (PD),[22] was performed to ensure equivalent sample preparation. All PCR reactions utilized 1.5 mM $MgCl_2$ and 40 cycles.

Real-time PCR for MafA, Foxa2, and Nkx6.1 was performed using SYBR Green I dye (Sigma, St. Louis, MO) according to manufacturer's protocols in the MJ Research Opticon DNA Engine real-time thermal cycler. See TABLE 1.

Cell Culture and Encapsulation

Cells were cultured in DMEM (low glucose) with 10% FBS. Cell aggregates were prepared as previously described.[16] Ten μL of packed βlox5 cell aggregates were inserted into a TheraCyte macroencapsulation device,[24] transplanted subcutaneously, and left for 5 weeks. The devices containing transplanted cells—including adjacent skin, vascular bed, and fibrosis—were then dissected from the site of implantation. The specimens were fixed over night at 4°C in 4% paraformaldehyde in PBS, dehydrated, embedded in paraffin, sectioned in 10-μm slices, and mounted on glass slides. The slides were stained with hematoxylin/eosin for microscopy.

Gene Array Studies

AffymetrixU95 GeneChips were utilized according to manufacturer protocols and analyzed using GeneSpring Software (Silicon Genetics).

RESULTS AND DISCUSSION

As stated above, we have been studying two cell lines, TRM-6 and βlox5, that are committed to the δ and β cell lineages, respectively. TRM-6 expresses somatostatin in response to PDX-1 expression.[16] While βlox5 can be induced to differentiate and exhibit glucose-responsive insulin secretion in response to expression of PDX-1, promotion of cell-cell contact, and activation of the GLP1R, induction of differentiation is complex and difficult. Moreover, βlox5 exhibits instability in its capacity to differentiate, similar to many other insulinoma cell lines that tend to lose insulin expression over time. To study the basis for the differential lineage commitment of TRM-6 and βlox5, as well as to understand the nature of the unstable differentiation of βlox5, the expression of markers of β cell differentiation has been analyzed.

Nkx6.1

Because βlox5 and TRM-6 differ dramatically in their lineage commitment and response to manipulations such as PDX-1 expression, the expression status of other markers of β cells was studied. Nkx6.1 is a homeodomain transcription factor that plays an important role in β cell development downstream of the Nkx2.2 factor.[25] In the adult pancreas, it is expressed solely in β cells, making it an excellent β cell marker. As demonstrated by quantitative RT-PCR, Nkx6.1 is expressed at high levels in βlox5 (FIG. 2), consistent with its origin from purified β cells. It is present at extremely low levels in TRM-6, which is committed to the δ cell lineage. Thus, the expression pattern of Nkx6.1 in the cell lines is consistent with what is known about Nkx6.1 expression in pancreatic islets, providing important verification of the origin of βlox5 from a β cell. Unlike PDX-1, which causes substantial inhibition of proliferation in βlox5 and to a lesser extent in TRM-6, Nkx6.1 does not seem to affect growth in culture. Also unlike PDX-1, which is lost during the process of cell line formation, Nkx6.1 expression is retained, demonstrating that continued expression of PDX-1 is not required for Nkx6.1 expression. Finally, the fact that the retroviral vector used to create the cell line will only infect dividing cells provides further

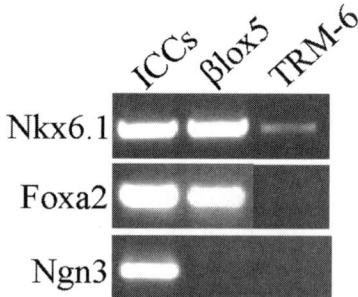

FIGURE 2. RT-PCR analysis of Nkx6.1, Foxa2, and Ngn3. RT-PCR was performed as described in the MATERIALS AND METHODS section and demonstrated that βlox5 expresses high levels of Nkx6.1 and Foxa2. Neither βlox5 nor TRM-6 expresses the Ngn3 gene, which is restricted to endocrine precursors.

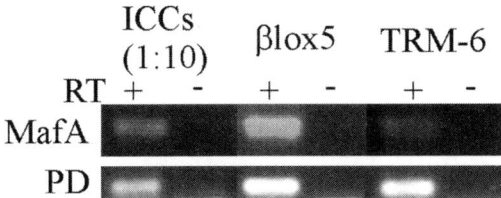

FIGURE 3. RT-PCR analysis of MafA expression in βlox5 and TRM-6. βlox5, but not TRM-6, expresses high levels of MafA, which has been identified as the RIPE3b1 insulin promoter binding factor. Because the MafA gene does not contain introns, reactions were done in the presence and absence of reverse transcriptase (RT).

proof of the ability of β cells to replicate in response to hepatocyte growth factor and extracellular matrix, as first proposed by Hayek and coworkers.[26]

MafA (RIPE3b1)

One of the most important elements in the insulin promoter is the RIPE3b1 element. By electrophoretic mobility shift assay (EMSA), it was demonstrated that βlox5, but not TRM-6, expressed a factor that bound to that element.[18] However, until recently, the identity of the factor that binds to the RIPE3b1 element in β cells was unknown. It has now been recognized as MafA, a transcription factor that plays important roles in growth and differentiation.[27] To determine whether the expression pattern of MafA is consistent with the previously obtained EMSA data, RT-PCR was performed for MafA (FIG. 3). βlox5, but not TRM-6, expresses high levels of MafA, consistent with the EMSA data and the identification of MafA as the RIPE3b1 binding factor in β cells.

Foxa2 (HNF3β)

One of the earliest markers of endodermal development is Foxa2 (formerly known as HNF3β). Foxa2 plays a critical role in the development of foregut endoderm. It regulates the expression of other HNFs and also has been reported to activate PDX-1 expression. In the mature pancreas, it is expressed in exocrine cells as well as in the islet in β and α cells. Expression of Foxa2 in δ cells has not been explicitly studied. In the course of performing Affymetrix GeneChip analyses on human pancreatic cell lines, we found that Foxa2 was expressed in βlox5, but not in TRM-1, a cell line derived from epithelial cells of the 18-week-gestation human fetal pancreas,[15] or TRM-6 (FIG. 4). To confirm this result, RT-PCR analysis was performed, with findings that were consistent with the GeneChip analysis (FIG. 2).

Ngn3

The transcription factor Ngn3 plays a critical role in pancreatic endocrine cell differentiation. Essentially all endocrine cells pass through an Ngn3-positive phase, and the Ngn3 knockout mouse lacks endocrine cells. However, in the adult pancreas, Ngn3 is absent. Neither βlox5 nor TRM-6 expresses Ngn3 (FIG. 2). This suggests that they are both derived from cells that have passed through the developmental phase where Ngn3 is expressed.

GLP1R

While βlox5 required addition of a GLP1R agonist, exendin-4, to induce β cell differentiation,[18] TRM-6, a cell line from human fetal islets, does not change its hormone expression at all in response to exendin-4. To determine the reason for this, the expression of the GLP1R was assayed by RT-PCR. Consistent with the finding that TRM-6 does not respond to exendin-4, it does not express the GLP1R (FIG. 5A). While βlox5 does express the receptor, expression was extremely variable, being

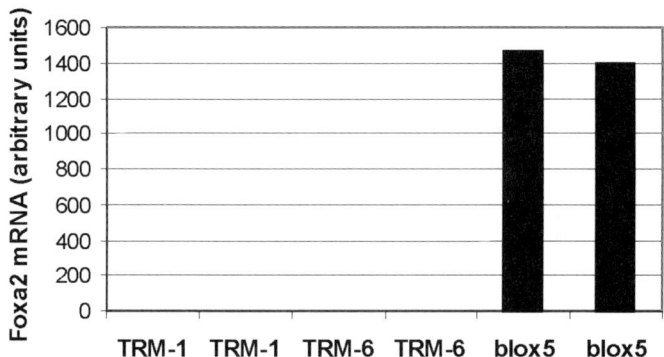

FIGURE 4. Foxa2 expression in TRM-1, TRM-6, and βlox5 cells. mRNA was prepared from two independent cultures of each cell line and analyzed on the Affymetrix U95A microarray. Foxa2 mRNA was absent from TRM-1 and TRM-6, but was present in βlox5 at an arbitrary intensity unit value of about 1400.

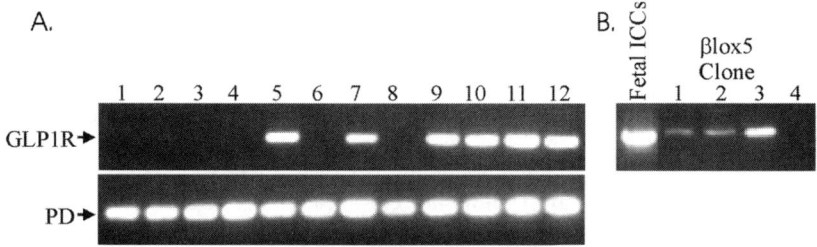

FIGURE 5. GLP1R expression. RT-PCR was performed using primers specific for the human GLP1R or the housekeeping gene, porphobilinogen deaminase (PD). **[A]** Lanes: (1) TRM-6/PDX-1 monolayer culture; (2) TRM-6/PDX-1 aggregates; (3) TRM-6 monolayer culture infected with a control retroviral vector not expressing PDX-1; (4) TRM-6/PDX-1/ BETA2 monolayer culture; (5) human pancreas, positive control; (6) Jurkat T cell line, negative control; (7) human fetal liver; (8) human adult liver; (9) human kidney; (10) human brain; (11) human heart; (12) human lung. **[B]** Four clones of βlox5 exhibiting variable expression of the GLP1R.

almost undetectable in some clones of βlox5 (FIG. 5B). This suggests that loss of GLP1R or another gene upstream of the GLP1R may be responsible for the loss of differentiation potential in βlox5.

Because of the interest in using hepatocytes as a source of cells that can differentiate along the β cell lineage,[28] we also examined the expression of the GLP1R in liver. It has already been reported that the GLP1R is not expressed in adult rat liver. However, no information on GLP1R expression in human liver is available. RT-PCR analysis of human fetal and adult liver revealed that GLP1R is highly expressed in fetal liver, but completely absent from adult liver (FIG. 5A). The presence of the GLP1R in fetal, but not adult, liver could have implications for the ability of hepatocytes from fetal versus adult liver to transdifferentiate into pancreatic endocrine cells.

Encapsulation of the βlox5 Human β Cell Line

Ultimately, it is anticipated that a human β cell line will be developed that can be transplanted into patients with diabetes. Because of the substantial difficulties in developing such cell lines, it is likely that a universal donor cell line will be used for transplantation into many patients. Thus, each patient will receive an allograft. Furthermore, patients with type 1 diabetes face the additional problem of recurrent autoimmune destruction of the grafted cells. To avoid this problem and to minimize the need for potent systemic immunosuppressive drugs, various encapsulation methods have been proposed.

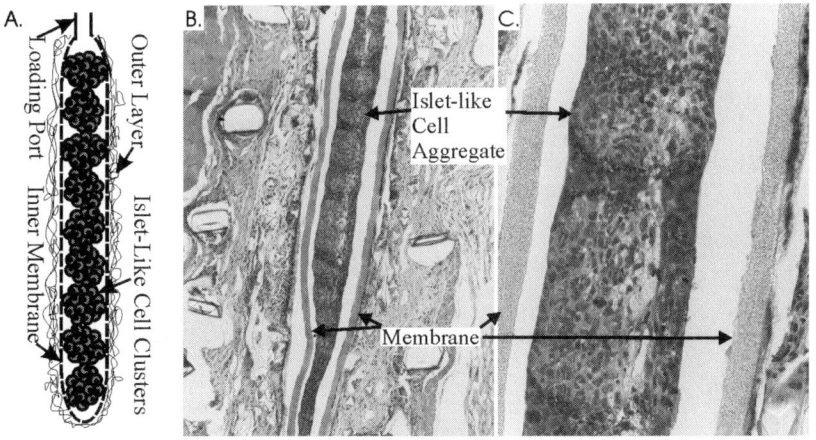

FIGURE 6. TheraCyte macroencapsulation device. **(A)** Schematic diagram. The device consists of a loose mesh outer layer that encourages cell ingrowth and vascularization, a semipermeable inner membrane that excludes cells and large proteins such as immunoglobulins, and a loading port for cells. **(B, C)** βlox5 cells were aggregated into islet-like cell aggregates and inserted into the TheraCyte device. The device was placed subcutaneously in nude mice and left for 5 weeks, after which it was removed and sectioned for H&E staining. Original optical magnification: 50× for panel B and 200× for panel C.

To test the ability of human pancreatic cell lines to survive in the context of a macroencapsulation device, we placed aggregates of uninduced βlox5 cells into the TheraCyte macroencapsulation device and transplanted them subcutaneously in nude mice. After 5 weeks, the devices were removed, embedded in paraffin, and stained with H&E (FIG. 6). Encouragingly, the islet-like structure of the transplanted aggregated cells was well maintained, demonstrating the feasibility of using the device for cell lines such as ours, where cell-cell contact is essential for maintaining differentiated function.

ACKNOWLEDGMENTS

This work was supported by grants from the NIDDK (Nos. DK55065, DK55283, and DK61248) and PanCel. Fred Levine holds equity in PanCel. Bjorn Tyrberg is a Hillblom Research Fellow.

REFERENCES

1. SHAPIRO, A.M. *et al.* 2000. Islet transplantation in seven patients with type 1 diabetes mellitus using a glucocorticoid-free immunosuppressive regimen. N. Engl. J. Med. **343:** 230–238.
2. DEMETERCO, C. & F. LEVINE. 2001. Gene therapy for diabetes. Front. Biosci. **6:** D175–D191.
3. LUMELSKY, N. *et al.* 2001. Differentiation of embryonic stem cells to insulin-secreting structures similar to pancreatic islets. Science **292:** 1389–1394.
4. ASSADY, S. *et al.* 2001. Insulin production by human embryonic stem cells. Diabetes **50:** 1691–1697.
5. JIANG, Y. *et al.* 2002. Multipotent progenitor cells can be isolated from postnatal murine bone marrow, muscle, and brain. Exp. Hematol. **30:** 896–904.
6. TERADA, N. *et al.* 2002. Bone marrow cells adopt the phenotype of other cells by spontaneous cell fusion. Nature **416:** 542–545.
7. WURMSER, A.E. & F.H. GAGE. 2002. Stem cells: cell fusion causes confusion. Nature **416:** 485–487.
8. WAGERS, A.J. *et al.* 2002. Little evidence for developmental plasticity of adult hematopoietic stem cells. Science **297:** 2256–2259.
9. BONNER-WEIR, S. & A. SHARMA. 2002. Pancreatic stem cells. J. Pathol. **197:** 519–526.
10. MIRALLES, F. *et al.* 1999. Characterization of beta cells developed *in vitro* from rat embryonic pancreatic epithelium. Dev. Dyn. **214:** 116–126.
11. RAMIYA, V.K. *et al.* 2000. Reversal of insulin-dependent diabetes using islets generated *in vitro* from pancreatic stem cells. Nat. Med. **6:** 278–282.
12. BONNER-WEIR, S. *et al.* 2000. *In vitro* cultivation of human islets from expanded ductal tissue. Proc. Natl. Acad. Sci. USA **97:** 7999–8004.
13. GUZ, Y., I. NASIR & G. TEITELMAN. 2001. Regeneration of pancreatic beta cells from intra-islet precursor cells in an experimental model of diabetes. Endocrinology **142:** 4956–4968.
14. LARDON, J., I. ROOMAN & L. BOUWENS. 2002. Nestin expression in pancreatic stellate cells and angiogenic endothelial cells. Histochem. Cell. Biol. **117:** 535–540.
15. WANG, S. *et al.* 1997. Isolation and characterization of a cell line from the epithelial cells of the human fetal pancreas. Cell Transplant. **6:** 59–67.
16. ITKIN-ANSARI, P. *et al.* 2000. PDX-1 and cell-cell contact act in synergy to promote delta-cell development in a human pancreatic endocrine precursor cell line. Mol. Endocrinol. **14:** 814–822.
17. HALVORSEN, T.L., G. LEIBOWITZ & F. LEVINE. 1999. Telomerase activity is sufficient to allow transformed cells to escape from crisis. Mol. Cell. Biol. **19:** 1864–1870.

18. DUFAYET DE LA TOUR, D. et al. 2001. β-cell differentiation from a human pancreatic cell line *in vitro* and *in vivo*. Mol. Endocrinol. **15:** 476–483.
19. DUFAYET DE LA TOUR, D. et al. 2000. Glucose-responsive insulin secretion from a human pancreatic β-cell line. Diabetes **49:** A31.
20. HALVORSEN, T. et al. 2000. *In vivo* glucose-responsive insulin secretion from a human pancreatic β-cell line. Diabetes **49:** A32.
21. BEATTIE, G.M. et al. 1999. Sustained proliferation of PDX-1+ cells derived from human islets. Diabetes **48:** 1013–1019.
22. SHIMIZU, H., C. SHIMIZU & J.C. BURNS. 1994. Detection of novel RNA viruses: morbilliviruses as a model system. Mol. Cell. Probes **8:** 209–214.
23. LAN, M. et al. 1999. mRNA profiling of pancreatic islets isolated from persistent hyperinsulinemic hypoglycemia of infancy (nesidioblastosis) reveals low amylin gene expression. Diabetes **48:** A246.
24. RAFAEL, E. et al. 2000. Longitudinal studies on the microcirculation around the TheraCyte immunoisolation device, using the laser Doppler technique. Cell Transplant. **9:** 107–113.
25. SANDER, M. et al. 2000. Homeobox gene Nkx6.1 lies downstream of Nkx2.2 in the major pathway of beta-cell formation in the pancreas. Development **127:** 5533–5540.
26. HAYEK, A. et al. 1995. Growth factor/matrix-induced proliferation of human adult beta-cells. Diabetes **44:** 1458–1460.
27. OLBROT, M. et al. 2002. Identification of beta-cell-specific insulin gene transcription factor RIPE3b1 as mammalian MafA. Proc. Natl. Acad. Sci. USA **99:** 6737–6742.
28. FERBER, S. et al. 2000. Pancreatic and duodenal homeobox gene 1 induces expression of insulin genes in liver and ameliorates streptozotocin-induced hyperglycemia [see comments]. Nat. Med. **6:** 568–572.

Islet Cell Autoimmunity and Transplantation Tolerance: Two Distinct Mechanisms?

TODD PEARSON,[a] THOMAS G. MARKEES,[b] DAVID V. SERREZE,[a,b,c]
MELISSA A. PIERCE,[c] LINDA S. WICKER,[d] LAURENCE B. PETERSON,[e]
LEONARD D. SHULTZ,[a,b,c] JOHN P. MORDES,[b] ALDO A. ROSSINI,[a,b,f]
AND DALE L. GREINER[a,b]

[a]*Program in Immunology and Virology, University of Massachusetts Medical School, Worcester, Massachusetts, USA*

[b]*Department of Medicine, University of Massachusetts Medical School, Worcester, Massachusetts, USA*

[c]*The Jackson Laboratory, Bar Harbor, Maine 04609, USA*

[d]*Juvenile Diabetes Research Foundation/Wellcome Trust Diabetes and Inflammation Laboratory, University of Cambridge, Cambridge, United Kingdom*

[e]*Department of Pharmacology, Merck Research Laboratories, Rahway, New Jersey, USA*

[f]*Program in Molecular Medicine, University of Massachusetts Medical School, Worcester, Massachusetts, USA*

> ABSTRACT: Recent advances in islet transplantation have enabled physicians to cure type 1 autoimmune diabetes, but at the cost of lifelong immunosuppression with its attendant side effects and long-term health risks. To eliminate the need for immunosuppression, researchers have developed methods for inducing tolerance to transplanted allografts. Tolerance-based transplantation using costimulation blockade has proven remarkably successful in many animal model systems. The most widely used animal model system for studying islet transplantation in type 1–like autoimmune diabetes is the NOD mouse. Unfortunately, this strain has proven resistant to costimulation blockade–based transplantation tolerance protocols that are successful in chemically diabetic mice given islet grafts. It has been assumed that resistance to transplantation tolerance in the NOD mouse is (1) related to autoimmunity directed against its pancreatic β cells, (2) a consequence of that autoimmunity, and (3) under the control of the same genes that control autoimmunity. In this review, we provide arguments to challenge these assumptions. We describe a new animal model and a new conceptual framework based on data indicating that the mechanisms responsible for resistance to transplantation tolerance and β cell autoimmunity are not identical. We believe that the recent discoveries we describe will have important implications for the development of tolerance-based transplantation therapies and their translation from the laboratory to the clinic.
>
> KEYWORDS: NOD mice; transplantation tolerance; costimulation blockade; CD154; type 1 diabetes

Address for correspondence: Aldo A. Rossini, M.D., Diabetes Division, University of Massachusetts Medical School, Two Biotech, Suite 218, 373 Plantation Street, Worcester, MA 01605. Voice: 508-856-3800; fax: 508-856-4093.
aldo.rossini@umassmed.edu

INTRODUCTION

Diabetes mellitus comprises a group of disorders characterized by hyperglycemia.[1] Most cases are classified as type 1 or type 2.[2] Both types can cause debilitating symptoms, predispose to infection, devastate pregnancy, and lead to many secondary complications. Type 1 diabetes is an autoimmune disease caused by T cell–mediated destruction of pancreatic beta cells. It occurs most commonly during childhood and results in absolute insulin deficiency. Patients with type 1 diabetes require exogenous insulin for survival, but insulin therapy never achieves perfect glucose regulation, and secondary complications of diabetes inevitably develop. The only alternative is transplantation of replacement beta cells, which would be curative.

Segmental pancreas transplantation can achieve normal glucose regulation and insulin independence, but requires major surgery and immunosuppression and has a substantial rate of postsurgical complications.[3] Transplantation of islets isolated from the pancreas would clearly be preferable because it is much less invasive. Successful islet transplantation for type 1 diabetes was first reported in 1990,[4] but until recently success rates were very low.

In 2000, however, researchers in Edmonton, Canada, demonstrated that transplantation of islets using a new regimen of preparation and immunosuppression could cure type 1 diabetes with a success rate that appeared to rival that of segmental pancreas transplantation.[5,6] Promising results for more than 30 patients were reported at the 2002 Meeting of the American Diabetes Association, and we have transplanted 2 patients using this protocol at our institution.

These successes have been encouraging, but islet transplantation to cure type 1 diabetes continues to require immunosuppressive drugs. These are medications with both detrimental side effects and potential long-term health risks. Although allograft recipients comprise a uniquely motivated group of patients, overall medication non-compliance rates reportedly vary from 20% to 50%.[7] In addition, many of these drugs have deleterious effects on the function of beta cells.[8] New formulations and treatment schedules have made immunosuppression safer and more effective than in the past, but diabetic patients considering pancreas or islet transplantation are still forced to choose between the risks of hyperglycemia and its complications on the one hand, and the risks and side effects of lifelong systemic immunosuppression on the other. Because of the risks, transplantation to ameliorate diabetes is primarily reserved for patients who have extremely labile glycemic control and severe recurrent hypoglycemia, or who have renal failure and need a kidney transplant. To make islet transplantation safe and more acceptable, research in transplantation is focused on developing alternatives to immunosuppression, most notably the induction of transplantation tolerance.[9]

MODELING AUTOIMMUNE DIABETES AND TRANSPLANTATION TOLERANCE IN SMALL ANIMALS

Rationale for Small Animal Models

The pathology and genetic basis of type 1 diabetes in humans have been studied extensively, but understanding of type 1 diabetes remains incomplete. The disease is under polygenic control and penetrance is modified by environmental factors; identifying at risk individuals is difficult.[10] In addition, studying disease in humans in general and children in particular poses serious ethical limitations, especially when considering a therapeutic intervention like an experimental transplantation procedure. Fortunately, reliable animal model systems are available that allow us to analyze the pathogenesis of autoimmune diabetes,[11] the induction of transplantation tolerance,[9] and the special problem of tolerance induction in the setting of autoimmunity.[12]

NOD Mouse Model of Type 1–like Diabetes Mellitus

The two best-characterized animal models of type 1 diabetes are the BioBreeding (BB) rat and the nonobese diabetic (NOD) mouse. The diabetic syndromes of the BB rat and NOD mouse have been reviewed extensively.[11,13–15] Both species have been used for studies of autoimmune pathogenesis and islet transplantation. Because the NOD mouse has both a well-defined genetic basis and readily available genetically modified stocks, we have chosen to study the problem of transplantation tolerance in the setting of autoimmunity in this model.

NOD mice develop insulitis when 4 to 5 weeks old. By 7 months of age, 90% of female and 60% of male mice become diabetic.[11] Diabetes in NOD mice is an autoimmune disorder mediated by autoreactive T cells. Immune defects in NOD mice that may have counterparts in humans with type 1 diabetes include defects in regulatory $CD4^+CD25^+$ T cells and NKT cells. Defects in $CD4^+CD25^+$ T cells may also lead to resistance to transplantation tolerance induction.[16] Deficiencies in NKT cell function are reportedly present in identical twins and triplets with type 1 diabetes and absent in their discordant siblings,[17] but the role of such defects in diabetes pathogenesis has been questioned.[18] Additional immune system defects in NOD mice include a lack of hemolytic complement, defects in NK cells, abnormalities in APC function, and an abnormal T cell population.[19]

To identify the immune defects responsible for autoimmunity in NOD mice, investigators have utilized a genetic approach. More than 27 diabetes susceptibility (*Idd*) loci have been identified,[11] and many genes important in immune system function map to these loci.[20] To date, the only non-MHC diabetes susceptibility gene identified in the NOD mouse is β2-microglobulin,[21] which dimerizes with MHC class I heavy chains; the other genes remain to be identified.[11]

Modeling Costimulation Blockade–Based Transplantation Tolerance

The transplantation of pancreata[3] and islets[22] using immunosuppression are clinical procedures that were prototyped in animals. Development of transplantation strategies that do not require immunosuppression is similarly based on animal experimentation. Findings that translate reproducibly from animals to humans are based on a detailed understanding of the mechanisms responsible for immune responses.[15]

Several transplantation tolerance protocols prolong allograft survival in normal inbred strains of mice.[9] The strategies typically involve blockade of (1) TCR-MHC/peptide interaction, (2) costimulatory CD40-CD154 interaction, or (3) CD80/86-CD28 interaction. These protocols can be used either to prevent activation of alloreactive peripheral T cells (peripheral tolerance) or to establish hematopoietic chimerism (central tolerance).[9]

In our laboratory, we have developed a two-element protocol that consists of a single transfusion of donor spleen cells (a donor-specific transfusion or DST) and a brief course of anti-CD154 mAb.[9] We hypothesize that this protocol operates through the following mechanism: (1) donor-origin resting APCs first engage the TCR of alloantigen-specific T cells; (2) anti-CD154 mAb then prevents ligand engagement of CD40 on the resting APCs, (3) thereby preventing the upregulation of B7 costimulatory molecules, MHC class II, and cytokine production. This protocol results in permanent islet and prolonged skin allograft survival in normal mouse strains[9] and nonhuman primates.[23] We have determined that the mechanism requires the elimination of alloreactive $CD8^+$ T cells from the circulation in a CTLA-4-dependent manner, the presence of $CD4^+$ T cells, and the secretion of IFNγ, but not IL-4 or IL-10.[24,25]

Costimulation Blockade–Based Transplantation Tolerance Induction in NOD Mice

Having documented the efficacy of tolerance induction for islet transplantation in chemically diabetic mice, the next logical step was to determine its applicability in NOD mice that develop autoimmune diabetes. The results were disappointing. Studies performed by us[12] and others[26] demonstrated that syngeneic and allogeneic islet grafts are rapidly destroyed in spontaneously diabetic NOD mice when treated with protocols that induce permanent islet graft survival in strains not prone to autoimmunity. Given that more than 100 therapies can protect NOD mice from diabetes,[27] the failure to induce transplantation tolerance in this strain was remarkable.

The outcome raised the question of whether the rejection of transplanted islets was due to inability to induce allotolerance or ongoing autoimmunity. Tolerance induction experiments in prediabetic male NOD mice using skin allografts, a tissue that is not the target of autoimmune attack in this model, suggested that the NOD mouse has a generalized defect in its response to transplantation tolerance induction.[12]

Does Autoimmunity Prevent Costimulation Blockade–Based Transplantation Tolerance?

A common belief is that the generalized defect in transplantation tolerance in the NOD mouse is a result of and/or controlled by the same genes that predispose it to autoimmunity (FIG. 1). This assumption has seemed reasonable because many transplantation interventions target parts of the immune system that are abnormal in NOD mice or are known to map to *Idd* loci. Examples include CTLA-4, which is often a target of tolerance-based protocols. We propose that the resistance of NOD mice to costimulation blockade–based transplantation tolerance and autoimmune diabetes are two distinct defects, possibly controlled by distinct genetic mechanisms.

Using **Idd** Congenic Strains to Analyze the Resistance of NOD Mice to Costimulation Blockade–Based Transplantation Tolerance

Congenic inbred NOD strains bearing diabetes resistance alleles at one or a few loci and reciprocal congenic strains harboring NOD-derived *Idd* susceptibility alleles on a normal background have been generated and studied extensively.[11,20,28] These stocks have allowed investigators to dissect the contribution of individual loci to the

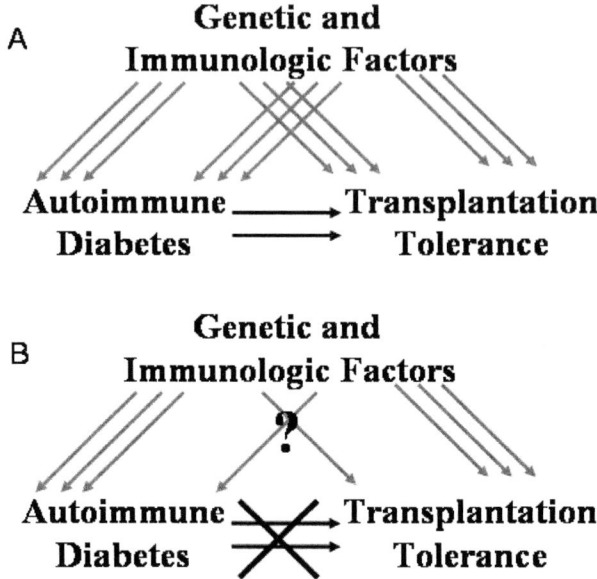

FIGURE 1. (**A**) This diagram depicts the traditionally held assumption that resistance to transplantation tolerance in NOD mice is a result of ongoing autoimmunity and/or controlled by the same genetic and immunologic factors that mediate type 1 diabetes. (**B**) A new way of thinking about autoimmunity and transplantation tolerance in the NOD mouse. Our new data suggest that the ongoing autoimmune process does not cause resistance to transplantation tolerance induction. Further studies are required to determine if the genetic basis of the two phenotypes, autoimmunity and transplantation tolerance, overlap or are completely distinct.

polygenic disease process. The congenic introgression of small numbers of resistance alleles to the NOD background can profoundly alter diabetes susceptibility. Such congenic stocks can be virtually diabetes-free. *Idd1*, which includes the NOD $H2^{g7}$ MHC haplotype on chromosome 17, is the most powerful susceptibility locus and is orthologous to *IDDM1* in humans.[11,20] *Idd1* is necessary, but not sufficient, for the development of type 1 diabetes in the mouse; NOD mice congenic for a non-$H2^{g7}$ haplotype and non-NOD strains that express the $H2^{g7}$ haplotype are both completely protected from disease.[11,20,28] Extending this paradigm to transplantation tolerance induction, we have shown that neither the congenic introgression of a non-NOD *H2* haplotype nor the reciprocal introgression of the NOD $H2^{g7}$ on the C57BL/6 background was able to restore or abrogate transplantation tolerance induction to skin allografts, respectively.[12]

NOD Congenic Mice Genetically Protected from Autoimmune Diabetes Remain Resistant to Transplantation Tolerance

To test the hypothesis that autoimmune diabetes and transplantation tolerance are controlled by overlapping sets of genes, we studied NOD *Idd* congenic strains. We hypothesized that if the two phenotypes are controlled by the same genes, then

TABLE 1. Qualitative summary of unpublished quantitative skin allograft survival data

Graft recipient	Partial list of candidate *Idd* loci	Diabetes[a]	Allograft survival[b]
C57BL/6	—	0	Prolonged
NOD/Lt	—	90	Short
NOD.B10*Idd9*	*Cd30, Cd137, Tnfr2*	3	Short
NOD.B6*Idd3*	*Il2, Il-21, Fgf2*	20	Short
NOD.B10*Idd5*	*Idd5.1*: *Cd152, Cd28, Casp8, Flip*; *Idd5.2*: *Cxcr2, Il-8r*	40	Short
NOD.B6*Idd3*B10*Idd5*	See *Idd3* and *Idd5* above	1	Short
C57BL/6.NODclt	See *Idd5.1* and *Idd5.2* above	0	Prolonged
C57BL/6.NODc6	*nkrp1* (NKR-P1 complex)	0	Prolonged
(NOD × C57BL/6)F1	Heterozygous at all loci	0	Short

[a]Diabetes prevalence in females at 7 months of age.
[b]Skin allograft survival in mice treated with DST plus anti-CD154 mAb as described: short, median survival time (MST) < 32 days; prolonged, MST > 75 days.

genetic attenuation of type 1 diabetes susceptibility in NOD congenic stocks should abrogate resistance to transplantation tolerance. The null hypothesis (the two defects are controlled by different genetic loci or a greater number of *Idd* resistance alleles are required for transplant tolerance) was that genetically improving islet self-tolerance and preventing diabetes should not concomitantly improve the response of NOD mice to transplantation tolerance induction.

We tested this hypothesis using NOD congenic strains bearing the most protective *Idd* loci and, conversely, C57BL/6 mice bearing the highest susceptibility *Idd* loci.[29] These congenic strains and their prevalence of diabetes at age 7 months are listed in TABLE 1. Also shown is the relative duration of skin allograft survival in these mice after treatment with DST plus anti-CD154 mAb, our costimulation blockade protocol for tolerance induction. As expected, skin allograft survival was prolonged on tolerized C57BL/6 mice and short on tolerized NOD mice (TABLE 1).[12,29] Surprisingly, NOD mice bearing very protective *Idd* loci remained resistant to tolerance induction and rejected skin allografts rapidly.[29] These included, for example, the NOD.B6 *Idd3* B10 *Idd5* and NOD.B10 *Idd9* stocks, which have rates of spontaneous diabetes of 1% and 3% (TABLE 1), respectively. Other NOD *Idd* congenic strains responded similarly (TABLE 1). Complementing the NOD congenic data, skin allograft survival on reciprocal C57BL/6 stocks harboring NOD-derived *Idd* susceptibility loci was comparable to that observed in wild-type C57BL/6 mice (TABLE 1).[29] Overall, these data demonstrate that the defective transplantation tolerance observed in the NOD mouse is not dependent on concurrent active autoimmunity or a consequence of autoimmune beta cell destruction.

In regard to the genetic control of autoimmunity versus the genetic control of tolerance induction to skin grafts, these data can be interpreted at least two ways. First, the genes that mediate the breakdown of self-tolerance leading to diabetes in the NOD mouse may be distinct from those that mediate resistance to transplantation tolerance. Alternatively, self-tolerance and transplantation tolerance may be controlled by the same genetic pathways, but at different "set points". The latter interpretation implies that one or a few *Idd* loci can profoundly alter diabetes prevalence, whereas a larger cohort of resistance loci or some unique combination of loci is required to induce transplantation tolerance.

(NOD × C57BL/6)F1 Hybrids Are Resistant to Transplantation Tolerance Induction

It is possible to argue that the diabetes-resistant NOD congenic strains resisted transplantation tolerance because of an underlying occult autoimmune process that led to overt diabetes in only a small number of individuals. To address this possibility, we generated (NOD × C57BL/6)F1 mice. These F1 mice are completely resistant to diabetes, even when a C57BL/6.$H2^{g7}$ parent is used to generate hybrid progeny homozygous for the diabetogenic MHC $H2^{g7}$ haplotype. Additionally, these hybrids are heterozygous for all *Idd* loci, the majority of which are NOD recessive susceptibility loci,[11,20] thereby providing us with a mouse with a highly self-tolerant state in which to study transplantation tolerance induction. Surprisingly, we observed that skin allograft survival in tolerized (NOD × C57BL/6)F1 mice was brief (TABLE 1). Thus, rendering an NOD-related strain completely free from diabetes by having it heterozygous at all *Idd* loci was not sufficient to restore transplantation tolerance. The fact that the autoimmune phenotype and the transplantation tolerance phenotype are differentially inherited in (NOD × C57BL/6)F1 hybrids suggests that an ongoing autoimmune process, even one with low penetrance as measured by diabetes, is not responsible for the failure of tolerance induction in NOD mice.

We next asked which of the immune defects in NOD mice described above are expressed in (NOD × C57BL/6)F1 mice, given that both are resistant to tolerance induction. In preliminary studies, we discovered that both dendritic cell maturation and the response of $CD4^+$ and $CD8^+$ T cells to costimulation blockade are defective in (NOD × C57BL/6)F1 mice, as they are in NOD mice. In contrast, however, we also observed that defects in macrophage maturation, previously postulated to be associated with the resistance of NOD mice to transplantation tolerance,[12] appear to be normal in (NOD × C57BL/6)F1 mice. In addition, natural killer cell activity, defective in NOD mice, is normal in (NOD × C57BL/6)F1 mice (T. Pearson, unpublished observations). Hence, at least two immune defects (in macrophages and NK cells) have been dissected away from the resistance of NOD mice to transplantation tolerance.

To assess whether the genes that determine autoimmunity and resistance to transplantation tolerance are distinct or overlapping, we are performing a genome-wide scan. We are generating N2 generation mice by backcrossing (NOD × C57BL/6)F1 mice to the tolerance-susceptible C57BL/6 strain; these N2 mice are then treated with DST and anti-CD154 mAb and the duration of skin allograft survival is measured. Identification of the quantitative trait loci (QTLs) that control the duration of graft survival will allow us to localize dominant NOD-derived genes and to determine if these coincide with the location of previously defined *Idd* genes or if new genes are resolved. We may discover new chromosomal regions that contain genes that control only the transplantation tolerance defect of NOD mice, but it is equally likely that these new regions may contain previously unknown dominant NOD-derived *Idd* genes. Previous *Idd* mapping strategies using the diabetes-resistant C57BL/10 and C57BL/6 strains involved an F1 backcross to the NOD strain in which dominant

NOD *Idd* susceptibility genes could not have been detected.[20] The genome scan strategy is particularly advantageous in comparison with testing existing *Idd* congenic strains for tolerance induction because it is unbiased. Using it, we will eventually be able to map and narrow the chromosomal intervals that control transplantation tolerance.

IMPLICATIONS FOR THE FUTURE OF TOLERANCE-BASED ISLET TRANSPLANTATION

Understanding the relationship between transplantation tolerance and autoimmunity represents an important area of research with implications for curing type 1 diabetes by islet transplantation. The assumption that autoimmunity and transplantation tolerance in NOD mice are controlled by the same genes may be incorrect, and our current research is directed at answering this question.

An immediate implication of the current findings concerns the way in which investigators evaluate tolerance induction protocols eventually intended for the clinic. If those protocols are evaluated in the NOD mouse, it must be asked if the defect in transplantation tolerance seen in these animals represents a defect that is likely to be encountered in people with type 1 diabetes or if it is a unique abnormality restricted to this mouse model. If the latter should prove true, this raises questions about the utility of the NOD mouse for modeling costimulation blockade–based transplantation tolerance induction in type 1 diabetes. Alternatively, the genome-wide scan for transplantation tolerance QTLs may lead to the identification of human orthologues, much like the *Idd-IDDM* orthologous diabetes loci. In this event, we envision the development of more advanced therapies that take into account the specific *IDDM* alleles, transplantation tolerance alleles, and *HLA* haplotype when a person with type 1 diabetes is evaluated for a curative islet graft in the clinic.

REFERENCES

1. ROSSINI, A.A. & J.P. MORDES. 1994. Diabetes mellitus. *In* Office Practice of Medicine, pp. 558–590. Saunders. Philadelphia.
2. GABIR, M.M., R.L. HANSON, D. DABELEA *et al.* 2000. The 1997 American Diabetes Association and 1999 World Health Organization criteria for hyperglycemia in the diagnosis and prediction of diabetes. Diabetes Care **23:** 1108–1112.
3. SUTHERLAND, D.E.R., R.W.G. GRUESSNER & A.C. GRUESSNER. 2001. Pancreas transplantation for treatment of diabetes mellitus. World J. Surg. **25:** 487–496.
4. SCHARP, D.W., P.E. LACY, J.V. SANTIAGO *et al.* 1990. Insulin independence after islet transplantation into type I diabetic patient. Diabetes **39:** 515–518.
5. SHAPIRO, A.M.J., J.R.T. LAKEY, E.A. RYAN *et al.* 2000. Islet transplantation in seven patients with type 1 diabetes mellitus using a glucocorticoid-free immunosuppressive regimen. N. Engl. J. Med. **343:** 230–238.
6. RYAN, E.A., J.R.T. LAKEY, B.W. PATY *et al.* 2002. Successful islet transplantation—continued insulin reserve provides long-term glycemic control. Diabetes **51:** 2148–2157.
7. LAEDERACH-HOFMANN, K. & B. BUNZEL. 2000. Noncompliance in organ transplant recipients: a literature review. Gen. Hosp. Psychiatry **22:** 412–424.
8. LOHMANN, T., C. LIST, P. LAMESCH *et al.* 2000. Diabetes mellitus and islet cell specific autoimmunity as adverse effects of immunosuppressive therapy by FK506/Tacrolimus. Exp. Clin. Endocrinol. Diabetes **108:** 347–352.

9. ROSSINI, A.A., D.L. GREINER & J.P. MORDES. 1999. Induction of immunological tolerance for transplantation. Physiol. Rev. **79:** 99–141.
10. LIU, E. & G.S. EISENBARTH. 2002. Type 1A diabetes mellitus–associated autoimmunity. Endocrinol. Metab. Clin. North Am. **31:** 391–410.
11. MORDES, J.P., D.V. SERREZE, D.L. GREINER & A.A. ROSSINI. 2003. Animal models of autoimmune diabetes mellitus: a fundamental and clinical text. In press.
12. MARKEES, T.G., D.V. SERREZE, N.E. PHILLIPS et al. 1999. NOD mice have a generalized defect in their response to transplantation tolerance induction. Diabetes **48:** 967–974.
13. MORDES, J.P., R. BORTELL, H. GROEN et al. 2001. Autoimmune diabetes mellitus in the BB rat. In Animal Models of Diabetes: A Primer. Vol. 2, pp. 1–41. Harwood Academic Pub. Amsterdam.
14. SERREZE, D.V. & E.H. LEITER. 2001. Genes and pathways underlying autoimmune diabetes in NOD mice. In Molecular Pathology of Insulin Dependent Diabetes Mellitus, p. 31. Karger. New York.
15. GREINER, D.L., A.A. ROSSINI & J.P. MORDES. 2001. Translating data from animal models into methods for preventing human autoimmune diabetes mellitus: *caveat emptor* and *primum non nocere*. Clin. Immunol. **100:** 134–143.
16. HARA, M., C.I. KINGSLEY, M. NIIMI et al. 2001. IL-10 is required for regulatory T cells to mediate tolerance to alloantigens *in vivo*. J. Immunol. **166:** 3789–3796.
17. WILSON, S.B., S.C. KENT, K.T. PATTON et al. 1998. Extreme Th1 bias of invariant $V\alpha24J\alpha Q$ T cells in type 1 diabetes. Nature **391:** 177–181.
18. LEE, P.T., A. PUTNAM, K. BENLAGHA et al. 2002. Testing the NKT cell hypothesis of human IDDM pathogenesis. J. Clin. Invest. **110:** 793–800.
19. LEITER, E.H. 1998. NOD mice and related strains: origins, husbandry, and biology. In NOD Mice and Related Strains: Research Applications in Diabetes, AIDS, Cancer, and Other Diseases, pp. 1–36. Landes. Austin.
20. TODD, J.A. & L.S. WICKER. 2001. Genetic protection from the inflammatory disease type 1 diabetes in humans and animal models. Immunity **15:** 387–395.
21. HAMILTON-WILLIAMS, E.E., D.V. SERREZE, B. CHARLTON et al. 2001. Transgenic rescue implicates β_2-microglobulin as a diabetes susceptibility gene in nonobese diabetic (NOD) mice. Proc. Natl. Acad. Sci. USA **98:** 11533–11538.
22. RYAN, E.A., J.R.T. LAKEY, R.V. RAJOTTE et al. 2001. Clinical outcomes and insulin secretion after islet transplantation with the Edmonton protocol. Diabetes **50:** 710–719.
23. ELSTER, E.A., H. XU, D.K. TADAKI et al. 2001. Treatment with the humanized CD154-specific monoclonal antibody, hu5C8, prevents acute rejection of primary skin allografts in nonhuman primates. Transplantation **72:** 1473–1478.
24. IWAKOSHI, N.N., T.G. MARKEES, N.A. TURGEON et al. 2001. Skin allograft maintenance in a new synchimeric model system of tolerance. J. Immunol. **167:** 6623–6630.
25. MARKEES, T.G., N.E. PHILLIPS, E.J. GORDON et al. 1998. Long-term survival of skin allografts induced by donor splenocytes and anti-CD154 antibody in thymectomized mice requires $CD4^+$ T cells, interferon-gamma, and CTLA4. J. Clin. Invest. **101:** 2446–2455.
26. MOLANO, R.D., T. BERNEY, H. LI et al. 2001. Prolonged islet graft survival in NOD mice by blockade of the CD40-CD154 pathway of T-cell costimulation. Diabetes **50:** 270–276.
27. ATKINSON, M. & E.H. LEITER. 1999. The NOD mouse model of insulin dependent diabetes: as good as it gets? Nat. Med. **5:** 601–604.
28. YUI, M.A., K. MURALIDHARAN, B. MORENO-ALTAMIRANO et al. 1996. Production of congenic mouse strains carrying NOD-derived diabetogenic genetic intervals: an approach for the genetic dissection of complex traits. Mamm. Genome **7:** 331–334.
29. PEARSON, T., T.G. MARKEES, L.S. WICKER et al. 2003. NOD congenic mice genetically protected from autoimmune diabetes remain resistant to transplantation tolerance induction. Diabetes **52:** 321–326.

Characterization of Early Developments in the Splenic Leukocyte Transcriptome of NOD Mice

I. C. GERLING, C. ALI, AND N. LENCHIK

Department of Medicine, University of Tennessee Health Science Center, and Research Service, Veterans Affairs Medical Center, Memphis, Tennessee, USA

ABSTRACT: Transcriptome analysis is a powerful tool to characterize changes in leukocyte gene expression patterns and reveal very early molecular abnormalities in tissue. Herein, we report on characterization of the very earliest abnormalities in the transcriptome of leukocytes from young "prepathologic" NOD and NON female mice.

KEYWORDS: diabetes; NOD; transcriptome; autoimmune; T cell

INTRODUCTION

The very earliest histological signs of autoimmunity in NOD females occur at approximately 4 weeks of age.[1] We hypothesized that defects associated with initiation of these pathological events may show up in the molecular signatures of spleen leukocytes. We have previously reported on changes in the spleen leukocyte proteome of young NOD and NON females.[2] Herein, we report on characterization of the very earliest abnormalities in the transcriptome of leukocytes from young "prepathologic" NOD and NON females.

METHODS

We isolated spleen leukocytes from NOD and NON females at 2 and 4 weeks of age. Each of the 4 samples consisted of a pool of cells from 5 individual animals. Spleen leukocytes were isolated on a Histopaque gradient (Sigma, MO), treated with a red blood cell lysing buffer, and washed, and the total RNA was isolated using a trireagent (Invitrogen, CA).

A core facility at our institution conducted characterization of the spleen cell transcriptomes using the MG_U7Aav2 chip from Affymetrix (www.affymetrix.com). This chip allows highly reproducible measurements of expression levels of 6000 known mouse genes and 6000 EST sequences. The quality of the data is ensured by using 32 different oligonucleotides (probe sets) for each gene/EST placed in different

Address for correspondence: Dr. Ivan C. Gerling, Ph.D., University of Tennessee Health Science Center, VAMC, Research 151, 1030 Jefferson Avenue, Memphis, TN 38104. Voice: 901-523-8990 (ext. 5088); fax: 901-577-7273.
igerling@utmem.edu

areas of the chip. Normalization of data, evaluation of quality of the data sets, and basic comparisons between data are conducted using software from Affymetrix. The MAS 5.0 software was used to individually compare the transcriptome data from the spleen sample of 4-week-old NOD females (NOD4wk) to each of the 3 other samples (NOD2wk, NON4wk, and NON2wk). For each of these 3 comparisons, we requested a list of all genes that were differentially expressed at a magnitude of no less than $1.0 \times \log 2$ and $p < 0.01$.

RESULTS

Each query for the 12,000 probe sets produced lists of 223–250 differentially expressed genes/ESTs. We consolidated the data further by producing a list of genes/ESTs differentially expressed in the same direction in all 3 comparisons (A3 pattern) or in 2 of the 3 comparisons, and with at least a 1.5-fold difference in the same direction for the remaining comparisons (A2 pattern). This produced a list of 24 probe sets following the A3 pattern and 33 probe sets following the A2 pattern. TABLE 1 shows the 15 "A3 pattern" and 22 "A2 pattern" probe sets that were uniquely increased in the 4-week-old NOD females. The table first gives the GenBank accession number that the probe set was constructed to match, then the expression level in each of the 4 samples, and finally the name of the gene product. If the probe set represents an expressed sequence tag (EST), we conducted a search of the EST against current databases using tBLASTx (www.ncbi.nlm.nih.gov) to identify matching genes.

The overall pattern of increased gene expression in NOD4wk indicates a strong activation of T cell immune responses compared to both NOD2wk and the NON females of either age (CD3, CD8, CD28, ZAP70). Specific TCR genes activated include Vβ8.2, V11.1d, a TCR specific for the A-chain of insulin, and a VDJ region of a TCR originally defined by its reactivity with pigeon cytochrome C (clone 7.9R.1F8). Although there were no clear indications of any generalized B cell activation, we did see two specific immunoglobulin genes increased in NOD4wk: one from a light chain variable region and one from an anti-DNA autoantibody.

There were no obvious patterns or functional grouping of the 20 probe sets that were downregulated in NOD4wk (data not shown). Thirty-five percent (7/20) of those probe sets represented unidentified ESTs, with only 1 of the 20 transcripts being unique for lymphocytes (IgD fragment).

CONCLUSIONS

We conclude that transcriptome analysis is a powerful tool to characterize changes in leukocyte gene expression patterns and reveal very early molecular abnormalities in tissue. Although some of the immune activation changes found were previously revealed by hypothesis-driven investigations, others were completely new and unexpected, and would be highly unlikely to ever have been discovered using the traditional hypothesis-driven approach.

TABLE 1. Genes with increased expression in leukocytes from 4-week-old NOD mice

GenBank acces. no.	Gene expression level				Name of gene product
	NOD4wk	NOD2wk	NON4wk	NON2wk	
U34881	212.0	11.9	11.1	21.4	CD8 α chain
M18228	795.2	262.4	148.4	52.7	CD3 γ chain
X02339	562.1	139.1	170.5	102.3	CD3 δ chain
AI019193	1332.3	424.5	423.3	254.3	EST: T cell transc. fact. 1
M16118	1216.0	328.2	446.0	43.0	α chain TCR anti-insulin
AF099808	2353.2	793.4	850.7	455.1	α chain TCR V11.1d
M26056	3470.8	913.8	1207.1	481.5	β chain TCR const. region
M20878	590.7	161.7	147.4	54.9	TCR VDJ clone 7.9R.1F8
X04653	1224.2	602.7	312.5	98.1	T cell act. prot. Ly-6E.1
U37543	416.3	51.5	69.7	7.5	CD6, T cell, B cell subset
L12367	355.1	219.0	99.6	45.1	CAP ad. cycl.–assoc. prot.
M12379	724.8	284.7	67.9	63.8	CD90 (Thy-1.2 glycoprot.)
M22531	199.9	85.5	21.4	16.3	Complement C1q B-ch.
AV336804	232.1	38.7	84.6	41.3	EST: PKC θ
AA182189	120.4	20.6	34.3	7.8	EST: no match
J04967	110.3	36.8	63.6	48.2	CD3 ζ chain
X61385	364.3	133.3	222.7	121.1	T cell transc. fact. 1
U04379	419.0	144.2	156.2	13.6	ZAP70, TCR ζ assoc.
AI386093	715.1	316.1	427.6	191.6	EST: ZAP70
L37871	178.2	102.2	128.3	46.5	TCR β ch. variable 8.2
L38444	301.4	94.5	164.3	98.0	T cell specific protein
D14042	400.5	158.4	259.4	122.6	T cell tyrosine kinase
M12056	1339.4	720.3	585.1	269.4	Lck, lymph. spec. kinase
M34563	162.7	36.0	97.0	46.3	CD28, T cell activation
AF014941	243.0	44.0	25.4	12.2	Cathepsin W
AF097357	198.9	4.9	79.5	16.9	KLRG1
M15177	399.6	244.0	135.2	102.9	CD5
U55585	1301.9	342.8	275.0	95.1	Anti-DNA antibody
M86751	150.6	71.9	55.8	42.5	Ig light variable region
M63630	549.2	207.1	359.2	211.5	IRG-47
V00727	2309.9	668.9	1296.2	609.2	C-FOS
M84487	430.9	258.5	161.9	121.7	VCAM1
AB020808	466.3	268.8	220.9	156.1	Toll-like receptor 6
AF000236	99.5	57.8	54.4	18.7	Chemokine orphan rec. 1
M90388	1107.9	311.0	522.8	719.0	70Z-PEP
X92523	183.8	87.8	36.1	96.5	Calpain 3
AF085219	1232.6	826.7	629.8	487.4	α-Diacylglycerol kinase

NOTE: A list of the transcripts (listed by GenBank assession no. corresponding to the probe set) found at increased levels in pooled spleen leukocytes from 4-week-old NOD females (NOD4wk) compared to 2-week-old NOD and NON females of either age. Expression levels are given in normalized fluorescent units. The first 15 transcripts are genes for which transcript levels in NOD4wk were significantly increased ($p < 0.01$) at >1.5-fold compared to all other samples. In the remaining 22 samples, 1 of the 3 comparisons were not significant, although the value was >1.5-fold higher in NOD4wk.

REFERENCES

1. THOMAS, H.E. & T.W. KAY. 2000. Beta cell destruction in the development of autoimmune diabetes in the non-obese diabetic (NOD) mouse. Diabetes Metab. Res. Rev. **16**(4): 251–261.
2. GERLING, I.C. *et al.* 2002. Characterization of proteome developments in peripheral leukocytes of young NOD female mice [abstract]. Diabetes **51**(suppl. 2): A285.

Autoimmune Diabetes in the NOD Mouse: An Essential Role of Fas-FasL Signaling in β Cell Apoptosis

DIEGO G. SILVA,[a,b] LUIS SOCHA,[a,b] BRETT CHARLTON,[b] WILLIAM COWDEN,[b] AND NIKOLAI PETROVSKY[a,b]

[a]*Autoimmunity Research Unit, The Canberra Hospital, Canberra, Australia*

[b]*John Curtin School of Medical Research, Canberra, Australia*

ABSTRACT: Despite evidence that both Fas and FasL can be expressed in pancreatic islets, there has been considerable controversy regarding the potential role of Fas signaling in autoimmune β cell death. Using the HIPFasL model, we have been able to demonstrate that, in the presence of an inflammatory infiltrate, FasL-expressing β cells are exquisitely sensitive to Fas-mediated apoptosis and that this can be blocked by preventing FasL-Fas interaction. This points to a highly important role of Fas-FasL interaction in autoimmune β cell death.

KEYWORDS: Fas ligand; autoimmunity; type 1 diabetes; NOD; apoptosis

INTRODUCTION

Autoimmune diabetes of the NOD mouse is characterized by destruction of pancreatic β cells by a process of programmed cell death, also called apoptosis.[1] Multiple signaling pathways can lead to apoptosis, mainly working through activation of cell surface molecules such as the TNF and Fas receptors, both of which belong to the TNF receptor superfamily. Binding of Fas (CD95) to its ligand (FasL) triggers a series of downstream events including activation of the caspase pathway and this ultimately leads to DNA fragmentation and apoptotic cell death. Despite evidence, as detailed below, that both Fas and FasL can be expressed in pancreatic islets, there has been considerable controversy regarding the potential role of Fas signaling in autoimmune β cell death. Fas is expressed by mouse and human β cells after stimulation with inflammatory cytokines (e.g., IFN-γ, IL-1, and/or TNF-α).[2–4] FasL is also present on islet cells[5,6] and, by dual labeling studies, has been shown to be expressed by β cells of diabetic NOD mice and nondiabetic C57BL/6 mice.[7] FasL is also expressed by islet-infiltrating inflammatory cells and by islet α cells.[5]

Address for correspondence: Professor Nikolai Petrovsky, Head, Autoimmunity Research Unit, The Canberra Hospital, P.O. Box 11, Woden ACT 2606, Australia. Voice: +612-62442595; fax: +612-62603372.

nikolai.petrovsky@anu.edu.au

HIPFasL TRANSGENIC MICE

In confirmation of the importance of Fas-FasL interaction in the development of autoimmune diabetes, NOD mice where FasL is transgenically expressed on the β cell surface (HIPFasL mice) demonstrate pronounced β cell destruction and accelerated diabetes.[2,8a] HIPFasL mice demonstrate a mononuclear cell islet infiltrate with associated β cell destruction, similar to the picture seen in spontaneous diabetes of the NOD mouse.[8b] Diabetes was not seen when the HIPFasL transgene was crossed onto various nondiabetes-prone strains including C57BL/6 mice, indicating that the NOD background was necessary for the FasL transgene to mediate diabetes.[8b] Similarly, HIPFasL mice with the SCID mutation, which have no T cells, were also protected against diabetes. The above findings suggest that the FasL transgene only mediates β cell death in the context of an inflammatory cell islet infiltrate such as occurs in all NOD mice even in the absence of overt diabetes.

SUSCEPTIBILITY OF HIPFasL ISLETS TO IMMUNE DESTRUCTION *IN VIVO*

From the above results, we hypothesized that HIPFasL β cells have an increased susceptibility to apoptosis, but only in the event of exposure of HIPFasL β cells to an inflammatory environment capable of upregulating β cell Fas expression. Coexpression of Fas and FasL would then rapidly lead to β cell suicide or fratricide. This would explain why HIPFasLSCID mice, which have no insulitis or T cell–derived cytokines, do not develop diabetes.[8b] We decided, therefore, to test the relative susceptibility of HIPFasL and nontransgenic NOD islets to destruction when exposed to a mononuclear infiltrate after grafting into nondiabetic NOD mice. HIPFasL and nontransgenic NOD islets were grafted at either end of the kidney capsule of 70-day-old NOD mice. The kidneys were then removed 60 days later and the degree of preservation or destruction of the HIPFasL and nontransgenic NOD grafts compared. Macroscopically, NOD grafts were vascularized and showed a normal graft structure, whereas the HIPFasL grafts showed all the features of destructive insulitis with the graft site being swollen and the normal graft morphology lost (FIGS. 1a and 1c). While hematoxylin-and-eosin and insulin staining revealed mononuclear cellular infiltrate in both HIPFasL and NOD islet grafts, the HIPFasL islet grafts had evidence of widespread destruction with an intra-islet infiltrate and loss of islet architecture. By comparison, nontransgenic NOD grafts revealed minimal islet destruction (FIGS. 1b and 1d).

SUSCEPTIBILITY OF HIPFasL/NOD ISLETS TO CYTOKINE-INDUCED APOPTOSIS

The question then arose as to whether the cellular infiltrate in the islets was necessary for FasL-mediated β cell death or, alternatively, whether it is simply the cytokines produced by this infiltrate that were necessary. As Fas expression is known to be induced on β cells by incubation in IFN-γ and IL-1,[9] we next asked whether HIPFasL β cells were more susceptible to cytokine-induced apoptosis than NOD

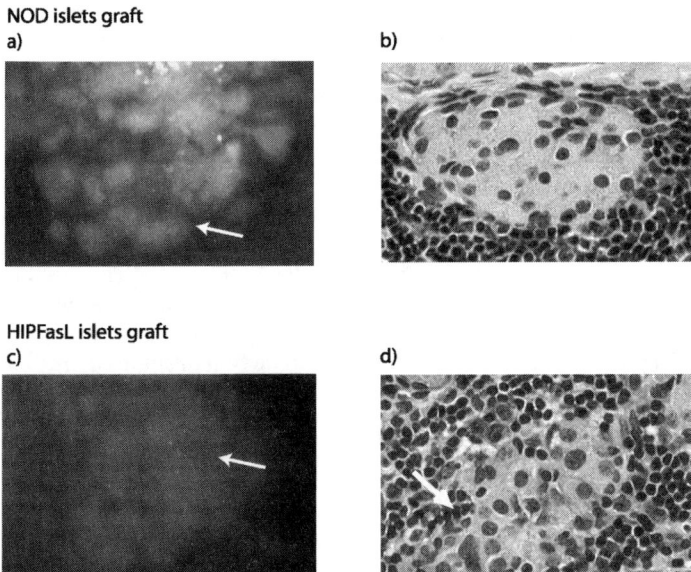

FIGURE 1. HIPFasL and NOD islets were cotransplanted under the kidney capsule of 70-day-old NOD mice and harvested 60 days later. Grafts from NOD donors (**a, b**) were clearly identified, with macroscopic (**a**) and microscopic (**b**) characteristics of nondestructive lesions. In contrast, HIPFasL islet grafts (**c, d**) showed signs of destructive lesions: grafts were cloudy and with no well-defined islets (**c**) and showed intra-islet infiltrate with islet destruction (**d**). The figure shows one representative animal.

β cell islets and, if so, whether this increased apoptosis could be blocked by FasL-neutralizing antibody. Islets were isolated from HIPFasL mice and nontransgenic NOD controls, and cultured at 30 islets/well for 24 h in the presence or absence of IL-1β and IFN-γ. The percentage of apoptotic HIPFasL β cells after 24 h of cytokine stimulation was approximately three times that of nontransgenic NOD β cells, indicating that β cells from HIPFasL-positive mice are indeed highly susceptible to cytokine-induced apoptosis compared to nontransgenic NOD β cells.[8b] Furthermore, the increased cytokine-induced apoptosis of HIPFasL β cells was prevented by the addition of neutralizing antibody to FasL (MFL3 clone), confirming that Fas-FasL interaction did underlie the observed increase of β cell apoptosis.[8b]

DISCUSSION

In autoimmune diabetes, islet β cells are chronically exposed to a milieu of inflammatory cytokines. In the NOD mouse, mononuclear invasion of the islets starts soon after weaning. The presence of this inflammatory environment markedly affects normal β cell biology, with increased or reduced expression of over 150 genes involved in a whole range of cellular processes,[10] including upregulation of cell surface receptors such as Fas. The presence of an inflammatory infiltrate is essential during the development of autoimmune diabetes as neither NOD nor HIPFasL mice carrying the SCID mutation develop diabetes.[8b]

Until recently, the mechanism by which the inflammatory infiltrate mediated β cell apoptosis remained uncertain, with Fas,[9,11] nitric oxide,[3,12,13] free radical stress,[14,15] and perforin[16–18] all being postulated to play a role. Studies by ourselves[8] and others[19,20] have increasingly emphasized the importance of Fas-mediated β cell apoptosis in NOD autoimmune diabetes. Using the HIPFasL model, we have been able to demonstrate that, in the presence of an inflammatory infiltrate, FasL-expressing β cells are exquisitely sensitive to Fas-mediated apoptosis and that this can be blocked by preventing FasL-Fas interaction with FasL-neutralizing antibody. Also, the effect of this inflammatory infiltrate can be reproduced with the cytokines, IFN-γ and IL-1, which together upregulate β cell Fas expression. Together, this evidence points to a highly important role of Fas-FasL interaction in autoimmune β cell death. Clearly, like so many other body systems, there is likely to be some redundancy built into the system such that other β cell death pathways are also likely to be relevant to autoimmune diabetes, albeit to a lesser degree than Fas. However, it does stress the importance of interrupting the Fas signaling pathway if autoimmune β cell death is to be prevented. We are now interested in looking at potential synergistic effects of blocking multiple apoptosis pathways including Fas in combination to see whether this is even more effective in preventing β cell death than blocking Fas alone.

ACKNOWLEDGMENTS

This work was supported by the Canberra Hospital Salaried Specialists Private Practice Fund.

REFERENCES

1. KURRER, M.O., S.V. PAKALA, H.L. HANSON & J.D. KATZ. 1997. Beta cell apoptosis in T cell–mediated autoimmune diabetes. Proc. Natl. Acad. Sci. USA **94:** 213.
2. CHERVONSKY, A.V., Y. WANG, F.S. WONG et al. 1997. The role of Fas in autoimmune diabetes. Cell **89:** 17.
3. STASSI, G., R. DE MARIA, G. TRUCCO et al. 1997. Nitric oxide primes pancreatic beta cells for Fas-mediated destruction in insulin-dependent diabetes mellitus. J. Exp. Med. **186:** 1193.
4. SUAREZ-PINZON, W., O. SORENSEN, R.C. BLEACKLEY et al. 1999. Beta-cell destruction in NOD mice correlates with Fas (CD95) expression on beta-cells and proinflammatory cytokine expression in islets. Diabetes **48:** 21.
5. SIGNORE, A., A. ANNOVAZZI, E. PROCACCINI et al. 1997. CD95 and CD95-ligand expression in endocrine pancreas of NOD, NOR, and BALB/c mice. Diabetologia **40:** 1476.
6. LOWETH, A.C., G.T. WILLIAMS, R.F. JAMES et al. 1998. Human islets of Langerhans express Fas ligand and undergo apoptosis in response to interleukin-1beta and Fas ligation. Diabetes **47:** 727.
7. REDD, S., S. GINN & J.M. ROSS. 2002. Fas and Fas ligand immunolocalization in pancreatic islets of NOD mice during spontaneous and cyclophosphamide-accelerated diabetes. Histochem. J. **34:** 1.
8. (a) PETROVSKY, N., D. SILVA, L. SOCHA et al. 2002. The role of Fas ligand in beta cell destruction in autoimmune diabetes of NOD mice. Ann. N.Y. Acad. Sci. **958:** 204;

(b) SILVA, D., N. PETROVSKY, L. SOCHA *et al.* 2003. Mechanisms of accelerated immune-mediated diabetes resulting from islet beta-cell expression of a FAS ligand transgene. J. Immunol. **170:** 4996.
9. THOMAS, H.E., R. DARWICHE, J.A. CORBETT & T.W. KAY. 1999. Evidence that beta cell death in the nonobese diabetic mouse is Fas independent. J. Immunol. **163:** 1562.
10. CARDOZO, A.K., M. KRUHOFFER, R. LEEMAN *et al.* 2001. Identification of novel cytokine-induced genes in pancreatic beta-cells by high-density oligonucleotide arrays. Diabetes **50:** 909.
11. SU, X., Q. HU, J.M. KRISTAN *et al.* 2000. Significant role for Fas in the pathogenesis of autoimmune diabetes. J. Immunol. **164:** 2523.
12. THOMAS, H.E. & T.W. KAY. 2000. Beta cell destruction in the development of autoimmune diabetes in the non-obese diabetic (NOD) mouse. Diabetes Metab. Res. Rev. **16:** 251.
13. ZUMSTEG, U., S. FRIGERIO & G.A. HOLLANDER. 2000. Nitric oxide production and Fas surface expression mediate two independent pathways of cytokine-induced murine beta-cell damage. Diabetes **49:** 39.
14. WEST, I.C. 2000. Radicals and oxidative stress in diabetes. Diabetes Med. **17:** 171.
15. SUAREZ-PINZON, W.L., C. SZABO & A. RABINOVITCH. 1997. Development of autoimmune diabetes in NOD mice is associated with the formation of peroxynitrite in pancreatic islet beta-cells. Diabetes **46:** 907.
16. KAY, T.W., H.E. THOMAS, L.C. HARRISON & J. ALLISON. 2000. The beta cell in autoimmune diabetes: many mechanisms and pathways of loss. Trends Endocrinol. Metab. **11:** 11.
17. YOON, J.W. & H.S. JUN. 2001. Cellular and molecular pathogenic mechanisms of insulin-dependent diabetes mellitus. Ann. N.Y. Acad. Sci. **928:** 200.
18. KREUWEL, H.T. & L.A. SHERMAN. 2001. The role of Fas-FasL in CD8+ T-cell-mediated insulin-dependent diabetes mellitus (IDDM). J. Clin. Immunol. **21:** 15.
19. MAHIOU, J., U. WALTER, F. LEPAULT *et al.* 2001. *In vivo* blockade of the Fas-Fas ligand pathway inhibits cyclophosphamide-induced diabetes in NOD mice. J. Autoimmun. **16:** 431.
20. SUAREZ-PINZON, W.L., R.F. POWER & A. RABINOVITCH. 2000. Fas ligand-mediated mechanisms are involved in autoimmune destruction of islet beta cells in non-obese diabetic mice. Diabetologia **43:** 1149.

Fas and Fas Ligand Immunoexpression in Pancreatic Islets of NOD Mice during Spontaneous and Cyclophosphamide-Accelerated Diabetes

SHIVA REDDY[a,b] AND JACQUELINE M. ROSS[c]

[a]*School of Biological Sciences,* [b]*Department of Pediatrics, and* [c]*Department of Anatomy with Radiology, University of Auckland, Auckland, New Zealand*

ABSTRACT: During insulin-dependent diabetes mellitus, beta cell destruction may involve activation of the Fas–Fas ligand (Fas-FasL) system. Here, we employed dual-label immunohistochemistry to examine the intra-islet expression, distribution, and cellular sources of Fas and FasL in the NOD mouse. Pancreatic tissues were studied during spontaneous diabetes (days 21, 40, and 90) and following acceleration of diabetes with cyclophosphamide (days 0, 4, 7, 11, and 14 after cyclophosphamide administration). Our results show that FasL was expressed constitutively in most beta cells of NOD mice and in nondiabetes-prone mice, but not in glucagon or somatostatin cells or in islet inflammatory cells. It paralleled the loss of insulin immunolabeling with advancing disease. Immunolabeling for Fas was first observed in extra-islet macrophages and those close to the islet in NOD and nondiabetes-prone mice. During spontaneous and cyclophosphamide diabetes, it was observed in a higher proportion of islet infiltrating macrophages than in CD4 and CD8 cells. In the cyclophosphamide group, Fas expression in intra-islet CD4 and CD8 cells showed an increase close to the onset of diabetes. At days 11 and 14, several intra-islet macrophages with immunolabeling for Fas also coexpressed interleukin-1β and inducible nitric oxide synthase. Fas was not detected in beta cells and other endocrine cells during spontaneous and cyclophosphamide diabetes. We show constitutive expression of FasL in beta cells in the NOD mouse and predominant expression of Fas in intra-islet macrophages and to a lesser extent in T cells prior to diabetes onset. The role of Fas-FasL in beta cell destruction in the NOD mouse requires further clarification.

KEYWORDS: Fas; FasL; NOD mouse; diabetes; islets

INTRODUCTION

The molecular mechanisms of beta cell destruction during insulin-dependent diabetes mellitus (IDDM) remain elusive. Fas (CD95/APO-1) is a 36-kDa protein that can initiate apoptosis when it is cross-linked with specific agonistic antibodies

Address for correspondence: S. Reddy, Ph.D., Senior Research Fellow, School of Biological Sciences, University of Auckland, Private Bag 92019, Auckland, New Zealand. Voice: +64-9-3737599 (ext. 82917); fax: +64-9-3737486.
 s.reddy@auckland.ac.nz

or with Fas ligand (FasL or CD95L).[1] Fas-FasL engagement can activate a complex apoptotic signal via a conserved intracellular "death domain". The apoptotic signal comprises an ordered program of molecular steps including the activation of initiator and effector caspases.[2]

Studies examining the expression of Fas and FasL and their colocalization within the pancreatic islets during IDDM are limited. *In vitro* studies have shown that various cytokines such as interleukin-1-beta (IL-1β), interferon-gamma (IFN-γ), and tumor necrosis factor-alpha (TNF-α) can induce Fas expression in isolated islets and in beta cells.[3,4] The presence of FasL within islet cells of the NOD mouse has been a subject of debate. It has been shown in glucagon cells in one study, but was not seen in any islet endocrine cell in a more recent study.[5,6] Here, we have examined the expression of Fas and FasL in the NOD mouse during spontaneous diabetes and following acceleration of disease with cyclophosphamide (Cy) by dual-label immunohistochemistry. We have correlated their expression with advancing disease.

METHODS

Female NOD mice were randomly allocated into group 1 and group 2 (18 mice per group) and maintained on standard mouse chow and water. At day 95, all but 3 mice from group 2 were injected intraperitoneally with Cy (300 mg/kg body weight), while mice from group 1 were injected with diluent (sterile water). Pancreatic tissues were removed at days 0, 4, 7, 11, and 14 after administration of Cy or diluent. Pancreas was also collected from female NOD mice at days 21, 40, and 90 (3 mice per age group) and from 3 female CD-1 and C57BL/6 mice at days 21 and 90. Frozen sections were examined by immunohistochemistry for the presence of Fas and FasL, in conjunction with insulin, glucagon, somatostatin, macrophages, CD4 and CD8 cells, inducible nitric oxide synthase (iNOS), or IL-1β.

RESULTS

Diabetes developed in 3 out of 6 mice at day 14 given Cy, while none developed the disease in group 1 (control group).

FasL was immunodetected in a majority of beta cells from NOD mice at days 21, 40, and 90 and also in beta cells of nondiabetes-prone mice (FIGS. 1a–c). It was also colocalized with insulin in the remaining beta cells in mice given Cy and was not expressed in islet inflammatory cells. FasL immunolabeling at day 0 (Cy group) was similar to the age-matched spontaneous group. At days 4, 7, 11, and 14 (Cy group), FasL staining persisted in beta cells, but was absent in intra-islet immune cells (FIGS. 1d–f). At day 14, only a few CD4 cells were FasL-positive.

Fas immunolabeling in islet endocrine cells of female NOD, CD-1, and C57BL/6 mice was absent. However, some immunolabeling was observed in a few macrophages distributed in the sinusoidal and perivascular areas and occasionally in close apposition to islets. At day 90, Fas expression in the NOD mouse was seen in the insulitis region and was present predominantly in macrophages and in some CD4 and CD8 cells. Fas immunolabeling was absent in islet endocrine cells.

In the Cy group, Fas expression was observed predominantly in macrophages and to a lesser extent in a proportion of CD4 and CD8 cells. At day 4, when there was

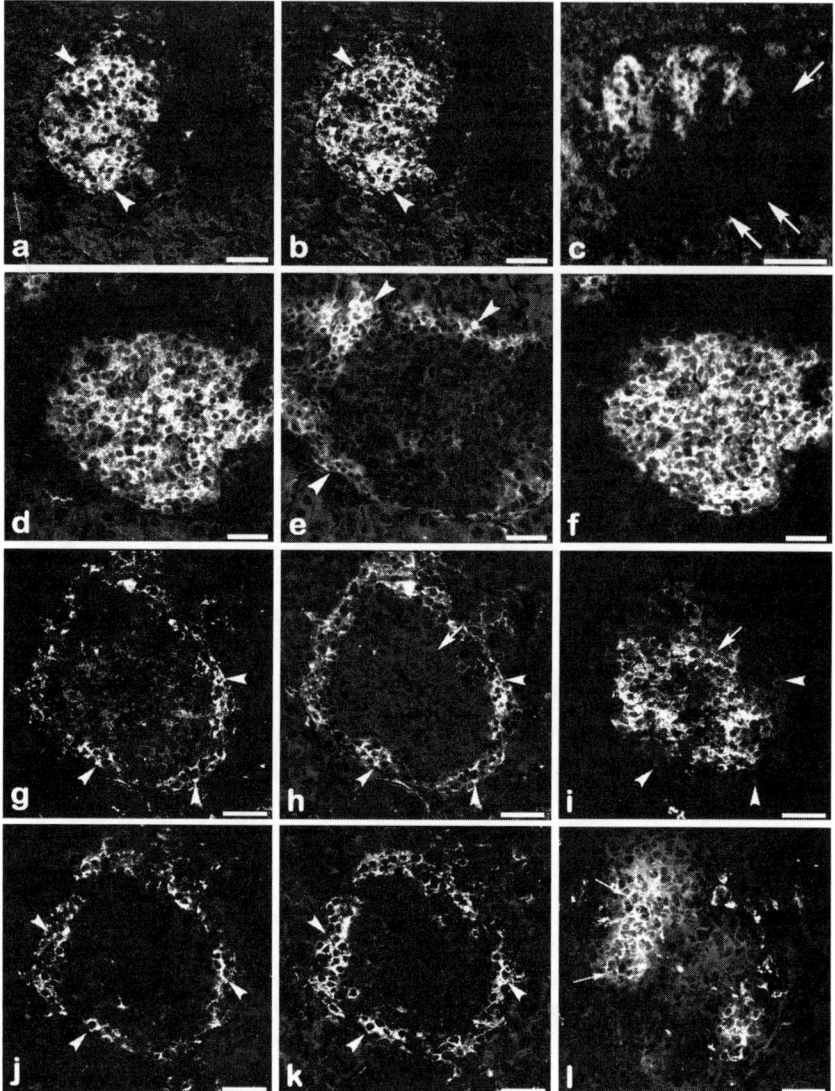

FIGURE 1. Photomicrographs of pancreatic islets from NOD mice immunolabeled for FasL, Fas, and IL-1β: **(a)** day 40 islet showing FasL; **(b)** same islet dual-labeled for insulin; arrowheads point to insulin cells that are FasL-positive; **(c)** day 90 islet showing FasL expression in remaining beta cells; arrows point to the insulitis region that is FasL-negative; **(d–f)** day 14 Cy group showing an islet triple-labeled for FasL **(d)**, macrophages **(e)**, and insulin **(f)**; arrowheads in **(e)** point to macrophages that are FasL-negative; **(g–l)** day 14 Cy group showing an islet triple-labeled for Fas **(g)**, macrophages **(h)**, and insulin **(i)**; arrowheads point to macrophages that are positive for Fas and negative for insulin; arrows in **(h)** and **(i)** point to insulin cells that are Fas-negative; **(j, k)** an islet dual-labeled for Fas **(j)** and CD8 cells **(k)**; arrowheads point to Fas-positive CD8 cells; **(l)** an islet labeled for IL-1β; arrows point to IL-1β cells that coexpress Fas. Scale bars: 30 μm, except **(c)** which is 50 μm.

minimum insulitis, Fas expression was confined to a few macrophages, but increased at day 7 and maximally at days 11 and 14. At this stage, Fas immunolabeling was more intense than at the earlier time points and was predominantly expressed in macrophages and in a proportion of CD4 and CD8 cells (FIGS. 1g–k). A proportion of macrophages coexpressed Fas and IL-1β, and Fas and iNOS (FIG. 1l).

DISCUSSION

This study shows that FasL is expressed constitutively in beta cells of NOD mice from at least day 21. A previous report has shown the presence of this protein in glucagon cells.[5] A more recent study failed to detect FasL in beta cells isolated from NOD mice, analyzed by flow cytometry.[6] These discrepancies may have been due to the use of anti-FasL of different specificities. In the latter study, there may been some loss of FasL from beta cells during islet isolation and separation into single cells. Our observations correlate with recent immunohistochemical and biochemical findings in normal human pancreas.[7] More recent immunohistochemical and *in situ* hybridization approaches also show the presence of FasL in human pancreas.[8] However, in recently diagnosed human diabetic pancreas, Fas expression has been shown in beta cells and FasL in immune cells.[9]

In our study, the strong expression of Fas in intra-islet immune cells during spontaneous and Cy-induced diabetes corroborates previous findings.[5,6,10] Although Fas immunolabeling in beta cells was not detected, it is possible that those beta cells that expressed Fas are cleared rapidly following ligation with FasL expressed by adjacent beta cells. In other studies, Fas expression in mouse beta cells *in vivo* has been shown only after employing various disease-amplifying models or *in vitro* following cytokine stimulation. This study suggests that the role of the Fas-FasL system in beta cell destruction in the NOD mouse requires further examination.

REFERENCES

1. NAGATA, S. 1994. Fas and Fas ligand; a death factor and its receptor. Adv. Immunol. **57:** 129–144.
2. CHANDRA, J. *et al.* 2001. Role of apoptosis in pancreatic β-cell death in diabetes. Diabetes **50**(suppl. 1): S44–S47.
3. YAMADA, K. *et al.* 1996. Mouse islet cell lysis mediated by IL-1-induced Fas. Diabetologia **39:** 1306–1312.
4. SUAREZ-PINZON, W. *et al.* 1999. β-cell destruction in NOD mice correlates with Fas (CD95) expression on β-cells and proinflammatory cytokine expression in islets. Diabetes **48:** 21–28.
5. SIGNORE, A. *et al.* 1997. CD95 and CD95-ligand expression in endocrine pancreas of NOD, NOR, and BALB/c mice. Diabetologia **40:** 1476–1479.
6. THOMAS, H.E. *et al.* 1999. Evidence that β cell death in the non-obese diabetic mouse is Fas independent. J. Immunol. **163:** 1562–1569.
7. LOWETH, A.C. *et al.* 1998. Human islets of Langerhans express Fas ligand and undergo apoptosis in response to interleukin-1β and Fas ligation. Diabetes **47:** 727–732.
8. MAEDLER, K. *et al.* 2001. Glucose induces β-cell apoptosis via up-regulation of the Fas receptor in human islets. Diabetes **50:** 1683–1690.
9. MORIWAKI, M. *et al.* 1999. Fas and Fas ligand expression in inflamed islets in pancreas sections of patients with recent-onset type 1 diabetes mellitus. Diabetologia **42:** 1332–1340.
10. CHERVONSKY, A.V. *et al.* 1997. The role of Fas in autoimmune diabetes. Cell **89:** 17–24.

Type 1 Diabetes in Swedish Bank Voles (*Clethrionomys glareolus*): Signs of Disease in Both Colonized and Wild Cyclic Populations at Peak Density

BO NIKLASSON,[a] BIRGER HÖRNFELDT,[b] ERIK NYHOLM,[b] MATTHIAS NIEDRIG,[c] OLIVER DONOSO-MANTKE,[c] HANS R. GELDERBLOM,[c] AND ÅKE LERNMARK[d]

[a]*Apodemus AB, Grevgatan 38, SE-114 53 Stockholm, Sweden*

[b]*Department of Ecology and Environmental Science, Umeå University, S-901 87 Umeå, Sweden*

[c]*Robert Koch-Institut, Nordufer 20, 13353 Berlin, Germany*

[d]*Department of Medicine, R. H. Williams Laboratory, University of Washington, Seattle, Washington 98195, USA*

> ABSTRACT: Colonized bank voles (*Clethrionomys glareolus*) originating from Sweden developed type 1 diabetes. Animals became polydipsic, glucosuric, and hyperglycemic and gradually developed a lethal ketoacidosis. Pancreas in animals with end-stage disease showed total destruction of islet cells. Interestingly, also a high proportion of wild bank voles in cyclic populations that were trapped at (or close to) the cyclic population density peak frequently showed high blood glucose levels and pathological glucose tolerance test. Extensive islet destruction was not seen in wild bank voles at the time of capture, but did develop in some of the animals over a time period of two months. Diabetes in both colonized and wild bank voles was associated with Ljungan virus (LV). LV could be isolated from the pancreas of diabetic bank voles and antigen detected at the site of tissue damage by immunohistochemistry. In addition, picornavirus-like particles were visualized in the islets of diabetic voles using thin-section transmission electron microscopy.
>
> KEYWORDS: bank vole; type 1 diabetes; picornavirus; Ljungan virus

It has recently been shown that bank voles (*Clethrionomys glareolus*) in Denmark developed signs of diabetes.[1] Bank voles trapped in the wild and brought to the laboratory showed no signs of diabetes immediately after being trapped, but a high proportion of these animals and their offspring developed polydipsia, polyuria, and glucosuria after a few months in captivity. Following these observations, another

---

Address for correspondence: Bo Niklasson, Apodemus AB, Grevgatan 38, S-114 53 Stockholm, Sweden. Voice: +46-8-663-23-83; fax: +46-708-23-23-11.
bo.niklasson@apodemus.se

recent study found that Danish bank voles do develop signs and symptoms similar to type 1 diabetes in humans with glucosuria, hyperglycemia (blood glucose levels decreased after administration of insulin), ketonuria, ketonemia, and hyperlipidemia.[2] Diabetic animals had also type 1 diabetes–associated GAD65, IA-2, and insulin autoantibodies. In addition, Ljungan virus (LV), a novel picornavirus recently isolated from both Swedish and Danish bank voles, was detected in cytopathic islet cells of bank voles with diabetes using immunohistochemistry (IHC).[2–5] It was also found that the frequency of animals developing diabetes could be manipulated by different regimes of stress.[6]

The aim of the present study was to investigate if type 1 diabetes also occurs in Swedish bank voles and to determine any association between diabetes in bank voles and LV. We especially wanted to determine if cyclic bank voles under natural stress at the high population density at cyclic peaks may develop diabetes in the wild.

COLONIZED BANK VOLES

Animals trapped both in the north (Västerbotten) and in the south (Småland, Skåne) of Sweden were taken to the laboratory and observed for several months. Animals of both sexes from the north as well as from the south developed diabetes. The disease occurred both in animals originally trapped in nature as well as in their offspring. Animals became polydipsic, glucosuric, and hyperglycemic and gradually

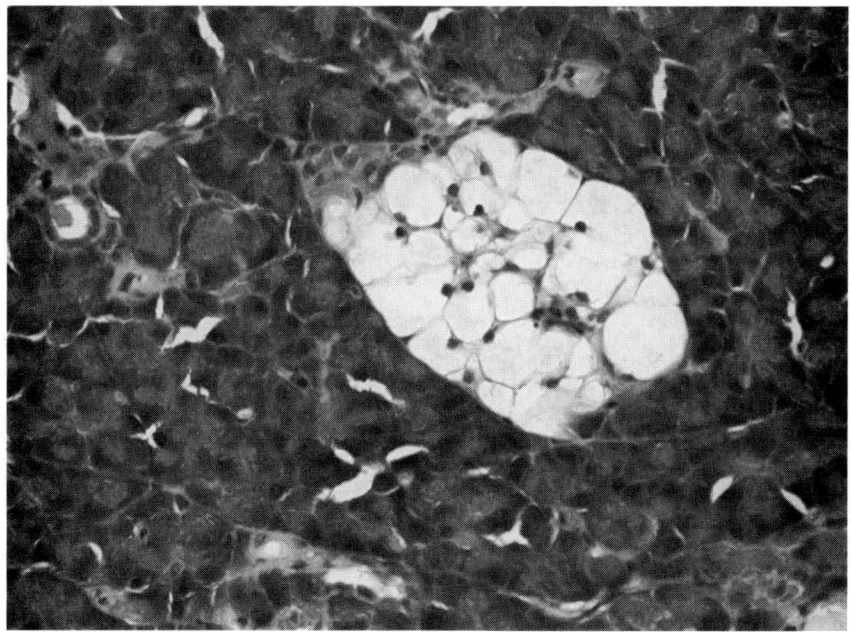

FIGURE 1. A typical vacuolization of an islet from an animal with end-stage diabetes disease. See text.

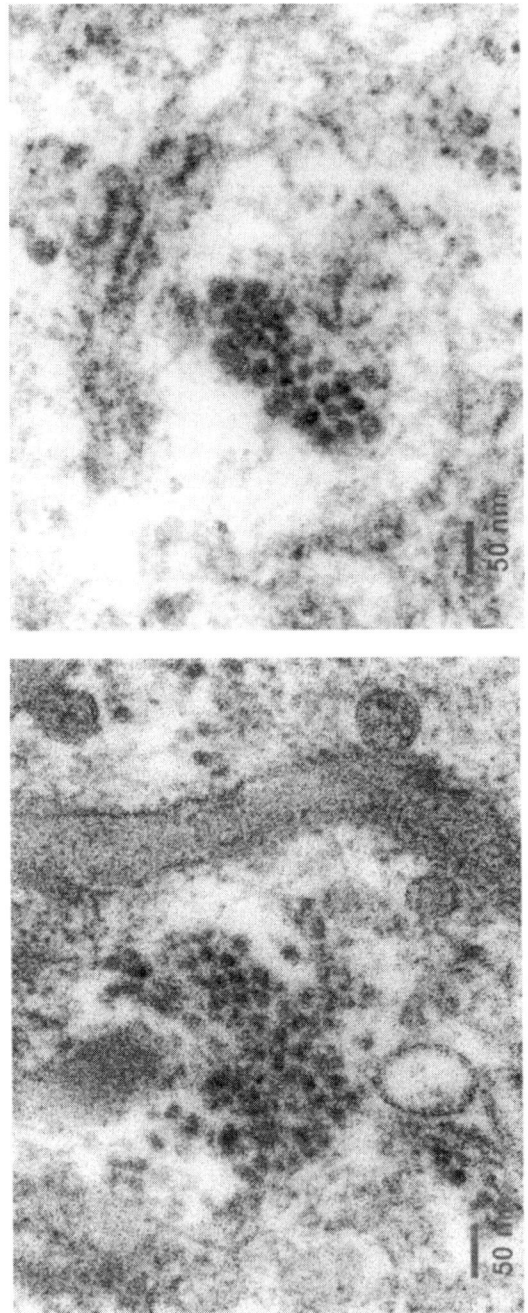

FIGURE 2. (Left) Thin section showing LV particles in an islet cell of the pancreas from a diabetic bank vole. The particles appeared in a small aggregate in the cytoplasm. The section thickness (about 50 nm) is bigger than the diameter of the virion (27 nm). [Magnification: ×40,000]. **(Right)** Thin section showing LV particles in an infected Vero B4 cell as reference. The virus particles were 27 nm in diameter, spherical with an almost featureless surface, and appeared in a small aggregate in the cytoplasm. [Magnification: ×40,000].

TABLE 1. Glucose tolerance test performed on colonized bank voles (*C. glareolus*) and tested just before receiving 2 g glucose per kg BW intraperitoneally and tested again at 15, 30, 90, and 120 min

Vole no.	Treatment	BG at 1 week before tol. test	BG time				
			0 min	15 min	30 min	90 min	120 min
1	Glucose	85	124	399	557	307	406
2	Glucose	180	84	424	>600	>600	582
3	Glucose	89	103	285	324	95	129
4	Glucose	107	97	226	153	106	103
5	NaCl	81	86	109	185	72	122

developed a lethal ketoacidosis. Pancreas in animals with end-stage disease showed total destruction of islet cells. FIGURE 1 show a typical vacuolization of an islet from an animal with end-stage diabetes disease. Pancreas from one bank vole with symptoms of diabetes and the islets of the pancreas staining LV-positive by IHC were analyzed by thin-section electron microscopy. LV-infected tissue culture was used as a positive control, and normal tissue culture and pancreas from a nondiabetes bank vole (IHC-negative) as a negative control. Clusters of particles with size and shape resembling picornavirus particles were found in the LV-infected tissue culture as well as in islet cells of the pancreas originating from the diabetic bank vole (FIG. 2). No such clusters were detected in the normal tissue culture or in the pancreas from a bank vole with no signs and symptoms of diabetes.

TABLE 1 shows the results from a glucose tolerance test on a selected number of nonsymptomatic animals. Based on the experience from other laboratory rodent models, we assumed that a blood glucose level above 200 mg/dL indicated a pathological finding. Animals 1 and 2 in TABLE 1 showed a clearly pathological glucose tolerance test. Animals 3 and 4 showed an increased blood glucose level at 15 and 30 min, respectively, but both animals normalized their values at 2 h. Animal 5 illustrated the increase that can be detected in an animal given normal saline and is likely to be caused by the stress induced by the handling such as repeated blood sampling.

BANK VOLES IN THE WILD

Although only one subspecies of *C. glareolus* is recognized throughout the Swedish mainland, a gradient exists in population stability. Populations of voles in southernmost Sweden are characterized as noncyclic, whereas populations in the north fluctuate on a 3- to 4-year cycle of abundance.[7,8] During peak abundance, voles may be >300 times more abundant than immediately after the rapid population decline typical in northern Sweden. We trapped animals in different locations in northern Sweden (Västerbotten County) from September 2001 to January 2002 when the cyclic small-rodent populations reached a density peak.[9]

A total of 188 bank voles were brought in alive from the field and tested for blood glucose (BG) using a Medisence precision PCx (Abbott Laboratories). Of these individuals, 50 (27%) had a BG level above 200 mg/dL, 30 (16%) had a BG level above 250 mg/dL, and 12 (6%) had a BG level above 350 mg/dL. Another 47 bank voles were taken to a temporary field laboratory. Animals were kept on normal diet (mouse pellets and water ad libitum) until they were subjected to a glucose tolerance test (2 g glucose administrated intraperitoneally), with BG tested only 60 min after administration of glucose. One group of 22 animals was tested within 24 h after being trapped, where 5 individuals (23%) had a BG value above 250 mg/dL and 2 (9%) had a value above 350 mg/dL. The remaining group of 25 bank voles was kept for 8 weeks and then subjected to the glucose tolerance test. Nine voles (36%) had a value above 250 mg/dL and 7 voles (28%) had a value above 350 mg/dL. The pathology of the pancreas was investigated on all 235 animals. End-stage diabetes with totally destroyed vacuolized islets was only seen in some individuals in the group kept in the laboratory for 8 weeks.

We conclude that Swedish bank voles develop type 1 diabetes with polydipsia, hyperglycemia, and lethal ketoacidosis. In contrast to earlier findings from Denmark, a significant frequency of the animals in the wild showed high blood glucose levels and, under the assumption that values from other rodent models are applicable also to the bank vole, many animals also showed a pathologic glucose tolerance test. Based on the Danish laboratory observations that stress influences the development of diabetes,[6] we suggest that the difference between bank voles in the wild in Sweden versus Denmark may be caused by a higher level of natural stress in cyclic versus noncyclic populations. Stress factors that are likely to differ between the two populations are the number of social contacts (with both conspecifics and other synchronously fluctuating small-rodent species), the number of predator contacts, and the amount of space and food per capita. A striking observation is the fact that no animal had any severe signs of diabetes at the time of trapping, although a high proportion of the bank voles tested showed signs of altered glucose metabolism. So far, such animals have only been seen under laboratory conditions. It is possible that animals with symptoms of diabetes are eliminated very fast in nature if not having free access to food and water and protection from predators, or that such individuals are not active enough to be trapped. If so, end-stage diabetes is therefore only seen under laboratory conditions.

Unfortunately, we have not been able to establish an LV free colony of animals and have thus not been able to determine the normal range of blood glucose in bank voles. It has also been impossible to fulfill Koch's postulate. However, the association between animals with disease and islet pathology as well as the association between tissue destruction and the presence of LV make LV a likely etiologic agent of type 1 diabetes in bank voles. We have previously shown a covariation of the incidence of type 1 diabetes in humans with the 3- to 4-year population density cycle of the bank vole (*Clethrionomys glareolus*) in Sweden.[10] Studies in humans are under way to determine if type 1 diabetes is a zoonotic disease caused by LV.

REFERENCES

1. SCHOENECKER, B., K.E. HELLER & T. FREIMANIS. 2000. Development of stereotypes and polydipsia in wild caught bank voles (*Clethrionomys glareolus*) and their laboratory-bred offspring: is polydipsia a symptom of diabetes mellitus? Appl. Anim. Behav. Sci. **68:** 349–357.

2. NIKLASSON, B., K.E. HELLER, B. SCHOENECKER et al. 2003. Development of type 1 diabetes in wild bank voles associated with islet autoantibodies and the novel Ljungan virus. Int. J. Exp. Diabetes Res. 4(1): 35–44.
3. NIKLASSON, B., L. KINNUNEN, B. HÖRNFELDT et al. 1999. A new picornavirus isolated from bank voles (Clethrionomys glareolus). Virology 255: 86–93.
4. JOHANSSON, S., B. NIKLASSON, J. MAIZEL et al. 2002. Molecular analysis of three isolates of Ljungan virus reveals a new, close-to-root lineage of the Picornaviridae with a cluster of two unrelated 2A proteins. J. Virol. 76: 8920–8930.
5. JOHANSSON, S., B. NIKLASSON, R.B. TESH et al. 2003. Molecular characterisation of M1146, an American isolate of Ljungan virus (LV), reveals the presence of a new LV genotype. J. Gen. Virol. 84: 837–844.
6. FREIMANIS, T., K.E. HELLER, B. SCHOENECKER & M. BILDSOE. 2003. Effects of preweaning stress on the development of type 1 diabetes in bank voles (Clethrionomys glareolus). Int. J. Exp. Diabetes Res. 4(1): 21–25.
7. HANSSON, L. & H. HENTTONEN. 1985. Gradients in density variations of small rodents: the importance of latitude and snow cover. Oecologia 67: 394–402.
8. HÖRNFELDT, B. 1994. Delayed density dependence as a determinant of vole cycles. Ecology 75: 791–806.
9. HÖRNFELDT, B. 2002. Environmental monitoring of small mammals [in Swedish] [http://www.eg.umu.se/personal/hornfeldt_birger/bh/sidor/index3.html].
10. NIKLASSON, B., B. HÖRNFELDT & B. LUNDMAN. 1998. Could myocarditis, insulin-dependent diabetes mellitus, and Guillain-Barré syndrome be caused by one or more infectious agents carried by rodents? Emerging Infect. Dis. 4: 187–193.

Defective Activation-Induced Cell Death in NOD T Lymphocytes

1,25-Dihydroxyvitamin D₃ Restores Defect

B. DECALLONNE AND C. MATHIEU

Laboratorium voor Experimentele Geneeskunde en Endocrinologie (LEGENDO), Katholieke Universiteit Leuven, Leuven, Belgium

ABSTRACT: The aim of this study was first to analyze strain differences in apoptosis resistance of NOD peripheral T lymphocytes in *in vitro* models of death by neglect and activation-induced cell death (AICD). Especially AICD is known to play a key role in peripheral tolerance, keeping autoimmune effector cells under control. Second, we studied the effects of *in vivo* treatment of NOD mice with 1α,25-dihydroxyvitamin D₃ [1α,25(OH)₂D₃], an immunomodulator known to prevent diabetes and insulitis in NOD mice, on *in vitro* T lymphocyte apoptosis resistance.

KEYWORDS: activation-induced cell death (AICD); 1α,25-dihydroxyvitamin D₃ [1α,25(OH)₂D₃]; apoptosis resistance; T lymphocytes

Resistance to apoptosis-inducing signals characterizes NOD T lymphocytes, allowing survival of potentially autoreactive cells.[1–3] Especially female NOD mice, exhibiting the highest diabetes incidence, are characterized by pronounced apoptosis resistance of T lymphocytes.[3]

The aim of this study was first to analyze strain differences in apoptosis resistance of NOD peripheral T lymphocytes in *in vitro* models of death by neglect and activation-induced cell death (AICD). Especially AICD is known to play a key role in peripheral tolerance, keeping autoimmune effector cells under control.[4] Second, we wanted to study the effects of *in vivo* treatment of NOD mice with 1α,25-dihydroxyvitamin D₃ [1α,25(OH)₂D₃], an immunomodulator known to prevent diabetes and insulitis in NOD mice,[5,6] on *in vitro* T lymphocyte apoptosis resistance.

Eight-week-old prediabetic female NOD, NOR, C57BL/6, and 1α,25(OH)₂D₃-treated NOD mice were used. 1α,25(OH)₂D₃ (5 μg/kg/2 days) was given intraperitoneally from 3 weeks of age onward. Splenic T lymphocytes (from $n = 2$ animals per experimental group) were isolated by nylon wool passage. T lymphocytes were resuspended at 2×10^6 cells/mL. For induction of death by neglect, T lymphocytes

---

Address for correspondence: Chantal Mathieu, M.D., Ph.D., Gasthuisberg, LEGENDO, Onderwijs & Navorsing N8, Herestraat 9, 3000 Leuven, Belgium. Voice: +32-16-34-60-30; fax: +32-16-34-59-34.

chantal.mathieu@med.kuleuven.ac.be

TABLE 1. TUNEL-positive T lymphocytes (expressed as mean ± SD)

	NOD	NOR	C57BL/6	NOD-vitD
Neglect	37 ± 6*	35 ± 5*	43 ± 8	39 ± 2
AICD	64 ± 10†	76 ± 3	72 ± 10	73 ± 9

NOTE: Results are expressed as the percentage of TUNEL-positive cells (mean ± SD of triplicate cultures from five separate experiments: *$p < 0.05$ vs. C57BL/6; †$p < 0.05$ vs. all (ANOVA and Fisher's LSD multiple comparison test).

were cultured 24 h in medium devoid of fetal calf serum. For induction of AICD, splenic T lymphocytes were cultured in medium with 10% fetal calf serum and concanavalin A (7.5 µg/mL) for 24 h, followed by rIL-2 (20 IU/mL) for 24 h and finally anti-CD3ε (10 µg/mL) + rIL-2 (20 IU/mL) for 24 h. TUNEL was used on harvested cells to detect apoptosis using flow cytometry. Results are expressed as the percentage of TUNEL-positive cells.

As shown in TABLE 1, death by neglect was defective in both NOD and diabetes-resistant NOR T lymphocytes compared to nonautoimmune C57BL/6 T lymphocytes. Interestingly, AICD was defective specifically in NOD T lymphocytes, suggesting a pathogenic role for this mode of cell death in diabetes development. Furthermore, *in vivo* treatment with $1\alpha,25(OH)_2D_3$ is able to restore *in vitro* AICD sensitivity of T cells. This enhanced peripheral AICD sensitivity by $1\alpha,25(OH)_2D_3$ can be the result of direct $1\alpha,25(OH)_2D_3$ action on peripheral T lymphocytes or indirect action via enhanced negative selection of apoptosis-resistant thymocytes,[3,7] or a combination of both. This issue is presently under investigation.

REFERENCES

1. COLUCCI, F., C. CILIO, K. LEIJON *et al.* 1996. Programmed cell death in the pathogenesis of murine IDDM: resistance to apoptosis induced in lymphocytes by cyclophosphamide. J. Autoimmun. **9:** 271–276.
2. RADOSEVIC, K., K. CASTEELS, C. MATHIEU *et al.* 1999. Splenic dendritic cells from the non-obese diabetic mouse induce a prolonged proliferation of syngeneic T cells: a role for an impaired apoptosis of NOD T cells? J. Autoimmun. **13:** 373–382.
3. CASTEELS, K., C. GYSEMANS, M. WAER *et al.* 1998. Sex difference in resistance to dexamethasone-induced apoptosis in NOD mice: treatment with $1,25(OH)_2D_3$ restores defect. Diabetes **47:** 1033–1037.
4. VAN PARIJS, L. & A.K. ABBAS. 1998. Homeostasis and self-tolerance in the immune system: turning lymphocytes off. Science **280:** 243–248.
5. MATHIEU, C., J. LAUREYS, H. SOBIS *et al.* 1992. 1,25-Dihydroxyvitamin D3 prevents insulitis in NOD mice. Diabetes **41:** 1491–1495.
6. MATHIEU, C., M. WAER, J. LAUREYS *et al.* 1994. Prevention of autoimmune diabetes in NOD mice by 1,25-dihydroxyvitamin D3. Diabetologia **37:** 552–558.
7. KISHIMOTO, H. & J. SPRENT. 2001. A defect in central tolerance in NOD mice. Nat. Immunol. **2:** 1025–1031.

The Role of Endoplasmic Reticulum Stress in Nonimmune Diabetes: NOD.k iHEL, a Novel Model of β Cell Death

L. SOCHA,[a,b] D. SILVA,[a,b] S. LESAGE,[c] C. GOODNOW,[c] AND N. PETROVSKY[a,b]

[a]*Autoimmunity Research Unit, The Canberra Hospital, Canberra, Australia*
[b]*John Curtin School of Medical Research, Canberra, Australia*
[c]*Medical Genome Center, John Curtin School of Medical Research, Canberra, Australia*

ABSTRACT: The final common pathway in diabetes development is β cell apoptosis. We herein describe a novel diabetes model based on transgenic NOD.k iHEL mice, wherein male mice develop diabetes due to nonimmune-mediated β cell death. Histology and electron microscopy confirm endoplasmic reticulum (ER) abnormalities that are consistent with endoplasmic stress caused by the HEL transgene. The NOD.k iHEL model may be particularly useful for studying mechanisms of β cell death secondary to ER stress and also for testing potential therapies designed to protect β cells from stress-induced apoptosis. The observation that only male NOD.k iHEL mice develop diabetes and exhibit ER abnormalities is intriguing and suggests these mice may be useful in deciphering the link between hyperandrogenism, insulin resistance, and diabetes.

KEYWORDS: β cell; diabetes; cell death; endoplasmic reticulum (ER) stress; NOD.k iHEL

INTRODUCTION

β cell apoptosis is now widely recognized to be the major final step in the development of both type 1 (autoimmune) and type 2 (nonimmune) diabetes. Increasingly, strategies to prevent diabetes development are focused on ways to prevent β cell apoptosis. Good animal models are required to help elucidate the mechanisms underlying β cell death and in which to test potential therapies that might prevent β cell death. NOD.k iHEL transgenic mice were created for the purpose of establishing a model to study how autoimmune susceptibility genes of nonobese diabetic (NOD) mice influence the acquisition of tolerance by organ-specific CD4 T cells.[1] The name of these mice is derived from two components, (i) iHEL and (ii) NOD.k. In these mice, hen egg lysozyme (HEL) is expressed on the pancreatic β cells and the NOD.k is a congenic NOD mouse where $H2^{g7}$ has been replaced by the $H2^k$ locus

Address for correspondence: Professor Nikolai Petrovsky, Head, Autoimmunity Research Unit, The Canberra Hospital, P.O. Box 11, Woden ACT 2606, Australia. Voice: +61-2-62443804; fax: +61-2-62603372.
  nikolai.petrovsky@anu.edu.au

of the class II molecule I-Ag7, which is a key diabetes susceptibility gene in the development of murine type 1 diabetes.[2] $H2^{g7}$ has a strong correlation to diabetes development in NOD mice[3] and genetic modifications at this locus protect NOD mice from diabetes.[4] NOD.k mice do not develop insulitis or diabetes, although they are more prone to thyroiditis than standard NOD mice.[5]

To create these mice, HEL DNA was ligated to the rat insulin promoter and the transmembrane domain of the major histocompatibility complex class I molecule (MHC class I) and inserted into the oocytes of C57BL/6 mice. This insert induces the cell surface expression of the HEL–MHC class I construct on islet β cells. To create double-transgenic mice, a second transgene was inserted, which consisted of DNA encoding for a T cell receptor (TCR) that specifically recognizes HEL protein presented on MHC $H2^k$. As expected, NOD.k iHEL TCR+ double-positive transgenic mice have a high incidence of autoimmune diabetes. Interestingly, some single transgenic iHEL-positive mice (iHEL-positive, but without the TCR transgene) also developed diabetes even though they do not have HEL-reactive lymphocytes. This review focuses on these NOD.k iHEL, TCR-negative mice (from now on referred to as NOD.k iHEL), which exhibit spontaneous diabetes, albeit only in male mice.

MATERIALS AND METHODS

NOD.k iHEL transgenic mice were bred at the Medical Genome Center, John Curtin School of Medical Research, Australian National University, as previously described by Lesage et al.[1] Urine test-tape was used to follow development of glucosuria at biweekly intervals or when the cage was wet. Mice with two successive positive results were bled, and a blood sugar of 10 mmol/L or greater was taken to confirm diabetes. Histology was performed on pancreas fixed with 10% formalin and stained with hematoxylin and eosin. Islet isolation was performed as described by Bowen et al.[6] for electron microscopy studies. Glucose tolerance tests (GTT) were performed to assess β cell function on mice fasted for 12 h. Glucose (2 mg/g) was injected intraperitoneally and blood glucose levels measured immediately before injection and 15, 30, 60, 120, and 240 min postinjection.

RESULTS

Sixty percent of male NOD.k iHEL–positive transgenic mice, but no female mice, develop diabetes at 24 weeks of age. This sexual dimorphism is supported by GTT data that show male, but not female, nondiabetic NOD.k iHEL–positive transgenic mice are glucose-intolerant. GTT were performed on four groups of mice ranging in age from 70 to 230 days old. Glucose levels at 60 min postchallenge were significantly higher in NOD.k iHEL–positive transgenic males (mean: 15.3; SD: 4.18; $p < 0.005$) compared to iHEL-positive transgenic females (mean: 9.78; SD: 4.66) and wild-type males (mean: 9.37; SD: 3.21) or females (mean: 8.23; SD: 1.97) (FIG. 1). Pancreas sections of male NOD.k iHEL–positive transgenic mice stained with H & E showed islet cells with basophilic cytoplasm and elongated nuclei. Islets were free of mononuclear infiltrates, suggesting that diabetes in this model is not immune-mediated unlike double-transgenic mice (FIG. 2).

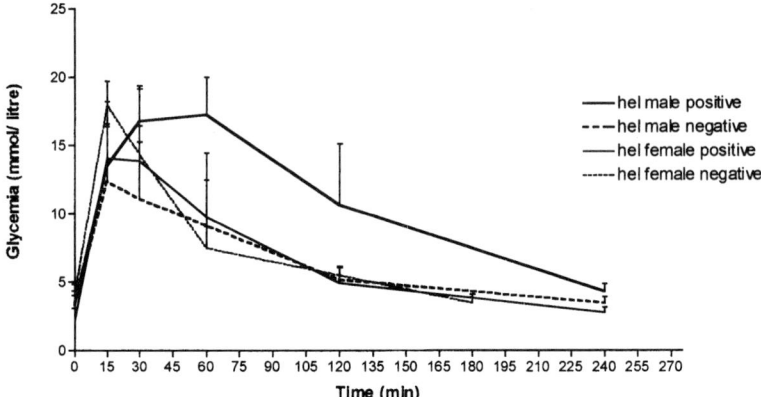

FIGURE 1. Glucose tolerance test results in groups of male and female nondiabetic NOD.k iHEL and control NOD.k mice.

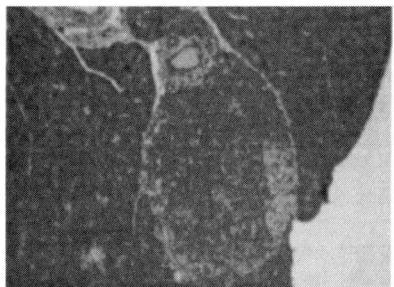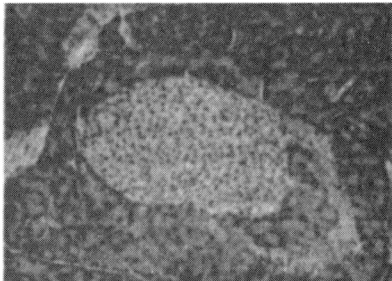

FIGURE 2. Islet histology of NOD.k iHEL single-transgenic (*left*) or double (TCR) transgenic (*right*) mice. The double-transgenic mice show a prominent islet inflammatory infiltrate, which is absent in the single-transgenic mice.

Electron microscopy (EM) revealed reduced β cell mass in male NOD.k iHEL mice with noticeable β cell apoptosis. Remaining β cells exhibited a dilated endoplasmic reticulum (ER) and a markedly reduced number of insulin secretory granules (FIG. 3). Male and female NOD.k mice, and female NOD.k iHEL mice, had normal β cells on EM with no organelle abnormalities and normal numbers of insulin granules.

DISCUSSION

NOD.k iHEL mice present as a novel model of nonautoimmune β cell death. We hypothesize that β cell death in this model is triggered by ER stress consequent upon expression of the HEL transgene in the NOD background. The tendency for only male

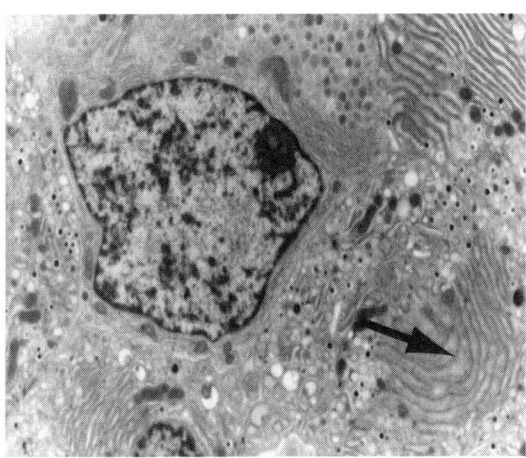

FIGURE 3. Electron microscopy of islet of male NOD.k iHEL transgenic mice (35 days old). Extensive ER dilatation (*arrow*) of β cells, with no signs of lymphocytic infiltrate.

mice to be affected may reflect increased expression of the HEL transgene in male mice due to a sex-linked increased activity of the rat insulin promoter in these mice.

ER dilatation can be due to ingress of water or trapping of secretory products in the ER, with a buildup of secretory products reflecting either an accelerated rate of protein synthesis, a defect in the transport system such as mechanical or enzymatic abnormality in the rough ER that handles the egress of proteins, or the production of an abnormal product with which the normal transport system is unable to cope.[7] This results in ER stress, which is defined as an imbalance between the load of client proteins on the ER and the ER's ability to process the load.[8,9] In general, the cellular response to ER stress has a number of functional consequences. The first is upregulation of the secretory pathway's capacity to process client proteins, for example, by upregulation of ER chaperones such as Bip/GRP78 and GRP94.[10] The second is repression of protein biosynthesis aimed at lowering the load of client proteins, for example, by phosphorylation by pancreatic ER kinase (PERK) of eukaryotic translation initiation factor 2 of its α subunit (eIF2α), which in turn inhibits the initiation step in protein biosynthesis.[11–13] The third is degradation of misfolded proteins on the ER, for example, transportation of the misfolded proteins from the ER to the cytosol where ubiquitin-conjugating enzymes target them for degradation by the 26S proteasome.[14,15] The last is programmed cell death, for example, via induction of the transcription factor CHOP or GADD153[14,16] and induction of ER-associated caspase 12.[17–19] Each of these pathways has been demonstrated to play a role in the development of diabetes.[20]

We hypothesize, therefore, that diabetes in male NOD.k iHEL mice is a result of transgene-mediated ER stress resulting in β cell apoptosis. A major question then is why only male mice are affected. This would suggest a gender-specific factor operating to increase the level of ER stress in male NOD.k iHEL mice or, alternatively, that male NOD.k iHEL mice are more susceptible to programmed cell death mediated by ER stress. Although neither human type 1 nor type 2 diabetes exhibits gender-specific differences in incidence, there is some evidence of a role of testosterone in β cell dysfunction. One study reported serum testosterone to be higher in female diabetic patients than in female nondiabetic controls, with a correlation between testosterone and C-peptide levels.[21] Serum testosterone and free testosterone levels have also been shown to be elevated in adolescents with diabetes when compared to healthy, sex- and pubertal stage–matched controls.[22] Furthermore, women with polycystic ovarian syndrome and associated hyperandrogenism have an increased risk of developing type 2 diabetes. In a study using Wistar rats (a common rat strain that normally does not develop diabetes), it was demonstrated that testosterone has a direct effect upon islet function and increases insulin gene expression and release.[23] It is thus possible that male NOD.k iHEL have higher HEL transgene expression due to a gender-specific increase in the activity of the rat insulin promoter driving the transgene. The greater production of β cell HEL in male NOD.k iHEL mice may then be sufficient to overload the ER, resulting in ER stress and triggering of β cell apoptosis.

Additional studies are clearly required to fully address issues underlying the role of ER stress in human diabetes. The novel NOD.k iHEL model may be particularly useful for studying these mechanisms and also for testing potential therapies designed to protect β cells from stress-induced apoptosis. Finally, the NOD.k iHEL model may assist in deciphering the link between hyperandrogenism, insulin resistance, and diabetes.

ACKNOWLEDGMENTS

L. Socha and D. Silva are recipients of scholarships from the JCSMR, Australian National University. D. Silva is also a recipient of a scholarship from the Canberra Hospital Salaried Specialists' Private Practice Fund. We would like to thank the electron microscopy service at The Canberra Hospital for their kind assistance.

REFERENCES

1. LESAGE, S., S.B. HARTLEY, S. AKKARAJU *et al.* 2002. Failure to censor forbidden clones of CD4 T cells in autoimmune diabetes. J. Exp. Med. **196:** 1175.
2. HATTORI, M., J.B. BUSE, R.A. JACKSON *et al.* 1986. The NOD mouse: recessive diabetogenic gene in the major histocompatibility complex. Science **231:** 733.
3. RAMMENSEE, H.G., T. FRIEDE & S. STEVANOVIIC. 1995. MHC ligands and peptide motifs: first listing. Immunogenetics **41:** 178.
4. JOHNSON, E.A., P. SILVEIRA, H.D. CHAPMAN *et al.* 2001. Inhibition of autoimmune diabetes in nonobese diabetic mice by transgenic restoration of H2-E MHC class II expression: additive, but unequal, involvement of multiple APC subtypes. J. Immunol. **167:** 2404.
5. DAMOTTE, D., E. COLOMB, C. CAILLEAU *et al.* 1997. Analysis of susceptibility of NOD mice to spontaneous and experimentally induced thyroiditis. Eur. J. Immunol. **27:** 2854.
6. BOWEN, K.M., L. ANDRUS & K.J. LAFFERTY. 1980. Successful allotransplantation of mouse pancreatic islets to nonimmunosuppressed recipients. Diabetes **29**(suppl. 1): 98.
7. FEROZE, G.N. 1997. Ultrastructural Pathology of the Cell and Matrix. Oxford University Press. London/New York/Washington.
8. RON, D. 2002. Proteotoxicity in the endoplasmic reticulum: lessons from the Akita diabetic mouse. J. Clin. Invest. **109:** 443.

9. RON, D. 2002. Translational control in the endoplasmic reticulum stress response. J. Clin. Invest. **110:** 1383.
10. KAUFMAN, R.J. 2002. Orchestrating the unfolded protein response in health and disease. J. Clin. Invest. **110:** 1389.
11. BROSTROM, C.O. & M.A. BROSTROM. 1998. Regulation of translational initiation during cellular responses to stress. Prog. Nucleic Acid Res. Mol. Biol. **58:** 79.
12. ZHANG, P., B. MCGRATH, S. LI et al. 2002. The PERK eukaryotic initiation factor 2 alpha kinase is required for the development of the skeletal system, postnatal growth, and the function and viability of the pancreas. Mol. Cell. Biol. **22:** 3864.
13. HARDING, H.P., Y. ZHANG, A. BERTOLOTTI et al. 2000. Perk is essential for translational regulation and cell survival during the unfolded protein response. Mol. Cell **5:** 897.
14. OYADOMARI, S., A. KOIZUMI, K. TAKEDA et al. 2002. Targeted disruption of the Chop gene delays endoplasmic reticulum stress-mediated diabetes. J. Clin. Invest. **109:** 525.
15. MORI, K. 2000. Tripartite management of unfolded proteins in the endoplasmic reticulum. Cell **101:** 451.
16. OYADOMARI, S., K. TAKEDA, M. TAKIGUCHI et al. 2001. Nitric oxide–induced apoptosis in pancreatic beta cells is mediated by the endoplasmic reticulum stress pathway. Proc. Natl. Acad. Sci. USA **98:** 10845.
17. MORISHIMA, N., K. NAKANISHI, H. TAKENOUCHI et al. 2002. An endoplasmic reticulum stress-specific caspase cascade in apoptosis: cytochrome c–independent activation of caspase-9 by caspase-12. J. Biol. Chem. **277:** 34287.
18. NAKAGAWA, T., H. ZHU, N. MORISHIMA et al. 2000. Caspase-12 mediates endoplasmic-reticulum-specific apoptosis and cytotoxicity by amyloid-beta. Nature **403:** 98.
19. DIAZ-HORTA, O., A. KAMAGATE, A. HERCHUELZ & F. VAN EYLEN. 2002. Na/Ca exchanger overexpression induces endoplasmic reticulum–related apoptosis and caspase-12 activation in insulin-releasing BRIN-BD11 cells. Diabetes **51:** 1815.
20. OYADOMARI, S., E. ARAKI & M. MORI. 2002. Endoplasmic reticulum stress-mediated apoptosis in pancreatic beta-cells. Apoptosis **7:** 335.
21. ZIETZ, B., A. CUK, S. HUGL et al. 2000. Association of increased C-peptide serum levels and testosterone in type 2 diabetes. Eur. J. Intern. Med. **11:** 322.
22. MEYER, K., J. DEUTSCHER, M. ANIL et al. 2000. Serum androgen levels in adolescents with type 1 diabetes: relationship to pubertal stage and metabolic control. J. Endocrinol. Invest. **23:** 362.
23. MORIMOTO, S., C. FERNANDEZ-MEJIA, G. ROMERO-NAVARRO et al. 2001. Testosterone effect on insulin content, messenger ribonucleic acid levels, promoter activity, and secretion in the rat. Endocrinology **142:** 1442.

Defective Maturation of Myeloid Dendritic Cell (DC) in NOD Mice Is Controlled by IDD10/17/18

RUIHUA PENG, K. BATHJAT, Y. LI, AND M. J. CLARE-SALZLER

Department of Pathology, Immunology, and Laboratory Medicine, University of Florida, Gainesville, Florida, USA

ABSTRACT: We previously demonstrated that adoptive transfer of NOD pancreatic lymph node (PLN) DC protected recipients from diabetes. Our recent studies showed that the tolerogenic DC population presented islet antigens and were mature myeloid DC that did not produce IL-12, suggestive of exhausted or fully mature DC. Extensive characterization of the DC population *in vivo* in NOD and control mice demonstrated a specific deficiency of PLN tolerogenic DC in older mice. These findings suggest autoimmunity might arise in NOD mice secondary to deficient maturation of myeloid DC to a tolerogenic state. To address this issue, we characterized maturation and function at development of bone marrow–derived myeloid DC from NOD and several control strains. We found that NOD DC were highly resistant to several maturation stimuli and maintained an immature phenotype (average % immature DC: 75% in NOD versus 15% in B6, $p < 0.01$). A survey of congenic NOD mice with various NOD diabetes susceptibility loci demonstrated that the IDD10/17/18 region on chromosome 3 controlled approximately 50% of the NOD DC maturation defect. The defect also affected NOD DC that underwent phenotypic maturation. These cells appeared to arrest in a "maturing" phase as they produced 5- to 7-fold more IL-12 than control strains and significantly less IL-10. The cytokine defect was completely corrected in NOD IDD10/17/18 mice. In addition, the IDD10/17/18 locus limited DC accumulation in islets and significantly increased tolerogenic DC in the PLN. Together, the above findings suggest that polygenic regulation of DC maturation defects in NOD mice promotes islet inflammation while limiting the generation of tolerogenic DC.

KEYWORDS: IDD10/17/18; dendritic cell (DC); pancreatic lymph node (PLN); NOD mice; bone marrow; maturation defect

INTRODUCTION

Previous studies by Serreze and others demonstrated a defect in the development and function of myeloid lineage cells in the NOD mouse.[1,2] As myeloid cells give rise to important APC populations, the defects in these cells may impact upon the development of effector and regulatory T cell responses.

We previously demonstrated that the transfer of NOD pancreatic lymph node (PLN) dendritic cells (DC) strongly protected recipient mice from the development of diabetes through the generation of regulatory cells.[3,4] These studies, however, did not address the identity of tolerogenic DC nor did they provide an explanation for their apparent failure in the NOD host.

In the following study, we set out to determine the identity of the tolerogenic DC population and to determine why tolerogenic DC fail in the NOD host.

MATERIALS AND METHODS

Mice

C57BL/6, NOD, and IDD10/17/18 female mice, 5 to 8 weeks of age, were obtained from the mouse colony at the University of Florida College of Medicine.

Culture of Bone Marrow–Derived DC

Myeloid DC from bone marrow were developed according to the established method.

Phenotyping of Bone Marrow–Derived DC

The myeloid DC generated from different strains of mice were characterized by four-color flow cytometry.

Measurement of Cytokines

ELISA was used for examination of cytokines secreted by DC.

RESULTS AND DISCUSSION

Phenotypic Maturation Defect of NOD Bone Marrow–Derived DC

Myeloid DC developed from NOD bone marrow failed to mature and upregulate CD86 and MHC class II in response to the stimulation of either LPS or anti-CD40 antibody (25% mature DC). In contrast, B6 bone marrow–derived DC readily matured and upregulated CD86 and MHC class II after stimulation by LPS or anti-CD40 (85% mature DC). We also analyzed several NOD congenic strains for the DC differentiation defect. Of all the congenic mice tested, we found that only bone marrow–derived DC from NOD IDD10/17/18 mice responded in an enhanced manner to the same maturation stimuli (52% mature DC). These findings indicate that NOD myeloid DC manifest significant maturation defect, which is regulated by factors encoded by genes within the IDD10/17/18 susceptibility loci.

Functional Maturation Defects of NOD DC Can Be Completely Normalized by IDD10/17/18 Loci

To evaluate the function of NOD DC, we established mixed lymphocyte responses (MLR) with allogeneic CD4+ T cells. We found that NOD DC were poor stimulators of allogeneic T cell proliferation and cytokine production (IL-2, IL-4, IFN-γ) in comparison to B6 DC. We also assessed whether defects in the maturation process of NOD DC likewise affected DC that do mature. We isolated mature NOD DC and found that, in comparison to B6 DC, they produced 5- to 10-fold more IL-12 and significantly lower levels of IL-10 following stimulation with LPS. In contrast, DC from NOD IDD10/17/18 mice produced levels of IL-12 and IL-10 that were nearly identical to B6 DC. The above results indicate that NOD DC that matured in bone marrow culture arrest in a maturing stage in which DC preferentially produce IL-12 and little IL-10. Finally, immunohistochemical analysis of IDD10/17/18 pancreata demonstrated limited DC accumulation in islets and significantly increased numbers of tolerogenic DC in the PLN in comparison to NOD. These findings suggest that IDD10/17/18 loci play an important role in regulating DC maturation.

REFERENCES

1. LANGMUIR, P.B. et al. 1993. Bone marrow abnormalities in the non-obese diabetic mouse. Int. Immunol. **5:** 169–177.
2. SERREZE, D.V. et al. 1993. Hematopoietic stem-cell defects underlying abnormal macrophage development and maturation in NOD/Lt mice: defective regulation of cytokine receptors and protein kinase C. Proc. Natl. Acad. Sci. USA **90:** 9625–9629.
3. CLARE-SALZLER, M.J. et al. 1992. Prevention of diabetes in nonobese diabetic mice by dendritic cell transfer. J. Clin. Invest. **90:** 741–748.
4. NAUMOV, Y.N. et al. 2001. Activation of CD1d-restricted T cells protects NOD mice from developing diabetes by regulating dendritic cell subsets. Proc. Natl. Acad. Sci. USA **98:** 13838–13843.

Absence of the T-bet Gene Coding for the Th1-Related Transcription Factor Does Not Affect Diabetes-Associated Phenotypes in Balb/c Mice

EVIE MELANITOU,[a] EDWIN LIU,[a] DONGMEI MIAO,[a] LIPING YU,[a] LAURIE H. GLIMCHER,[b] AND GEORGE EISENBARTH[a]

[a]*Barbara Davis Center for Childhood Diabetes, University of Colorado Health Science Center, Denver, Colorado 80262, USA*

[b]*Department of Immunology and Infectious Diseases, Harvard School of Public Health, Boston, Massachusetts 02115, USA*

> ABSTRACT: The T-box expressed in T cells gene (T-bet) is a member of the T-box family of transcription factors. T-bet-deficient mice show normal lymphoid development, but exhibit profound defects in their Th1-mediated immune responses. As the balance between Th1- and Th2-mediated immune responses plays a role in autoimmune-prone diseases, we have investigated the diabetes-related insulin autoantibody (IAA) and cellular immune responses (insulitis), in the absence of Th1 lineage commitment, in T-bet KO Balb/c mice, after immunization with the B9–23 insulin peptide. We have therefore investigated whether absence of the T-bet gene influences diabetes-related phenotypes in Balb/c T-bet KO mice.
>
> KEYWORDS: T-bet; Balb/c mice; B9–23 insulin peptide; immune response

INTRODUCTION

The T-box expressed in T cells gene (T-bet) is a member of the T-box family of transcription factors.[1] It regulates the lineage commitment in CD4 T helper lymphocytes in part by activating the T_H1 cytokine interferon-γ (IFN-γ).[2] While Th1 cells produce IFN-γ and are important in macrophage activation as well as inflammatory and autoimmune reactions, Th2 cells produce cytokines such as interleukin-4 (IL-4) and IL-10 and are mainly involved in controlling humoral and allergic immune responses.[3] Tight control of Th1 immunity is essential in preventing immunopathology. T-bet-deficient mice show normal lymphoid development, but exhibit profound defects in their Th1-mediated immune responses.[2] CD4 T cells and natural killer T cells of T-bet-deficient mice produce reduced amounts of IFN-γ, whereas

---

Address for correspondence: Evie Melanitou, Ph.D., Dr.Sc., Barbara Davis Center for Childhood Diabetes, University of Colorado Health Science Center, 4200 East 9th Avenue, Box B-140, Denver, CO 80262. Voice: 303-315-7108; fax: 303-315-4892.
    eviemel@pasteur.fr

Ann. N.Y. Acad. Sci. 1005: 187–191 (2003). © 2003 New York Academy of Sciences.
doi: 10.1196/annals.1288.024

cytotoxic CD8+ T cells show unaltered IFN-γ production, indicating a key role for T-bet in controlling IFN-γ production by CD4, but not CD8 T cells.[2] T-bet knockout (KO) alleles have been placed in the Balb/c genetic background by backcrossing onto the Balb/c strain.[2]

As the balance between Th1- and Th2-mediated immune responses plays a role in autoimmune-prone diseases, we have investigated the diabetes-related insulin autoantibody (IAA) and cellular immune responses (insulitis), in the absence of Th1 lineage commitment, in T-bet KO Balb/c mice, after immunization with the B9–23 insulin peptide. Proinsulin/insulin[4–6] and B9–23 have been extensively studied as islet autoantigens.[7] The sequence of the B9–23 peptide is identical in mice and humans, and T cell responses can be demonstrated in both species. Treatment of NOD mice with B9–23 induces IAA and insulitis and protects from diabetes.[8] In addition, in Balb/c mice, B9–23 in combination with poly-IC (polyinosinic-polycytidilic acid), a viral RNA mimic, induces IAA and insulitis, but not diabetes.[8–10] We have therefore investigated whether absence of the T-bet gene influences diabetes-related phenotypes in Balb/c T-bet KO mice.

METHODS

Balb/c.*tgn*.T-bet^{KO} mice have been generated by Laurie Glimcher's group by backcrossing the initial KO mouse into the Balb/c genetic background until BC8 generation.[2] Genotyping of the littermates was performed as described.[11] Animals at 4 weeks of age were treated subcutaneously with 100 μg of B9–23 in incomplete Freund's adjuvant (IFA) (day 1). Poly-IC (7.5 μg/g body weight) was also administered intraperitoneally on days 1–5 and 8–14. IAA was measured in the serum at 4 weeks and up to 12 weeks of age by a 96-well filtration plate micro-IAA-assay as described.[9,12] Histological and immunohistochemical analysis of pancreas was performed by fixation of portions of the tissue in 10% formalin, paraffin-embedded and stained with hematoxylin and eosin as previously described.[9]

RESULTS AND DISCUSSION

The T-bet Gene Is Not Required for IAA Responses after Immunization

Balb/c wild-type (+/+), KO mice for the T-bet gene (–/–), as well as mice heterozygous for the KO allele (+/–) were immunized with B9–23 insulin peptide and/or poly-IC. IAA concentrations in serum were monitored before and after treatment. B9–23 and B9–23 together with poly-IC induced IAA in all three groups of mice (FIG. 1). No gender differences were observed as male and female animals showed similar responses (data not shown). Therefore, the absence of the Th1-regulating transcription factor does not affect B cell responses after immunization with this self-peptide. A role for the T-bet gene has been reported in the regulation of IgG class switching, especially to IgG2a.[13] In fact, T-bet-deficient B lymphocytes demonstrated impaired production of IgG2a, IgG2b, and IgG3 and are unable to generate germ line or IgG2a transcripts in response to IFN-γ.[13] In a murine model of lupus, absence of T-bet led to a reduction in autoantibody production, hypergammaglobulinemia, immune complex–mediated renal disease, and impaired IgG2a production.[13] Thus, a role has been attributed to the T-bet gene in controlling B cell–mediated autoimmunity. It is interesting to note that IAAs, naturally occurring or after immunization, are mainly of the IgG1 subclass, which corresponds to the Th2 type. We have assessed the immunoglobulin subclass of IAA in the T-bet KO mice after immunization with B9–23 and confirmed the IgG1 subclass (data not shown). Therefore, the IgG1 subclass of IAA in response to immunization with the B9–23 peptide is not affected by the absence of the T-bet gene.

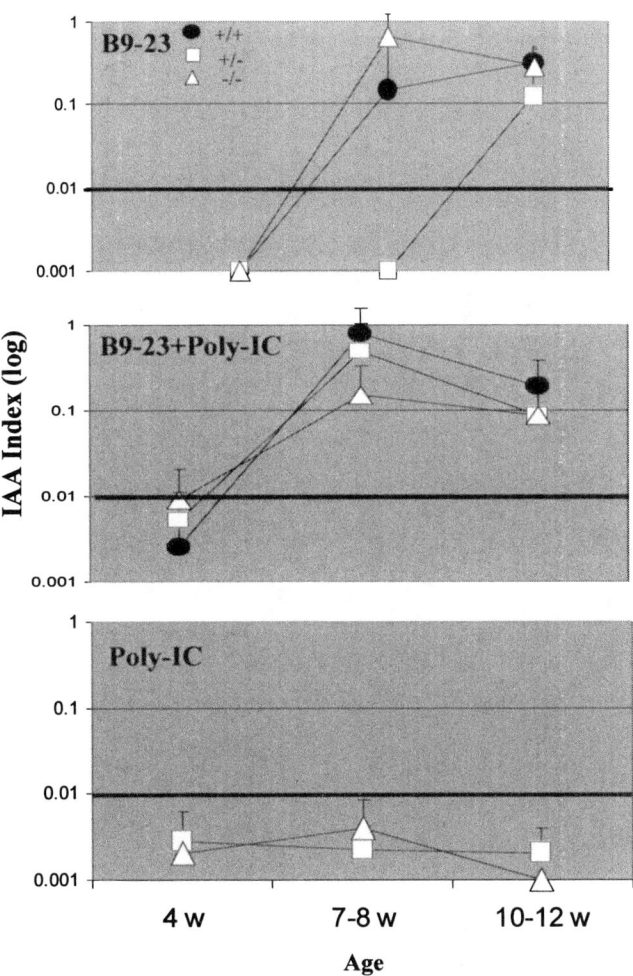

FIGURE 1. Mean values of IAA induction after immunization of male and female Balb/c.*tgn*.T-bet[KO] mice (each experimental point corresponds to 4 or 5 animals). Total number of animals: 35.

TABLE 1. Summary of autoimmune diabetes subphenotypes after immunization

Mouse strain	Treatment	IAA	Insulitis	Diabetes	Ref.
NOD	B9–23	+	+	no	8, 10
Balb/c	B9–23	+	no	no	10
Balb/c	B9–23 + poly-IC	+	+	no	9
Balb/c	Poly-IC	no	no	no	9
Balb/c.tgn.T-bet^{KO*}	B9–23	+	no	no	
Balb/c.tgn.T-bet^{KO*}	B9–23 + poly-IC	+	+	no	
Balb/c.tgn.T-bet^{KO*}	Poly-IC	no	no	no	

NOTE: +, present; no, absent; *similar data obtained for T-bet +/+, +/−, and −/− mice.

Absence of the T-bet Gene Does Not Influence the Progression to Insulitis after Immunization

Balb/c mice in addition to the NOD strain have been extensively studied for their responses to immunization.[9,10] As already mentioned, in this H-2^d permissive genetic background, immunostimulation results not only in the production of IAA, but also in the presence of insulitis (summarized in TABLE 1). However, for this later phenotype, daily injections of poly-IC are required together with antigen stimulation. Although the mechanisms underlying this induced phenotype might be different from the spontaneous appearance of insulitis, observed in the NOD mouse, it is noteworthy that H-2^b mice do not develop any response after B9–23 immunization.[9] It was of interest to examine if the absence of T-bet gene in the Balb/c mice could be a determinant for the appearance of insulitis after immunization with the combination of B9–23 and poly-IC as previously characterized in Balb/c mice. Animals positive for IAA were sacrificed at 10 and 16 weeks of age, and their pancreata assessed for histology and CD4 and CD8 staining. As summarized in TABLE 1, the combination of B9–23 and poly-IC results in insulitis similarly in all three genotypes studied (wild-type +/+, heterozygous +/−, and homozygous −/− for the T-bet KO). Therefore, impairment of CD4 Th1 cells due to the absence of the T-bet gene does not affect the progression to insulitis, the first prerequisite phenotype for autoimmune diabetes. It has been debated that early stages of diabetes might require the presence of CD8+ T cells rather than CD4+ T cells, which might be responsible for the final stages of autoimmune destruction.[14] Since the T-bet transcription factor influences the production of IFN-γ from the CD4 T cells, but does not affect CD8 T cells, its absence might not influence the progression to insulitis. However, generalization of this observation is speculative as the presented data correspond to an induced model and the influence of the T-bet gene to autoimmune diabetes should also be assessed for the spontaneous phenotype in NOD mice lacking the T-bet gene.

In summary, the T-box transcription factor T-bet gene regulating Th1 lineage commitment is not required for IAA responses nor for insulitis after immunization with B9–23 insulin peptide and poly-IC in the Balb/c mice.

ACKNOWLEDGMENTS

E. Melanitou is on sabbatical leave from the Pasteur Institute, Paris, France. L. H. Glimcher was supported by grants from the NIH and the Juvenile Diabetes Foundation International.

REFERENCES

1. SZABO, S.J., S.T KIM, G.L. COSTA et al. 2000. A novel transcription factor, T-bet, directs Th1 lineage commitment. Cell **100:** 655–669.
2. SZABO, S.J., B.M. SULLIVAN et al. 2002. Distinct effects of T-bet in Th1 lineage commitment and IFN-γ production in CD4 and CD8 T cells. Science **295:** 338–342.
3. MOSMANN, T.R. & R.L. COFFMAN. 1989. Th1 and Th2 cells: different patterns of lymphokine secretion lead to different functional properties. Annu. Rev. Immunol. **7:** 145–173.
4. ZHANG, Z.J., L. DAVIDSON, G. EISENBARTH & H.L. WEINER. 1991. Suppression of diabetes in nonobese diabetic mice by oral administration of porcine insulin. Proc. Natl. Acad. Sci. USA **88:** 10252–10256.
5. MUIR, A., A. PECK, M. CLARE-SALZLER et al. 1995. Insulin immunization of nonobese diabetic mice induces a protective insulitis characterized by diminished intraislet interferon-gamma transcription. J. Clin. Invest. **95:** 628–634.
6. WONG, F.S., J. KARTUNEN, C. DUMONT et al. 1999. Identification of an MHC class I–restricted autoantigen in type 1 diabetes by screening an organ-specific cDNA library. Nat. Med. **5:** 1026–1031.
7. WEGMANN, D.R., M. NORBURY-GLASER & D. DANIEL. 1994. Insulin-specific T cells are a predominant component of islet infiltrates in prediabetic NOD mice. Eur. J. Immunol. **24:** 1853–1857.
8. LIU, E., N. ABIRU, H. MORIYAMA et al. 2002. Induction of insulin autoantibodies and protection from diabetes with subcutaneous insulin B:9–23 peptide without adjuvant. Ann. N.Y. Acad. Sci. **958:** 224–227.
9. MORIYAMA, H., L. WEN, N. ABIRU et al. 2002. Induction and acceleration of insulitis/diabetes in mice with a viral mimic and an insulin self-peptide. Proc. Natl. Acad. Sci. USA **99:** 5539–5544.
10. ABIRU, N., A.K. MANIATIS, L. YU et al. 2001. Peptide and major histocompatibility complex specific breaking of humoral tolerance to native insulin with the B9–23 peptide in diabetes-prone and normal mice. Diabetes **50:** 1274–1281.
11. NEURATH, M.F., B. WEIGMANN, S. FINOTTO et al. 2002. The transcription factor T-bet regulates mucosal T cell activation in experimental colitis and Crohn's disease. J. Exp. Med. **195:** 1129–1143.
12. YU, L., D. ROBLES, N. ABIRU et al. 2000. Early expression of antiinsulin autoantibodies of humans and the NOD mouse: evidence for early determination of subsequent diabetes. Proc. Natl. Acad. Sci. USA **97:** 1701–1706.
13. PENG, S.L., S.J. SZABO & L.H. GLIMCHER. 2002. T-bet regulates IgG class switching and pathogenic autoantibody production. Proc. Natl. Acad. Sci. USA **99:** 5545–5550.
14. DILORENZO, T.P., R.T. GRAZER, T. ONO et al. 1998. Major histocompatibility complex class I–restricted T cells are required for all but the end stages of diabetes development in nonobese diabetic mice and use a prevalent T cell receptor alpha chain gene rearrangement. Proc. Natl. Acad. Sci. USA **95:** 12538–12543.

Immunolocalization of Caspase-3 in Pancreatic Islets of NOD Mice during Cyclophosphamide-Accelerated Diabetes

SHIVA REDDY,[a,b] JOSHUA BRADLEY,[a] AND JACQUELINE M. ROSS[c]

[a]*School of Biological Sciences,* [b]*Department of Pediatrics, and* [c]*Department of Anatomy with Radiology, University of Auckland, Auckland, New Zealand*

ABSTRACT: Apoptosis may be a major mechanism of beta cell loss during insulin-dependent diabetes mellitus. Caspase-3 is a key enzyme involved in the terminal steps of this death process. Here, the intra-islet expression of caspase-3 in the NOD mouse was examined immunohistochemically following acceleration of the disease with cyclophosphamide. Female NOD mice were treated at day 95 with cyclophosphamide, and caspase-3 expression in pancreatic sections was studied at days 0, 4, 7, 11, and 14 and compared with age-matched control tissue. In the treated group at day 0, caspase-3 labeling was seen in several peri-islet macrophages and only extremely rarely in beta cells. At day 4, only a few beta cells weakly expressed the enzyme. From day 7, caspase-3 expression began to increase in intra-islet macrophages and reached a peak at days 11 and 14, when a small number of CD4 and CD8 T cells also showed positive labeling. Beta cell expression of caspase-3 at days 11 and 14 was rare. At this stage, several intra-islet immune cells with positive labeling for the enzyme coexpressed either Fas or interleukin-1β. Only a small proportion of intra-islet caspase-3 cells showed apoptotic nuclei judged by terminal deoxynucleotidyl transferase–mediated dUTP nick end labeling (TUNEL). We conclude that, during cyclophosphamide-accelerated diabetes, the predominant caspase-3 immunolabeling in intra- and extra-islet macrophages suggests that apoptosis of macrophages may be an important mechanism for their elimination. The virtual absence of caspase-3 immunolabeling in most beta cells even during the height of beta cell loss supports the need for developing other markers of early beta cell apoptosis in the NOD mouse.

KEYWORDS: caspase-3; NOD mouse; islets; beta cell death

INTRODUCTION

Studies in the NOD mouse *in situ* suggest that beta cell death may occur by apoptosis.[1] Islets in culture exposed to various cytokines also undergo apoptosis.[2] During this process, a group of proteolytic enzymes known as caspases are activated from their precursor forms into active catalytic species. Thus, activated initiator

---

Address for correspondence: S. Reddy, Ph.D., Senior Research Fellow, School of Biological Sciences, University of Auckland, Private bag 92019, Auckland, New Zealand. Voice: +64-9-3737599 (ext. 82917); fax: +64-9-3737486.
s.reddy@auckland.ac.nz

caspases can convert inactive procaspase-3 to active caspase-3, a key enzyme involved in the terminal apoptotic cascade of cell death.[3,4] In the NOD mouse, the expression of active caspase-3 within the islets, its role in mediating beta cell apoptosis, and its temporal relationship with the development of IDDM remain unclear. Here, we have examined pancreatic islets of NOD mice following disease acceleration with cyclophosphamide (Cy) for the expression of active caspase-3 by dual-label immunohistochemistry.

METHODS

Female NOD mice were allocated at random into two groups (group 1 and group 2; 18 mice per group) and maintained on standard mouse chow and water. At day 95, all but 3 mice from group 2 were injected intraperitoneally with Cy (300 mg/kg body weight), while mice from group 1 (control group) received sterile water as diluent. Animals were sacrificed at days 0, 4, 7, 11, and 14 and the pancreas examined by immunohistochemistry. The cellular source of caspase-3 was studied by coimmunolabeling sections with antibodies to insulin, CD4 and CD8 cells, macrophages, interleukin-1β (IL-1β), or Fas. Sections were also analyzed by terminal deoxynucleotidyl transferase–mediated dUTP nick end labeling (TUNEL) to detect apoptotic cells.

RESULTS

In the control group (group 1), an increasing number of caspase-3-positive cells were observed in the exocrine, perivascular, and peri-islet areas and were colocalized in macrophages (FIGS. 1a and 1b). Beta cells were generally devoid of caspase-3 despite the presence of significant insulitis. In islets with an absence of or with minimum insulitis, only occasional beta cells contained weak labeling for caspase-3.

In the Cy group, a changing pattern of caspase-3 labeling was observed. At day 4, weak labeling for the enzyme was occasionally seen in some beta cells only and in a minority of islets. At day 7, an increasing number of macrophages in peri-islet areas expressed the enzyme. At day 11, there was a marked increase in the number of macrophages, positive for the enzyme. Such macrophages were located in the peri- and intra-islet areas and occasionally in the perivascular and exocrine space (FIGS. 1c and 1d). At this stage, some CD4 cells were positive for the enzyme, while CD8 cells were negative. At day 11, most infiltrated islets containing insulin were devoid of caspase-3 (FIGS. 1e and 1f). At day 14, there was a marked increase in both the intensity and number of caspase-3-positive cells within the intra-islet and exocrine regions. Caspase-3-positive cells corresponded to mostly macrophages and occasionally CD4 and CD8 cells (FIGS. 1g and 1h). However, several macrophages were devoid of caspase-3 immunolabeling.

A proportion of intra-islet macrophages positive for caspase-3 also coexpressed IL-1β and Fas.

At days 11 and 14 (Cy group), only a minority of caspase-positive cells showed TUNEL-positive nuclei. Apoptotic nuclei were also observed in caspase-3-negative cells mainly in the insulitis region. Beta cell apoptotic nuclei judged by TUNEL were rare (FIGS. 1i and 1j).

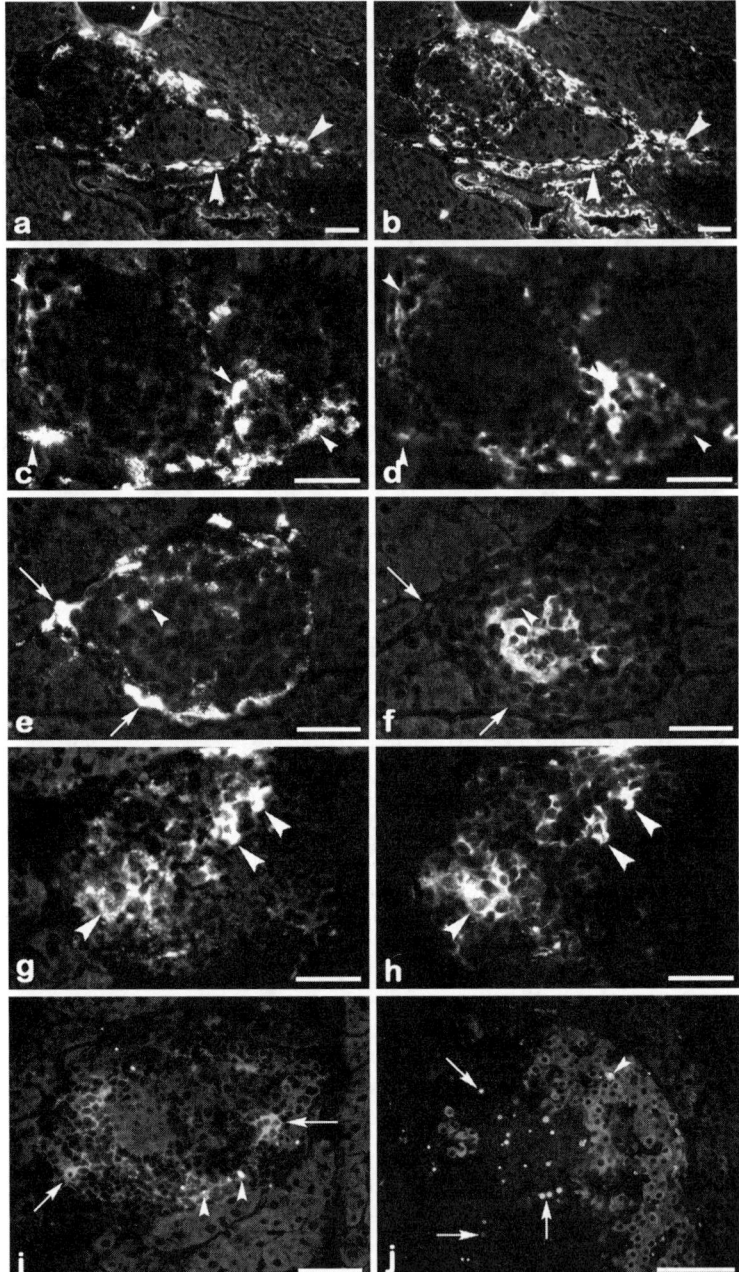

FIGURE 1. Photomicrographs of pancreatic islets from Cy-treated NOD mice showing the expression of caspase-3. **(a, b)** Day 0, showing an islet dual-labeled for caspase **(a)** and macrophages **(b)**. Arrowheads point to peri-islet macrophages positive for caspase. **(c–f)** Day 11 islet dual-labeled for caspase **(c)** and macrophages **(d)**. Arrowheads point to macro-

DISCUSSION

During IDDM, beta cell death may be executed by apoptosis.[2] However, experimental evidence for this process *in vivo* remains weak. Although various distinct signals may initiate beta cell apoptosis, they may enter a common "execution" pathway of apoptosis involving the catalytic conversion of procaspase-3 to active caspase-3. Thus, the presence of active caspase-3 may be an important surrogate marker of beta cell death during apoptosis.

In the day 95 NOD mouse, caspase-3 was observed in several macrophages in the peri-islet areas and was only rarely seen in beta cells. This pattern of mainly macrophage-specific expression of the enzyme was also seen in later stages of Cy-induced diabetes. These observations support the view that macrophages may die at or near the site of inflammation and may be a mechanism of regulating or reducing macrophage populations following resolution of inflammation.[5,6] The much smaller numbers of CD4 and CD8 cells positive for caspase-3 in islets at days 11 and 14 suggest that some T cells may also die by apoptosis within the islets. These observations are in agreement with previous studies.[7,8] In this study, the absence of a significant number of caspase-3-positive beta cells suggests that dying beta cells are cleared rapidly. Since the presence of caspase-3 and apoptotic nuclei represent late stages of the cell death pathway and since the frequency of apoptotic beta cells is extremely low *in situ*, other cell biological or molecular detection tools are necessary in identifying those beta cells that have embarked on the early pathway of irreversible apoptotic death during IDDM.

REFERENCES

1. O'BRIEN, B.A. *et al.* 1997. Apoptosis is the mode of beta-cell death responsible for the development of IDDM in the non-obese diabetic (NOD) mouse. Diabetes **46:** 750–757.
2. EIZIRIK, D.L. & T. MANDRUP-POULSEN. 2001. A choice of death—the signal transduction of immune-mediated beta-cell apoptosis. Diabetologia **44:** 2115–2133.
3. THORNBERRY, N.A. & Y. LAZEBNIK. 1998. Caspases: enemies within. Science **281:** 1312–1316.
4. MATHIS, D. *et al.* 2001. β-cell death during progression to diabetes. Nature **414:** 792–798.
5. TIDBALL, J.G. & B.A. ST. PIERRE. 1996. Apoptosis of macrophages during the resolution of muscle inflammation. J. Leukocyte Biol. **59:** 380–388.
6. LAN, H.Y. *et al.* 1997. Macrophage apoptosis in rat crescentic glomerulonephritis. Am. J. Pathol. **151:** 531–538.
7. AUGSTEIN, P. *et al.* 1998. Apoptosis and beta cell destruction in pancreatic islets of NOD mice with spontaneous and cyclophosphamide-accelerated diabetes. Diabetologia **41:** 1381–1388.
8. KIM, Y-H. *et al.* 1999. Apoptosis of pancreatic β-cells detected in accelerated diabetes of NOD mice: no role for Fas–Fas ligand in autoimmune diabetes. Eur. J. Clin. Immunol. **29:** 455–465.

---

phages that express caspase. **(e, f)** Islet dual-labeled for caspase **(e)** and insulin **(f)**. Arrows point to caspase-labeled cells that are insulin-negative, while arrowheads point to a few beta cells that are weakly labeled for caspase. **(g, h)** Day 14 islet dual-labeled for caspase **(g)** and macrophages **(h)**. Arrowheads point to macrophages with strong labeling for caspase. **(i)** Day 11 islet dual-labeled for caspase and by TUNEL. Arrowheads point to caspase-positive cells also positive by TUNEL, while arrows point to caspase-positive cells that are negative by TUNEL. **(j)** Day 11 islet dual-labeled for insulin and by TUNEL. Arrows point to numerous TUNEL-positive nuclei that are in the insulitis region, while most beta cells are TUNEL-negative, except one beta cell (arrowhead). Scale bars: 40 µm.

Congenic Mapping and Candidate Sequencing of Susceptibility Genes for Type 1 Diabetes in the NOD Mouse

HIROSHI IKEGAMI, TOMOMI FUJISAWA, SUSUMU MAKINO, AND TOSHIO OGIHARA

Department of Geriatric Medicine, Osaka University Graduate School of Medicine, Osaka 565-0871, Japan

ABSTRACT: Inheritance of type 1 diabetes is polygenic with a major susceptibility gene located in the major histocompatibility complex (MHC). In addition to MHC-linked susceptibility, a number of susceptibility genes have been mapped outside the MHC in both humans and animal models. In order to localize and identify susceptibility genes for type 1 diabetes, we have developed a series of congenic strains in which either susceptibility intervals from the NOD mouse, a mouse model of type 1 diabetes, were introgressed onto control background genes or protective intervals from control strains were introgressed onto NOD background genes. NOD.CTS-*H-2* congenic mice, which possess recombinant MHC with NOD alleles at class II A and E genes, which are candidates for *Idd1*, revealed that *Idd1* consists of multiple components, one in class II (*Idd1*) and the other adjacent to, but distinct from, *Idd1* (*Idd16*). Phenotypes of NOD.IIS-*Idd3* congenic mice, which share the same alleles at both *Il2* and *Il21* as the NOD mouse, were indistinguishable from the NOD parental strain, indicating that both *Il2* and *Il21* are candidates for *Idd3*. In contrast, NOD.IIS-*Idd10* congenic mice, which share the same alleles at *Fcgr1*, a previous candidate for *Idd10*, as the NOD mouse, were protected from type 1 diabetes, suggesting that *Fcgr1* may not be responsible for the *Idd10* effect. These data suggest that the use of strain colony closely related to a disease model to find the same candidate mutation on different haplotypes and make congenic strains with this recombinant chromosome, termed ancestral haplotype congenic mapping, is an effective strategy for fine mapping and identification of genes responsible for complex traits.

KEYWORDS: type 1 diabetes; NOD mouse; major histocompatibility complex (MHC); susceptibility gene; interleukin-2; interleukin-21

INTRODUCTION

Type 1 diabetes is caused by autoimmune destruction of insulin-producing beta cells of the pancreas. Inheritance of type 1 diabetes is polygenic with a major sus-

Address for correspondence: Dr. Hiroshi Ikegami, Department of Geriatric Medicine, Osaka University Graduate School of Medicine, 2-2, Yamada-oka, Suita, Osaka 565-0871, Japan. Voice: +81-6-6879-3852; fax: +81-6-6879-3859.
ikegami@geriat.med.osaka-u.ac.jp

ceptibility gene located in the major histocompatibility complex (MHC). In addition to MHC-linked susceptibility, a number of susceptibility genes have been mapped outside the MHC in both humans and animal models.

In order to localize and identify susceptibility genes for type 1 diabetes, we have developed a series of congenic strains in which either susceptibility intervals from the NOD mouse, a mouse model of type 1 diabetes, were introgressed onto control background genes or protective intervals from control strains were introgressed onto NOD background genes.

MHC-LINKED SUSCEPTIBILITY

In the NOD mouse, the strongest susceptibility gene, *Idd1*, has been mapped to the MHC region on mouse chromosome 17.[1,2] NOD mice congenic for the MHC from control laboratory strains or even from NOD-related strains such as NON and NCT were completely resistant to insulitis and type 1 diabetes,[3–7] indicating that the NOD MHC is necessary for the development of type 1 diabetes. The NOD MHC, however, is not sufficient for the development of type 1 diabetes because control strains, such as C57BL/6, congenic for the NOD MHC do not develop type 1 diabetes.[6,8]

MHC-LINKED SUSCEPTIBILITY IN CLASS II REGION

To further localize the MHC-linked susceptibility gene, we have studied the phenotypes and genotypes of the MHC region in the NOD and its related strains derived from the same closed colony, Jcl:ICR, as the NOD mouse. Among the NOD-related strains studied, we identified three strains, CTS, ILI, and IOI, that share the same unique class II MHC with the NOD mouse (TABLE 1). These strains have the same genotypes at the class II Ab gene and the same phenotypes of I-A molecules as the NOD mouse and lack I-E expression as in the NOD mouse.[9–11] Since class II A and E genes encoding class II I-A and I-E molecules have been strong candidates for *Idd1*,[1,9] these strains are important in that the MHC of these strains potentially confers susceptibility to type 1 diabetes. The lack of type 1 diabetes in these strains despite the presence of a potentially susceptible MHC may be due to lack of non-MHC susceptibility genes as in the case of control strains congenic for the NOD MHC.

In order to prove that the same class II MHC detected in these NOD-related strains can confer susceptibility to type 1 diabetes, we developed a new congenic strain in which the MHC from an NOD-related strain, the CTS mouse, was introgressed onto NOD background genes. The MHC of the CTS mouse is suitable for this kind of study because the CTS MHC is identical to the NOD MHC in the class II region, but different from the NOD MHC outside of the class II MHC.[9–11] In contrast to the complete protection against type 1 diabetes observed in NOD strains congenic for the MHC from control strains or NOD-related NON and NCT strains,[6,7] NOD mice congenic for the CTS MHC, NOD.CTS-*H-2*, developed type 1 diabetes, indicating that the CTS MHC confers susceptibility to type 1 diabetes.[12] Since the CTS mouse has the same class II MHC as the NOD mouse with different flanking markers from the NOD mouse, the data suggest that the class II MHC of the NOD mouse is responsible for the MHC-linked susceptibility, *Idd1*.

TABLE 1. Alleles at loci on chromosome 17 in NOD-related strains shared with the NOD mouse

cM	Locus	NOD	NON	CTS	ILI	IOI
11.0	D17Mit44	■	□	□	□	□
18.44	K	■	□	□	■	■
18.63	Ob	■	□	■	■	■
18.64	Ab	■	□	■	■	■
18.66	Eb	■	□	■	■	■
18.94	Hsp70-1	■	■	■	■	■
19.021	D17Mit13	■	■	□	■	□
19.059	Lta	■	■	□	■	□
19.060	Tnf	■	■	□	■	□
19.09	D	■	□	□	■	□
21.95	D17Mit105	■	□	□	□	□

NOTE: Closed boxes show NOD alleles and open boxes show non-NOD alleles.

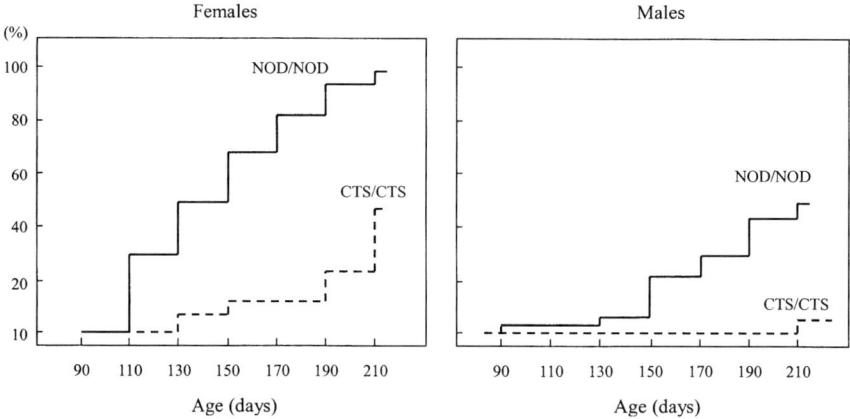

FIGURE 1. Cumulative incidence of type 1 diabetes in NOD.CTS-*H-2* congenic mice.

MHC-LINKED SUSCEPTIBILITY CONSISTS OF MULTIPLE COMPONENTS

Although the NOD.CTS-*H-2* strain developed type 1 diabetes, the incidence of type 1 diabetes was much lower than that in the NOD parental strain (FIG. 1), indicating that the CTS MHC confers susceptibility to type 1 diabetes, but its effect is not as strong as that in the NOD parental strain.[12] These data suggest that MHC-linked susceptibility consists of multiple components, and the CTS MHC contains part of, but not all of, the components. Since the CTS MHC is identical to the NOD MHC in the class II A and E region, but is different from the NOD MHC outside of this region, another gene adjacent to, but distinct from, *Idd1* in the class II region is necessary for full expression of the MHC-linked susceptibility. This gene, termed *Idd16*, is now localized to a less than 11 cM segment of the MHC.[12,13] Subsequent studies from other groups using different congenic strains have confirmed these findings,[14] and multiple components of MHC-linked susceptibility have also been found in humans.[15,16]

CANDIDATE GENES FOR *IDD16*

Among candidate genes for *Idd16* is the *Tnf* gene in the class III region, encoding tumor necrosis factor α (TNFα). The endogenous TNFα level has been reported to be lower in the NOD mouse than in other mouse strains,[17] and administration of TNFα was reported to prevent insulitis and diabetes in the NOD mouse.[17,18] To clarify the contribution of *Tnf* to the *Idd16* effect, we determined haplotypes in the *Tnf* region as well as nucleotide sequences of all exons and the complete upstream region of *Tnf* in NOD and its related strains. The CTS mouse had different alleles at *Tnf* and adjacent loci from the NOD mouse. Although the protein-coding region of *Tnf* in the CTS mouse was identical to that in the NOD mouse,[12] the 5′ upstream region was different from that in the NOD mice.[19] In particular, a C to A substitution at position 3408 in the CTS mouse creates a new GATA family binding site, which may be responsible for the lower incidence of type 1 diabetes in the NOD.CTS-*H-2* congenic strain despite the presence of the same class II MHC as in the NOD mouse.

Among haplotypes determined in NOD-related strains, the NON mouse was found to share the same haplotypes in the class III region with the NOD mouse, but different flanking markers from the NOD mouse (TABLE 1). Consistent with this, Lund *et al.* reported that the class III region of the NON mouse appeared to be identical to that in the NOD mouse using RFLPs detected by Southern hybridization with class III gene probes.[20] Sequence analysis of *Tnf*, a candidate for *Idd16*, revealed that the NON mouse shares the same sequence with the NOD mouse.[12,19] To further study the contribution of *Tnf* to the *Idd16* effect, an NOD strain congenic for MHC from the NON mouse, NOD.NON-*H-2*, was established. Although NON MHC homozygotes were completely resistant to type 1 diabetes, about 20% of MHC heterozygotes developed type 1 diabetes, indicating that the NON MHC confers susceptibility to type 1 diabetes in a heterozygous state. Extensive insulitis was observed in these mice, suggesting an autoimmune nature of diabetes, although the age at onset was considerably later (9–18 months of age) than that in the NOD parental strain. The identical *Tnf* sequence in the NON mouse as in the NOD mouse and the development of type 1 diabetes in NOD.NON-*H-2* heterozygotes suggest that *Tnf* may contribute to type 1 diabetes susceptibility and may be responsible for the *Idd16* effect.

Since the NON mouse expresses surface I-E molecules in contrast to the lack of I-E in the NOD mouse, the data indicate that I-E-positive NOD mice can develop type 1 diabetes, which is in clear contrast to complete protection by the expression of I-E molecules in transgenic NOD mice.[21] Consistent with our data, Podolin *et al.* reported the development of insulitis and diabetes in some of the I-E-positive NOD congenic mice.[5] These data suggested that expression of I-E molecules at a physiological level as in the case of congenic strains does not completely protect against type 1 diabetes in the NOD mouse. Since MHC heterozygotes in the NOD.NON-*H-2* congenic strain possess only one dose of the NOD MHC in combination with the NON MHC, which provides resistance to type 1 diabetes in homozygous state, the development of type 1 diabetes in MHC heterozygotes suggests that the NOD MHC is not completely recessive in conferring susceptibility and the NON MHC, which is different from the NOD MHC at class II A and E loci with the presence of I-E, is not completely dominant in providing resistance to type 1 diabetes. Consistent with these observations, Wicker *et al.* reported the development of type 1 diabetes in MHC heterozygotes in crosses of NOD with C57BL/10 mice, and proposed that the MHC-linked gene in this strain combination may be dominant with low penetrance.[22]

STRONG LINKAGE ON CHROMOSOME 3 IS DUE TO MULTIPLE SUSCEPTIBILITY GENES ON THE SAME CHROMOSOME

Among non-MHC genes, *Idd3* on chromosome 3 is one of the strongest susceptibility genes. *Idd3* was initially mapped to the central part of chromosome 3 near a marker, *D3Nds1*, by a genome scan in a large number of backcross animals between NOD and C57BL/10 mice congenic for the NOD MHC (B10.*H-2^{g7}*) (FIG. 2).[23] Subsequent studies using NOD mice congenic for different segments of chromosome 3 from control B6 or B10 strains, however, revealed that no susceptibility gene exists in the *D3Nds1* region, where peak linkage was initially detected, and that the initial localization of *Idd3* was caused by the combined effect of multiple independent loci on the same chromosome (FIG. 2).[24–26] At least four independent loci, *Idd3*, *Idd10*, *Idd17*, and *Idd18*, have been shown to contribute to susceptibility to type 1 diabetes and to the strong linkage initially detected in the central part of chromosome 3.

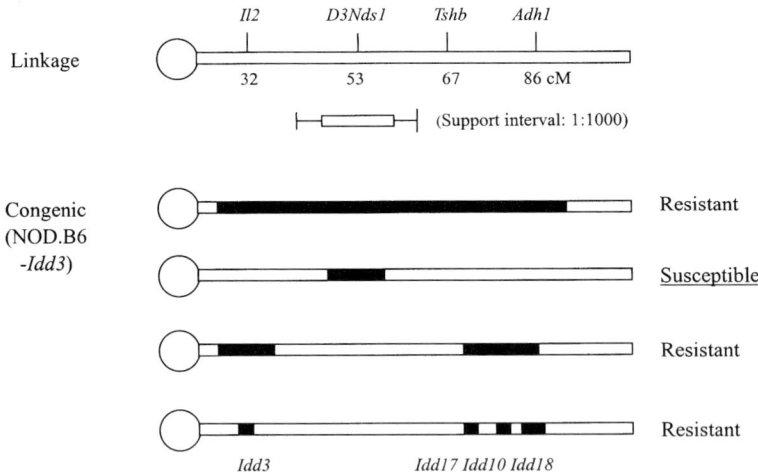

FIGURE 2. Multiple susceptibility genes on mouse chromosome 3: (■) B6-derived chromosomal region; (□) NOD-derived chromosomal region.

IL2 IS A CANDIDATE GENE FOR *IDD3*

Among these loci, *Idd3* has been mapped to a 780-kb region of chromosome 3 by Wicker, Lyons, and coworkers using a series of congenic strains, in which different segments of chromosome 3 from control B6 or B10 strain were introgressed onto NOD background genes.[24,27,28] A strong candidate gene, *Il2*, encoding cytokine interleukin-2 (IL2), is located in this *Idd3* interval. The *Il2* sequence of the NOD mouse was reported to be allelically variant from that of control B6 or B10 strain, leading to amino acid substitutions, insertions, and deletions.[29] Subsequent studies, however, failed to show functional differences in IL2 between NOD and control B6 or B10 strain, except a difference in the glycosylation pattern of the IL2 molecule.[30]

To demonstrate that the NOD allele of *Il2* confers susceptibility to type 1 diabetes, we screened nucleotide sequences of *Il2* in NOD-related strains.[31] Among seven strains screened, four strains were found to have the same *Il2* allele as the NOD mouse,[31] indicating that the NOD allele of *Il2* is common in NOD-related strains and suggesting that the NOD allele of *Il2* was contained in the original Jcl:ICR colony and segregated into NOD and these strains. One of these strains, IIS, was shown to be a naturally occurring recombinant strain with the same *Il2* region as the NOD mouse, but different flanking markers from the NOD mouse. Using these markers as selection markers, we introgressed the *Il2* region of the IIS mouse onto the genetic background of the NOD mouse, and a congenic strain, NOD.IIS-*Il2*, was established by using a marker-assisted "speed" congenic strategy.[32] Phenotypes of NOD.IIS-*Il2* were indistinguishable from those in the NOD parental strain, indicating that the *Il2* region of the IIS mouse confers susceptibility to type 1 diabetes. Since the *Il2* sequence of the IIS was identical to that in the NOD mouse, the data support the notion that the NOD allele of *Il2* is responsible for the *Idd3* effect.

Recent studies, however, suggested that another candidate gene, *Il21*, encoding a cytokine interleukin-21 (IL21) is also located in the *Idd3* interval adjacent to *Il2*.[33] To study the contribution of *Il21* to susceptibility to type 1 diabetes, we compared nucleotide sequences of NOD and its related strains with those in control strains. The NOD sequence was allelically variant from control sequences in a number of positions. A preliminary study of the alleles at *Il2* and *Il21* loci in NOD-related strains suggested that *Il2* and *Il21* are in strong linkage disequilibrium, making a haplotype with NOD alleles in both genes. These data suggest that both *Il2* and *Il21* are candidate genes for *Idd3*. Genetic and functional studies in NOD-related and unrelated strains are now under way to clarify the contribution of *Il21* to the *Idd3* effect.

CANDIDATE GENE ANALYSIS OF *IDD10*

As mentioned above, *Idd3* was originally defined as a broad peak of linkage in the central part of chromosome 3.[23] Subsequent studies with congenic strains, however, revealed that *Idd3* was encoded by two distinct chromosome 3 loci, one located in the centromeric region and the other, *Idd10*, located in the telomeric region of chromosome 3. A candidate gene, *Fcgr1*, which encodes the high-affinity Fc receptor for IgG, was also mapped to the *Idd10* region. The NOD sequence of *Fcgr1* was reported to be allelically variant from the control B10 sequence, with 17 amino acid differences and deletion of 75% of the cytoplasmic tail, resulting in a reduction in the turnover of cell surface receptor–antibody complexes.[34]

To clarify whether or not *Fcgr1* is responsible for the *Idd10* effect, we searched for the same *Fcgr1* sequence as in NOD in NOD-related strains. Among the seven NOD-related strains studied, four strains were found to have the same *Fcgr1* alleles as the NOD mouse, indicating that the NOD allele of *Fcgr1* is common in NOD-related strains. One of these strains, IIS, was shown to have a naturally occurring recombinant with the same allele at *Fcgr1* as the NOD, but different flanking markers from the NOD mouse. Using this recombinant chromosome, we established NOD mice congenic for the *Idd10* region, NOD.IIS.*Idd10*. Despite the presence of the same *Fcgr1* allele as the NOD mouse, the incidence of type 1 diabetes in NOD.IIS.*Idd10* congenic mice was lower than that in the NOD parental strain, suggesting that the NOD allele of *Fcgr1* may not confer susceptibility to type 1 diabetes and that another gene adjacent to, but distinct from, *Fcgr1* may be responsible for the *Idd10* effect. Consistent with this, Podorin *et al.* demonstrated in their studies using NOD mice congenic for the *Idd10* region from the B6 strain that *Idd10* was localized to a 10 cM region distal to *Fcgr1*, excluding *Fcgr1* as a candidate for *Idd10*.[21] The original *Idd10* is now found to comprise three linked loci, *Idd10*, *Idd17*, and *Idd18* (FIG. 2),[24-26] indicating the importance of the congenic mapping strategy in genetic dissection of complex traits.

ANCESTRAL HAPLOTYPE CONGENIC MAPPING

As shown in fine mapping of *Idd1* and *Idd3*, congenic mapping is an effective strategy for genetic dissection of complex traits. In complex traits, genes responsible for the disease are not necessarily located in the region where peak linkage is observed, but strong susceptibility mapped can be due to a combined effect of multiple genes, as in the case of *Idd1* and *Idd16* as well as *Idd3*, *10*, *17*, and *18*. In addition to classical congenic mapping, the use of strains closely related to a disease model to find the same candidate mutation as the disease model on different haplotypes and make congenic strains with this recombinant chromosome, termed ancestral haplotype congenic mapping,[12] is an effective mapping strategy as shown in the fine mapping of *Idd1*, *Idd3*, and *Idd10*. Information on susceptibility genes for type 1 diabetes and the functions of gene products will make it possible to establish effective methods for the prediction, prevention, and cure of type 1 diabetes.

ACKNOWLEDGMENTS

We thank M. Moritani for her skillful technical assistance. This study was supported by a Grant-in-Aid for Scientific Research on Priority Areas (to H. Ikegami), a Grant-in-Aid for Scientific Research (to H. Ikegami), a Grant-in-Aid for Exploratory Research (to H. Ikegami), and a Grant-in-Aid for Encouragement of Young Scientists (to T. Fujisawa) from the Ministry of Education, Science, Sports, Culture, and Technology of Japan.

REFERENCES

1. HATTORI, M., J. BUSE, R. JACKSON et al. 1986. The NOD mouse: recessive diabetogenic gene in the major histocompatibility complex. Science **231**: 733–735.
2. WICKER, L.S., B.J. MILLER, L.Z. COKER et al. 1987. Genetic control of diabetes and insulitis in the nonobese diabetic (NOD) mouse. J. Exp. Med. **165**: 1639–1654.
3. PROCHAZKA, M., D. SERREZE, S. WORTHEN et al. 1989. Genetic control of diabetogenesis in NOD/Lt mice: development and analysis of congenic stocks. Diabetes **38**: 1446–1455.
4. WICKER, L., M. APPEL, F. DOTTA et al. 1992. Autoimmune syndromes in major histocompatibility complex (MHC) congenic strains of nonobese diabetic (NOD) mice: the NOD MHC is dominant for insulitis and cyclophosphamide-induced diabetes. J. Exp. Med. **176**: 67–77.
5. PODOLIN, P., A. PRESSEY, N. DELARATO et al. 1993. I-E$^+$ nonobese diabetic mice develop insulitis and diabetes. J. Exp. Med. **178**: 793–803.
6. IKEGAMI, H. & S. MAKINO. 1993. Genetic susceptibility to insulin-dependent diabetes mellitus: from NOD mice to humans. In Lessons from Animal Diabetes IV, pp. 39–50. Smith-Gordon. London.
7. IKEGAMI, H., S. MAKINO & T. OGIHARA. 1996. Molecular genetics of insulin-dependent diabetes mellitus: analysis of congenic strains. In Lessons from Animal Diabetes VI, pp. 33–46. Birkhauser. Boston
8. WICKER, L., J. TODD & L. PETERSON. 1995. Genetic control of autoimmune diabetes in the NOD mouse. Annu. Rev. Immunol. **13**: 179–200.
9. IKEGAMI, H., S. MAKINO, M. HARADA et al. 1988. The cataract Shionogi mouse, a sister strain of the nonobese diabetic mouse: similar class II, but different class I gene products. Diabetologia **31**: 254–258.
10. IKEGAMI, H., G. EISENBARTH & M. HATTORI. 1990. Major histocompatibility complex–linked diabetogenic gene of the nonobese diabetic mouse: analysis of genomic DNA amplified by the polymerase chain reaction. J. Clin. Invest. **85**: 18–24
11. IKEGAMI, H., Y. KAWAGUCHI, H. UEDA et al. 1993. MHC-linked diabetogenic gene of the NOD mouse: molecular mapping of the 3′ boundary of the diabetogenic region. Biochem. Biophys. Res. Commun. **192**: 677–682.
12. IKEGAMI, H., S. MAKINO & E. YAMATO. 1995. Identification of a new susceptibility locus for insulin-dependent diabetes mellitus by ancestral haplotype congenic mapping. J. Clin. Invest. **96**: 1936–1942.
13. BABAYA, N., H. IKEGAMI, Y. KAWAGUCHI et al. 2000. Congenic mapping and functional analysis of a second component of the MHC-linked diabetogenic gene (*Idd16*). Int. J. Diabetes **8**: 1–7.
14. HATTORI, M., E. YAMATO, N. ITOH et al. 1999. Homologous recombination of the MHC class I K region defines new MHC-linked diabetogenic susceptibility gene(s) in nonobese diabetic mice. J. Immunol. **163**: 1721–1724.
15. FUJISAWA, T., H. IKEGAMI, Y. KAWAGUCHI et al. 1995. Class I HLA is associated with age-at-onset of IDDM, while class II HLA confers susceptibility to IDDM. Diabetologia **38**: 1494–1496.
16. NEJENTSEV, S., Z. GOMBOS, A-P. LAINE et al. 2000. Non-class II HLA gene associated with type 1 diabetes maps to the 240-kb region near HLA-B. Diabetes **49**: 2217–2221.
17. SATOH, J., H. SEINO, T. ABO et al. 1989. Recombinant human tumor necrosis factor α suppresses autoimmune diabetes in nonobese diabetic mice. J. Clin. Invest. **84**: 1345–1348.
18. JACOB, C.O., S. AISO, S. MICHIE et al. 1990. Prevention of diabetes in nonobese diabetic mice by tumor necrosis factor (TNF): similarities between TNF-alpha and interleukin 1. Proc. Natl. Acad. Sci. USA **87**: 968–972.
19. BABAYA, N., H. IKEGAMI, T. FUJISAWA et al. 2002. Sequence analysis of *Tnf* as a candidate for *Idd16*. Autoimmunity **35**: 63–66.
20. LUND, T., S. SHAIKH, E. KENDALL et al. 1993. RFLP analysis of the MHC class III region defines unique haplotypes for the non-obese diabetic, cataract Shionogi and the non-obese non-diabetic mouse strains. Diabetologia **36**: 727–733.
21. NISHIMOTO, H., H. KIKUTANI, K. YAMAMURA et al. 1987. Prevention of autoimmune insulitis by expression of I-E molecules in NOD mice. Nature **328**: 432–434.

22. WICKER, L.S., B.J. MILLER, P.A. FISCHER et al. 1989. Genetic control of diabetes and insulitis in the nonobese diabetic mouse: pedigree analysis of a diabetic H-$2^{nod/b}$ heterozygote. J. Immunol. **142**: 781–784.
23. TODD, J.A., T. AITMAN, R. CORNALL et al. 1991. Genetic analysis of autoimmune type 1 diabetes mellitus in mice. Nature **351**: 542–547.
24. WICKER, L., J. TODD, J-B. PRINS et al. 1994. Resistance alleles at two non-major histocompatibility complex–linked insulin-dependent diabetes loci on chromosome 3, *Idd3* and *Idd10*, protect nonobese diabetic mice from diabetes. J. Exp. Med. **180**: 1705–1713.
25. PODOLIN, P., P. DENNY, C. LORD et al. 1997. Congenic mapping of the insulin-dependent diabetes (*Idd*) gene, *Idd10*, localizes two genes mediating the *Idd10* effect and eliminate the candidate Fcgr1. J. Immunol. **159**: 1835–1843.
26. PODOLIN, P., P. DENNY, N. ARMITAGE et al. 1998. Localization of two insulin-dependent diabetes (*Idd*) genes to the *Idd10* region on mouse chromosome 3. Mamm. Genome **9**: 283–286.
27. DENNY, P., C.J. LORD, N.J. HILL et al. 1997. Mapping of the IDDM locus *Idd3* to 0.35 cM interval containing the interleukin-2 gene. Diabetes **46**: 695–700.
28. LYONS, P., N. ARMITAGE, F. ARGENTINA et al. 2000. Congenic mapping of the type 1 diabetes locus, *Idd3*, to a 780-kb region of mouse chromosome 3: identification of a candidate segment of ancestral DNA by haplotype mapping. Genome Res. **10**: 446–453.
29. GHOSH, S., S.M. PALMER, N.R. RODRIGUES et al. 1993. Polygenic control of autoimmune diabetes in nonobese diabetic mice. Nat. Genet. **4**: 404–409.
30. PODOLIN, P.L., M.B. WILUSZ, R.M. CUBBON et al. 2000. Differential glycosylation of interleukin-2, the molecular basis for the NOD *Idd3* type 1 diabetes gene? Cytokine **12**: 477–482.
31. IKEGAMI, H., T. FUJISAWA, S. MAKINO et al. 2002. Genetic dissection of type 1 diabetes susceptibility gene, *Idd3*, by ancestral haplotype congenic mapping. Ann. N.Y. Acad. Sci. **958**: 325–328.
32. IKEGAMI, H. & S. MAKINO. 2001. The NOD mouse and its related strains. *In* A Primer on Animal Models of Diabetes, pp. 43–62. Harwood Academic Pub. Amsterdam.
33. PARRISH-NOVAK, J., S.R. DILLON, A. NELSON et al. 2000. Interleukin 21 and its receptor are involved in NK cell expansion and regulation of lymphocyte function. Nature **408**: 57–63.
34. PRINS, J-B., J.A. TODD, N.R. RODRIGUES et al. 1993. Linkage on chromosome 3 of autoimmune diabetes and defective Fc receptor for IgG in NOD mice. Science **260**: 695–698.

Establishing Insulin 1 and Insulin 2 Knockout Congenic Strains on NOD Genetic Background

JOHANNA PARONEN, HIROAKI MORIYAMA, NORIO ABIRU, KAMILA SIKORA, EVIE MELANITOU, SUNANDA BABU, FEI BAO, EDWIN LIU, DONGMEI MIAO, AND GEORGE S. EISENBARTH

Barbara Davis Center for Childhood Diabetes, University of Colorado Health Sciences Center, Denver, Colorado, USA

ABSTRACT: As insulin is a major autoantigen in autoimmune diabetes and because the insulin gene region locus in humans has been linked to diabetes risk, we have bred insulin gene knockouts onto the NOD mouse. Mice differ from humans in terms that they express two nonallelic genes of insulin. Insulin 2 is the murine homologue of the human insulin gene and is located on mouse chromosome 7. Insulin 1 is thought to have evolved by a gene duplication event, lacks the second intron of the insulin 2 gene, and is located on mouse chromosome 19. The differential thymic expression of the insulin gene may be important for central tolerance induction. Here, we present the initial establishment of congenic knockouts and characterization of the congenic intervals corresponding to insulin 1 and insulin 2 knockout genes on mouse chromosome 19 and 7, respectively.

KEYWORDS: insulin; knockout; speed congenic; microsatellite marker

INTRODUCTION

As insulin is a major autoantigen in autoimmune diabetes and because the insulin gene region locus in humans has been linked to diabetes risk, we have bred insulin gene knockouts onto the NOD mouse. Mice differ from humans in terms that they express two nonallelic genes of insulin. Insulin 2 is the murine homologue of the human insulin gene and is located on mouse chromosome 7. Insulin 1 is thought to have evolved by a gene duplication event, lacks the second intron of the insulin 2 gene, and is located on mouse chromosome 19. In the thymus, the two genes differ dramatically in terms of mRNA expression, with much greater thymic insulin 2 mRNA and protein.[1–3] This differential thymic expression of the insulin gene may be important for central tolerance induction. It has been shown that mice having low thymic insulin levels present detectable peripheral T cell reactivity to insulin, whereas

Address for correspondence: George S. Eisenbarth, Barbara Davis Center for Childhood Diabetes, University of Colorado Health Sciences Center, Denver, CO 80262. Voice: 303-315-4891; fax: 303-315-4892.
george.eisenbarth@uchsc.edu

no such reactivity is observed in wild-type mice with normal insulin levels in the thymus.[3] In agreement with this, *aire*-deficient mice (a mouse model of autoimmune polyendocrine syndrome type-1) show a specific loss or reduction in the thymus of ectopic transcription of genes encoding peripheral antigens. This is hypothesized to lead to loss of tolerance and emergence of autoimmunity, although *aire* mice did not develop insulitis.[4] In addition, the two insulin molecules differ in their sequence— by two amino acids in the B chain and by three amino acids in the C peptide—and this could play a role in maintaining peripheral tolerance to these molecules. Here, we present the initial establishment of congenic knockouts and characterization of the congenic intervals corresponding to insulin 1 and insulin 2 knockout genes on mouse chromosome 19 and 7, respectively.

METHODS AND RESULTS

Construction of Speed Congenic Mice for Ins1 and Ins2 KO

The original insulin knockouts (*Ins1* KO, *Ins2* KO) were produced by J. Jami in D3 embryonal stem cells from 129S1/SvImJ mice and were further microinjected into C57BL/6 blastocysts and kept on C57BL/6 genetic background.[5] We bred these two knockout strains into NOD genetic background initially using a speed congenic approach. Briefly, mice from the BC1 [(KO × NOD) × NOD] generation have been selected for further breeding upon the presence of two NOD alleles at major *Idd* loci by using polymorphic microsatellite markers for screening. Genetic intervals corresponding to *Idd* loci have been fixed with two "NOD" alleles as follows: *Idd1*/chr17 D17*Mit34*; *Idd2*/chr9 D9*Mit25*; *Idd3*/chr3 D3*Mit95*; *Idd4*/chr11 D11*Mit245* and D11*Mit219*; *Idd5*/chr1 D1*Mit18*; *Idd6*/chr6 D6*Mit339*; *Idd7*/chr7 D7*Mit20*; *Idd8&12*/chr14 D14*Mit222*; *Idd9&11*/chr4 D4*Mit59*; *Idd10*/chr3 D3*Mit103*; *Idd13*/chr2 D2*Mit17* and D2*Mit395*; *Idd14*/chr13 D13*Mit61*. Further congenic breeding has been achieved by successive backcrossing of speed congenic males with NOD females. The current mice are at backcross 9 for the insulin 1 KO strain and at backcross 10 for the insulin 2 KO strain, having fixed NOD *Idd* loci (*Idd* 1–14) by backcross 3 for insulin 1 KO and backcross 4 for insulin 2 KO strains.

KO genes have been selected at each generation as follows: The construction of the insulin 2 KO gene includes a segment of the LacZ gene. LacZ-specific primers (see TABLE 1) have been designed to follow by PCR the inheritance of this KO gene to the BC progenies. Concerning the detection of the insulin 1 gene KO, two different approaches have been used: one based on selection of heterozygous animals with microsatellite markers located proximally (D19*Mit54*) and distally (D19*Mit37*) to the insulin KO locus; the second consisted of using neo gene markers since the neo gene was used in the *Ins1* KO construct. However, initially, amplification by PCR of the neo gene was revealed to be inefficient for following the presence of the *Ins1* KO gene, but later another set of neo primers[6,7] (see TABLE 1) allowed the detection with a better efficiency of the transmission of the *Ins1* KO gene locus into the congenic generations. It has been recently found that the D19*Mit54* microsatellite marker is finally assigned to the distal part of chromosome 19 and is actually next to the other marker D19*Mit37*. As our selection of the *Ins1* KO gene has been based on two different approaches, the presence of the *Ins1* KO in the congenic strain was assured.

TABLE 1. Primers

Primer	Sequence	Denaturation	Annealing	Extension	Cycle	Size (bp)
Ins1 KO-neo1	5'-GCTATTCGGCTATGACTGGG-3' 5'-GAAGGCGATAGAAGGCGATG-3'	94°C for 30 s	65°C for 30 s	72°C for 30 s	30	706
Ins1 KO-neo2	5'-CCTTGCGCAGCTGTGCTCGACGTTG-3' 5'-GCCGCATTGCATCAGCCATGATGA-3'	94°C for 30 s	65°C for 30 s	72°C for 30 s	30	~150
Ins2 KO-lacZ	5'-GGCAGAGAGGAGGTGCTTTG-3' 5'-ATTGACCGTAATGGGATAGG-3'	94°C for 45 s	53°C for 45 s	72°C for 60 s	35	287
Ins1 and 2 wt	5'-GGCTTCTTCTACACACCCA-3' 5'-CAGTAGTTCTCCAGCTGGT-3'	94°C for 45 s	53°C for 45 s	72°C for 60 s	35	*Ins1*: 675 *Ins2*: 169
Ins1 wt	5'-ATGTCCAATGAGTGCTTTCT-3' 5'-AGCTCCAGTTGTTCCACTTGT-3'	94°C for 45 s	53°C for 45 s	72°C for 60 s	35	592
Ins2 wt	5'-GGCAGAGAGGAGGTGCTTTG-3' 5'-AGAAAACCAGGGTAGTTAGC-3'	94°C for 45 s	53°C for 45 s	72°C for 60 s	35	466

NOTE: *Ins1* KO-neo1 data from ref. 6; *Ins1* KO-neo2 data from ref. 7; wt, wild type; KO, knockout.

Confirmation of the Presence of the Disrupted Insulin Genes in the NOD.tgn.^{insKO} Mice

Additional confirmation of the presence of insulin 1 or 2 KO genes was obtained by PCR amplification detecting disruption of the two insulin wild genes (see TABLE 1). Reciprocally, only insulin 2 wild-type alleles were present in *Ins1* KO homozygous mice, and only insulin 1 alleles were present in *Ins2* KO homozygous mice.

Characterization of the Genetic Intervals in the Ins1 and Ins2 KO Congenic Strains

By detailed microsatellite typing (with ABI 377), we were able to assess recombinants occurring around the insulin KO locus at each backcross in the two knockout strains. Several microsatellite markers (8 markers for chr 19 and 6 for chr 7; FIG. 1) were used to map the whole chromosome at distances of ~10 cM. In the insulin 1 KO strain, the proximal segment surrounding the insulin gene was starting to be replaced by NOD alleles already by backcross 5; also, by backcross 7 in one of the breeders for further generations, the segment was all NOD heritage down to position 47 cM, only 2 cM from the KO. At the distal site of the KO and especially at the telomere

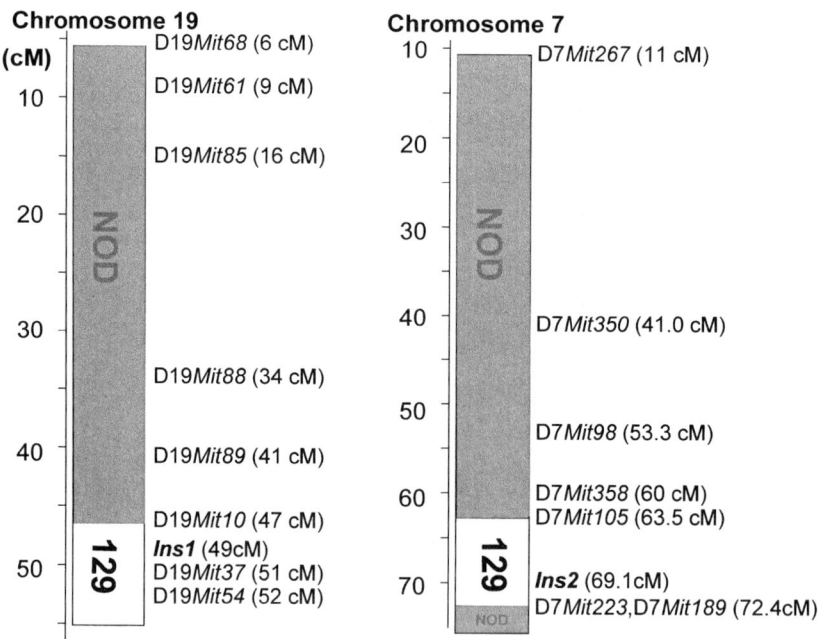

FIGURE 1. Map of the congenic intervals on chromosomes 19 (insulin 1) and 7 (insulin 2) in the NOD.tgn.^{insKO} mice. All microsatellite markers shown in the figure distinguish NOD and 129 strains. The maximum interval of chromosome 19 from the 129 strain between the insulin 1 gene region and the telomere was determined to be less than 8 cM and the maximum interval of chromosome 7 from the 129 strain to be less than 8.9 cM.

of chromosome 19, it was difficult to find good microsatellite markers (i.e., markers polymorphic between the NOD and 129 alleles). At backcross 8, the mice still carry a 129 allele at positions 51 cM (D19*Mit37*) and 52 cM (D19*Mit54*), but this is understandable because (as mentioned before) we initially used these two microsatellite markers for selection of the KO gene. Backcross 9 mice have not been fine mapped yet. In the insulin 2 KO strain, the proximal segment was replaced by NOD alleles down to position 63.5 cM by backcross 7. This position is 5.6 cM from the insulin 2 KO gene (69.1 cM). At the telomere of chr 7 (D7*Mit223*, 72.4 cM), backcross 7 and 8 mice still had a 129 allele; however, by backcross 9, a recombinant event had occurred replacing this segment by NOD alleles. We could not easily find polymorphic markers on chr 7 distinguishing NOD from 129 alleles between positions 63.5 cM and 72.4 cM, and this seems to point to a fact that 129S1/SvImJ and NOD mice are probably closely related strains (this also noted when fine mapping chr 19). The maximum interval of chr 19 from the 129 strain between the insulin 1 gene region and the telomere was thus determined to be less than 8 cM (NOD homozygous at 47 cM confirmed with D19*Mit10* typing) and the maximum interval of chr 7 from the 129 strain surrounding the insulin 2 gene (position 69.1 cM) to be less than 8.9 cM (NOD homozygous at 63.5 cM and 72.4 cM confirmed with D7*Mit105* and D7*Mit223* typing) (FIG. 1). This detailed microsatellite typing also allowed us to select mice for producing intercross KO homozygous mice. At the moment, intercross mating is carried out at backcross 5 and 8 for establishing insulin 1 KO homozygous colony and at backcross 8 and 10 for insulin 2 KO homozygous colony.

CONCLUSIONS AND PERSPECTIVES

We have constructed congenic lines carrying *Ins1* or *Ins2* KO alleles in an NOD genetic background and have restricted the genetic intervals corresponding to each gene KO to less than 10 cM in an NOD homozygous background (99.6%). This should allow us to test the influence of these genes on diabetogenesis. Because 129 genomic sequences are still carried within ~10 cM of each *Ins* KO genetic interval, two other speed congenic strains have been started by introducing a normal (no KO) 129 donor segment surrounding the insulin gene and matching to KO intervals on chromosomes 19 (insulin 1) and 7 (insulin 2) into the NOD receiver strain. This approach will let us rule out any neighboring gene effect from the 129 strain on the incidence of autoimmune diabetes. Twelve out of 14 NOD *Idd* loci are already fixed in the BC2 generation. Repetitive backcrosses to NOD will be performed with breeder selection based on the presence of a 129-derived allele for chr 19 or 7 and the progeny will then be followed for diabetes. These lines will be valuable for assessing the implication of the insulin gene(s) in the pathogenesis of immune-mediated diabetes.

ACKNOWLEDGMENTS

This research was supported by the National Institutes of Health (Nos. DK32082, AI39213, DK55969, DK62718, AI50864, AI95380, DK32493, DK32493, DK50970, and AI46374), the Diabetes Endocrine Research Center (No. P30 DK57516), the Clinical Research Centers (Nos. MO1 RR00069 and MO1 RR00051), the American

Diabetes Association, the Juvenile Diabetes Foundation, the Children's Diabetes Foundation (to G. S. Eisenbarth), the Academy of Finland, the Finnish Cultural Foundation, the Foundation of Pediatric Research (to J. Paronen), a postdoctoral fellowship from the Juvenile Diabetes Research Foundation (to H. Moriyama), and an American Diabetes Association mentor-based fellowship (to N. Abiru).

REFERENCES

1. HEATH, V.L., N.C. MOORE et al. 1998. Intrathymic expression of genes involved in organ specific autoimmune disease. J. Autoimmun. **11:** 309–318.
2. PLEAU, J.M., A. ESLING et al. 2001. Pancreatic hormone and glutamic acid decarboxylase expression in the mouse thymus: a real-time PCR study. Biochem. Biophys. Res. Commun. **283:** 843–848.
3. CHENTOUFI, A.A. & C. POLYCHRONAKOS. 2002. Insulin expression levels in the thymus modulate insulin-specific autoreactive T-cell tolerance: the mechanism by which the IDDM2 locus may predispose to diabetes. Diabetes **51:** 1383–1390.
4. ANDERSON, M.S., E.S. VENANZI et al. 2002. Projection of an immunological self-shadow within the thymus by the Aire protein. Science **298:** 1395–1401.
5. DUVILLIE, B., N. CORDONNIER et al. 1997. Phenotypic alterations in insulin-deficient mutant mice. Proc. Natl. Acad. Sci. USA **94:** 5137–5140.
6. SERREZE, D.V., H.D. CHAPMAN et al. 1996. B lymphocytes are essential for the initiation of T cell–mediated autoimmune diabetes: analysis of a new "speed-congenic" stock of NOD.Igu^{null} mice. J. Exp. Med. **184:** 2049–2053.
7. SHLOMCHIK, M.J., M.P. MADAIO et al. 1994. The role of B cells in lpr/lpr-induced autoimmunity. J. Exp. Med. **180:** 1295–1306.

Relationship between β Cell Mass of NOD Donors and Diabetes Development of NOD-scid Recipients in Adoptive Transfer System

SATORU YAMADA,[a,b] AKIRA SHIMADA,[b] KEIICHI KODAMA,[b] JIRO MORIMOTO,[b] RYUJI SUZUKI,[b] YOICHI OIKAWA,[b] JUNICHIRO IRIE,[b] AND TAKAO SARUTA[b]

[a]*Department of Internal Medicine, Kitasato Institute Hospital, Tokyo, Japan*

[b]*Department of Internal Medicine, Keio University School of Medicine, Tokyo, Japan*

ABSTRACT: Background—There is controversy about the way the β cell mass is reduced in type 1 diabetes. One view is that a gradual fall in β cell mass begins soon after the onset of insulitis. Another view is that a sudden wave of β cell destruction occurs just before the onset of diabetes. To clarify how the β cell mass is reduced, we performed adoptive transfer experiments and examined the relationship between the pancreatic status of NOD donors and the time taken to transfer diabetes into NOD-scid recipients. Methods—We killed 18-week-old female NOD mice ($n = 20$), removed their spleen, and transferred splenocytes into 5-week-old female NOD-scid mice ($n = 60$). The relationship between the pancreatic status of donors and the time taken to transfer diabetes into recipients was assessed. As pancreatic status, we measured insulin content and severity of insulitis. Results—There was no linear correlation between the pancreatic status of donors and the time taken to transfer diabetes into recipients. NOD donors who needed 7 or more weeks to transfer diabetes in NOD-scid recipients had similar levels of insulin content or severity of insulitis as those of NOD donors who could not transfer diabetes. On the other hand, NOD donors who needed 6 or less weeks to transfer diabetes in recipients had similar levels of insulin content or severity of insulitis as those of diabetic NOD mice. Conclusions—According to our observations, β cell mass seems to be preserved until just before the onset of diabetes and decreased dramatically within a few weeks.

KEYWORDS: NOD mouse; insulitis; β cell mass; adoptive transfer; type 1 diabetes

BACKGROUND

Several trials on the prevention of type 1 diabetes have shown that prevention is more difficult than previously thought.[1] Therefore, we consider that accurate understanding of the disease process in type 1 diabetes is important. Thus far, the issue of β cell mass reduction in the prediabetic period remains controversial and two

Address for correspondence: Akira Shimada, M.D., Ph.D., Department of Internal Medicine, Keio University School of Medicine, 35 Shinanomachi, Shinjuku-ku, Tokyo 160-8582, Japan. Voice: +81-3-5363-3797; fax: +81-3-5269-3219.
asmd@sc.itc.keio.ac.jp

hypotheses have been proposed. One view is that a gradual fall in β cell mass begins soon after the onset of insulitis.[2] Another view is that a sudden wave of β cell destruction occurs just before the onset of diabetes.[3] The method of prevention of type 1 diabetes onset would be affected by which of these models is appropriate. Thus, in the present study, to evaluate the change of β cell mass in the prediabetic stage, we investigated the β cell mass of NOD mice, transferred their splenocytes to NOD-scid mice, and assessed the relation between β cell mass of NOD donors and the time taken for diabetes transfer into NOD-scid recipients.

MATERIALS AND METHODS

The spleen and pancreas were removed from 16- to 18-week-old female NOD mice ($n = 20$). After teasing them apart into a single cell suspension, the cell suspension from 1 donor NOD mouse was injected intraperitoneally into 3 NOD-scid recipients (2×10^6 cells/recipient). When at least 1 NOD-scid recipient developed diabetes, the donor splenocytes were assessed as diabetogenic and the donor NOD mouse was considered "diabetes-prone". On the other hand, when no NOD-scid recipient developed diabetes within 14 weeks posttransfer, the donor NOD mouse was considered "nondiabetes-prone" in this study. NOD-scid recipients were examined for glycosuria twice a week using Tes Tape (Eli Lilly, Indianapolis, IN). The mice with glycosuria were bled, and plasma glucose levels were determined using a Glutest-ace meter (Arkray Co., Kyoto, Japan). Mice with two consecutive plasma glucose readings (48 h or more apart) of >250 mg/dL were considered diabetic. Each pancreas removed was divided into two portions. Half of the pancreas was fixed with 10% formaldehyde and embedded in paraffin. At least three levels, 50 μm apart, were cut for staining with hematoxylin-eosin. The severity of insulitis of all observable islets was assessed and all insulitis scores were averaged in each mouse. After weighing, the other half of the pancreas was minced. After mincing, insulin was extracted from the pancreas according to a previous report.[4]

RESULTS

In our adoptive transfer system, 27 of 60 NOD-scid recipients developed diabetes within 14 weeks after transfer. We examined the association between the insulin content of donor NOD mice and the time taken for diabetes transfer in the "NOD to NOD-scid" adoptive transfer system. According to Rohane *et al.*, the onset of diabetes of donor NOD can be estimated from the time of diabetes onset posttransfer of donor splenocytes into NOD-scid recipients.[5] Therefore, if the reduction of β cell mass occurs gradually in the disease process of type 1 diabetes, insulin content should correlate linearly with the time taken for diabetes transfer to NOD-scid recipients. However, insulin content did not correlate linearly with the time taken for diabetes transfer to NOD-scid recipients; that is, a gradual fall of insulin content was not observed. In fact, insulin content of "diabetes-prone" donor NOD mice whose transferred splenocytes induced diabetes in NOD-scid recipients at 7 weeks posttransfer was almost the same as that of "nondiabetes-prone" NOD donors; that is, these "diabetes-prone" NOD donors were considered to be in the "benign" phase

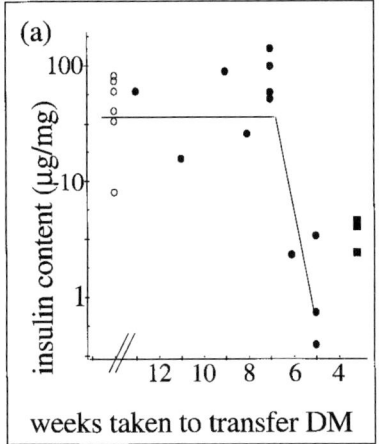
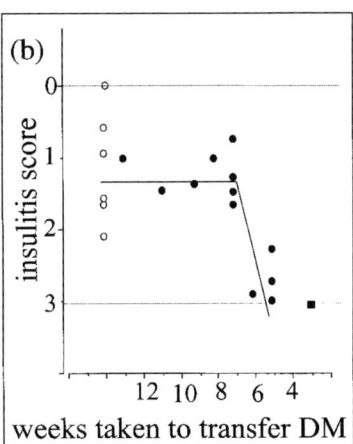

FIGURE 1. Pancreatic status [insulin content (**a**) and severity of insulitis (**b**)] of donor NOD mice and time taken for diabetes transfer in "NOD to NOD-scid" adoptive transfer system. Pancreatic status of donor NOD mice whose splenocytes took 5–6 weeks to transfer diabetes to NOD-scid recipients (= "malignant" donors) was almost the same as that of diabetic donors (■). On the other hand, pancreatic status of donor NOD mice whose splenocytes took 7 or more weeks to transfer diabetes to NOD-scid recipients (= "benign" donors) was almost the same as that of "nondiabetes-prone" NOD donors (○). Taken together, a marked reduction of insulin content (= β cell mass) within 1–2 weeks was suggested.

(= "benign" donors). On the other hand, insulin content of donor NOD mice whose transferred splenocytes induced diabetes in NOD-scid recipients at 5–6 weeks posttransfer was almost the same as that of diabetic donor NOD mice; that is, these "diabetes-prone" NOD donors were considered to be in the "malignant" phase (= "malignant" donors). Taken together, there was a large difference in insulin content between the "benign" and "malignant" donor groups. From these data, a marked reduction of insulin content (= β cell mass) within 1–2 weeks was suggested [5–6 ("malignant") vs. 7 ("benign") weeks posttransfer] (FIG. 1a). We also examined the association between the severity of insulitis of NOD donors and the time taken for diabetes transfer to NOD-scid recipients. Similarly, the severity of insulitis of donor NOD mice was not inversely correlated with the time taken for diabetes transfer of donor splenocytes to NOD-scid recipients (FIG. 1b). Again, it was suggested that the reduction of β cell mass did not occur gradually.

CONCLUSIONS

In the relationship between insulin content (and severity of insulitis) of donor NOD and the time taken for diabetes onset after transfer in the "NOD to NOD-scid" adoptive transfer system, we did not find a linear association. Because diabetic splenocytes took 3–6 weeks to transfer diabetes to NOD-scid recipients, we can assume that it takes at least 3–6 weeks for NOD donor splenocytes to reexpand in the recipients. Thus, the fact that NOD-scid recipients developed diabetes at 7 weeks after transfer from an NOD donor with preserved insulin content (= "benign" donor) suggests that the β cell mass must be preserved until just before the onset of diabetes. We hope these observations will lead to a good understanding of type 1 diabetes and the development of an effective method of prevention.

REFERENCES

1. DIABETES PREVENTION TRIAL–TYPE 1 DIABETES STUDY GROUP. 2002. Effect of insulin in relatives of patients with type 1 diabetes mellitus. N. Engl. J. Med. **346:** 1685–1691.
2. EISENBARTH, G.S. 1986. Type 1 diabetes mellitus: a chronic autoimmune disease. N. Engl. J. Med. **314:** 1360–1368.
3. SHIMADA, A. *et al.* 1996. β-cell destruction may be a late consequence of the autoimmune process in nonobese diabetic mice. Diabetes **45:** 1063–1067.
4. KENNY, A.J. 1955. Extractable glucagon of human pancreas. J. Clin. Endocrinol. Metab. **15:** 1089–1105.
5. ROHANE, P.W. *et al.* 1995. Islet-infiltrating lymphocytes from prediabetic NOD mice rapidly transfer diabetes to NOD-scid/scid mice. Diabetes **44:** 550–554.

Hen Egg White Lysozyme Vaccination Induces Acute Shock in NOD Mice

DUMITRU D. BRANISTEANU,[a] LUTGART OVERBERGH,[b] BRIGITTE DECALLONNE,[b] AND CHANTAL MATHIEU[b]

[a]*Department of Endocrinology, University of Medicine and Pharmacy "Gr. T. Popa" Iasi, Iasi, Romania*

[b]*Laboratorium voor Experimentele Geneeskunde en Endocrinologie (LEGENDO), Katholieke Universiteit Leuven, Leuven, Belgium*

> ABSTRACT: To investigate whether vaccination could induce lethal shock and which mechanisms are involved in this phenomenon, we tested a panel of autoantigens or diabetes-irrelevant peptides or proteins in nonobese diabetic (NOD), Balb/c, and C57Bl/6 mice. Of the antigens tested, only nondiabetogenic hen egg white lysozyme induced a severe form of shock exclusively in NOD mice. The mechanism involved is suggestive of a Th_2-mediated anaphylactic reaction possibly connected to activation of PAF and triggering of DIC.
>
> KEYWORDS: hen egg white lysozyme; NOD mice; shock; platelet-activating factor; diabetes; vitamin D

Several recent reports described the appearance of allergic or anaphylactic reactions subsequent to autoantigen vaccination in animal models of autoimmune diabetes mellitus[1] or multiple sclerosis,[2–4] questioning the safety of this immune-modulating strategy in preventing the onset of T helper 1 (Th_1)–mediated diseases. To investigate whether vaccination could induce lethal shock and which mechanisms are involved in this phenomenon, we tested a panel of autoantigens or diabetes-irrelevant peptides or proteins in nonobese diabetic (NOD), Balb/c, and C57Bl/6 mice. Eight-week-old mice were immunized by injection of 100 μg antigen (hen egg white lysozyme [HEL], GAD65, insulin B, hsp65, proteolipid protein, ovalbumin, tetanus toxin), emulsified at a 1:1 concentration in complete Freund's adjuvant (Difco Laboratories, Detroit, MI), in the hind foot pads and reinjected with the same antigen 3 weeks later.

Of all the antigens tested, only nondiabetogenic HEL induced a severe form of shock exclusively in NOD mice (TABLE 1). Administration of $1,25(OH)_2D_3$ (a hormone known to favor a differentiation shift toward Th_2)[5] at a dose of 5 μg/kg/2 days, starting from 3 weeks of age, further increased shock severity in NOD mice (increase

Address for correspondence: Chantal Mathieu, M.D., Ph.D., Gasthuisberg, LEGENDO, Onderwijs & Navorsing, Herestraat 49, 3000 Leuven, Belgium. Voice: +32-16-34-60-30; fax: +32-16-34-59-34.

chantal.mathieu@med.kuleuven.ac.be

TABLE 1. Shock incidence and severity in various groups of mice rechallenged with HEL and pretreated ip with 1,25(OH)$_2$D$_3$ (+) or only with the vehicle (peanut oil, –)

Mouse strain	1,25-D$_3$	Rescue therapy	Shock incidence (from total)	Shock severity Lethal	Shock severity Reversible
NOD	–	–	11/11	3 (27%)	8
	+	–	17/17	14 (82%)	3
	–	DEX	0/8	0	0
	+	DEX	0/8	0	0
	–	WEB2086	6/8	0	6
	+	WEB2086	6/8	0	6
Balb/c	–	–	0/9	0	0
	+	–	9/9	0	9
C57Bl/6	–	–	0/9	0	0
	+	–	0/9	0	0

NOTE: Certain groups of NOD mice were submitted to rescue therapy with dexamethasone (DEX) or WEB2086.

in lethality incidence from 27% to 82%, $p < 0.0001$) and led to the appearance of reversible shock signs also in Balb/c mice, while C57Bl/6 mice remained shock-resistant (TABLE 1).

The mRNA levels of IL-13 (Th$_2$-specific cytokine involved in anaphylaxis)[6] measured by real-time PCR before HEL boost injection were significantly higher in spleen of NOD mice than in shock-resistant C57Bl/6 mice (38.1 ± 7.8 vs. 18 ± 2.2 IL-13 mRNA/actin × 10^{-6}, $p < 0.05$). IL-13 was further increased by administration of 1,25(OH)$_2$D$_3$ in NOD mice (63.4 ± 6.9 IL-13 mRNA/actin × 10^{-6}, $p < 0.05$), but not in C57Bl/6 mice (13 ± 4.9 IL-13 mRNA/actin × 10^{-6}, ns). Serum total IgE levels (Th$_2$-dependent immunoglobulin involved in anaphylactic reactions),[7] measured by ELISA before boost injection, were higher in NOD mice (mean OD of 690 ± 130 in NOD mice vs. 338 ± 47 in C57Bl/6 mice, $p < 0.05$). 1,25(OH)$_2$D$_3$ administration further increased IgE levels only in NOD mice (mean OD of 950 ± 104, $p < 0.05$), but not in C57Bl/6 mice (mean OD of 376 ± 36, ns). IgE hence displayed a parallel evolution with IL-13, suggesting a causal relationship, as previously described.[7]

Because the shock induced in NOD mice was suggestive of disseminated intravascular coagulation (DIC), we further investigated a possible role of platelet-activating factor (PAF) as a shock mediator. The expression of PAF receptor was higher in spleen of NOD mice than in C57Bl/6 mice (96.3 ± 15 × 10^{-2} vs. 39.8 ± 11 × 10^{-2} PAF receptor mRNA/actin, $p < 0.05$), suggesting a hypersensitivity to PAF in HEL-sensitized NOD mice. PAF receptor expression in NOD mice was further increased by therapy with 1,25(OH)$_2$D$_3$ (from 96.3 ± 15 × 10^{-2} to 155 ± 22 × 10^{-2}, $p < 0.05$), raising the possibility of a Th$_2$-dependent hypersensitivity to PAF.

The involvement of both immune effectors and PAF in the etiology of HEL-induced shock was further indicated by the efficacy of rescue therapy with dexamethasone, 50 μg ip, 48, 24, and 2 h before the HEL booster injection, and

WEB2086 (PAF receptor antagonist, Boehringer Mannheim, Germany; kind gift from Prof. Vermylen, University of Leuven, Leuven, Belgium), 500 µg ip, 10 min before booster injection, respectively (TABLE 1).

In conclusion, NOD mice are highly susceptible to lethal shock upon immunization with HEL. The mechanism involved is suggestive of a Th_2-mediated anaphylactic reaction possibly connected to activation of PAF[8] and triggering of DIC. In the case of Th_1-mediated autoimmune diseases, balancing the immune system toward Th_2 differentiation might increase the risk of unwanted anaphylactic effects. Extreme caution should therefore be taken in using any kind of immune-modulating strategies of T helper differentiation in order to prevent excessive Th_2-dependent reactions.

REFERENCES

1. LIU, E., H. MORIYAMA, N. ABIRU et al. 2002. Anti-peptide autoantibodies and fatal anaphylaxis in NOD mice in response to insulin self-peptides B:9–23 and B:13–23. J. Clin. Invest. **110:** 1021–1027.
2. PEDOTTI, R., D. MITCHELL, J. WEDEMEYER et al. 2001. An unexpected version of horror autotoxicus: anaphylactic shock to a self-peptide. Nat. Immunol. **2:** 216–222.
3. KAPPOS, L., G. COMI, H. PANITCH et al. 2002. The Altered Peptide Ligand in Relapsing MS Study Group: Induction of a non-encephalitogenic type 2 T helper-cell autoimmune response in multiple sclerosis after administration of an altered peptide ligand in a placebo-controlled, randomized phase II trial. Nat. Med. **6:** 1176–1182.
4. SILVERSTEIN, A.M. 2001. Autoimmunity versus horror autotoxicus: the struggle for recognition. Nat. Immunol. **2:** 279–281.
5. MATHIEU, C. & L. ADORINI. 2002. The coming of age of 1,25-dihydroxyvitamin D(3) analogs as immunomodulatory agents. Trends Mol. Med. **8:** 174–179.
6. FALLON, P.G., C.L. EMSON, P. SMITH & A.N. MCKENZIE. 2001. IL-13 overexpression predisposes to anaphylaxis following antigen sensitization. J. Immunol. **166:** 2712–2716.
7. CORRY, D.B. & F. KHERADMAND. 1999. Induction and regulation of the IgE response. Nature **402:** B18–B23.
8. SNYDER, F. 1995. Platelet-activating factor and its analogs: metabolic pathways and related intracellular processes. Biochim. Biophys. Acta **1254:** 231–249.

In Vivo Expression of B:9–23 Peptide/I-A^{g7} Complex May Abrogate the Inhibition of Diabetes Induced by RGD-Fiber-Mutant Adenovirus in NOD Mice

NORIO ABIRU,[a] FUYAN SUN,[a] EIJI KAWASAKI,[a] HIRONORI YAMASAKI,[b] KATSUYA OSHIMA,[b] YUJI NAGAYAMA,[c] HIROYUKI MIZUGUCHI,[d] TAKAO HAYAKAWA,[d] DONGMEI MIAO,[e] EDWIN LIU,[e] GEORGE S. EISENBARTH,[e] AND KATSUMI EGUCHI[b]

[a]*Unit of Metabolism/Diabetes and Clinical Nutrition,* [b]*Department of Internal Medicine 1, and* [c]*Department of Pharmacology 1, Nagasaki University School of Medicine, Nagasaki, Japan*

[d]*Division of Biological Chemistry and Biologicals, National Institute of Health Sciences, Tokyo, Japan*

[e]*Barbara Davis Center for Childhood Diabetes, University of Colorado Health Sciences Center, Denver, Colorado, USA*

> ABSTRACT: Insulin B chain peptide B:9–23 given to NOD mice decreases the development of diabetes, and phase II trials of an altered peptide ligand of B:9–23 are under way in humans. We have created a gene for the NOD MHC class II β chain, covalently linked to the B:9–23 peptide. B lymphoma cells transfected with the gene stimulated NOD islet–derived B:9–23 reactive T cell clones *in vitro*. In this study, we generated an RGD-fiber-mutant adenovirus vector encoding the covalent B:9–23 peptide/I-A^{g7} gene (Ad-RGD-B:9–23) to test whether *in vivo* expression of the gene could protect NOD mice from diabetes. NOD female mice were injected intramuscularly with 5×10^8 PFU of Ad-RGD-B:9–23 and empty RGD-adenovirus vector. A single administration of the empty vector did not alter the expression of insulin autoantibodies, but delayed the onset of diabetes in NOD mice. In contrast, Ad-RGD-B:9–23 immunization induced an early expression of insulin autoantibodies, but did not change the disease occurrence compared to control NOD mice. Our results suggest that adenovirus infection could confer protection from diabetes in NOD mice. The *in vivo* expression of covalent B:9–23 peptide/class II complex by adenovirus gene transfer might activate anti-insulin autoimmunity, resulting in abrogation of the inhibition of diabetes induced by an RGD-fiber-mutant adenovirus vector.
>
> KEYWORDS: B:9–23 peptide; NOD mice; RGD-fiber-mutant adenovirus; insulin

Address for correspondence: Katsumi Eguchi, M.D., First Department of Internal Medicine, Nagasaki University School of Medicine, 1-7-1 Sakamoto, Nagasaki 852-8501, Japan. Voice: +81-95-849-7260; fax: +81-95-849-7270.
eguchi@net.nagasaki-u.ac.jp

INTRODUCTION

It has been previously shown that insulin B chain peptide B:9–23 protects NOD mice from diabetes when given subcutaneously with incomplete Freund's adjuvant (IFA).[1] With this vaccine, NOD mice express significantly higher and prolonged insulin autoantibodies (IAA) associated with protection from disease.[2] We have previously created a modified I-A^{g7} gene covalently linked to B:9–23 peptide sequence. B cell lymphoma lines transfected with this construct were excellent presenting cells for all NOD islet–derived B:9–23 reactive T cell clones studied.[3] In this study, we generated an adenovirus vector encoding the covalent B:9–23 peptide/I-A^{g7} gene (Ad-RGD–covalent B:9–23) to test whether *in vivo* expression of the gene could protect NOD mice from diabetes. Arg-Gly-Asp (RGD)–fiber-mutant adenovirus vector was used for an efficient transduction into dendritic cells (DC) via an RGD-alpha(v) integrin–dependent, CAR-independent cell entry pathway.[4]

RESEARCH DESIGN AND METHODS

The construction of the expression vector pCR3.1-Uni for generation of the NOD MHC class II β chain (I-Aβ^{g7}), covalently linked to the B:9–23 peptide, has been described previously.[3] The fragment of I-Aβ^{g7}/B:9–23 peptide was ligated into RGD-fiber-mutant adenovirus vector carrying GFP (Ad-RGD-GFP) cDNA by an *in vitro* ligation method with a shuttle vector, pHMCMV6. Recombinant adenovirus expressing I-Aβ^{g7}/B:9–23 (designated Ad-RGD–covalent B:9–23) was propagated in 293 HEK cells and purified as described previously.[4] Ad-RGD-GFP was used as a negative control. Female NOD mice (CLEA Japan Inc., Tokyo, Japan) at 4 weeks of age were divided into three groups. The mice in group 1 were injected in the thigh muscle with 5×10^8 particles of Ad-RGD–covalent B:9–23 in 100 μL PBS at 4 weeks of age. The mice in group 2 received Ad-RGD-GFP in 100 μL PBS. Group 3 was an unvaccinated control group that received 100 μL PBS only. Serum IAA was measured prior to vaccination at 4 weeks and then at 6, 8, and 12 weeks of age thereafter by radioassay. Blood glucose was monitored every other week starting at 12 weeks with the GLUTEST SENSOR blood glucose meter (Sanwa Kagaku Kenkyusho Co., Nagoya, Japan) and mice were considered diabetic after two consecutive blood glucose values above 250 mg/dL.

RESULTS

Ad-RGD–covalent B:9-23 treated NOD mice expressed IAA more often than Ad-RGD-GFP treated mice (4/5 vs. 2/9 at 8 weeks, $p < 0.05$). The mean IAA level was 0.06 ± 0.07 at 8 weeks in Ad-RGD–covalent B:9-23 treated mice. The expressions of IAA in Ad-RGD–covalent B:9–23 treated mice were transient and the positive IAA disappeared or decreased at 12 weeks of age. No significant difference of IAA expression was observed between Ad-RGD-GFP and PBS treated NOD mice (FIG. 1A). The incidence of diabetes of the NOD mice was followed until 30 weeks. Interestingly, 55.5% of the Ad-RGD-GFP treated mice were diabetes-free at 30 weeks and the mice showed a significant delay in the progression of clinical diabetes

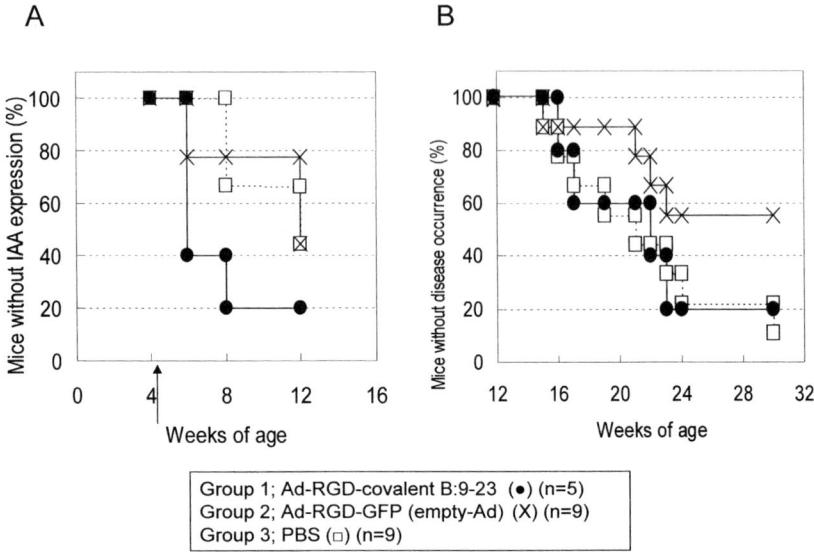

FIGURE 1. Life table analysis for the expression of insulin autoantibodies (**A**) and for the development of diabetes (**B**). The NOD female mice were intramuscularly injected at 4 weeks of age with Ad-RGD–covalent B:9–23 (●), Ad-RGD-GFP (×), and PBS (□).

compared to PBS treated mice. For Ad-RGD–covalent B:9–23 and PBS treated mice, 11% and 20% were diabetes-free at 30 weeks, respectively. An administration of Ad-RGD–covalent B:9–23 did not alter the occurrence of diabetes in NOD mice compared to PBS control mice (FIG. 1B).

DISCUSSION

As reported by Casares *et al.*, it is likely that soluble multimers of peptide bound to MHC class II proteins may be useful therapeutic reagents for type 1 diabetes.[5] In this study, we studied an adenovirus expressing vector encoding the B:9–23 peptide gene bound to NOD MHC class II gene to test whether *in vivo* expression of the gene could protect NOD mice from diabetes. Surprisingly, a single administration of RGD-fiber-mutant adenovirus vectors not containing the cDNA can suppress the development of diabetes in NOD mice. The protection is not complete, but the single injection of the vector did result in only 44.5% diabetes incidence at 30 weeks. Recent reports demonstrated that adenovirus vector, especially RGD-fiber-mutant adenovirus, induces the maturation of murine DC.[6] Maturated myeloid DC cultured with GM-CSF and IL-4 have been shown to prevent diabetes in NOD mice by adoptive transfer.[7] *In vivo* maturation of DC induced by adenovirus administration may be associated with inhibition of diabetes in our study. Four out of 5 mice treated with Ad-RGD–covalent B:9–23 expressed IAA after 4 weeks of administration, indicating that adenovirus gene transfer could express B:9–23 peptide/class II complex on antigen-presenting cells *in vivo*. Contrary to our expectation, the covalent B:9–23 peptide/I-A^{g7} gene abrogated the inhibitory effect of diabetes development induced by an empty adenovirus administration. We have demonstrated previously that administration of a viral mimic (poly-IC) and B:9–23 peptide to BALB/c mice induced insulitis.[8] Diabetes was induced in RIP-B7-1 transgenic mice with H-2^d following poly-IC. Of note, disease induction was accelerated with B:9–23 immunization.[8] As illustrated by the current study, there is the possibility that a "double hit" by a virus infection and an insulin self-peptide gene may accelerate a pathogenic T cell response rather than a regulatory (protective) T cell response in NOD mice. A trial is under way in humans using an altered peptide ligand of insulin peptide B:9–23 by the company Neurocrine. For prevention trials in prediabetic subjects, we have to consider the obvious potential danger that self-peptide "vaccines" for autoimmunity may stimulate the immune system and worsen the process disease.

ACKNOWLEDGMENTS

This work was supported by grants from the Japan Society for the Promotion of Science (No. 13922142) and the Japan Diabetes Foundation (No. 14-55).

REFERENCES

1. DANIEL, D. & D.R. WEGMANN. 1996. Protection of nonobese diabetic mice from diabetes by intranasal or subcutaneous administration of insulin peptide B-(9–23). Proc. Natl. Acad. Sci. USA **93:** 956–960.
2. ABIRU, N. *et al.* 2001. Peptide and MHC-specific breaking of humoral tolerance to native insulin with the B:9–23 peptide in diabetes-prone and normal mice. Diabetes **50:** 1274–1281.
3. ABIRU, N. *et al.* 2000. Dual overlapping peptides recognized by insulin peptide B:9–23 reactive T cell receptor AV13S3 T cell clones of the NOD mouse. J. Autoimmun. **14:** 231–237.
4. OKADA, N. *et al.* 2001. Efficient gene delivery into dendritic cells by fiber-mutant adenovirus vectors. Biochem. Biophys. Res. Commun. **282:** 173–179.
5. CASARES, S. *et al.* 2002. Down-regulation of diabetogenic CD4+ T cells by a soluble dimeric peptide–MHC class II chimera. Nat. Immunol. **3:** 383–391.
6. OKADA, N. *et al.* 2001. Efficient antigen gene transduction using Arg-Gly-Asp fiber-mutant adenovirus vectors can potentiate antitumor vaccine efficacy and maturation of murine dendritic cells. Cancer Res. **61:** 7913–7919.
7. FEILI-HARIRI, M. *et al.* 2002. Regulatory Th2 response induced following adoptive transfer of dendritic cells in prediabetic NOD mice. Eur. J. Immunol. **32:** 2021–2030.
8. MORIYAMA, H. *et al.* 2002. Induction and acceleration of insulitis/diabetes in mice with a viral mimic (polyinosinic-polycytidylic acid) and an insulin self-peptide. Proc. Natl. Acad. Sci. USA **99:** 5539–5544.

Abnormal Peripheral Blood Dendritic Cell Populations in Type 1 Diabetes

RUIHUA PENG, Y. LI, K. BREZNER, SALLY LITHERLAND, AND M. J. CLARE-SALZLER

Department of Pathology, Immunology, and Laboratory Medicine, University of Florida, Gainesville, Florida 32608, USA

ABSTRACT: Type 1 diabetes (T1D) is a T cell–mediated disease. Various DC populations play important roles in initiating and directing T cell responses and thus may be critical for T1D pathogenesis. We thus examined peripheral blood DC1 and DC2 populations by flow cytometry in healthy controls, subjects at risk for T1D, new-onset patients, and established T1D patients. We found a significant increase in the number of DCs (including DC1 and DC2) in at-risk subjects and those with new-onset T1D versus healthy controls and established T1D patients (ANOVA; $p < 0.0001$). Analysis of DC1 and DC2 subsets in these same groups demonstrated a significant decrease in the ratio of DC1 and DC2 in subjects at risk and new-onset and established T1D patients in contrast with healthy controls ($p < 0.0001$). Both subsets of peripheral blood DCs from T1D patients expressed significantly higher levels of HLA-DR than healthy controls. Peripheral blood mononuclear cells from T1D patients secreted significantly higher amounts of IFN-α than controls, and IFN-α production correlated inversely with the DC1/DC2 ratio. This study demonstrates a marked increase in peripheral blood DC numbers that occurs during a time of active autoimmunity in at-risk subjects and patients with new-onset T1D, but is lost in established diabetes. However, the abnormal distribution of peripheral blood DC populations appears to be a persistent phenotype in all stages of T1D.

KEYWORDS: type 1 diabetes (T1D); T cells; peripheral blood; dendritic cells

INTRODUCTION

Type 1 diabetes (T1D) is an autoimmune disease mediated by autoreactive T cells against β cells.[1] Because dendritic cells (DCs) play an essential role in initiating and directing T cell responses, we chose to study peripheral blood DC subsets in T1D. It has been reported that human peripheral blood contains two subsets of DCs, DC1 and DC2.[2] DC1 are myeloid DCs that upon maturation upregulate MHC class II, costimulatory molecules, and IL-12 production, and promote Th1 response. In contrast, DC2, designated plasmacytoid DCs because of their morphological features, generally are thought to promote Th2 response. However, additional reports suggest

Address for correspondence: Dr. Michael J. Clare-Salzler, Department of Pathology, Immunology, and Laboratory Medicine, University of Florida, P.O. Box 100275, Gainesville, FL 32607. Voice: 352-392-9885; fax: 352-392-5393.
salzler@ufl.edu

that DC2 under certain conditions prime Th1 response.[3] This may occur under the condition of high amounts of IFN-α production by DC2. In this study, we attempted to determine whether there are abnormalities in the number or function of DC subsets in subjects at risk for T1D and new-onset and established T1D patients in comparison with healthy controls.

MATERIALS AND METHODS

Patients and Normal Control Subjects

Blood samples from human subjects under informed consent were obtained from the University of Florida. Thirty-nine cases of subjects at risk for T1D, 8 subjects with new-onset (within 3 months of diagnosis) T1D, 31 cases of established T1D, and 40 healthy controls were analyzed.

Flow Cytometry Assay for Peripheral Blood DCs

Peripheral blood DCs were characterized using a method previously reported[4] with limited modifications.

PBMC IFN-α Production

The production of IFN-α by peripheral blood mononuclear cells (PBMCs; 8×10^6 cells) with or without depletion of DC2 were cultured with or without flu virus (10 HPA/mL) in 1 mL medium with IL-3 (10 ng/mL) for 24 h. IFN-α in the supernatants was measured by specific ELISA. In some experiments, DC2 were depleted with BDCA-2 antibody.

RESULTS

Characterization of DC Subsets in Peripheral Blood

We examined peripheral blood DC1 (lin–/DR+/CD11c+/CD123–) and DC2 (lin–/DR+/CD11c–/CD123+) by flow cytometry in healthy controls, subjects at risk, new-onset T1D patients, and patients with established T1D. Panels A and B in FIGURE 1 show a sample of a T1D patient and a normal control, respectively. We found a significant increase in the number of DCs in at-risk subjects and those with new-onset T1D versus healthy controls and established T1D patients (ANOVA; $p < 0.0001$). We also demonstrated a significant decrease in the ratio of DC1/DC2 in subjects at risk, new-onset patients, and established T1D patients in contrast with healthy controls. Both subsets of peripheral blood DCs from all T1D subjects expressed higher levels of HLA-DR than healthy controls (ANOVA; $p < 0.0001$).

IFN-α Production by PBMCs from T1D Patients

We found that the unmanipulated PBMCs from at-risk subjects, new-onset T1D patients, or established T1D patients secreted significantly higher amounts of IFN-α compared with normal controls ($p < 0.0001$). After depletion of DC2 with BDCA-2

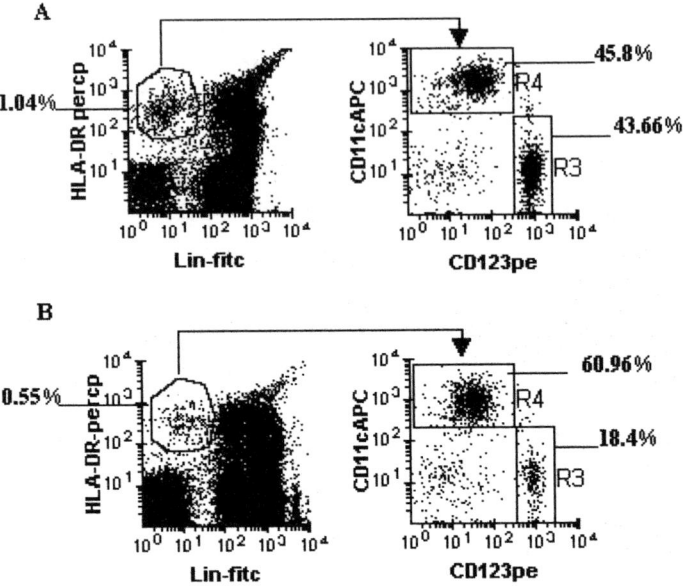

FIGURE 1. Distribution and phenotypes of DC1 and DC2 in peripheral blood. The peripheral blood myeloid (DC1; lin−/DR+/CD11c+/CD123−) and plasmacytoid (DC2; lin−/DR+/CD11c−/CD123+) DC populations were examined by flow cytometry in healthy controls, subjects at risk, new-onset patients, and patients with established T1D: **(A)** a representative of samples from T1D patients; **(B)** a sample from normal controls.

antibodies, the production of IFN-α was reduced 15-fold, indicating that IFN-α was produced by DC2 in PBMCs. In addition, statistical analysis demonstrated that IFN-α production correlated inversely with the DC1/DC2 ratio (T1D subjects correlation coefficient = 0.763, $p < 0.0001$; healthy controls: correlation coefficient = 0.7652, $p < 0.0001$).

SUMMARY

A marked increase in peripheral blood DC number (DR+/lin− cells) occurs during a time of active autoimmunity in at-risk subjects and those with new-onset T1D, but not in controls or established T1D subjects. The abnormal distribution of peripheral blood DC1/DC2 subsets, however, appears to be a persistent phenotype in all stages of T1D. In at-risk subjects and patients with new-onset T1D, both types of DCs have higher levels of HLA-DR, suggesting that DCs are more activated than those in normal controls. The capacity for IFN-α production in response to virus is significantly higher in the PBMCs of subjects where increased numbers of DC2 are found. Our findings suggest that the abnormality of DC subsets in T1D patients may play an important role in pathogenesis of T1D.

REFERENCES

1. DURINOVIC-BELLO, I. 1998. Autoimmune diabetes: the role of T cells, MHC molecules, and autoantigens. Autoimmunity **27:** 159–177.
2. BANCHEREAU, J. & R.M. STEINMAN. 1998. Dendritic cells and the control of immunity. Nature **392:** 245–252.
3. GROUARD, G. et al. 1997. The enigmatic plasmacytoid T cells develop into dendritic cells with interleukin (IL)-3 and CD40-ligand. J. Exp. Med. **185:** 1101–1111.
4. CELLA, M. et al. 2000. Plasmacytoid dendritic cells activated by influenza virus and CD40L drive a potent Th1 polarization. Nat. Immunol. **1:** 305–310.

Characterization of Dendritic Cells in Humans with Type 1 Diabetes

KELLY L. SUMMERS,[a,b] MARGARET T. BEHME,[c] JEFFERY L. MAHON,[c] AND BHAGIRATH SINGH[a,b]

[a]*John P. Roberts Research Institute, London, Ontario N6A 5C1, Canada*

[b]*Department of Microbiology and Immunology, University of Western Ontario, London, Ontario N6A 5C1, Canada*

[c]*Departments of Medicine and Epidemiology, London Health Sciences Center, London, Ontario N6A 5C1, Canada*

ABSTRACT: The characterization of dendritic cells (DCs) in diabetes has primarily examined *in vitro*–generated DCs. In this study, we have compared the composition and phenotype of naturally occurring DCs within the peripheral blood of subjects with type 1 diabetes, latent-onset autoimmune diabetes in adults, and nondiabetic controls. We find that circulatory DC subsets exist in normal frequencies and phenotypic states in diabetic patients. *In vivo*, DCs were located around the pancreatic islets in type 1 diabetic patients, but were absent in pancreatic tissue of normal controls. These findings provide new insight toward understanding the pathological role of DCs in type 1 diabetes.

KEYWORDS: dendritic cell subsets; humans; peripheral blood; pancreas; type 1 diabetes; LADA

INTRODUCTION

Dendritic cells (DCs) have opposing roles because they are capable of inducing immune responses against foreign antigens, as well as tolerance to self-antigens.[1] Animal models of type 1 diabetes (T1D) demonstrate that DCs drive an immunogenic response;[2–4] however, the rationale remains unclear. Various factors have been proposed, including defective DC numbers, altered DC subset ratios, and abnormal maturation/activation states; however, the details are conflicting between studies.[2–6]

These inconsistencies are likely attributed to differences in the DC populations between studies. Few studies on DCs in diabetes have examined directly isolated DCs. Instead, most reports both in animal models of diabetes[2–4] and in humans[5,6] describe DCs generated *in vitro* by incubating monocytes or bone marrow cells in cytokines for extended periods of time. This procedure activates cells and promotes the selective differentiation of myeloid DCs. Clearly, DCs generated in culture are not representative of naturally occurring DCs.

Address for correspondence: Dr. Kelly L. Summers, Department of Microbiology and Immunology, University of Western Ontario, London, Ontario N6A 5C1, Canada. Voice: 519-661-3483; fax: 519-661-3499.
ksummers@uwo.ca

We compared the maturation state, activation state, frequency, and subset ratio of naturally occurring DCs in the peripheral blood of patients with T1D, latent-onset autoimmune diabetes in adults (LADA), and nondiabetic healthy controls. We also examined for the presence of DCs in pancreatic tissue obtained from subjects with T1D and nondiabetic controls.

METHODS

Subjects

Nine patients with T1D (age: 38.4 ± 8.3 years; duration: 16.1 ± 10.5 years [mean ± SD]; all positive for antibodies to ICA512; 5 of 9 positive for antibodies to GAD65) and five patients with LADA (age: 37.8 ± 16.8 years; duration: 1.5 ± 1.3 years; all positive for type 2 diabetes and antibodies to GAD65 and/or ICA512) were recruited from a parallel study. Seven healthy volunteers were recruited as controls. Informed consent was received from each subject.

Analysis of DCs in the Blood

Venous peripheral blood was obtained from each subject and drawn into EDTA tubes. Whole blood was labeled directly with a combination of monoclonal antibodies to allow determination of the frequency of DCs, the ratio of DC subsets, and the activation state of each DC subset. Cells were analyzed using four-color flow cytometry on a BD FACS Calibur. DCs were defined as cells lacking expression of the lineage-specific markers, CD3, CD14, CD16, CD19, and CD57, while coexpressing the HLA-DR molecule. Myeloid DCs were defined as $CD11c^+$ DCs. Lymphoid DCs were defined as $CD11c^-$ DCs.

Analysis of DCs in the Pancreatic Tissue

Formaldehyde-fixed blocks of pancreatic tissue from cadavers with T1D or nondiabetic controls were obtained from archives in the Pathology Department at the London Health Sciences Center (London, Ontario, Canada). Tissue sections were stained using standard immunohistological techniques. In brief, paraffinized tissue was labeled with monoclonal antibodies against DC-specific antigens (P55, S100) or an isotype control after antigen retrieval, detected by alkaline phosphatase, and developed using DAB substrate.

RESULTS

The total number of DCs per liter of blood was similar between subjects with T1D ($1.7 \times 10^7 \pm 0.5 \times 10^7$), LADA ($1.6 \times 10^7 \pm 0.7 \times 10^7$), and controls ($2.2 \times 10^7 \pm 0.9 \times 10^7$; FIG. 1). The percentages of myeloid DC and lymphoid DC subsets within the total DC population, respectively, were also similar between subjects with T1D (61.4% ± 12.2%; 38.6% ± 12.2%), LADA (51.7% ± 18.1%; 48.3% ± 18.1%), and controls (62.3% ± 12.5%; 37.7% ± 12.5%; FIG. 1).

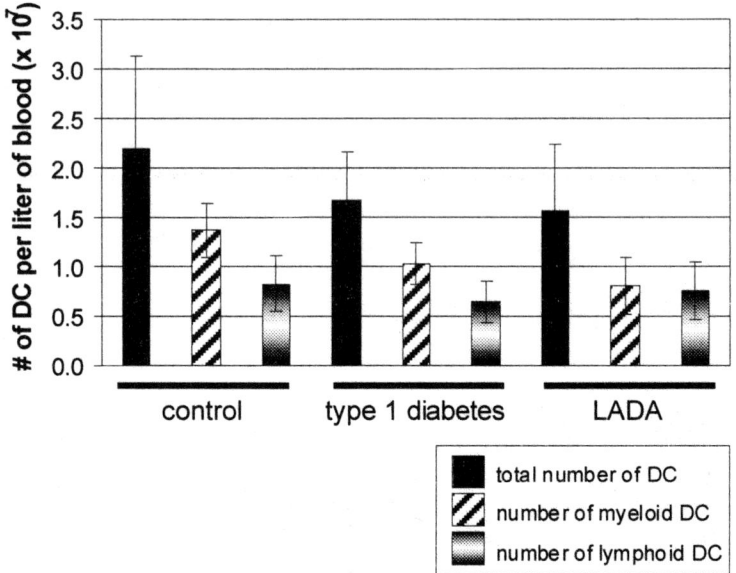

FIGURE 1. The numbers of circulatory total DCs, myeloid DCs, and lymphoid DCs are similar between nondiabetic controls and subjects with T1D and LADA. Mean ± SD.

Both DC subsets existed in a resting state within the blood from each group, as defined by the uniform absence of the CD83 activation marker. Similarly, there were no differences in the surface expression of costimulator molecules on DC subsets between the groups. In all cases, myeloid DCs lacked expression of 4-1BB ligand and CD40, expressed the CD86 molecule, and showed variable density expression of the CD80 molecule. Lymphoid DCs consistently lacked surface expression of all costimulator molecules examined.

DCs were found within the pancreatic tissue of subjects with T1D. In each case, they were located in the exocrine tissue around the islets, but not within the islets. In contrast, DCs were not found in the pancreatic tissue from nondiabetic controls.

DISCUSSION

We show that naturally occurring DCs within the blood of patients with T1D and LADA circulate in normal numbers, exist in a normal resting state, and consist of similar proportions of myeloid DC and lymphoid DC subsets. This does not support previously described differences in DC yield or phenotype between normal and diabetic subjects,[6] which is likely explained by the use of unmanipulated DCs versus *in vitro*–generated DCs.[6] The presence of DCs within the pancreas of subjects with T1D indicates that β cell destruction may be facilitated either directly or indirectly by DCs that have migrated into the pancreas.

ACKNOWLEDGMENTS

This work was supported by the Juvenile Diabetes Research Foundation and the Canadian Institute of Health Research.

REFERENCES

1. SHORTMAN, K. & Y. LIU. 2002. Mouse and human dendritic cell subtypes. Nat. Rev. **2:** 151–161.
2. FEILI-HARIRI, M. & P.A. MOREL. 2001. Phenotypic and functional characteristics of bone marrow–derived DC from NOD and non-diabetes-prone strains. Clin. Immunol. **98:** 133–142.
3. STRID, J. et al. 2001. A defect in bone marrow derived dendritic cell maturation in the nonobese diabetic mouse. Clin. Exp. Immunol. **123:** 375–381.
4. MARLEAU, A. & B. SINGH. 2002. Myeloid dendritic cells in non-obese diabetic mice have elevated costimulatory and T helper-1–inducing abilities. J. Autoimmun. **19:** 23–35.
5. JANSEN, A., M. VAN HAGEN & H.A. DREXHAGE. 1995. Defective maturation and function of antigen-presenting cells in type 1 diabetes. Lancet **345:** 491–492.
6. TAKAHASHI, K., M.C. HONEYMAN & L.C. HARRISON. 1998. Impaired yield, phenotype, and function of monocyte-derived dendritic cells in humans at risk for insulin-dependent diabetes. J. Immunol. **161:** 2629–2635.

NKT Cell Frequency in Japanese Type 1 Diabetes

YOICHI OIKAWA,[a] AKIRA SHIMADA,[a] SATORU YAMADA,[a]
YOSHIKO MOTOHASHI,[a] YOSHINORI NAKAGAWA,[a] JUN-ICHIRO IRIE,[a]
TARO MARUYAMA,[b] AND TAKAO SARUTA[a]

[a]*Department of Internal Medicine, Keio University School of Medicine, Tokyo 160-8582, Japan*

[b]*Department of Internal Medicine, Saitama Social Insurance Hospital, Saitama 336-0002, Japan*

ABSTRACT: A numerical and functional deficit of natural killer T (NKT) cells has been reported to be associated with the pathogenesis of Caucasian patients with type 1 diabetes. However, a conflicting finding of a higher frequency of NKT cells (Valpha24+ Vbeta11+ T cells) was observed in islet-associated Ab+ and Ab– Japanese "classic" type 1 diabetes. Here, we combined the data of NKT cell frequency in Ab+ and Ab– "classic" type 1 diabetic patients and then analyzed the relationship between NKT cell frequency and disease activity.

KEYWORDS: type 1 diabetes; NKT cell

A numerical and functional deficit of natural killer T (NKT) cells has been reported to be associated with the pathogenesis of white patients with type 1 diabetes.[1,2] However, we recently reported a conflicting finding that a higher frequency of NKT cells (Valpha24+ Vbeta11+ T cells) was observed in islet-associated antibody (GAD and/or IA-2)–positive (Ab+) and antibody-negative (Ab–) Japanese "classic" type 1 diabetes.[3] In this study, we combined the data of NKT cell frequency in Ab+ and Ab– "classic" type 1 diabetic patients, these subjects were stratified by disease duration, and then we analyzed the relationship between NKT cell frequency and disease activity.

MATERIALS AND METHODS

Peripheral blood samples were obtained from 164 Japanese diabetic patients and 67 healthy subjects (39 males, 28 females; age, 40.5 ± 14.3 years) with informed consent for use in this study. The diabetic patients were classified into three categories as follows: "classic" type 1 diabetes ($n = 78$; 41 males, 37 females; age, 40.6 ± 17.1

Address for correspondence: Yoichi Oikawa, M.D., Department of Internal Medicine, Division of Endocrinology and Metabolism, Keio University School of Medicine, 35 Shinanomachi, Shinjuku-ku, Tokyo 160-8582, Japan. Voice: +81-3-3353-1211 (ext. 62383); fax: +81-3-5269-3219.
y-oikawa@mvc.biglobe.ne.jp

years; disease duration, 4.0 ± 4.5 years; HbA1c, 8.4 ± 1.9%); latent autoimmune diabetes in adults (LADA) (n = 26; 19 males, 7 females; age, 51.3 ± 12.1 years; disease duration, 6.7 ± 5.6 years; HbA1c, 8.4 ± 1.9%); and type 2 diabetes (n = 60; 33 males, 27 females; age, 61.3 ± 10.1 years; disease duration, 9.8 ± 6.7 years; HbA1c, 7.1 ± 1.4%). Moreover, classic type 1 diabetic patients were divided into the following two groups: *recent-onset* type 1 (disease duration, <3 years; n = 45) and *established* type 1 diabetes (disease duration, ≥3 years; n = 33). We measured the frequency of peripheral Valpha24+ Vbeta11+ CD3+ triple-positive cells (as representatives of NKT cells) with a three-color flow cytometer. Results are presented as the mean ± SE. A difference in NKT cell frequency was analyzed using the Bonferroni-Dunn test. The correlation between NKT cell frequency and disease duration (or age) was analyzed by Spearman's rank order correlation test.

RESULTS AND CONCLUSIONS

It is intriguing that recent-onset (Ab+ and Ab– combined) classic type 1 diabetic patients showed a significantly higher NKT cell frequency than those with established (Ab+ and Ab– combined) classic type 1 diabetes (0.165 ± 0.022% vs. 0.069 ± 0.011%; $p < 0.0001$), LADA patients ($p < 0.0001$), type 2 diabetic patients ($p < 0.0001$), and healthy subjects ($p < 0.0001$; FIG. 1). Moreover, an inverse correla-

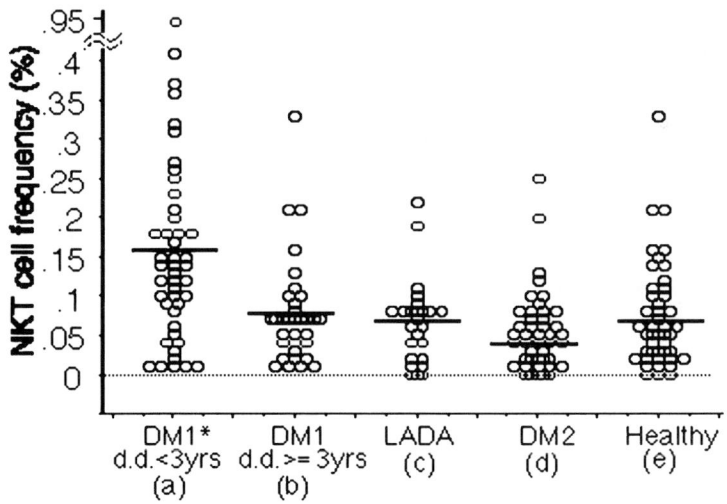

FIGURE 1. Peripheral NKT cell frequency in classic type 1 diabetes (DM1), LADA, type 2 diabetes (DM2), and healthy subjects. Peripheral NKT cells were significantly increased in recent-onset (disease duration [d.d.], <3 years) classic type 1 diabetes (a) as compared with other types of diabetes (b, c, d) and healthy subjects (e). Horizontal lines indicate the mean of NKT cell frequency; *$p < 0.0001$ (compared with groups b, c, d, and e).

tion between NKT cell frequency and disease duration was observed in classic type 1 diabetes ($r = -0.423$; $p = 0.0002$). Considering our previous report,[3] these findings indicate that a higher frequency of NKT cells was observed in recent-onset classic type 1 diabetes, irrespective of the positivity of islet-associated autoantibodies.

We demonstrated here the striking finding that NKT cells were significantly increased in Japanese type 1 diabetes, especially in recent-onset (Ab+ and Ab− combined) classic type 1 diabetes, and this conflicts with previous reports.[1,2] A difference in onset age (child or adult) and/or disease duration could account for the discrepancy between their reports and ours, although we cannot exclude the possibility of a difference in genetic background and, especially, the definition of NKT cell markers. In a future study, we must evaluate NKT cell frequency by using other surrogate NKT cell markers, such as CD1d tetramers loaded with α-galactosylceramide. Moreover, we would like to measure the cytokine profile of the increasing NKT cells to clarify their roles in the pathogenesis of type 1 diabetes.

It is generally considered that higher disease (insulitis) activity is expected in type 1 diabetes with shorter disease duration[4] because a severe beta cell mass reduction is suspected in cases of established (long-standing) type 1 diabetes. Although there is no general consensus on a useful marker to assess "disease activity" of type 1 diabetes thus far, we have shown here a high frequency of NKT cells in recent-onset classic type 1 diabetes. This observation raises the possibility that the increased NKT cells may reflect active disease (or insulitis) status in classic type 1 diabetes. Because there is no report of an increment in NKT cells among other autoimmune diseases in humans thus far, we would like to emphasize that high NKT cell frequency in peripheral blood is a unique finding in recent-onset classic type 1 diabetes, and measurement of NKT cell frequency in peripheral blood may be useful to assess the disease activity of classic type 1 diabetes.

REFERENCES

1. WILSON, S.B. et al. 1998. Extreme Th1 bias of invariant Valpha24JalphaQ T cells in type 1 diabetes. Nature **391:** 177–181.
2. KUKREJA, A. et al. 2002. Multiple immuno-regulatory defects in type-1 diabetes. J. Clin. Invest. **109:** 131–140.
3. OIKAWA, Y. et al. 2002. High frequency of valpha24(+) vbeta11(+) T-cells observed in type 1 diabetes. Diabetes Care **25:** 1818–1823.
4. SHIMADA, A. et al. 2001. Elevated serum IP-10 levels observed in type 1 diabetes. Diabetes Care **24:** 510–515.

IL-6 Modulates Hyperglycemia-Induced Changes of Na+ Channel Beta-3 Subunit Expression by Schwann Cells

DUSANKA S. SKUNDRIC,[a,b] RUJUAN DAI,[a] AND PHILIP MATAVERDE[a]

[a]*Department of Neurology, Division of Neuroimmunology,*
[b]*Department of Immunology and Microbiology,*
Wayne State University, Detroit Medical Center, Detroit, Michigan, USA

> ABSTRACT: Our data show the suppressive effect of hyperglycemia on expression of voltage-gated Na+ channel β3 subunit by Schwann cells as well as the protection of β3 expression by treatment with IL-6. Our findings have direct relevance for therapy of diabetic neuropathy.
>
> KEYWORDS: Schwann cell; diabetic neuropathy; IL-6; Na+ channel beta subunits; hyperglycemia; rat

INTRODUCTION

Diabetic sensory-motor polyneuropathy is a chronic complication of insulin-dependent diabetes mellitus (IDDM). It develops as a result of both hyperglycemia-induced metabolic changes and microangiopathy.[1] Improper function of voltage-gated Na+ and K+ channels and Na+/K+ ATPase occurs very early in patients with type 1 diabetes and results in decreased conduction velocity of the peripheral nerve.[2,3] In the sciatic nerve, voltage-gated Na+ channels are clustered at the nodes of Ranvier, which are formed by Schwann cells. Nodal regions are also enriched in cell adhesion molecules (CAMs), some of which are believed to facilitate clustering of Na+ channels at these sites.[4] Structure of the voltage-gated Na+ channel includes a central pore-forming α subunit, with a major role in impulse conduction, and two β subunits, which serve as channel modulators and CAMs. Three different β subunits (β1, β2, and β3) are described in mammals. Extracellular domains of all three β subunits are highly conserved and share structural homology with immunoglobulin (Ig) domain, similar to CAMs. Ig-like domain of the β3 subunit has the highest degree of similarity with P_0 glycoprotein, a myelin protein with established function as a CAM in the peripheral nerve.[5] IL-6 is a proinflammatory and neuropoietic cytokine. IL-6, IL-6R, and activated components of its signaling pathway are constitutively expressed in normal rats and downregulated in sciatic nerves of BB/W rats with type 1 diabetes.[6,7]

Address for correspondence: Dusanka S. Skundric, M.D., Ph.D., Department of Neurology, School of Medicine, Wayne State University, 421 East Canfield, 3141 Elliman Building, Detroit, MI 48201. Voice: 313-993-4002; fax: 313-577-7552.
skundric@cmb.biosci.wayne.edu

Neuropoietic properties of IL-6 include neuroprotective effect on dorsal root ganglia/neuron cocultures[8] and stimulation of P_0 expression, leading to Schwann cell (SC) attachment to axons.[9]

MATERIALS AND METHODS

Schwann Cell Culture

Rat SC line S16 was generated by and obtained from R. Quarles (NIH, Bethesda, MD).[10] After thawing, 10^6 cells were seeded onto poly-D-lysine-coated 35-mm petri dishes and maintained in Dulbecco's minimum essential medium (DMEM) until reaching confluence. Cells then were detached by the treatment with 2.5% trypsin (Invitrogen, Carlsbad, CA) for 3–5 min, washed, and seeded onto new precoated petri dishes, similar to as described by Goda et al.[10] Confluent SC cultures after two passages were used for experiments. Experimental hyperglycemia was achieved by culturing cells in serum-free DMEM, containing 25 mM glucose for 96 h. In a separate experiment, rat IL-6 (2 ng/mL; R&D Systems, Minneapolis, MN) was added to high-glucose (25 mM) serum-free DMEM at the beginning of the 96-h culture period. Control SCs were cultured in serum-free DMEM containing 5 mM glucose. After the 96 h of culture, cells were trypsinized, washed, snap-frozen, and kept at −70°C until RNA isolation.

Real-Time PCR

RNA was isolated by Trizol Reagent (Gibco-BRL, Grand Island, NY). Total RNA was reverse-transcribed similarly as described.[11] Real-time PCR was done on the LightCycler System, using LightCycler–Fast Start DNA Master SYBR Green I (Roche, Mannheim, Germany). In brief, the PCR mix consisted of LightCycler–Fast Start DNA Master SYBR Green I mix (final concentration: ×1), $MgCl_2$ (4 mM), primers (0.5 µM each; Sigma Genosys, St. Louis, MO), and cDNA (4 µg). In the negative control, the template DNA was replaced with PCR-grade water. Cycling was performed as follows: denaturation at 95°C for 30 s, annealing at 55°C for 5 s, elongation at 72°C for 10 s, for a total of 45 cycles. Rat-specific primers were β-actin: 5′ TGCCCTGAGTGTTTCTTGTG, 3′ CCCTCATAGATGGGCACAGT; and Na+ channel β3 subunit: 5′ TAGCCCAGTGGGTAAAATGC; 3′ CCTGGAGCTTGC-CAAGTAAG.

RESULTS AND DISCUSSION

The S16 rat SC line was selected because of its unique properties to express adhesion proteins, neural cell adhesion molecule L1, laminin, myelin-associated glycoprotein, and P_0 glycoprotein without presence of axons.[12] Given the highest structural homology between β3 subunit and P_0 glycoprotein, which serves as a CAM, we first investigated expression of β3 subunit by S16 cells, its regulation by experimental hyperglycemia, and modulation by IL-6.

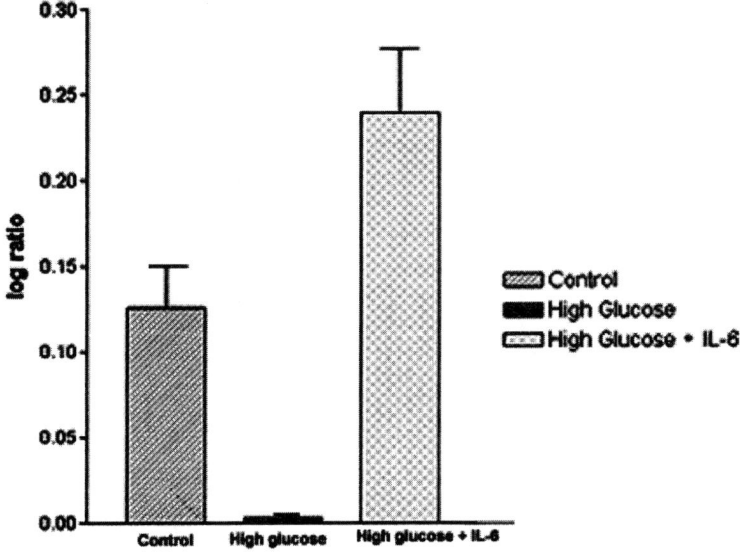

FIGURE 1. Expression levels of voltage-gated Na+ channel β3 subunit in cultured rat S16 cell line. Expression levels of β3 subunit are presented as log values of the ratio calculated from comparison to β-actin expression levels in the same sample. Each value presents the mean from three separate cell culture experiments. β3 subunit–specific mRNA is constitutively expressed in control S16 SC line, cultured in serum-free medium containing 5 mM glucose. It is significantly downregulated after 96 h of SC culture in high glucose (25 mM). Addition of IL-6 (2 ng/mL) to high-glucose culture medium protects from hyperglycemia-induced changes.

The Na+ channel β3 subunit was found constitutively expressed in the S16 SC line. Constitutive expression of Na+ channel β2 subunit and glial Na+ channel was also found at lower levels compared with β3.[7] After the 96 h of experimental hyperglycemia, constitutive levels of β3 subunit were significantly decreased, reaching the borderline of detectable values. Levels of β3 subunit–specific mRNA displayed an approximately tenfold change in high-glucose cultured SCs compared with constitutive levels (FIG. 1). When SCs were cultured in high glucose with addition of IL-6, gene expression levels of β3 subunit were unaffected by hyperglycemia. Moreover, IL-6 treatment led to approximately twofold higher expression levels of β3 subunit compared with constitutive levels. We found some protective effect of IL-6 on β2 subunit and glial Na+ channel expression in high-glucose cultured S16 cells.[7] However, the most pronounced protective effect of IL-6 was observed on β3 subunit expression. These *in vitro* results correspond well to our findings of significant downregulation of Na+ channel β subunits in the sciatic nerve at early stages of the diabetic neuropathy in the BB/W rat.[7] Concomitant with this downregulation of Na+ channel subunits, we found downregulation of IL-6R and abrogation of IL-6 signaling through signal transducer and transcription activator 3, in the sciatic nerve, early after the onset of diabetes.[7]

Our data show (1) suppressive effect of hyperglycemia on expression of voltage-gated Na+ channel β3 subunit by Schwann cells and (2) protection of β3 expression by treatment with IL-6. Our findings have direct relevance for therapy of diabetic neuropathy.

ACKNOWLEDGMENTS

We thank Richard H. Quarles (NIH, Bethesda, MD) for providing us with the S16 rat Schwann cell line. We are thankful to Detroit Veterans Affairs Medical Center Research Services for allowing the use of their LightCycler real-time PCR machine. This work was funded by a Career Development Award from the American Diabetes Association (No. 255FR) to D. S. Skundric.

REFERENCES

1. CAMERON, N.E. & M.A. COTTER. 1997. Metabolic and vascular factors in the pathogenesis of diabetic neuropathy. Diabetes **46**(suppl. 2): S31.
2. BEHSE, X. et al. 1977. Nerve biopsy and conduction studies in diabetic neuropathy. J. Neurol. Neurosurg. Psychiatry **40**: 1072.
3. SIMMONS, Z. & E.L. FELDMAN. 2002. Update on diabetic neuropathy. Curr. Opin. Neurol. **15**: 595–603.
4. SCHERER, S.S. & E.J. ARROYO. 2002. Recent progress on the molecular organization of myelinated axons. J. Peripheral Nerv. Syst. **7**: 1–12.
5. ISOM, L. 2002. The role of sodium channels in cell adhesion. Front. Biosci. **7**: 12–23.
6. SKUNDRIC, D.S., B. BEALMEAR & R.P. LISAK. 1997. IL-1, IL-6, and TNF upregulate gene expression of each other in cultured Schwann cells (SC). J. Neurochem. (Suppl.) **69**: S152D.
7. SKUNDRIC, D.S., R.J. DAI, P. MATAVERDE et al. 2002. Role of IL-6 in modulation of Na^+ and K^+ transport at early stages of diabetic neuropathy. Diabetes Metab. Res. Rev. **18**(suppl. 4): S23.
8. EDOFF, K. & H. JERREGARD. 2002. Effects of IL-1beta, IL-6, or LIF on rat sensory neurons co-cultured with fibroblast-like cells. J. Neurosci. Res. **67**: 255–263.
9. HAGGIAG, S., P.L. ZHANG, G. SLUTZKY et al. 2001. Stimulation of myelin gene expression in vitro and sciatic nerve remyelination by interleukin-6 receptor–interleukin-6 chimera. J. Neurosci. Res. **64**: 564–574.
10. GODA, S., J. HAMMER, D. KOBILER & R.H. QUARLES. 1991. Expression of the myelin-associated glycoprotein in cultures of immortalized Schwann cells. J. Neurochem. **56**: 1354–1361.
11. TODA, K., J.A. SMALL, S. GODA & R.H. QUARLES. 1994. Biochemical and cellular properties of three immortalized Schwann cell lines expressing different levels of the myelin-associated glycoprotein. J. Neurochem. **63**: 1646–1657.
12. SKUNDRIC, D.S., B. BEALMEAR & R.P. LISAK. 1997. Induced upregulation of IL-1, IL-1RA, and IL-1R type I gene expression by Schwann cells. J. Neuroimmunol. **74**: 9–18.

Glucose-Responsive Expression of the Human Insulin Promoter in HepG2 Human Hepatoma Cells

BRANT R. BURKHARDT,[a] SCOTT A. LOILER,[b,c] JO ANNE ANDERSON,[a] MICHAEL S. KILBERG,[d] JAMES M. CRAWFORD,[a] TERENCE R. FLOTTE,[b,c] KEVIN S. GOUDY,[a] TAMIR M. ELLIS,[a] AND MARK ATKINSON[a]

[a]*Department of Pathology,* [b]*Department of Pediatrics,* [c]*Powell Gene Therapy Center,* [d]*Department of Biochemistry and Molecular Biology, University of Florida, Gainesville, Florida, USA*

ABSTRACT: The concept of insulin production afforded by hepatic gene therapy retains promise as a potential therapy for type 1 diabetes, but the approach has been limited by the need for strict transgene regulation in response to fluctuating levels of both glucose and insulin. Furthermore, while hepatocytes contain various glucose-responsive elements, they lack the appropriate regulated secretory system necessary for insulin release, thereby necessitating the requirement for transcriptional regulation of hepatic insulin production under the direction of a glucose-responsive promoter. To address this, we have evaluated several glucose-responsive promoters that may be used successfully for hepatic insulin production via recombinant adeno-associated virus (rAAV) therapy. Our results suggest that the human insulin promoter represents a strong candidate as a robust, glucose-responsive promoter for regulated hepatic insulin production.

KEYWORDS: diabetes; insulin; transfection; promoter

INTRODUCTION

Treatment of type 1 diabetes by exogenous insulin therapy can be very effective at glycemic control. However, multiple daily insulin injections do not achieve strict blood glucose regulation and can cause extreme patient discomfort.[1,2] Stringent glycemic control is vital to preventing the onset of diabetic complications.[3] Therefore, a more effective and safe treatment is needed to achieve regulated insulin release in response to glucose levels. Type 1 diabetes is an ideal candidate for gene therapy because of the lack of production of a single protein (insulin), yet this concept has been limited because of questions of metabolic regulation, gene delivery, and site of production. The liver represents an excellent surrogate organ for insulin production because it contains several glucose-sensing and responsive elements,

Address for correspondence: Mark Atkinson, Department of Pathology, University of Florida, Gainesville, FL 32610. Voice: 352-392-0048; fax: 352-392-8464.
atkinson@ufl.edu

Ann. N.Y. Acad. Sci. 1005: 237–241 (2003). © 2003 New York Academy of Sciences.
doi: 10.1196/annals.1288.035

including glucose transporter-2 (GLUT2) and glucokinase (GK), and thus is highly responsive to changing glucose concentrations.[4,5] One major caveat for impairing hepatic insulin production via gene therapy is that hepatocytes lack a regulated insulin secretory system that is present in pancreatic β cells. Hence, for hepatic insulin gene therapy to be effective, regulated insulin production has to be controlled at the transcriptional level. To address this problem, we have evaluated several glucose-responsive promoters that may be used successfully for hepatic insulin production via recombinant adeno-associated virus (rAAV) therapy. Our results suggest that the human insulin promoter represents a strong candidate as a robust, glucose-responsive promoter for regulated hepatic insulin production.

MATERIALS AND METHODS

Amplification and Cloning of the Rat Glucose 6-Phosphatase (RG6P), Mouse Fructose 1,6-Bisphosphatase (MF16BP), and Human Insulin Promoters (HIP)

Liver genomic DNA was extracted from a nonobese diabetic (NOD) mouse and a Fisher 344 rat by the DNeasy tissue kit (Qiagen). The PCR amplification of the 1377-bp RG6P (−1309 to +68 of G6Pase gene) and 1238-bp MF16BP (−1140 to +98 of MF16BP gene) promoters was performed using primers synthesized by Geno-Mechanix (Alachua, FL). The primers used for PCR amplification of the RG6P promoter were published previously by other investigators and slightly modified for our cloning purposes.[6] The primers used for the MF16BP were forward primer 1140SstF [5′-GC<u>GAGCTC</u>CTTTCTTTCCTGGTGTCTGTGTG-3′]; and reverse primer 98XhoIR [5′-GG<u>CTCGAG</u>GTGGCTAAAGGTGCTGACTAAAGGTG-3′]. Additional sequences (*Sst*I and *Xho*I as underlined above) were added to the end of each promoter for cloning into the pGL3-basic luciferase plasmid (Promega) for subsequent transient transfections. The HIP was received as an 8.2-kb plasmid containing a 2096-bp region of the HIP, driving the luciferase and enhanced yellow fluorescent fusion protein, all flanked by inverted terminal repeats in the backbone of rAAV2. Each construct was verified by sequencing using ABI 373 Prism Dye Terminator Cycle Sequencing (Perkin-Elmer), and large-scale plasmid DNA purifications were done by using the Qiagen Endofree Maxiprep kit (Qiagen).

Cell Culture and Transfections

Approximately 2×10^5 HepG2, or 2×10^4 BNL-CL2, and H4IIE cells were plated onto 24-well plates and maintained in Minimum Essential Medium containing L-glutamine (Cellgro), 10% FBS (Gibco-BRL), nonessential amino acids (×1; Gibco-BRL), and penicillin (100 units/mL)/streptomycin (100 μg/mL; Gibco-BRL). After a 24-h incubation period, 0.9 μg of promoter-reporter construct and 0.1 μg of pRL-TK (Promega) were transfected in each well using 12 μg of Superfect transfection reagent (Qiagen). The pRL-TK plasmid was cotransfected as a transfection efficiency control. Three hours after transfection, these cells were washed with 1× PBS and cultured in fresh medium for 16 h. Each construct was transfected in either duplicate or triplicate. Each experiment included the pGL3-basic promoterless construct that was transfected in separate wells to measure the background luciferase expression.

In addition, the pGL3-control plasmid (pGL3-C) (Promega) containing the SV40 promoter also was transfected in separate wells to serve as a positive control. After a 16-h incubation period, cells were washed twice with 1× PBS and lysed in 200 μL of Passive Lysis Buffer (Promega). Luciferase activity of the promoter constructs and the pRL-TK construct was measured sequentially by using the Dual-Luciferase Reporter Assay System (Promega). Luciferase activity was measured for 10 s after a 2-s delay using a Monolight 2010 luminometer (Analytical Luminescence Laboratory). Variation in transfection efficiency was normalized by dividing the promoter construct luciferase activity by the pRL-TK luciferase activity. Promoter activity is presented as luciferase expression relative to that of the promoterless pGL3-basic plasmid.

RESULTS

We tested a series of promoters that could, in theory, be glucose-responsive and have a high level of gene expression in hepatocytes. To evaluate basal promoter activity in various hepatocyte cell lines, we transfected the HIP, MF16BP, and RG6P constructs in duplicate into BNL-CL2 (mouse hepatocyte), H4IIE (rat hepatoma), and HepG2 (human hepatoma) cell lines. To account for transfection efficiency, we cotransfected the pRL-TK plasmid in all wells. In all hepatocyte cell lines tested, the HIP had the highest promoter activity (FIGS. 1A and 1B) among the experimental constructs tested, with the exception of the pGL3-C plasmid in H4IIE and HepG2 cells. In BNL-CL2 cells, the HIP demonstrated a 22- and 31-fold higher promoter activity than both the RG6P and MF16BP promoters (FIG. 1A), respectively. In addition, the HIP had a 3.7- and 4.3-fold higher promoter activity than the RG6P and MF16BP promoters in H4IIE cells (FIG. 1B), respectively. In HepG2 human hepatoma cells, the HIP and pGL3-C constructs provided the only detectable luciferase expression (data not shown). To determine whether the HIP was also glucose-responsive, we tested the HIP in increasing concentrations of glucose in both HepG2 and BNL-CL2 cells (FIG. 1C). Increasing concentrations of glucose resulted in an increase in luciferase expression as determined by the HIP. Maximum glucose responsiveness of the HIP was observed between 0 and 22 mM glucose concentrations with a 7-fold increase in promoter activity ($p < 0.05$, ANOVA). An increase in glucose concentration from 11 to 22 mM induced a 3.5-fold increase in promoter activity ($p < 0.05$, ANOVA). However, in contrast, glucose concentration had no effect on HIP-driven promoter expression in BNL-CL2 cells (data not shown).

DISCUSSION

Our data have shown that the HIP provides robust gene expression in multiple hepatocyte cell lines. In addition, the HIP is also glucose-responsive in the HepG2 human hepatoma cell line. These findings are in sharp discordance with other studies wherein the HIP has been characterized as a β cell–specific promoter.[7] The reasons for this discrepancy may be many and include our use of transient transfections and hepatocyte cell lines. Previous studies have evaluated the HIP through the use of transgenic mouse models that test the integrated HIP. Thus, the HIP may be capable

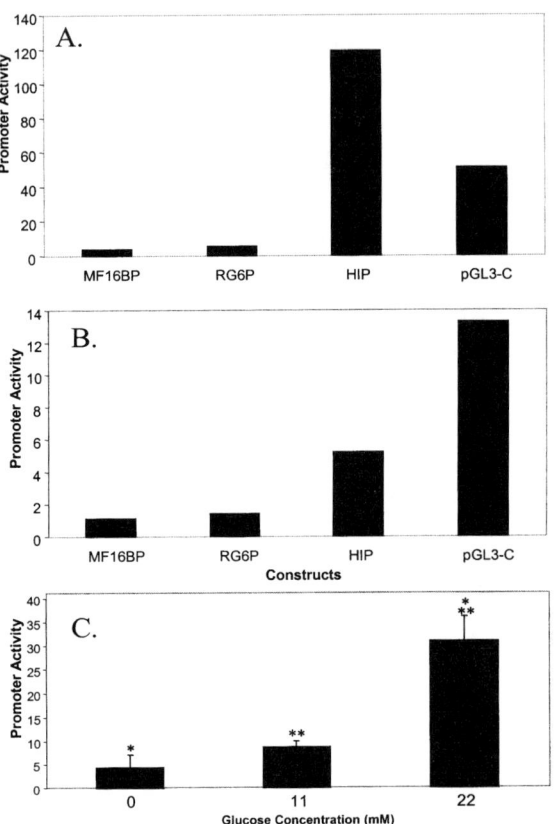

FIGURE 1. Expression of the HIP in hepatocyte cell lines. Transient transfections of the MF16BP, RG6P, and HIP constructs were performed in BNL-CL2, H4IIE, and HepG2 hepatocyte cell lines. Promoter activity is expressed as a ratio of the luciferase expression above the promoterless pGL3-basic construct. Transfection efficiency was accounted for by cotransfecting with the pRL-TK plasmid. The pGL3-control (pGL3-C) plasmid also was transfected as a measure of overall transfection efficiency. **(A)** Transfection of BNL-CL2 cells. Reporter constructs were transfected in duplicate, and promoter expression is expressed as the mean luciferase activity. **(B)** Transfection of H4IIE cells. **(C)** Transfection of the HIP in HepG2 cells with increasing concentrations of glucose. The data (means ± SEM) are shown from two independent experiments with each construct transfected in triplicate. Statistically significant differences ($p < 0.05$, ANOVA) are denoted by like symbols of a single asterisk or double asterisks.

of gene expression in hepatocyte cell lines without the regulation of chromatin structure or the overabundance of transcriptional factors found in transformed cell lines. Nonetheless, our purpose for utilizing the HIP would be for rAAV hepatic insulin gene therapy for the treatment of type 1 diabetes and, because the rAAV can typically remain episomal, this may allow for gene expression outside β cells. Yang et al. recently demonstrated that the rat insulin 1 gene promoter and a cytomegalovirus immediate-early promoter were capable of a glucose-responsive and insulin-inhibitory response in both Huh-7 hepatoma cells and the livers of streptozocin-treated mice.[8] Overall, our data show that the HIP also functions in multiple hepatocyte cell lines, indicating the possibility of similar transcriptional activation pathways between hepatocytes and β cells. Finally, the HIP may provide robust and rapid autoregulation of insulin via hepatic insulin gene therapy for type 1 diabetes.

REFERENCES

1. DIABETES CONTROL AND COMPLICATION TRIAL RESEARCH GROUP (DCCT). 1993. The effect of intensive treatment on the development and progression of long-term complications in insulin-dependent diabetes mellitus. N. Engl. J. Med. **329:** 977–986.
2. GAUTIER, J.F. et al. 1996. Are the implications of the Diabetes Control and Complication Trial (DCCT) feasible in daily clinical practice? Diabetes Metab. **22:** 415–419.
3. ATKINSON, M.A. & G.S. EISENBARTH. 2001. Type 1 diabetes: new perspectives on disease pathogenesis and treatment. Lancet **358:** 221–229.
4. GOULD, G.W. & G.D. HOLMAN. 1993. The glucose transporter family: structure, function, and tissue specific expression. Biochem. J. **295:** 329–341.
5. LYNEDJIAN, P.B. 1993. Mammalian glucokinase and its gene. Biochem. J. **293:** 1–13.
6. WOO, S.L.C. et al. 2000. Glucose-stimulated and self-limiting insulin production by glucose 6-phosphatase promoter drive insulin expression in hepatoma cells. Gene Ther. **7:** 1802–1809.
7. SELDEN, R.F. et al. 1986. Regulation of human insulin gene expression in transgenic mice. Nature **321:** 525–528.
8. YANG, Y.W., Y.C. HSIEH & C.K. CHAO. 2002. Glucose-modulated transgene expression via recombinant adeno-associated virus. Pharm. Res. **19:** 968–975.

Interleukin-6 Protects MIN6 β Cells from Cytokine-Induced Apoptosis

HYEWON PARK, YUHERN AHN, CHUNG-KYU PARK, HEE-YONG CHUNG, AND YONGSOO PARK

Division of Endocrinology and Metabolism, Department of Internal Medicine and Microbiology, Hanyang and Seoul National University, Seoul, Korea

ABSTRACT: Host nonspecific β cell injury by cytokines has been implicated in the process of early islet graft dysfunction. Islet transplant destruction by cytokines released from inflammatory cells that infiltrate the graft is thought to be mainly mediated by NF-κB-dependent nitric oxide (NO) production by the islet. In this study, we aimed to evaluate the role of IL-6 in making a β cell resistant to cytokine-induced apoptosis by decreasing the NF-κB-dependent NO production and compared the result with that of the expression of a dominant negative inhibitor of NF-κB (DN NF-κB). Incubation of MIN6 cells with IL-1β, IFN-γ, and TNF-α (cytomix) increased production of nitrites, with increased expression of iNOS mRNA. When treated with cytomix, the DN NF-κB–transfected mutant demonstrated significantly less nitrite production and apoptosis than parent MIN6. NO production was effectively blocked by IL-6 as well as by N-monomethyl-L-arginine (L-NMMA). Inhibition of the NO production led to decreased rate of apoptosis accompanied by downregulation of the proapoptotic molecule Bax and increased expression of the antiapoptotic molecule Bcl-2 and Bcl-x_L. These data indicate that cytokine-induced cell death in the MIN6 β cell line involves mechanisms that are, in part, NF-κB- and NO-dependent. Inhibition of the NO production by the incubation of the MIN6 cells by the pretreatment of IL-6 or L-NMMA is cytoprotective and can be used as a substitute for the expression of DN NF-κB.

KEYWORDS: IL-6; NF-κB; NO; apoptosis

INTRODUCTION

More than a million people have received diagnoses of type 1 diabetes mellitus (T1DM) in the United States. Recent advances in the developments of immunosuppressive regimens have lead to the first real success in human islet transplantation.[1] Donated islets, however, remain sensitive to host immune responses, and the number of islets required for successful transplant is still high. A further understanding of the immunobiology of the transplanted islets will identify therapeutic targets for improving posttransplant graft viability. Autoimmune destruction caused by the reactivation of the dormant autoreactive T lymphocytes is one of the mechanisms

Address for correspondence: Yongsoo Park, M.D., Department of Internal Medicine, Hanyang University Hospital, 249-1 Kyomun-dong, Kuri, Kyunggi-do 471-020, Korea. Voice: +82-31-560-2239; fax: +82-31-553-7369.
parkys@hanyang.ac.kr

mediating the immunological rejection. Rejection of transplanted islets also involves the classic allospecific T cell immune responses. In contrast with other solid organ transplant systems, host nonspecific immune responses are even more critically important mechanisms of early islet graft destruction. Infiltration of the transplanted islets by macrophages results in early graft failure. Cytokines released by these macrophages including IL-1β, IFN-γ, and TNF-α have been identified as the intercellular mediators of the early decrease in transplanted islet viability. These cytokines have been proposed to induce intraislet β cell death by apoptosis after binding their cell surface receptors. This detrimental cytokine injury is thought to be mainly mediated by NF-κB-dependent nitric oxide (NO) production by the islet.[2] The current study aimed to investigate the role of another multifunctional cytokine IL-6 in making a β cell resistant to cytokine-induced apoptosis by decreasing the NF-κB-dependent NO production, and we compared the result with that of the expression of a dominant negative inhibitor of NF-κB (DN NF-κB).

MATERIALS

Cell Culture

A murine β cell line established from an insulinoma obtained by targeted expression of the simian virus 40 T antigen gene in transgenic mouse, MIN6 cell was maintained in Dulbecco's Modified Eagle Medium (high glucose) (DMEM; Gibco-BRL, Grand Island, NY) with 10% heat-inactivated fetal calf serum (FCS), 100 U/mL penicillin, and 100 µg/mL streptomycin at 37°C in 5% CO_2. A mutant cell line transfected by a DN NF-κB was grown at 37°C in 5% CO_2 in DMEM, 15% FCS, 28 mM glucose, Pen/Strep, and 2 mM of the selective antibiotic puromycin (Sigma, St. Louis, MO).

Transfection

Unless otherwise stated, all molecular cloning procedures were performed by standard protocols, and reagents were of analytical grade and purchased from Sigma. Suppression of the NF-κB gene in the MIN6 cell was done using retroviral transduction. IκBαM (a flag-tagged DN gene) cDNA was synthesized and cloned into MFG.ires.puro retroviral vector. MIN6 cells were transduced with the vectors and the expression was detected by Western blot.

Cytokine Treatment

MIN6 or mutant cells were taken from culture flasks in their normal culture medium, split, and replated onto a 6-well culture plate at a concentration of 2×10^6 cells per well and grown in normal growth medium at 37°C in 5% CO_2 for 72 h. Cells then were washed with plain DMEM three times and preincubated for 24 h with the presence or absence of 100 ng/mL mouse IL-6 in normal growth medium. Cells then were washed with plain DMEM three times and incubated for 24, 48, and 72 h in 2 mL of one of three treatment media: (1) normal growth medium, (2) normal growth medium containing 50 U/mL IL-1β, 1000 U/mL IFN-γ, and 1000 U/mL TNF-α; or (3) normal growth medium with cytokines plus 1 mM *N*-monomethyl-L-arginine (L-

NMMA; Calbiochem, La Jolla, CA). Cytokines used for these studies were recombinant mouse cytokines obtained from R&D Systems (Minneapolis, MN). At the end of that incubation, 100 µL of the incubation medium was removed and taken for nitrite assay. The cells then were taken off the plate for flow cytometric analysis, and RNA and protein extraction.

Nitrite Assay

Because nitrite is one of the stable by-products of NO production and a reliable indicator of the level of NO production in a cell system, the production NO was assessed by measuring the amount of nitrite accumulated in the supernatants, using a colorimetric reaction with the Griess reagent (Promega). In brief, 50 µL of each standard and sample to be analyzed was added to wells in 96-well nonculture plates in duplicate. A 50-µL sulfanilamide solution was added to all wells, and the plates then were incubated for 10 min in the dark at room temperature. Then, 50 µL of an NED solution was added to all wells, and the plate was incubated for another 10 min in the dark at room temperature. Nitrite then was determined by absorbance at 550 nm on a spectrophotometric reader (Molecular Devices, Menlo Park, CA).

Apoptosis and Related Molecules

The degree of cell death was determined by flow cytometry. After culture, the plated cells were collected from the plate, washed in 1× PBS, resuspended in 200 µL 0.1% Triton X-100 in PBS, and incubated at room temperature for 15 min. Ten µL of propidium iodide (10 mg/mL; Clonetech, Palo Alto, CA) was then added. The resultant suspension was allowed to stand at room temperature for 5 min, and cells were analyzed by flow cytometry on a linear scale (Becton Dickinson). Apoptotic cells were those appearing within the distinct sub-G1 peak in which the DNA condensation and fragmentation associated with apoptosis result in decreased PI staining.

Total RNA was extracted from 2×10^6 cells with Trizol (Gibco-BRL) according to the manufacturer's directions. First-strand cDNA synthesis was performed, using 1 µg of each RNA sample primed with oligo(dT) primer (Gibco-BRL) in a 20-µL reaction volume with 400 U of Moloney murine leukemia virus reverse-transcriptase (Gibco-BRL). All PCRs were performed on a portion (1 µL) of each cDNA mixture in a 10-µL reaction volume containing 0.2 pM of each upstream and downstream primer, 5 U of Taq polymerase (Takara, Japan), 0.25 mM each deoxynucleoside triphosphate, 15 mM $MgCl_2$, and 1× reaction buffer. The primers specific for Bcl-2, Bax-α, and β-actin were used.[3] All products were analyzed by 2% agarose gel electrophoresis.

The plated cells were collected, resuspended, and sonicated in 100 µL of lysis buffer (50 mM Tris-HCl, pH 7.5, 5 mM EDTA, 150 mM NaCl, 1% Triton X-100, and 1 mM proteinase inhibitor) and incubated on ice for 30 min. The extracts were sedimented in a microcentrifuge for 30 min at 4°C. The supernatant solution represented whole-cell extract; 50 µg of this protein was analyzed by SDS-PAGE (12% gel) and subsequently transferred to a polyvinylidine difluoride membrane. The membrane was incubated with monoclonal mouse anti-Bcl-2, Bcl-x_L, α-tubulin (Santa Cruz Biotechnology), and polyclonal rabbit anti-Bax (Cell Signaling Technology). Secondary antibodies were incubated with the membranes at 1:1000 dilutions for 1 h at room temperature. The membranes were washed four times with 1× TBS for a total of 1 h and analyzed by enhanced chemiluminescence using ECL Western blotting detection reagents (Amersham), followed by exposure to X-ray film.

RESULTS

In vitro exposure of MIN6 cells to IL-1β, IFN-γ, and TNF-α for 2 days resulted in more increased production of nitrites than that for 3 days. This also was confirmed by the expression of iNOS mRNA expression (FIG. 1). Therefore, we examined the effects of cytokines on β cell apoptosis and the expression of the various apoptosis-related molecules before and 48 h after the incubation of cytokine mixture. Treatment of MIN6 with NO demonstrated a threshold of nitrite concentration (0.1 µM/well) below which the rate of apoptosis was essentially the same as baseline. The relative ability of the MIN6 cells to respond to cytokines in the absence of IL-6 was compared with that of the MIN6 in the presence of IL-6.[4] MIN6 responded to cytokine with increased production of nitrite, when exposed to the combination of IL-1β, IFN-γ, and TNF-α (cytomix). NO production was effectively blocked by the cotreat-

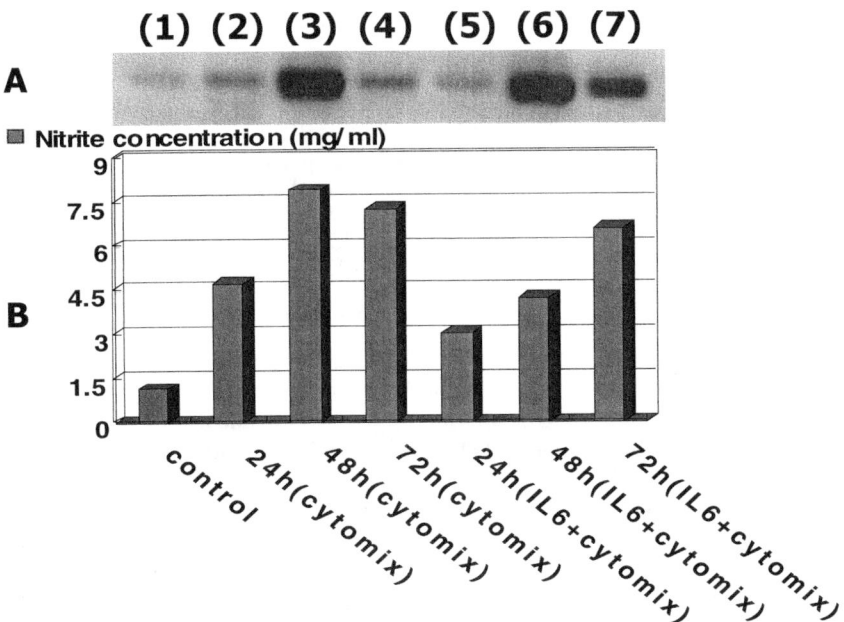

FIGURE 1. Cytokine-induced expression of inducible nitric oxide synthase (iNOS) and the resultant nitrite production in MIN6 with and without pretreatment of IL-6. Cells were preincubated for 24 h with the presence or absence of 100 ng/mL of mouse IL-6 in normal growth medium. Cells then were incubated for 24, 48, and 72 h in 2 mL of either of two treatment media: (1) normal growth medium or (2) normal growth medium containing 50 U/mL IL-1β, 1000 U/mL IFN-γ, and 1000 U/mL TNF-α. **(A)** Expression of the iNOS gene detected by RT-PCR. **(B)** Nitrite production measured by the Griess reaction.

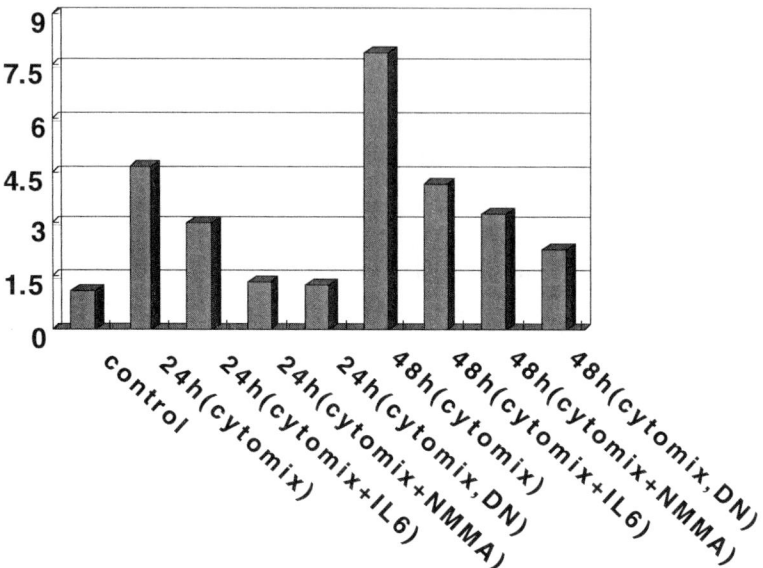

FIGURE 2. Cytokine-induced nitrite production in MIN6 with and without treatment of IL-6 and L-NMMA and a mutant cell line transfected by a DN inhibitor of the NF-κB gene. Cells were preincubated for 24 h with the presence or absence of 100 ng/mL of mouse IL-6 in normal growth medium. Cells then were incubated for 24, 48, and 72 in 2 mL of one of three treatment media: (1) normal growth medium; (2) normal growth medium containing 50 U/mL IL-1β, 1000 U/mL IFN-γ, and 1000 U/mL TNF-α; or (3) normal growth medium with cytokines plus 1 mM L-NMMA. Nitrite production was measured by the Griess reaction.

ment of IL-6 as well as by L-NMMA. Inhibition of the NO production achieved by the pretreatment of IL-6 or L-NMMA for 24 h before the incubation with the cytokine mix for 24 and 48 h demonstrated significantly less apoptosis (data not shown). However, the mutant (MIN6 cells transfected with the dominant negative form of NF-κB gene) produced significantly less nitrite production in response to cytokine stimulation (FIG. 2). Cotreatment with IL-6 or NO inhibitor resulted in a partial inhibition of apoptosis for MIN6 and no change in rates of death for the mutant.

MIN6 cells were subjected to the same 24-h incubation with the conventional growth media in the presence or absence of IL-6 and subsequently assayed for the expression of apoptosis-related molecules. The baseline expression levels of the apoptotic molecules changed into the antiapoptotic state taking into account that the relative ratio of proteins Bcl-2 (Bcl-x_L) and Bax increased after incubation with IL-6. This was also true after the cytomix exposure. Inhibition of the NO production led to decreased rate of apoptosis accompanied by a downregulation of the proapoptotic molecule Bax and increased expression of the antiapoptotic molecules Bcl-2 and Bcl-x_L (FIG. 3).

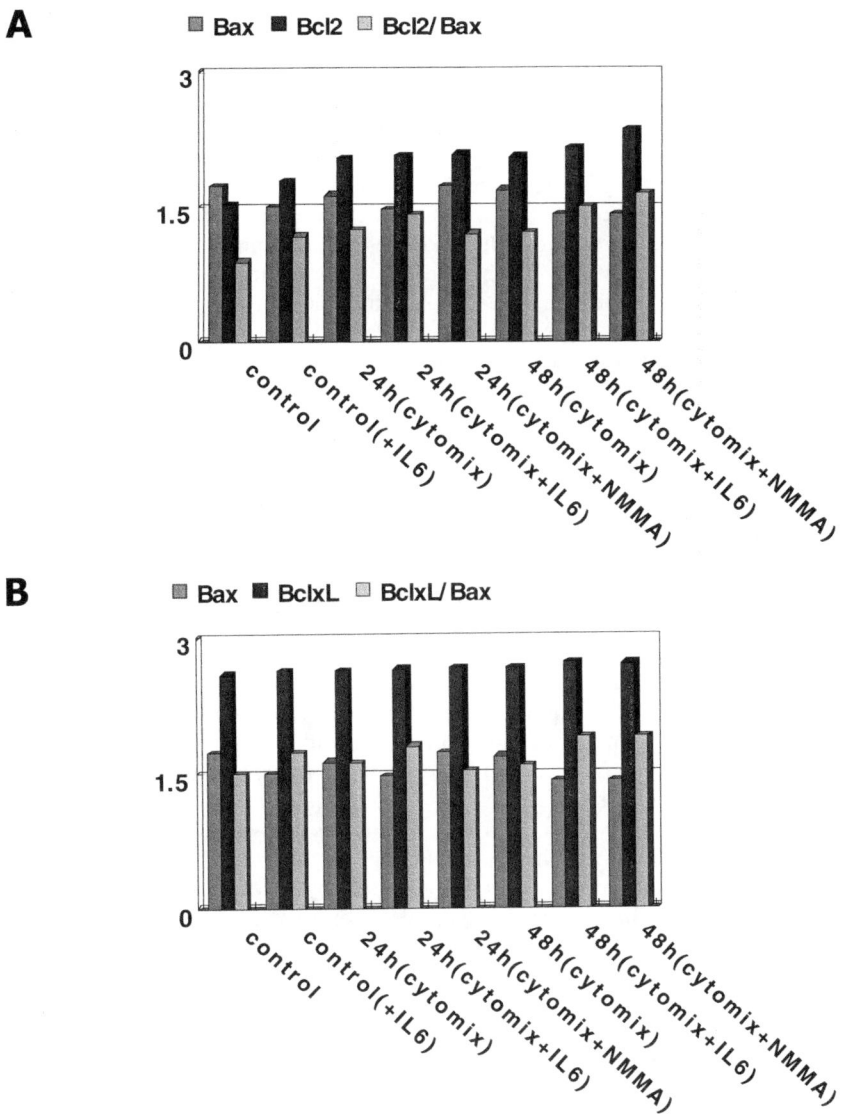

FIGURE 3. Bcl-2 (Bcl-x_L) and Bax protein expression in MIN6 with and without treatment of IL-6 and L-NMMA. **(A)** The relative band intensity of the Western blot applying whole-cell extract of MIN6 cells after the culture in each combination of treatment media using monoclonal mouse anti-Bcl-2 and polyclonal rabbit anti-Bax. **(B)** The relative band intensity of the Western blot applying MIN6 cells after the culture in each combination of treatment media using monoclonal mouse anti-Bcl-x_L and polyclonal rabbit anti-Bax.

DISCUSSION

Host nonspecific islet graft injury by cytokines released from inflammatory cells (macrophages) that infiltrate the transplant site is an important mechanism of early islet transplant dysfunction. Cytokines released by macrophages including IL-1β, IFN-γ, and TNF-α have been identified as the intercellular mediators of the early decrease in transplanted islet viability. These cytokines have been proposed to induce intraislet β cell death by apoptosis after binding their cell surface receptors. Our data indicate that cytokine-induced cell death in the MIN6 β cell line involves mechanisms that are, in part, NF-κB- and NO-dependent. Cytokine receptor binding at the cell surface activates intracellular kinases that phosphorylate IκB. Once phosphorylated, IκB releases NF-κB. The phosphorylation sites of IκB are known to be two amino-terminal serine residues. Genomic mutation affecting these phosphorylation sites results in the expression of a DN NF-κB.[5] Using this DN NF-κB, we inhibited the activation of the iNOS gene by inhibiting iNOS promoter binding of the NF-κB and thereby interrupted cellular production of NO and apoptosis.

We found that pretreatment of IL-6 inhibited the NO production. This inhibition is as effective as the cotreatment of L-NMMA, an inhibitor of iNOS. However, cotreatment with IL-6 or NO inhibitor resulted in a partial inhibition of apoptosis for MIN6 and no change in rates of death for the mutant. This indicates that there were, in fact, important NO-independent pathways to β cell apoptosis after cytokine injury. A mitochondrial-dependent, proapoptotic effect of NO has been described recently.[6] NO increased the mitochondrial membrane potential and modifies cytochrome c, thereby altering its structure and promoting its release from the mitochondria, which subsequently can activate caspase-3. In contrast, an antiapoptotic effect of NO has also been proposed where NO induces the *S*-nitrosylation of caspases, thereby preventing their activation and promoting resistance to Fas-mediated apoptosis.

IL-6 is a multifunctional cytokine exhibiting a wide array of biological effects. It regulates immune responses, hematopoiesis, and acute phase reactions. It plays a central role in host defense mechanisms.[4] In addition, IL-6 has been used as a marker of mononuclear cell activation. However, no one has investigated the role of IL-6 in protecting β cells from cytokine-induced apoptosis. IL-6 inhibited NO production and decreased the rate of apoptosis accompanied by a downregulation of the proapoptotic molecule Bax and increased expression of the antiapoptotic molecules Bcl-2 and Bcl-x_L. In human islets, the β cell is also subjected to many other apoptosis modifiers, such as various cytokines (e.g., IL-4, IL-6, IL-2, IL-10), circulating or membrane-bound molecules capable of triggering specific ligand-receptor interactions, and NO. We could not determine whether it is possible that pretreatment of IL-6 can protect the β cell from cytokine-induced apoptosis *in vivo*. Moreover, the true mechanism of β cell protection by IL-6 has to be investigated more thoroughly. In general, apoptotic β cell death induced by cytokines has been shown to be prevented by overexpression of Bcl-2. Our preliminary data of the islet protection study told us that not only IL-6, but also LIF and EGF, could increase the expression of Bcl-x_L taking that of Bax into account. From our data, IL-6 is as effective as L-NMMA in terms of cytoprotective influence and can be used as one of substitutes for the expression of DN NF-κB in β cells. Genetically engineered cell lines with genomic modifications targeted at improving cellular resistance to host immune responses could be one of the important potential sources of insulin-producing cells and could aid in developing that understanding of host-graft immunobiology in the transplanted islet. However, if a short-term incubation of islets with IL-6 before transplantation can replace the potential risk of reactivation of the virus, more efficient islet transplantation will improve the results of the posttransplant graft viability.

ACKNOWLEDGMENTS

This study was supported by a grant from the Korea Health 21 R&D Project, Ministry of Health and Welfare, Republic of Korea (HMP-01-PJ1-PG1-01CH09-0006).

REFERENCES

1. SHAPIRO, A. *et al.* 2000. Islet transplantation in seven patients with type I diabetes mellitus using a glucocorticoid free immunosuppression regimen. N. Engl. J. Med. **343:** 230–238.
2. FLODSTROM, M. *et al.* 1996. Cytokines activate the NF-κB and induce nitric oxide production in human pancreatic islets. FEBS Lett. **385:** 4–6.
3. DE CASTEELE, M. *et al.* 2002. Specific expression of Bax-ω in pancreatic β-cells is downregulated by cytokines before the onset of apoptosis. Endocrinology **143:** 320–326.
4. BENDA, B. *et al.* 2001. Interleukin-6 in islet xenograft rejection. Transplant. Int. **14:** 63–71.
5. LI, Z. *et al.* 1999. The I-κB kinase (I-κK) is essential for nuclear factor κB activation and prevention of apoptosis. J. Exp. Med. **189:** 1839–1845.
6. HORTELANO, S. *et al.* 1999. Nitric oxide induces tyrosine nitration and release of cytochrome c preceding an increase of mitochondrial transmembrane potential in macrophages. FASEB J. **13:** 2311–2317.

A Diabetes-Related Epitope of GAD65

A Major Diabetes-Related Conformational Epitope on GAD65

MARK A. MYERS,[a] GUSTAVO FENALTI,[a] ROBYN GRAY,[a] MARITA SCEALY,[a] JONATHAN C. TONG,[a] OSSAMA EL-KABBANI,[b] AND MERRILL J. ROWLEY[a]

[a]*Department of Biochemistry and Molecular Biology, Monash University, Clayton, Victoria, Australia*

[b]*Department of Medicinal Chemistry, Monash University, Parkville, Victoria, Australia*

ABSTRACT: The 65-kDa isoform of glutamic acid decarboxylase (GAD65) is a major autoantigen in type 1 diabetes, and most patients have serum antibodies reactive with conformational epitopes on the GAD65 molecule. The aims of this study were to prepare mutants of GAD65 to further localize the type 1 diabetes epitope in the region of the PEVKEK loop of GAD65 and to identify the particular amino acids within the epitope that are recognized by autoimmune diabetes sera.

KEYWORDS: glutamic acid decarboxylase; type 1 diabetes; autoantibodies; epitope mapping

INTRODUCTION

The 65-kDa isoform of glutamic acid decarboxylase (GAD65) is a major autoantigen in type 1 diabetes, and most patients have serum antibodies reactive with conformational epitopes on the GAD65 molecule. The actual epitopes have not been defined, and the closely related protein, GAD67, is rarely antigenic. In a previous study,[1] we used the human islet cell monoclonal antibody MICA3 to screen phage-displayed random peptide libraries to identify peptide mimotopes of the MICA3 epitope. Most peptide sequences among the phage clones reactive with MICA3 contained basic residues, particularly lysine. The sequences were mapped to a homology model of the pyridoxal phosphate binding domain of GAD65 to identify a possible epitope composed of three adjacent surface-exposed regions, each constituting a peptide "loop", and comprising amino acids 263–270 (loop 1), 285–296 (loop 2), and 315–334 (loop 3), that included the sequence $P_{269}EVKEK_{274}$. For the GAD65 mutant, $GAD65_{\Delta 258-270}$, in which the PEVKEK loop was removed, the reactivity of MICA3 was reduced by 70%,[1] and the reactivity of most diabetes sera was reduced by 80% or greater.[2] The aims of this study were to prepare mutants of GAD65 to

Address for correspondence: Merrill J. Rowley, Department of Biochemistry and Molecular Biology, Monash University, Clayton, Victoria 3800, Australia. Voice: +61-3-9905-1438; fax: +61-3-9905-4699.

merrill.rowley@med.monash.edu.au

TABLE 1. Summary of reactivity of diabetes sera with mutants

Mutant	Description	Reactivity,[a] median (range)	Frequency of reduction[b]
aa 255–257 RFK to AAA	Loop 1: removal of basic amino acids	92 (69–115)	33%
aa 263–265 KEK to AAA	Loop 1: removal of basic amino acids; difference between GAD65, GAD67	104 (37–133)	17%
aa 270–273 LPRL to APAA	Loop 1: difference between GAD65, GAD67; Leu 270 may be important for MICA3 binding	83 (56–102)	38%
aa 285–287 LKK to AAA	Loop 2: removal of basic amino acids	92 (69–115)	21%
aa 294–298 IGTDS to AAAAA	Loop 2: differences between GAD65, GAD67; T, D, S common among phage sequences	80 (33–122)	50%
aa 317–318 RR to AA	Loop 3: removal of basic amino acids; difference between GAD65, GAD67	96 (50–146)	17%

[a]Reactivity of 24 diabetes sera with mutant, expressed as a percentage of the reactivity with wild-type GAD65.
[b]Percentage of type 1 diabetes sera with reactivity with mutant < 80% of wild-type GAD65.

further localize the type 1 diabetes epitope in the region of the PEVKEK loop of GAD65 and to identify the particular amino acids within the epitope that are recognized by autoimmune diabetes sera.

METHODS

Molecular modeling of GAD65 and GAD67 using previously published coordinates for the pyridoxal phosphate binding domain of GAD65[3] was used to identify surface-exposed amino acids in the three regions and to identify regions of difference between the two isoforms. The selection of particular amino acids for mutagenesis was based on surface exposure, the presence of basic amino acids (particularly lysine), sequence differences between GAD65 and GAD67, and the presence of amino acids commonly selected by phage display. The mutants in the three regions are shown in TABLE 1.

The template cDNA was generated as a construct encoding residues 1–101 of GAD67 fused to residues 96–585 of GAD65. The encoded recombinant hybrid GAD67/65 reacts similarly to GAD65 in radioimmunoprecipitation assays with diabetes sera, but has favorable purification properties.[4] Amino acids were modified by site-directed alanine mutagenesis, using a QuickChange site-directed mutagenesis kit (Stratagene, La Jolla, CA) and appropriate oligonucleotides, and the mutants were confirmed by sequencing. Sera from 24 patients with type 1 diabetes that contained anti-GAD was tested for reactivity by radioimmunoprecipitation in the same assay using ^{35}S-labeled mutant or wild-type GAD65/65 expressed in rabbit reticulocyte lysate. The amount of antigen in each preparation was standardized using the monoclonal antibody GAD6 that reacts with a linear epitope in the C-terminal region of GAD65. Results were transformed to units of reactivity by defining the reactivity of ^{35}S-labeled antigen with GAD6 as 100 units. A given diabetes serum was considered to have reduced reactivity if the reactivity with the mutant was less than 80% of the reactivity with wild-type GAD67/65.

RESULTS

For the 24 diabetes sera tested, 5 showed no reduction of reactivity with any mutant and most of the remaining 19 sera had reduced activity with several mutants, consistent with reactivity with a conformational epitope extending across two or more loops. The results obtained are summarized in TABLE 1. In particular, reactivity for 12 of the sera (50%) was reduced with the loop 2 mutant aa 294–298 IGTDS to AAAAA, for 9 of the sera (38%) it was reduced with the loop 1 mutant aa 270–273 LPRL to APAA, and for 8 of the sera (33%) it was reduced with the loop 1 mutant aa 255–257 RFK to AAA.

CONCLUSIONS

Autoimmune diabetes sera contain polyclonal antibodies that react with an immunodominant conformational epitope of GAD65 comprising amino acids from three loops (one being from the PEVKEK loop) of the PLP domain of GAD65. However, there were individual-specific serologically defined differences for particular amino acids that constitute this epitope. Because these studies used diabetes sera that contain polyclonal antibodies to GAD65, the results provide strong evidence for a single immunodominant epitope surrounding the PEVKEK loop of GAD65 that is recognized by most type 1 diabetes sera.

REFERENCES

1. MYERS, M.A. *et al.* 2000. Conformational epitopes on the diabetes autoantigen GAD65 identified by peptide phage display and molecular modeling. J. Immunol. **165:** 3830–3838.
2. TONG, J.C. *et al.* 2002. The PEVKEK region of the pyridoxal phosphate-binding domain of GAD65 expresses a dominant B cell epitope for type 1 diabetes sera. Ann. N.Y. Acad. Sci. **958:** 182–189.
3. QU, K., D.L. MARTIN & C.E. LAWRENCE. 1998. Motifs and structural fold of the cofactor binding site of human glutamate decarboxylase. Protein Sci. **7:** 1092–1105.
4. LAW, R.H. *et al.* 1998. Expression in *Saccharomyces cerevisiae* of antigenically and enzymatically active recombinant glutamic acid decarboxylase. J. Biotechnol. **61:** 57–68.

SOX13 Autoantibodies Are Likely to Be a Supplementary Marker for Type 1 Diabetes in Korea

YONGSOO PARK, HYEWON PARK, EUNKYUNG YOO, AND DUKHEE KIM

Division of Endocrinology and Metabolism, Department of Internal Medicine and Pediatrics, Hanyang and Yonsei University, Seoul, Korea

ABSTRACT: The SOX13, one of the family of transcription factors that play key roles in organ development, is reported to be a diabetes autoantigen, islet cell antigen 12 (ICA12). Recently, a study of antibodies to SOX13 was conducted in patients with type 1 diabetes mellitus (T1DM) indicating that these antibodies potentially identified patients without antibodies to the major T1DM-associated autoantigens, insulin, GAD, or IA-2. We know that the prevalence of islet-specific autoantibodies (GAD, IA-2) in Korean patients is much lower than that in white patients. It may be possible that other autoantibodies that could be directed to as yet unknown antigen may play a role in Korean T1DM patients. To investigate this, we measured SOX13 autoantibodies applying a radioligand binding assay using *in vitro* transcribed and translated antigen in 188 T1DM patients (mean duration, 4.2 years) and 64 T2DM patients and compared the results with those of 101 healthy control subjects. SOX13 autoantibodies occurred at a significantly higher frequency among T1DM patients (55/188, 29.3%) than among T2DM patients (4/64, 6.2%) or healthy adult controls (1/101, 1%). The 55 patients with positive SOX13 antibodies had significantly shorter duration of diabetes than SOX13 antibody-negative patients (3.6 ± 2.8 vs. 4.5 ± 3.9 years; $p < 0.05$). We could detect a prevalence similar to control in patients with Hashimoto's thyroiditis (4.9%, $n = 101$) and rheumatoid arthritis (6.7%, $n = 89$). As a whole, 44 of the 55 patients with SOX13 antibodies had at least one or more other autoantibodies to the major T1DM-associated autoantigens. However, SOX13 antibodies were the only antibodies detected as positive in 1 of the 11 new-onset patients. We conclude, therefore, that these antibodies are likely to be one of several epitope-spreading responses to islet- or nonislet-specific autoantigens seen in the development of T1DM, and they may be used as a supplementary marker for investigating T1DM in Korea.

KEYWORDS: SOX13; autoantibodies; T1DM; Korea

INTRODUCTION

Type 1 diabetes mellitus (T1DM) is characterized by an absolute deficiency of insulin caused by destruction of the pancreatic β cells through an autoimmune mech-

Address for correspondence: Yongsoo Park, M.D., Department of Internal Medicine, Hanyang University Hospital, 249-1 Kyomun-dong, Kuri, Kyunggi-do 471-020, Korea. Voice: +82-31-560-2239; fax: +82-31-553-7369.

parkys@hanyang.ac.kr

anism. During the long prodromal period, three major specificities of diabetes-associated autoantibodies to pancreatic β cell antigens may arise and persist even after the disease has become clinically overt: autoantibodies to insulin, glutamic acid decarboxylase (GAD), and an islet tyrosine phosphatase–related molecule termed ICA512/IA-2 (IA-2).

The SOX13, one of the family of SRY-related HMG box protein transcription factors that play key roles in determining cell fate during organ development, has been suggested to be a diabetes autoantigen expressed in pancreatic islets, islet cell antigen 12 (ICA12). Recently, a study on the prevalence of the antibodies to SOX13 in new-onset T1DM patients suggested that these antibodies potentially identified patients without antibodies to the major T1DM-associated autoantigens, insulin, GAD, and IA-2.[1]

T1DM is much less frequent in Korea than in other countries with predominantly white populations. It has been suggested that there are marked differences in the prevalences of islet-specific autoantibodies between whites and Koreans, and there also have been some suggestions that SOX13 antibodies may be good markers for Asian adult-onset T1DM patients.[1–3] With the recent cloning and recombinant expression of novel islet autoantigens, it is possible to investigate whether the quantitative expression of one autoantibody is correlated with those of other autoantibodies.[4] To do this, we measured SOX13 autoantibodies applying a radioligand-binding assay using *in vitro* transcribed and translated antigen in ethnically distinct Korean T1DM and T2DM patients and compared the results with those of healthy controls.

MATERIALS

For this investigation, 188 cases of T1DM patients were selected randomly from the Korean Seoul Type 1 Diabetes Registry (incidence: 0.6/100,000/year):[5] 91 were male and 97 were female; their mean current age was 18.8 years (range, 3–38 years). Their mean age at diagnosis was 14.6 ± 9.3 years, with a mean duration of 4.2 ± 3.6 years. Patients with T1DM were subclassified according to the age of onset of the disease into childhood-onset (<15 years) or adult-onset (≥15 years), and according to whether the disease at the time of testing for autoantibodies was of new onset (<12 months) or long duration (≥12 months). Among them, 144 patients were childhood-onset and 44 were adult-onset. Only 35 patients were new-onset cases. We also recruited 64 Korean T2DM patients from a diabetic clinic of Hanyang University (M:F, 34:30; age, 42.8 ± 14.9 years). The criteria for classification of T1DM and T2DM were determined by the National Diabetes Data Group. Separately, we also recruited 101 cases of Hashimoto's thyroiditis patients (M:F, 25:76; age, 39.8 ± 13.9 years) and 89 rheumatoid arthritis patients (M:F, 30:59; age, 41.1 ± 14.1 years) from an endocrinologic and a rheumatologic clinic of Hanyang University, respectively. Also, 101 healthy control subjects were recruited (M:F, 51:50; age, 40.9 ± 13.4 years).

A human SOX13 (amino acids 66–604) cDNA subcloned into pET23b vector (Promega, Madison, WI) in addition to the human full-length GAD65 cDNA subcloned into pcDNA II vector (pEx9) and intracellular human IA-2 (amino acids 604–979) cDNA subcloned into PCRII vector (Invitrogen, San Diego, CA) were transcribed and translated *in vitro* in the presence of ^{35}S-methionine (Amersham International, Amersham, Bucks, United Kingdom; >1000 Ci/mmol) using the TNT-coupled rabbit reticulocyte system (Promega). The ^{35}S-labeled protein was separated from unincorporated label by gel filtration on Sephadex G25 columns (NAP5; Pharmacia, Uppsala, Sweden) before use in the radioligand-binding assay. The expressed SOX13 protein migrated as a 62-kDa component by autoradiography after separation by 8% SDS-PAGE. The SOX13 radioassay was performed using a 96-well plate format similar to that used for detecting the GAD and IA-2 autoantibodies.[4] The antibody levels were expressed as an index defined as [cpm in the unknown sample − negative control]/[positive control − negative control]. "Positive" was based on the 99th percentile of sera from 101 healthy control subjects, being an index of 0.218. The interassay CV in our SOX13 antibody assay was 6.5% ($n = 9$).

Results are presented in the form of mean ± SD. Comparisons between the groups were made by unpaired parametric tests (Student's t tests) and nonparametric tests (Mann-Whitney U tests). The χ^2 test was used for comparison of proportions, unless the expected frequency in any cell was less than 5, in which case Fisher's exact test was used. Spearman's rank correlation and nonparametric Spearman's univariate correlations were used to assess the relationship between levels of autoantibodies.

RESULTS

The frequencies of SOX13 autoantibodies in patients with T1DM and T2DM and controls are shown in FIGURE 1. SOX13 antibodies occurred at a significantly higher frequency among T1DM patients (55/188, 29.3%) than among T2DM patients (4/64,

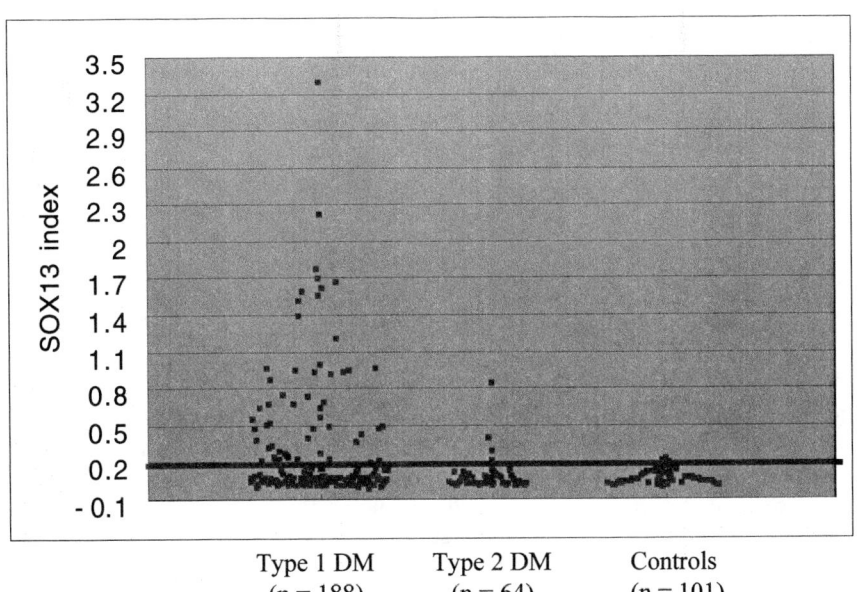

FIGURE 1. Differences in the prevalence of SOX13 autoantibodies in patients with type 1 and type 2 diabetes compared with controls.

TABLE 1. Differences of the clinical profile between SOX13 antibody-positive and antibody-negative patients

	SOX13 antibody (+)	SOX13 antibody (−)	p
Number	55	133	
Sex (M:F)	25:30	66:67	
Duration (years)	3.6 ± 2.8	4.5 ± 3.9	<0.05
Age (years)	17.5 ± 14.8	19.3 ± 15.0	
Age at diagnosis (years)	15.4 ± 15.5	15.0 ± 15.2	
Family history (%)	21.9	17.6	
GAD antibody (index)	0.16 ± 0.30	0.16 ± 0.38	
IA-2 antibody (index)	0.28 ± 0.40	0.16 ± 0.33	

6.2%) or in healthy adult controls (1/101, 1%). The 55 T1DM patients with positive SOX13 antibodies had significantly shorter duration of diabetes than SOX13 antibody-negative T1DM patients (3.6 ± 2.8 years vs. 4.5 ± 3.9 years, $p < 0.05$; TABLE 1). However, we could detect a prevalence similar to control in patients with Hashimoto's thyroiditis (4.9%, $n = 101$) and rheumatoid arthritis (6.7%, $n = 89$). As a whole, 11 of the 55 T1DM patients with SOX13 antibodies did not have any other autoantibodies to the major T1DM-associated autoantigens. The titer of SOX13 antibodies did not correlate with those of IA-2 or GAD antibodies.

To find their independent role in prediction of the T1DM development, we investigated the prevalence of SOX13 antibodies in 35 new-onset T1DM patients. In this new-onset subset of T1DM, the prevalences of IA-2, GAD, and SOX13 antibodies were 51% (18/35), 63% (22/35), and 31% (11/35), respectively. IA-2 and GAD antibodies were significantly associated with the presence of SOX13 antibodies. Among these new-onset T1DM patients, 74% had one or more and 54% had two or more of these autoantibodies. Only 1 patient of 35 new-onset T1DM patients did not have other autoantibodies. SOX13 antibodies were more prevalent in T1DM patients with antibodies to GAD or IA-2 (FIG. 2).

DISCUSSION

T1DM is more prevalent among white patients than among Asians. T1DM in white patients is attributed to autoimmune destruction of the pancreatic β cells as judged by the frequency of multiple antibodies, in aggregate nearly 100% in acute-onset cases with childhood-onset. Among Asians, especially with the adult-onset form of diabetes, the prevalence of T1DM and the frequency of autoantibodies in incident cases are lower than among white patients.[2,6] In Asians, there is a possibility of autoantibodies to islet-cell autoantigens other than those usually measured, insulin, GAD, and IA-2. One potential antigen, ICA12, was identified as the high mobility group (HMG) box transcription factor SOX13. The current study extends data on serological testing of autoantibodies to diabetes-relevant autoantigens in Korean T1DM patients by including data for antibodies to SOX13. In our Korean T1DM patients, the prevalence of SOX13 antibodies was 29–31% according to the

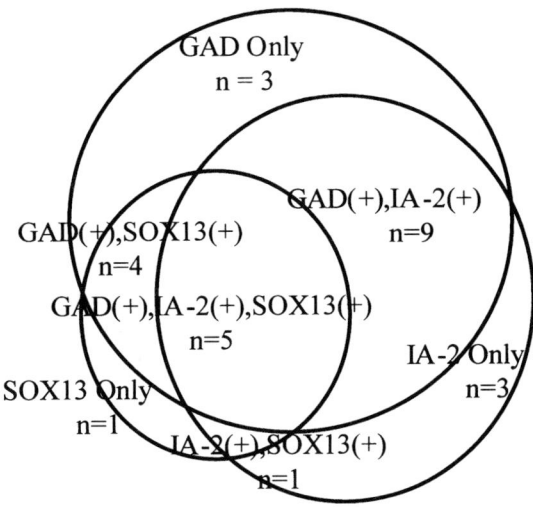

FIGURE 2. Clustering of autoantibodies in 35 new-onset type 1 diabetes patients with one or more of the autoantibodies. Each number in a circle denotes the number of patients positive for each combination of autoantibodies. IA-2, GAD, and SOX13 denote IA-2 autoantibodies, anti-GAD65 antibodies, and anti-SOX13 antibodies, respectively.

duration of diabetes. The SOX13 antibody-positive patients had shorter duration of diabetes. The prevalence of SOX13 antibodies appeared not to vary greatly according to the onset age of diabetes because it is 29.2% (42/144) in childhood-onset form and 29.5% (13/44) in adult-onset form. In Australian Europids with T1DM, 20% prevalence of SOX13 antibodies was noted, dependent on age and duration of diabetes.[2] Some Korean T1DM patients appeared to have the autoantibodies for SOX13 as an alternative to IA-2 or GAD autoantibodies. It may still be possible that other islet-specific or islet-nonspecific autoantibodies that could be directed to an as yet unknown antigen may play a role in Korean T1DM patients in the context of different HLA context.

In a subset of T1DM with new onset, the prevalences of IA-2, GAD, and SOX13 antibodies were 51% (18/35), 63% (22/35), and 31% (11/35), respectively. Although their prevalences appeared to be slightly lower than expected, IA-2 and GAD antibodies were significantly associated with the presence of SOX13 antibodies. Among new-onset T1DM patients, 74% had one or more and 54% had two or more of these autoantibodies. In our prior report of childhood-onset cases, we reported the prevalences of IA-2 in 75% and of GAD antibodies in 75% of new-onset T1DM patients (<1 year).[4] At that time, among T1DM patients, 69% had one or more and 43% had two or more of ICA, GAD, or IA-2 autoantibodies.

To find their independent role in prediction of the diabetes development, we investigated the prevalence of SOX13 antibodies in 35 new-onset T1DM patients.

Among new-onset cases, only 1 patient (2.9%, 1/35) was associated with only SOX13 antibody-positivity. SOX13 antibodies were more prevalent in patients with antibodies to GAD or IA-2. We conclude, therefore, that SOX13 antibodies are likely to be one of several epitope-spreading responses to islet- or nonislet-specific autoantigens seen in T1DM, and they may be used as a supplementary marker for investigating T1DM in Korea.

ACKNOWLEDGMENTS

This study was supported by grants from the Korea Health 21 R&D Project, Ministry of Health and Welfare, Republic of Korea (HMP-02-PJ1-PG3-21004-0003 and HMP-00-PJ3-PG6-GN07-0001).

REFERENCES

1. KASIMIOTIS, H. et al. 2001. Antibodies to SOX13 (ICA12) are associated with type 1 diabetes. Autoimmunity **33:** 95–101.
2. FIDA, S. et al. 2001. Antibodies to diabetes-associated autoantigens in Indian patients with type 1 diabetes: prevalence of anti-ICA512/IA-2 and anti-SOX13. Diabetes Res. Clin. Pract. **52:** 205–211.
3. GUPTA, M. et al. 2002. ICA12 autoantibodies are associated with non-DR3/non-DR4 in patients with latent autoimmune diabetes in adults from northern India. Ann. N.Y. Acad. Sci. **958:** 329–332.
4. PARK, Y. et al. 2001. Evaluation of the efficacy of the combination of multiple autoantibodies to islet-specific antigens in Korean type 1 diabetic patients. Acta Diabetol. **38:** 51–56.
5. KO, K. et al. 1994. The incidence of IDDM in Seoul from 1985 to 1988. Diabetes Care **17:** 1473–1475.
6. PARK, Y. et al. 1996. The low prevalence of immunogenetic markers in Korean adult-onset IDDM patients. Diabetes Care **19:** 241–245.

Development and Validation of a Radioligand Binding Assay to Measure Insulin Specific IgG Subclass Antibodies in Human Serum

D. FINCO-KENT,[a] A. MORRONE,[a] M. MOXNESS,[b] V. BEDIAN,[a] A. KRASNER,[a] J. FOLEY,[b] M. STENE,[b] AND T. KAWABATA[a]

[a]*Pfizer Incorporated, Groton, Connecticut, USA*

[b]*Esoterix Incorporated, Calabasas, California, USA*

ABSTRACT: The objective was to develop and validate a radioligand binding assay for insulin antibodies (IABs) of the IgG1, IgG2, IgG3, and IgG4 subclasses in human serum. The validation studies focused on determining specificity, capacity, linearity, sensitivity, and precision of each assay. It was seen that our assay for IAB IgG subclasses is specific and has sufficient capacity to measure each of the subclasses in human serum. Moreover, the linear region and limits of detection and quantitation for each assay are clearly determined.

KEYWORDS: insulin antibodies (IABs); radioligand binding (RLB) assay; IgG; specificity; capacity; linearity; sensitivity; precision; Sepharose beads

INTRODUCTION

The objective of the studies presented in this report was to develop and validate a radioligand binding (RLB) assay for insulin antibodies (IABs) of the IgG1, IgG2, IgG3, and IgG4 subclasses in human serum to meet the recommendations from the 1994 and 1996 International Conferences on Harmonization[1,2] and the U.S. FDA "Guidance for Industry, Bioanalytical Method Validation".[3] The IAB subclass assays were developed based on the method reported by Bonifacio et al.[4] This method uses biotinylated mouse monoclonal antibodies against each of the human IgG subclasses bound to streptavidin Sepharose beads.

The validation studies focused on determining specificity, capacity, linearity, sensitivity, and precision of each assay. Commercially available monoclonal antibodies against IgG subclasses are known to differ greatly in terms of specificity and affinity. Thus, as a starting point, the monoclonal antibodies recommended by the WHO-sponsored Human Immunoglobulin Subcommittee of the IUIS Standardization Committee were evaluated.[5] Because the IgG subclass IAB RLB assay requires that the antibody-labeled streptavidin beads have the capacity to capture all or most of the immunoglobulins of the desired subclass, validation studies that determine the optimal amount of beads were conducted. Positive serum samples containing high

Address for correspondence: Deborah Finco-Kent, Pfizer Incorporated, 1 Eastern Point Road, MS 8274-1234, Groton, CT 06340. Voice: 860-715-2071; fax: 860-715-3577.
deborah_finco-kent@groton.pfizer.com

levels of IABs were used to validate precision and linearity of the assay. Moreover, the limit of detection and quantitation were determined.

METHODS

Test serum is combined with charcoal-dextran and acidified (pH ~3.5) to dissociate bound insulin. After neutralization with NaOH, the charcoal with bound insulin is removed from the serum by centrifugation. Five μL of serum (duplicates) is then incubated with radiolabeled insulin (1470 μU/25 μL) for 72 h at 4°C. As a control for nonspecific binding, unlabeled insulin is added to a duplicate sample to compete with radiolabeled insulin for IAB binding. Biotinylated antihuman IgG1, IgG2, IgG3, and IgG4 bound to streptavidin Sepharose beads are added to appropriate tubes incubated at room temperature with shaking for 2 h. Specific insulin binding for each subclass is calculated by subtracting the NSB counts from the total counts of the corresponding sample tube. Specific counts are converted to μU of insulin based on the specific activity of the radiolabeled insulin used in the assay. Data are presented as IgG1, IgG2, IgG3, and IgG4 IAB binding in μU of insulin bound per mL of serum tested.

VALIDATION STUDIES

Validation studies were performed as described in METHODS unless otherwise indicated.

Specificity

To demonstrate the specificity of an antibody against a particular subclass and minimal cross-reactivity with the other three IgG subclasses, we evaluated radiolabeled myeloma IgG subclass proteins. Monoclonal anti-IgG subclass reagents were conjugated to the Sepharose beads at a concentration of 1 μg/μL of packed streptavidin Sepharose beads, diluted to a 50% slurry using Tris assay buffer. Each subclass specific reagent was tested against all four radiolabeled myeloma proteins for each subclass. After a 2-h incubation, the tubes were washed six times and the pellet was counted on a gamma counter. Counts obtained were reported as a percentage relative to the total counts of myeloma protein added to the tubes. Pharmingen rat anti-IgM was used as a negative control.

Capacity

To determine the volume of Sepharose beads needed to bind most or all of the desired IgG subclass in each serum sample, we tested IAB-positive serum for each subclass as described in METHODS using varying volumes of beads.

Linearity

To determine the linear region of each assay, we tested serial twofold dilutions of samples with high levels of IAB subclass antibodies.

Precision and Sensitivity

Intra-assay precision, level of quantitation (LOQ), and limit of detection (LOD) were determined. Interassay precision was determined by measuring three samples for eight times on different days. Intra-assay precision and LOQ were determined by measuring ten replicates of four serum samples on the same day. The LOQ was defined as the concentration in µU/mL at which the intra-assay %CV did not exceed 20%. The LOD was calculated as the concentration in µU/mL of the mean IAB-negative samples plus three standard deviations.

RESULTS

Specificity

Reagents with the greatest degree of specificity, least amount of cross-reactivity, and highest percentage of binding were selected for use. As an example of the studies, FIGURE 1 shows results for IgG1 monoclonal reagents from several different vendors. Zymed anti-IgG1 (clone HP6069), Pharmingen anti-IgG2 (clone G18-21),

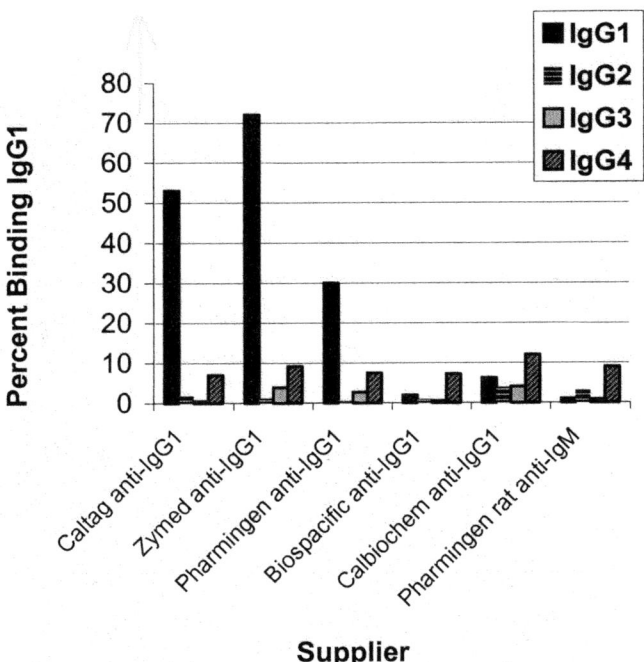

FIGURE 1. IgG1 specificity: Comparison of IgG1 reagents. Testing for specificity for IgG1 and cross-reactivity with other subclasses using radiolabeled myeloma proteins. Rat anti-IgM is a negative control.

and Southern Biotechnical Associates anti-IgG3 (clone HP6050) and anti-IgG4 (clone HP6025) were selected for use.

Capacity

The volume of monoclonal bound Sepharose beads required to bind most of the corresponding IgG subclass was determined to be 90 μL of anti-IgG1, 50 μL of anti-IgG2 and anti-IgG3, and 30 μL of anti-IgG4 (FIG. 2). Volumes less than 50 μL were not evaluated for anti-IgG2, nor was less than 30 μL evaluated for anti-IgG4.

Linearity

Linearity for each subclass was determined to be as follows: IgG1 from 1.4 to 29 μU/mL, IgG2 from 1.4 to 13 μU/mL, IgG3 from 3 to 83 μU/mL, and IgG4 from 2.5 to 27 μU/mL (FIG. 3). Samples containing levels of IgG2 higher than the upper end shown in FIGURE 3 were not available for testing and, thus, the linear region may be higher for IgG2.

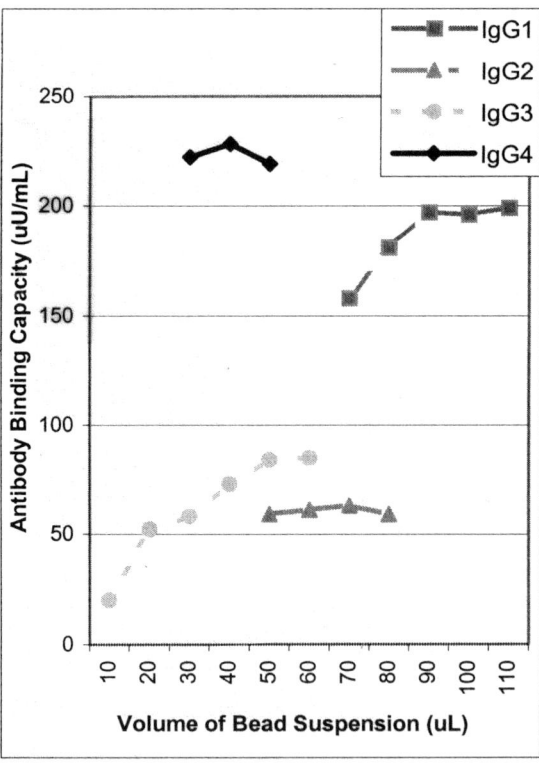

FIGURE 2. Capacity: IAB-positive serum was used to evaluate capacity for each subclass using different volumes of labeled steptavidin beads.

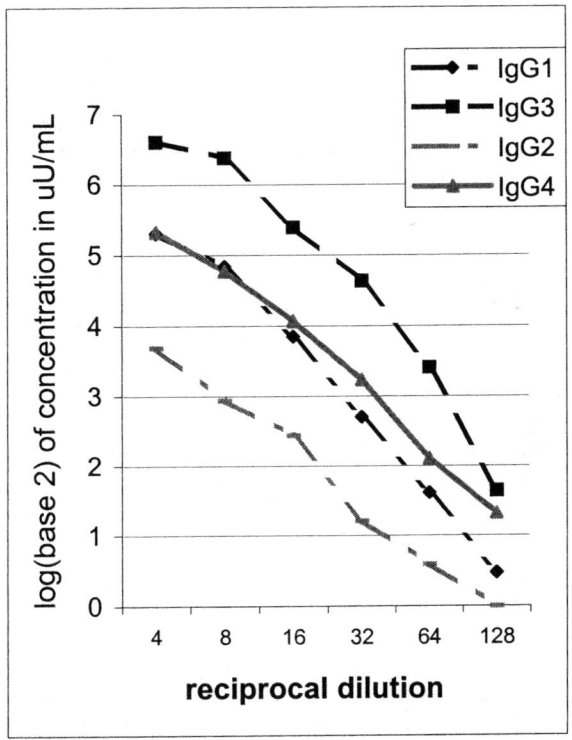

FIGURE 3. Linearity: IAB-positive samples serially diluted to determine the linear region of the assay.

Precision and Sensitivity

Intra-assay precision had a CV of less than 15%, whereas interassay precision had a CV of less than 20%. The LOQ values for IgG1, IgG2, IgG3, and IgG4 were 2.6, 1.4, 3.0, and 2.5 µU/mL, respectively. The limits of detection for IgG1, IgG2, IgG3, and IgG4 were 0.33, 0.07, 0.19, and 0.97 µU/mL, respectively.

CONCLUSIONS

The findings from this study demonstrate that our assay for IAB IgG subclasses is specific and has sufficient capacity to measure each of the subclasses in human serum. Moreover, the linear region and limits of detection and quantitation for each assay were clearly determined.

REFERENCES

1. INTERNATIONAL CONFERENCE ON HARMONIZATION (ICH). 1994. Test on Validations of Analytical Procedures. Issued as CPMP/ICH/381/95.
2. INTERNATIONAL CONFERENCE ON HARMONIZATION (ICH). 1996. Validation of Analytical Procedures: Methodology. Issued as CPMP/ICH/281/95.
3. U.S. FOOD AND DRUG ADMINISTRATION, CDER, CVM. 2001. Guidance for Industry, Bioanalytical Method Validation.
4. BONIFACIO, E. et al. 1999. Early autoantibody responses in prediabetes are IgG1 dominated and suggest antigen-specific regulation. J. Immunol. **163:** 525–532.
5. JEFFERIS, R. et al. 1985. Evaluation of monoclonal antibodies having specificity for human IgG sub-classes: results of an IUIS/WHO collaborative study. Immunol. Lett. **10:** 223–225.

Development and Validation of Radioligand Binding Assays to Measure Total, IgA, IgE, IgG, and IgM Insulin Antibodies in Human Serum

MICHAEL MOXNESS,[a] JIM FOLEY,[a] MARK STENE,[a] DEBORAH FINCO-KENT,[b] VAHE BEDIAN,[b] ALAN KRASNER,[b] AND THOMAS KAWABATA[b]

[a]*Esoterix Incorporated, Calabasas, California, USA*

[b]*Pfizer Incorporated, Groton, Connecticut, USA*

ABSTRACT: Radioligand binding assays for total and Ig classes of insulin antibodies (IAB) were developed and validated. For each assay, insulin-extracted serum samples were incubated with radiolabeled insulin in the presence and absence of high levels of unlabeled insulin to determine nonspecific binding and total binding, respectively. To measure total IAB, antibody-bound insulin was precipitated with a polyethylene glycol solution, washed, and counted in a gamma-counter. To measure IgG IAB, samples were treated with protein G–Sepharose beads, centrifuged, washed, and counted. For the measurement of IgA, IgE, and IgM IAB, IgG was removed from the samples and treated with anti-IgA, -IgE, or -IgM conjugated to Sepharose beads, centrifuged, washed, and counted. The acid/charcoal extraction of bound and unbound insulin from serum samples was optimized. Specificity and binding capacity of the protein G and antibody-bound beads were evaluated and optimized. The linear region of the total and IgG IAB assays was determined using serum samples containing high levels of insulin antibodies. The limit of quantitation, limit of detection, and precision for all the assays were also determined.

KEYWORDS: insulin antibodies; IgA; IgM; IgE; IgG; immunoglobulins

INTRODUCTION

Various immunoassays to measure insulin antibodies (IABs) have been developed for human serum; however, extensive validation of these methods has not been reported. To characterize the immune response to insulin, we developed solution-based radioligand binding assays to measure total (all Ig classes), IgA, IgE, IgG, and IgM IABs. The specificity, sensitivity, capacity, precision, and linear range of each assay were determined. In addition, the efficiency of endogenous insulin extraction was optimized.

Address for correspondence: Deborah Finco-Kent, Pfizer Incorporated, 1 Eastern Point Road, MS 8274-1234, Groton, CT 06340. Voice: 860-715-2071; fax: 860-715-3577.
 deborah_finco-kent@groton.pfizer.com

MATERIALS AND METHODS

Test and control sera first were acidified to dissociate bound insulin, and charcoal was added to adsorb the serum insulin. After neutralization, the charcoal with bound insulin was removed from the serum by centrifugation. The specific IABs were measured in duplicate in the insulin-free serum as described below. In addition, all samples also were incubated with excess unlabeled insulin in duplicate to measure nonspecific binding (NSB). The NSB counts were subtracted from the total binding counts and divided by the total counts to give results as μU of insulin bound per mL of serum.

Total IABs were incubated for 72 h at 4°C with radiolabeled insulin and precipitated with 11% PEG (final concentration). The pellets were washed with 11% PEG and counted with a gamma-counter.

IgG IABs were incubated for 72 h at 4°C with radiolabeled insulin and precipitated with protein G–Sepharose (2-h incubation). The pellets were washed once and counted on a gamma-counter.

Samples for IgA, IgE, and IgM analyses were first treated with protein G–Sepharose to deplete IgG and then incubated for 48 h with radiolabeled insulin at 4°C. Sepharose beads conjugated to anti-human IgA, IgE, or IgM were added and incubated for 24 h at 4°C. The beads were washed once and counted on a gamma-counter.

Optimization of Insulin Extraction Efficiency

Acidic conditions were needed to dissociate antibody-bound insulin during the extraction process. However, exposure to low pH altered sample Ig so that anti-Ig binding was decreased. Thus, a pH that will sufficiently dissociate insulin from antibody and yet not alter Ig structure was needed. The efficiency of insulin extraction at different pH was evaluated with radiolabeled insulin in pooled samples containing high levels of insulin antibodies. In addition, the binding of each antibody to

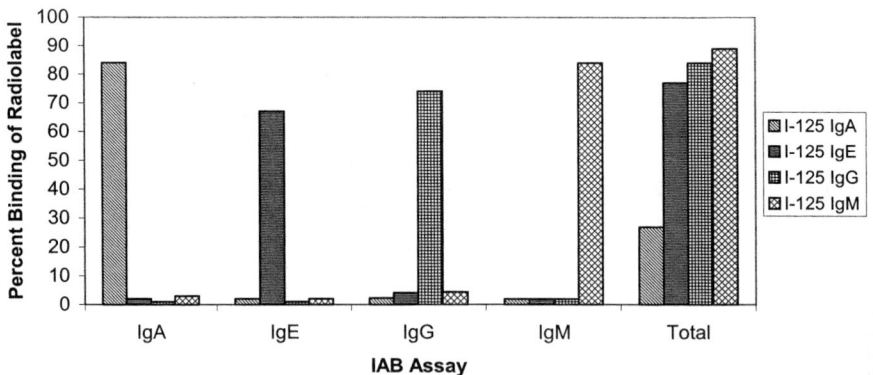

FIGURE 1. Radiolabeled IgA, IgE, IgG, and IgM were prepared and incubated with anti-IgA, IgE, and IgM antibodies linked to Sepharose. Protein G was used for the IgG IAB assay, and PEG precipitation was used for the total IAB assay. Percentage of each radiolabel precipitated is shown for each Ig specific assay.

the corresponding class of Ig was determined by using radiolabeled IgG, IgE, IgA, and IgM. An optimal pH of 3.7 was found to remove 95% of the insulin and allow 75% binding of each Ig class after the samples were neutralized.

Specificity

Radiolabeled (^{125}I) IgA, IgE, IgG, and IgM antibodies were prepared by the chloramine T method. For the IgA, IgE, and IgM IAB assays, each radiolabeled immunoglobulin was incubated with Sepharose-linked anti-immunoglobulin antibodies from various manufacturers. Specificity of each antibody selected is shown in FIGURE 1. To verify that IAB binding was specific for each class of immunoglobulin, we incubated a sample containing IgA, IgE, and IgM IABs in the presence of increasing amounts of unlabeled immunoglobulin. Decreased binding of IgA, IgE, and IgM IABs indicated that each assay was specific for its respective class of immunoglobulin. Each radiolabel also was precipitated with protein G to demonstrate the specificity of the IgG IAB assay. PEG precipitation (total IAB assay) showed almost complete precipitation of IgE, IgG, and IgM; however, only 25% of the radiolabeled IgA was precipitated (FIG. 1). Increasing PEG concentration increased the efficiency of IgA precipitation, but also increased precipitation of unbound insulin.

Capacity

Radiolabeled IgA, IgE, IgG, and IgM were incubated with increasing amounts of the corresponding unlabeled class of Ig. Sufficient capacity for Ig levels expected in human serum was demonstrated. A 20% slurry of agarose beads coupled with monoclonal antibodies from Medix Biochemica was used in the following quantities: 250 µL for IgA, 100 µL for IgE, and 150 µL for IgM. A 25% slurry of agarose beads coupled with protein G (100 µL) was used for IgG.

Assay Precision and Linearity

Three IAB samples were analyzed 20 times on the same day in the total and IgG assays to determine intra-assay precision. The coefficient of variation was less than 5% for the total IAB assay and less than 15% for the IgG assay. Two samples containing high levels of IABs also were serially diluted, and the linear range was determined to be between the dilutions that gave less than 20% bias from expected levels. The linear range of the total IAB assay was 1 to 12.5 µU of insulin bound per mL of serum, and for the IgG IAB assay it was 1.25 to 11.25 µU of insulin bound per mL of serum. Because samples containing high levels of IgA, IgE, and IgM IABs were not available, linearity and precision could not be determined for these assays.

Sensitivity

Samples containing low IAB levels for each class were assayed 20 times in one assay. The lowest binding capacity that had a coefficient of variation of less than 20% was determined to be the lower limit of quantitation. A sample containing no measurable IABs was measured 20 times in each assay. The mean antibody binding capacity at two standard deviations above the mean was defined as the limit of detection. The limit of detection and the lower limit of quantitation were 0.56 and

1.9 for total IABs, 0.67 and 13 for IgA IABs, 0.61 and 16 for IgE IABs, 0.57 and 2.0 for IgG, and 0.98 and 20 for IgM, respectively (presented as µU of insulin bound per mL of serum).

CONCLUSIONS

Optimizing the extraction pH to 3.7 resulted in an insulin extraction efficiency of 95% while maintaining the stability of the immunoglobulins for subsequent recognition by antibodies directed against IgA, IgE, IgM, and the IgG subclasses. Rigorous screening of monoclonal antibodies provided assays that are very specific for IgA, IgE, and IgM IABs as demonstrated by radiolabel binding of purified immunoglobulins and competitive inhibition with nonradiolabeled immunoglobulins. The precision, linear range, and sensitivity studies demonstrated that these assays are robust and reproducible for routine clinical work.

Induction of Diabetes-Related Autoantibodies below Cutoff for "Positivity" in Young Nondiabetic Children

HANNA HOLMBERG,[a,b] OUTI VAARALA,[a,b] KARIN FÄLTH-MAGNUSSON,[a] AND JOHNNY LUDVIGSSON[a]

[a]*Department of Molecular and Clinical Medicine, Division of Pediatrics,*
[b]*Clinical Research Center, Faculty of Health Sciences, Linköping University, Linköping, Sweden*

ABSTRACT: The aim was to study the natural course of diabetes-related autoantibodies at low concentrations, below "positivity", in a nondiabetic population followed up from infancy. Blood samples were taken from 205 children at 6 weeks, 6 months, 18 months, and 5 years of age. Autoantibodies against GAD_{65} (GADA), tyrosine phosphatase (IA-2A), and insulin (IAA) were determined by radioligand-binding assays. All children had detectable levels of GADA and approximately half had IA-2A, but only approximately 10% had detectable levels of IAA during the follow-up period. Many children developed IA-2A already at 6 months of age, similar concentrations were seen at 18 months, and then the levels of IA-2A decreased until 5 years of age. GADA were induced less often at 6 months of age, increased up to 18 months, and fluctuated at similar levels up to 5 years of age. IAA were detectable in so few children and at low levels, so no trend in natural course could be revealed. We conclude that there is a natural induction of humoral immune response to β cell autoantigens early in life. Our results suggest that the mechanisms of β cell tolerance to GAD and IA-2 differ in healthy children.

KEYWORDS: IA-2; GAD; insulin; healthy children; tolerance

INTRODUCTION

Healthy children react with antibody development against any exogenous antigen early in life, but with low concentrations of antibodies. Most of the children develop tolerance to foreign antigens, and no immune intolerance or allergic reaction occurs.[1] The interest for diabetes-related autoantibodies so far has been focused on the high concentrations of autoantibodies, defined as levels above, for example, the 97.5th percentile of a nondiabetic population. This kind of positivity for autoantibodies against β cell antigens, such as insulin, glutamic acid decarboxylase (GAD_{65}), and tyrosine phosphatase (IA-2), predicts type 1 diabetes. High levels of autoantibodies

Address for correspondence: Hanna Holmberg, Department of Molecular and Clinical Medicine, Division of Pediatrics, Clinical Research Center, Faculty of Health Sciences, Linköping University, SE-581 85 Linköping, Sweden. Voice: +46-13-222241; fax: +46-13-127465.
hanna.holmberg@imk.liu.se

against GAD_{65} (GADA) are found in 2–6% of first-degree relatives and in 1–3% of the healthy population.[2-4] The corresponding percentages for IA-2 autoantibodies (IA-2A) are 4–5% and 0–2%;[2-6] for insulin autoantibodies (IAA), they are 0–4% and 0–3%.[5,6]

However, there has been little discussion about the physiological induction of autoantibodies in healthy children and development of tolerance to β cell antigens. We therefore decided to study the natural course of diabetes-related autoantibodies at low concentrations below "positivity" in a nondiabetic population followed up from infancy.

MATERIALS AND METHODS

Subjects

The families of the children were recruited to a prospective study to investigate the effect of maternal diet during pregnancy on the development of atopic diseases in children. All children had an atopic family history.[7]

Half of the mothers were randomized into a diet group and avoided cow's milk during the third trimester; the others had a normal diet. Until 3 months of age, all children were exclusively breast-fed or received supplementary casein hydrolysate formula (Nutramigen). Venous blood samples were drawn from the children at 6 weeks, 6 months, 18 months, and 5 years of age. The sera were frozen at −20°C for later analysis. At least one blood sample was available from 205 children.

Methods

DNA for human GAD_{65} and IA-2 was extracted from plasmid-carrying *E. coli*. ^{35}S-incorporation in the product was estimated by precipitation with TCA.

Antigen was diluted in a Tris-HCl buffer to an activity of 20,000 cpm/50 µL. Serum samples were incubated with the antigen in a 1:25 dilution in duplicates, overnight on a shaker at 4°C. The following day, sample antigen mixture was incubated with Protein A–Sepharose in 96-well filter plates blocked with 1% bovine serum albumin in Tris-HCl buffer. After incubation, wells were washed with Tris-HCl buffer. After drying, scintillation fluid was added and the plates were counted in a Micro-Beta Tri-Lux counter. For all samples, mean and %CV were calculated. The results were expressed as concentrations of autoantibodies calculated in relation to the standard curve.

The cutoff for "positivity" was 36 WHO units for IA-2A and 101.5 WHO units for GADA. In the Diabetes Autoantibody Standardization Program in 2002, we had a specificity for GADA of 96% and for IA-2A of 100%, whereas the sensitivity was 82% for GADA and 54% for IA-2A. Intra-assay coefficient of variation was 5.2%, and interassay variation was 13–18%.

IAA was analyzed in sera by a radiobinding assay. Human insulin labeled with ^{125}I was diluted in a Tris-Tween buffer, pH 8.0, to an activity of 15,000 cpm/25 µL. Serum samples were incubated with insulin in a 1:4 dilution in duplicates on a deep-well plate at 4°C with shaking for 72 h. The sample antigen mixture was incubated with Protein A–Sepharose. After incubation, samples were washed with Tris-HCl and counted in a Micro-Beta Tri-Lux counter. For all samples, mean and %CV were calculated. The results were expressed as concentrations of autoantibodies calculated in relation to the homemade standard curve. Sera with insulin binding above 2 U/mL were tested in competition assay. Each sample was analyzed in quadruplicate. Specific bounds were calculated by subtraction of counts of excess unlabeled insulin from counts of labeled insulin. The detection limit of the method was 2 U/mL based on the accuracy of the standard curve. The cutoff for "positivity" was 6 U/mL. In the Diabetes Autoantibody Standardization Program in 2002, we had a specificity for IAA of 98%, whereas the sensitivity was 24%.

Statistics

Nonparametric tests were used. Calculations were performed with the statistical package SPSS 11.0 (SPSS Inc., Chicago, IL). Correlation between antibodies was analyzed with Spearman's rank correlation test. Comparisons of the levels of autoantibodies were analyzed by using the Wilcoxon test.

Ethics

The study was approved by the Human Research Ethics Committee of the Faculty of Health Sciences, Linköping University, Linköping, Sweden.

RESULTS

Low concentrations of diabetes-related autoantibodies, in most cases below the traditionally used cutoff limit for "positivity", were detected in all children (see FIGS. 1–3). GADA were detectable in 100% (196/196) of the children at 6 weeks of age, in 97.3% (186/191) at 6 months of age, in 99.5% (184/185) at 18 months of age,

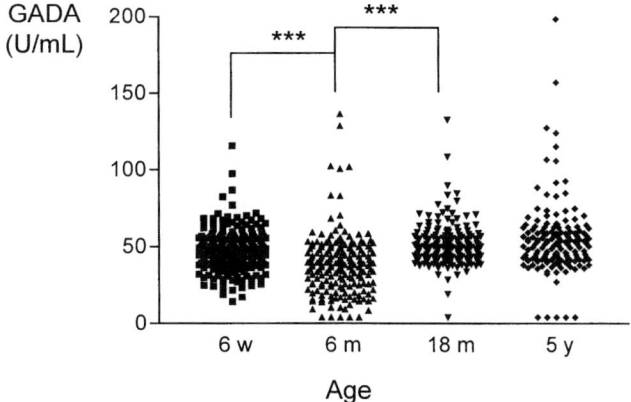

FIGURE 1. Fluctuation of the levels of GADA during the first 5 years of life (cutoff limit for GADA "positivity": 101.5 U/mL). The levels of GADA were compared in children of different age by the Wilcoxon test; ***$p < 0.001$.

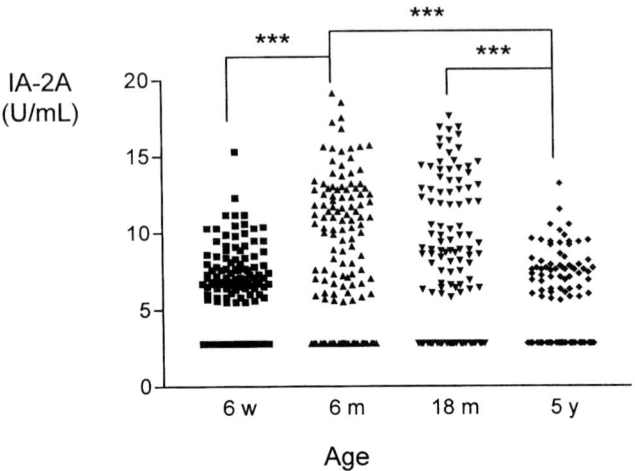

FIGURE 2. Fluctuation of the levels of IA-2A during the first 5 years of life (cutoff limit for IA-2A "positivity": 36.0 U/mL). The levels of IA-2A were compared in children of different age by the Wilcoxon test; ***$p < 0.001$.

and in 96.8% (152/157) at 5 years of age. Corresponding percentages for IA-2A were 46.9% (92/196), 52.2% (97/186), 44.3% (81/183), and 39.1% (61/156); for IAA, they were 6.1% (12/196), 8.6% (16/186), 11.1% (20/180), and 6.5% (10/154).

When using the cutoff for "positivity", 0.5% (1/196) were positive for GADA at 6 weeks, 2.1% (4/191) at 6 months, 1.1% (2/185) at 18 months, and 4.5% (7/157) at 5 years of age. For IAA, 3.6% (7/196) were positive at 6 weeks, 2.7% (5/186) at 6 months, 3.9% (7/180) at 18 months, and 1.3% (2/154) at 5 years of age. No children were positive for IA-2A.

The levels of GADA decreased from 6 weeks to 6 months of age ($p < 0.001$), increased up to 18 months ($p < 0.001$), and remained at the same level until the age of 5 years (FIG. 1). IA-2A increased from 6 weeks to 6 months of age ($p < 0.001$) and then decreased until the age of 5 years ($p < 0.001$) (FIG. 2). No significant changes in the levels of IAA were found (FIG. 3).

The levels of GADA and IA-2A correlated at 6 weeks of age ($p = 0.01$, $r = 0.18$) and at 6 months of age ($p = 0.001$, $r = 0.25$). At 6 months of age, the levels of IAA correlated with GADA ($p < 0.001$, $r = 0.26$), and at 5 years of age with IA-2A ($p = 0.001$, $r = 0.26$).

DISCUSSION

We found autoantibodies in all children very early in life. These concentrations are far below the cutoff traditionally used for "positivity", but the autoantibodies detected under the cutoff limit were inhibited effectively by homologous autoantigen, indicating antigen-specific autoantibodies (data not shown). The investigated popu-

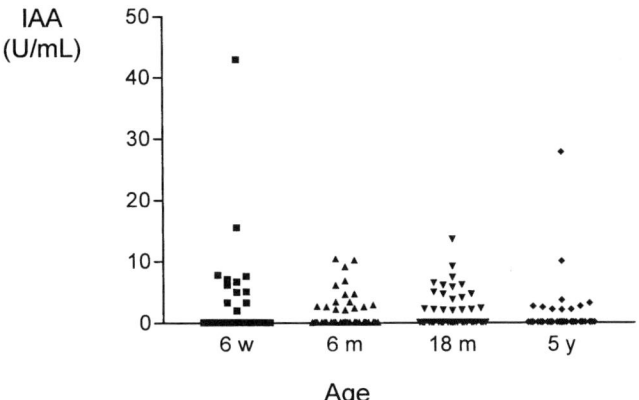

FIGURE 3. Fluctuation of the levels of IAA during the first 5 years of life (cutoff limit for IAA "positivity": 6.0 U/mL). The levels of IAA were compared in children of different age by the Wilcoxon test; ***$p < 0.001$.

lation is not a random healthy population because all children studied had heredity for atopy. However, because we have no reason to believe that children prone to atopy and Th-2 deviation should be more likely to develop autoantibodies, we believe that similar findings are to be expected in children without heredity for atopy. Neither have we reason to believe that avoidance of cow's milk proteins during the last trimester of pregnancy nor the first 3 months of life should increase tendency to develop autoantibodies.

The levels of autoantibodies at 6 weeks of age probably reflected the maternal IgG antibodies transferred via placenta.[8] The natural course of GADA, IA-2A, and IAA then showed different patterns during the first 5 years of life. We found IAA in quite few children, possibly because of low sensitivity of our method, and thus could not see any trend regarding natural course. IA-2A were detectable in approximately half of the children, increasing from 6 weeks to 6 months of age, but then decreasing toward 5 years of age. The increase in IA-2A between 6 weeks and 6 months of age reflected the child's own production of autoantibodies, followed by the development of tolerance, indicated by decreasing levels to 5 years of age. The levels of GADA decreased from 6 weeks to 6 months of age, indicating clearance of maternal GADA. Humoral immune response to GAD appeared later than response to IA-2, with a peak at 18 months, and the levels of GADA remained on average constant. It is possible that the mechanisms of tolerance differ between GAD and IA-2. The occurrence of GADA is not restricted to type 1 diabetes, but GADA are common also in other autoimmune conditions. IA-2A have good predictive value for type 1 diabetes in children as shown by several studies and could be considered less common and more specific autoantibodies for type 1 diabetes. Our findings suggest that the humoral immune response to IA-2 is induced during the first months of life, thus resulting in tolerance. B lymphocyte response to GAD seems to be induced later and levels of GADA increase with age in healthy children. This is in accordance with the finding that the frequency of GADA increases with age also in newly diagnosed patients with type 1 diabetes, opposite to IA-2A and IAA which show inverse correlation with age in type 1 diabetes.

ACKNOWLEDGMENTS

This study was generously supported by JDF-Wallenberg (K98-99JD-12813-01A), the Swedish Medical Research Council (MFR) (K99-72X-11242-05A), the Swedish Child Diabetes Foundation (Barndiabetesfonden), the Swedish Diabetes Association, the Söderberg Foundation, and the Novo Nordisk Foundation. We thank Gosia Smolinska for skillful technical assistance.

REFERENCES

1. GREENWOOD, R. & J. FRELINGER. 2001. Mechanisms of unresponsiveness: T- and B-cell mediated mechanisms of anergy. Adv. Exp. Med. Biol. **489:** 99–108.
2. KULMALA, P. et al. 1998. Prediction of insulin-dependent diabetes mellitus in siblings of children with diabetes. J. Clin. Invest. **101:** 327–336.
3. MARCIULIONYTE, D. et al. 2001. A comparison of the prevalence of islet autoantibodies in children from two countries with differing incidence of diabetes. Diabetologia **44:** 16–21.
4. SEISSLER, J. et al. 1996. Combined screening for autoantibodies to IA-2 and antibodies to glutamic acid decarboxylase in first degree relatives of patients with IDDM. Diabetologia **39:** 1351–1356.
5. LINDBERG, B. et al. 1999. Islet autoantibodies in cord blood from children who developed type I (insulin-dependent) diabetes mellitus before 15 years of age. Diabetologia **42:** 181–187.
6. STREBELOW, M. et al. 1999. Karlsburg type 1 diabetes risk study of a general population: frequencies and interactions of the four major type 1 diabetes–associated autoantibodies studied in 9419 schoolchildren. Diabetologia **42:** 661–670.
7. FÄLTH-MAGNUSSON, K. & N-I.M. KJELLMAN. 1987. Development of atopic disease in babies whose mothers were receiving exclusion diet during pregnancy—a randomized study. J. Allergy Clin. Immunol. **80:** 868–875.
8. HÄMÄLAINEN, A-M. et al. 2000. Postnatal elimination of transplacentally acquired disease-associated antibodies in infants born to families with type 1 diabetes. J. Clin. Endocrinol. Metab. **85:** 4249–4253.

Cow-Milk-Free Diet during Last Trimester of Pregnancy Does Not Influence Diabetes-Related Autoantibodies in Nondiabetic Children

JOHNNY LUDVIGSSON

Department of Molecular and Clinical Medicine, Division of Pediatrics, Faculty of Health Sciences, Linköping University, Linköping, Sweden

ABSTRACT: The aim was to study whether cow-milk-free diet during the last trimester of pregnancy influences the development of diabetes-related autoantibodies in nondiabetic children. We also examined the effect of later introduction of cow milk proteins and gluten. Blood samples were taken from 205 children at 6 weeks, 6 months, 18 months, and 5 years, whose mothers had been randomized to either a cow-milk-free diet or not during the last trimester of pregnancy. During the first 3 months of life, cow milk proteins were not fed to the children. Autoantibodies against GAD_{65} (GADA), tyrosine phosphatase (IA-2A), and insulin (IAA) were determined by a radioligand-binding assay. We found specific autoantibodies, although in low concentrations below the traditional cutoff for positivity in the children. The diet of the mother during pregnancy had no influence on development of autoantibodies, nor did duration of breast-feeding or time for introduction of gluten. Cow milk introduction between 3 and 6 months caused a transient increase in GADA at 6 months of age ($p < 0.05$). Children who developed atopic disease had significantly lower IA-2A at 6 months ($p < 0.001$).

KEYWORDS: cow milk; pregnancy; autoantibodies; type 1 diabetes; atopic disease

INTRODUCTION

The presence of abnormally high concentrations of autoantibodies against β cell antigens, such as insulin, glutamic acid decarboxylase (GAD_{65}), and tyrosine phosphatase (IA-2), as well as islet cell antibodies, are used as markers of type 1 diabetes.[1–3] These autoantibodies exist in high concentrations in approximately 1–3% of healthy people, but can be found in very low concentrations in most healthy children early in life as a natural response to autoantigens, usually followed by the development of tolerance.[4] In our search for the cause of the autoimmune reaction leading in some cases to diabetes, it may be helpful to study the effect of suspected

Address for correspondence: Johnny Ludvigsson, Department of Molecular and Clinical Medicine, Division of Pediatrics, Faculty of Health Sciences, Linköping University, SE-581 85 Linköping, Sweden. Voice: +46-13-221332; fax: +46-13-148265.
johnny.ludvigsson@lio.se

environmental factors on the development of low concentrations of autoantibodies, even below the traditional cutoff for positivity. Among the environmental triggers, early exposure to dairy products has been indicated as a potential risk factor for type 1 diabetes. A protective effect of breast-feeding has been suggested, and short duration of breast-feeding and early introduction of cow milk have been indicated as risk factors for type 1 diabetes.[5,6] Because the immune process might start already during pregnancy, when the fetus first meets the antigens the mother eats, we found it interesting to analyze whether a cow-milk-free diet during the last trimester of pregnancy influences the development of diabetes-related autoantibodies in children. We also examined the effect of later introduction of cow milk proteins and gluten.

RESEARCH DESIGN AND METHODS

Subjects

The children were recruited to a previously published prospective study of the effect of maternal diet on the development of atopic diseases in children. All children therefore had one or more family members with atopic disease.[6,7] Altogether, 210 pregnant women participated in the study. The mothers randomized into the diet group avoided cow milk during the third trimester, whereas the other mothers did not. Until 3 months of age, all the children were exclusively breast-fed or received supplementary casein hydrolysate formula (Nutramigen). The diet regimen was recorded with questionnaires at 6 weeks, 3 months, 6 months, 12 months, and 18 months of age.

Materials

Venous blood samples were drawn from the children at 6 weeks, 6 months, 18 months, and 5 years of age. After centrifugation, the sera were frozen at $-20°C$ for later analysis. At least one blood sample was available from 205 children. Autoantibodies against GAD_{65} (GADA), tyrosine phosphatase (IA-2A), and insulin (IAA) were determined by a radioligand-binding assay

The cutoff for positivity was 36 WHO units for IA-2A and 101.5 WHO units for GADA. In the Diabetes Autoantibody Standardization Program in 2002, we had a specificity for GADA of 96% and for IA-2A of 100%, whereas the sensitivity was 82% for GADA and 54% for IA-2A. Intra-assay coefficient of variation was 5.2% and interassay variation was 13–18%.

The detection limit of the method for IAA was 2 U/mL based on the accuracy of the standard curve. The cutoff for positivity was 6 U/mL. In the Diabetes Autoantibody Standardization Program in 2002, we had a specificity for IAA of 98%, whereas the sensitivity was 24%.

Statistics

Nonparametric tests were used. Calculations were performed with the statistical package SPSS 11.0 (SPSS Inc., Chicago, IL). Correlation between antibodies was analyzed with Spearman's rank correlation test. Comparisons of the levels of autoantibodies were analyzed by using the Wilcoxon test.

Ethics

The study was approved by the Human Research Ethics Committee of the Faculty of Health Sciences, Linköping University, Linköping, Sweden.

RESULTS

Low levels of diabetes-related autoantibodies, although in most cases below the cutoff for what is regarded as "positive", were detected in the children.[4] Low levels of GADA were detectable in 100% (196/196) of the children at 6 weeks, and then in 98–99% of the children during follow-up. IA-2A were detected in 52.2% (97/186) at 6 months of age, decreasing to 39.1% (61/156) at 5 years of age. Detectable levels of IAA were most commonly found at 18 months of age (11.1% [20/180]).

When using the cutoff for positivity based on the prediction of type 1 diabetes, we found that at most 3.8% (6/157) were positive for GADA at 5 years of age, and 3.9% (7/180) were positive for IAA at 18 months of age. No children were positive for IA-2A.

Maternal elimination of cow milk during the last trimester of pregnancy did not influence the levels of autoantibodies in children at any age. Neither did the length of total breast-feeding affect the levels of GADA, IA-2A, or IAA in the children, nor the time of introduction of gluten. Children who were exposed to cow milk before 6 months of age, but after 3 months of age, had higher levels of GADA at 6 months of age ($p < 0.05$) than children who had not been exposed to cow milk at that age. No association between cow milk exposure and IA-2A or IAA was found. The levels of IA-2A were higher at 18 months in children who had otitis media before 6 months of age than in children with no otitis media ($p = 0.05$). Children with atopy diagnosis at 18 months had lower levels of IA-2A at 5 years of age than children without atopy ($p < 0.001$).

DISCUSSION

The incidence of both type 1 diabetes and atopic diseases are increasing in Western societies, suggesting that the same or similar environmental factors may be involved in the development of the immune imbalance causing the diseases in children. Early introduction of cow milk proteins has been suspected to play an important role for both diseases and thus we found it relevant to study diabetes-related autoantibodies in children, although they had heredity for atopy. Furthermore, there is no reason to believe that their heredity for Th2 deviation should increase their tendency to develop autoantibodies and give false-positive results.

The levels of GADA, IA-2A, and IAA all showed different patterns of fluctuation during the first 5 years of life.[4] Maternal abstention from cow milk during the last trimester of pregnancy did not influence the level of autoantibodies, nor did the length of total breast-feeding.[8] However, exposure to cow milk between 3 and 6 months of age was associated with higher levels of GADA at 6 months of age. Children with atopic disease diagnosis at 18 months of age had lower levels of IA-2A at 5 years of age than children without atopic diseases in this study. It is possible that development of atopy and Th2-deviated immune response have inhibitory effects on the development of IgG class autoantibodies. Children with ear infections before 6 months of age had increased levels of IA-2A at 18 months compared to children without ear infections, which might be caused by an unspecific triggering of the immune system.

In conclusion, we find no indication that the development of diabetes-related autoantibodies is influenced by avoiding cow milk proteins during the last trimester of pregnancy, but introduction between 3 and 6 months gives a transient increase of GADA. Atopic disease with supposed Th2 deviation is accompanied by a more rapid decrease of IA-2A during childhood.

ACKNOWLEDGMENTS

Many thanks to Sonja Hellström and Hanna Holmberg, who determined autoantibodies; to Karin Fälth-Magnusson, who allowed use of her serum samples; and Outi Vaarala, who gave valuable comments. This study was generously supported by JDF-Wallenberg (K98-99JD-12813-01A), the Swedish Medical Research Council (MFR) (K99-72X-11242-05A), the Swedish Child Diabetes Foundation (Barndiabetesfonden), and the Söderberg Foundation.

REFERENCES

1. KULMALA, P. et al. 1998. Prediction of insulin-dependent diabetes mellitus in siblings of children with diabetes. J. Clin. Invest. **101:** 327–336.
2. SAVOLA, K.E. et al. 1998. IA-2 antibodies—a sensitive marker of IDDM with clinical onset in childhood and adolescence. Diabetologia **41:** 424–429.
3. VERGE, C.F. et al. 1998. Combined use of autoantibodies (IA-2ab, GADab, IAA, ICA) in type I diabetes: combinatorial islet autoantibody workshop. Diabetes **47:** 1857–1866.
4. HOLMBERG, H. et al. 2003. Induction of diabetes-related autoantibodies below cutoff for "positivity" in young nondiabetic children. This volume.
5. VIRTANEN, S.M. et al. 1994. Dietary factors in the aetiology of diabetes. Ann. Med. **26:** 469–478.
6. VIRTANEN, S.M. et al. 1998. Cow's milk consumption, disease-associated autoantibodies, and type 1 diabetes mellitus: a follow-up study in siblings of diabetic children—Childhood Diabetes in Finland Study. Diabetic Med. **15:** 730–738.
7. FÄLTH-MAGNUSSON, K. & N.-I.M. KJELLMAN. 1987. Development of atopic disease in babies whose mothers were receiving exclusion diet during pregnancy—a randomized study. J. Allergy Clin. Immunol. **80:** 868–875.
8. KOSTRABA, J.N. et al. 1993. Early exposure to cow's milk and solid foods in infancy, genetic predisposition, and risk of IDDM. Diabetes **42:** 288–295.

Difference in Gene Expression Profiles between Human CD4+CD25+ and CD4+CD25− T Cells

NIRUPMA PATI, SOUMITRA GHOSH, MARTIN J. HESSNER, HUOY-JII KHOO, AND XUJING WANG

Max McGee National Research Center for Juvenile Diabetes, Department of Pediatrics, Medical College and Children's Hospital of Wisconsin, Milwaukee, Wisconsin, USA

ABSTRACT: We studied the gene expression profiles of human CD4+CD25+ and CD4+CD25− T cells by using cDNA microarrays. Our preliminary results indicate that there are likely significant differences in the regulation of apoptosis, cell cycle, cytokine receptor, cell-cell interaction, and stress pathway genes between these two subtypes of T cells.

KEYWORDS: T cells; CD4+CD25+ T cells; CD4+CD25− T cells; gene expression; microarray

INTRODUCTION

To maintain immunological self-tolerance, self-reactive T cells are eliminated and regulated in thymus; otherwise, their activation can result in autoimmune disease.[1] It is known that regulatory CD4+CD25+ T cells in the periphery suppress self-reactive T cell activation and proliferation.[2] Furthermore, regulatory T cell number and alteration in function lead to autoimmune diseases including type 1 diabetes.[3] Murine models for type 1 diabetes have demonstrated that defects in both antigen presentation and regulatory (suppressor) CD4+CD25+ T cells play an important role in peripheral tolerance. Regulatory CD4+CD25+ T cells suppress proliferation of other T cells by inhibiting their IL-2 production. However, the exact mechanism of suppression is still unclear. Recent efforts[4] in mice have linked suppression with differential gene expression in CD4+CD25+ T cells. In this study, we investigated the differential gene expression in fresh regulatory CD4+CD25+ T cells and responder CD4+CD25− T cells in humans.

CELL FRACTIONATION, RNA ISOLATION, AND MICROARRAY STUDIES

Human peripheral blood monocytes were isolated from freshly drawn blood of healthy individuals by Ficoll Hypaque (Amersham Pharmacia) gradient centrifugation. The CD4+CD25−, CD4+CD25+ T cell populations were isolated (>97% purity)

Address for correspondence: Soumitra Ghosh, Max McGee National Research Center for Juvenile Diabetes, Department of Pediatrics, Medical College/Children's Hospital of Wisconsin, 8701 Watertown Plank Road, Milwaukee, WI 53226. Voice: 414-456-4901; fax: 414-456-6663.
sghosh@post.its.mcw.edu

by incubating 1×10^8 peripheral blood mononuclear cells with MACS CD4 and MACS CD25 magnetic microbeads (Miltenyl Biotech, Auburn, CA). Total RNA was isolated from cells using Trizol method. Five μg of total RNA was amplified with the Arcturus kit (Arcturus, Mountain View, CA). Comparative gene expression studies were performed between amplified mRNAs from CD25+ and CD25− T cells using our in-house MAC060 human cDNA arrays, which possess approximately 10,000 elements.[5,6] After hybridization, data were analyzed using Matarray.[7] Eight replicate hybridizations were made, with four of them reverse-labeled (dye switch) with respect to the other four, to control dye bias.

DATA FILTERING, NORMALIZATION, AND QUALITY CONTROL OF EXPERIMENTS

Microarrays are prone to noise and data variation. Therefore, we have built our microarray analysis platform with a strong emphasis on quality control and assurance before complex data mining.[5–7] Of the eight slides, two (one from each direction of dye labeling) were of significantly lower quality[7] and correlated poorly with the other replicates (Pearson's correlation coefficient < 0.6); they were thus discarded from further analysis. The remaining six hybridizations were of high quality, and all pairwise correlation coefficients of log ratios were above 0.80 for all genes and above 0.95 for differentially expressed genes. Data from these six slides were normalized using the Z-method,[5] and the mean log ratio for each gene was determined, weighted by the quality score q_{com}. The geometric mean of q_{com} from all replicates was calculated for each gene.[5] Before data mining, 30% of spots lowest in this final quality score were dropped.

STATISTICAL INFERENCE FOR DIFFERENTIALLY EXPRESSED GENES

Utilizing our reverse-labeled hybridization design, we estimated the null distribution by constructing null scores from the pairs of reverse-labeled replicates. Assuming there are m such pairs, for each pair we denote the two slides "a" and "b"; then, we determine the null score log R_n for every gene by log $R_n = (\log R_{1a} + \log R_{1b} + \ldots + \log R_{ma} + \log R_{mb})/2m$ and use the values to estimate the null distribution. FIGURE 1 shows the null hypothesis and ratio measurement distributions. A similar approach has been reported using paired (exact) replicates.[8] In comparison, reverse-labeled pairs have the advantage that the potential gene-dependent dye incorporation bias is automatically corrected and therefore should represent a closer approximate to true null distribution.

GENE PATHWAYS THAT ARE REGULATED DIFFERENTLY BETWEEN CD25+ AND CD25− CELLS

Based on our statistical evaluation, we examined in more detail genes that exhibited significant differential expression at $p \leq 0.05$. Some genes of interest were signifi-

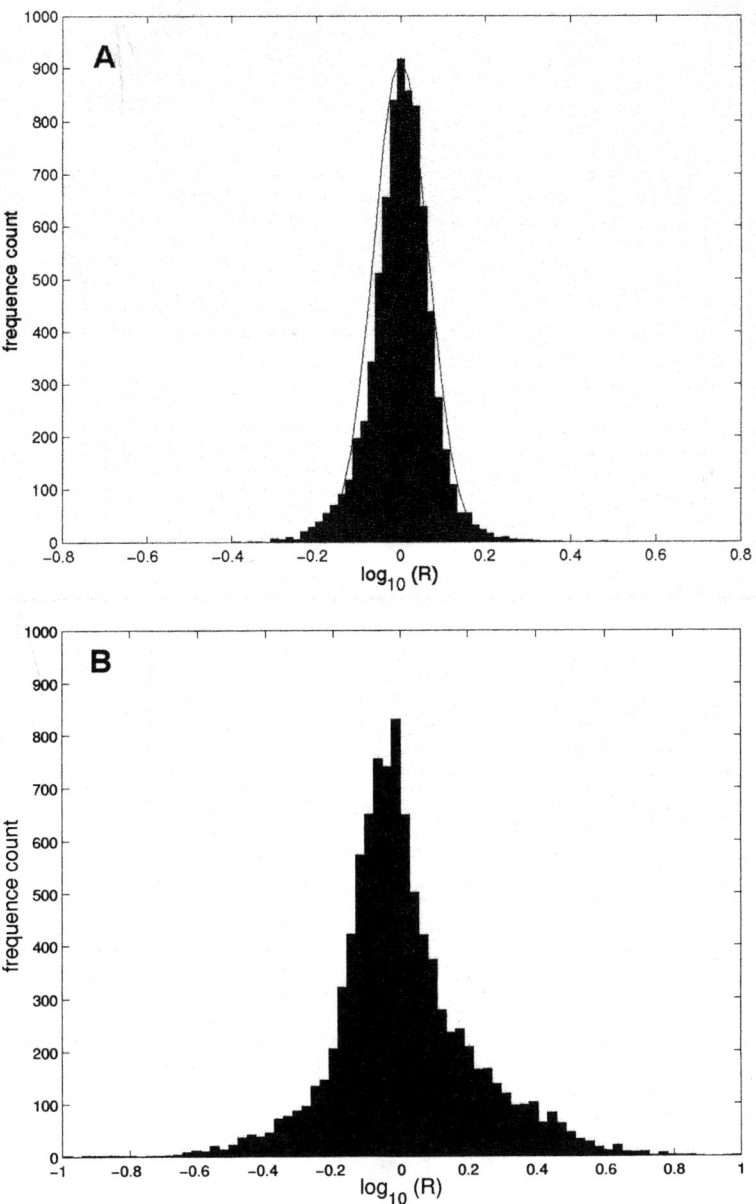

FIGURE 1. (**A**) Estimated null distribution. (**B**) Ratio measurement distribution. The *solid line* is the fitted result of a simple normal model by maximum likelihood algorithm. With the fitted model values, one then can decide the cutoff values for outliers according to a specified type I error rate, corrected by the Bonferroni factor.

TABLE 1. Number of genes in each functional group that are differentially expressed between CD25+ and CD25− T cells

Function	Apoptosis	Cell cycle	Cytokine receptor	Cell-cell interaction	Stress	Total
Total no. of genes	133	70	137	149	135	624
Up in CD25+	0	0	6	5	3	14
Up in CD25−	5	2	6	8	3	24

cantly upregulated in CD4+CD25+ T cells: SLAM, FK506 binding protein 5, CNOT2, leukocyte membrane antigen, Ubiquinol-cytc reductase, STAT4, Fyn, Ras homologue gene, TXK tyrosine kinase, and MAP kinase 9. In contrast, the following are upregulated in CD4+CD25− T cells: cell division cycle 25B, signal transducing adapter molecule, DOX1, and vJun. Among differentially expressed genes, we also examined the general difference in pathways regulating apoptosis, cell cycle, cytokine receptor, cell-cell interaction and stress, and key functions related to cell regulatory mechanisms. Using this knowledge, we tested whether gene expression profile differences between the two cell types could be merely by chance, given the a priori representation frequency of each group. In TABLE 1, we show the total number of genes available on our array for each category and the number of genes that have shown differential expression. We performed a χ^2 test and found that the observed numbers are significantly different from the numbers expected by chance ($\chi^2 = 10.27$, DF = 4, and $p < 0.05$). Therefore, we project that it is likely that the network of these five types of pathways are regulated differently between CD25+ and CD25− T cells.

DISCUSSION

In this study, we have shown evidence of regulatory differences between CD4+CD25+ and CD4+CD25− T cells in several major pathways. In particular, the results suggest that pathways regulating cytokine receptors and cell-cell interaction may be more active in CD4+CD25+ T cells than in CD4+CD25− T cells (TABLE 1). Genes of interest identified in this study were investigated further in type 1 diabetes patients (N. Pati et al., manuscript in preparation)

REFERENCES

1. OTA, K. et al. 1990. T-cell recognition of an immunodominant myelin basic protein epitope in multiple sclerosis. Nature **346:** 183–187.
2. SHEVACH, E.M. 2000. Regulatory T cells in autoimmmunity. Annu. Rev. Immunol. **18:** 423–449.
3. SAKAGUCHI, S. et al. 1995. Immunologic self-tolerance maintained by activated T cells expressing IL-2 receptor alpha-chains (CD25): breakdown of a single mechanism of self-tolerance causes various autoimmune diseases. J. Immunol. **155:** 1151–1164.
4. GAVIN, M.A. et al. 2002. Homeostasis and anergy of CD4(+)CD25(+) suppressor T cells in vivo. Nat. Immunol. **3:** 33–41.

5. WANG, X. et al. 2003. Quantitative quality control in microarray experiments and the application in data filtering, normalization, and false-positive rate prediction. Bioinformatics **19**(11): 1341–1347.
6. HESSNER, M., X. WANG, K. HULSE et al. 2003. Three-color cDNA microarrays: quantitative assessment through the use of fluorescein-labeled probes. Nucleic Acids Res. **31**(4): E14.
7. WANG, X., S. GHOSH & S-W. GUO. 2001. Quantitative quality control in microarray image processing and data acquisition. Nucleic Acids Res. **29**: E75–E82.
8. PAN, W., J. LIN & C.T. LE. 2002. How many replicates of arrays are required to detect gene expression changes in microarray experiments? A mixture model approach. Genome Biol. **3**(5): 0022.1–0022.10.

The Design of a Gene Chip for Functional Immunological Studies on a High-Quality Control Platform

JILL WAUKAU, PARTHAV JAILWALA, YOUMIN WANG, HUOY-JII KHOO, SOUMITRA GHOSH, XUJING WANG, AND MARTIN J. HESSNER

Max McGee National Research Center for Juvenile Diabetes, Department of Pediatrics, Medical College and Children's Hospital of Wisconsin, Milwaukee, Wisconsin, USA

ABSTRACT: We have created an immunology-related microarray chip containing primarily known genes with well-studied functional properties. By looking at known genes rather than expressed sequence tags, we hope to gain a better understanding of immunological pathways and how they work. The immunology gene chip contains genes from the following functional categories: T cell genes; B cell genes; dendritic cell genes; chemokine and cytokine genes; apoptosis genes; cell cycle genes; cell interaction genes; general hematology and immunology genes; and adhesion genes. We have also developed a novel three-color cDNA array platform in which arrays are directly visualized before hybridization, which allows us to select only high-quality chips for our experiments. In an effort to provide quantitative quality control for each array element as well as the entire chip, we have developed Matarray, a software package for image processing and data acquisition. With Matarray, we have built a quantitative data filtering and normalization scheme that has proved to be more efficient than the existing methods. The list of immunology chip genes is available from the authors.

KEYWORDS: Matarray; T cell; B cell; array; gene chip; expressed sequence tags

INTRODUCTION

The direction that immunology has taken in recent years has changed immensely. Far more emphasis is now placed on understanding the molecular mechanisms underlying cellular phenotypes. By unraveling pathways, we may be able to find better therapies for autoimmune and allergic diseases, in particular. Because most commercially available gene chips and clone libraries contain an abundance of expressed sequence tags (ESTs), we sought to enrich our chip for known genes with well-studied functional properties. This is the major difference between our chip and the lymphochip, which contains mainly ESTs and is heavily B cell–biased.[1] In this way, we hope to increase the information content of the long list of differentially expressed

Address for correspondence: Soumitra Ghosh, Max McGee National Research Center for Juvenile Diabetes, Department of Pediatrics, Medical College/Children's Hospital of Wisconsin, 8701 Watertown Plank Road, Milwaukee, WI 53226. Voice: 414-456-4901; fax: 414-456-6663.
sghosh@post.its.mcw.edu

genes that normally appear after the analysis of any gene expression experiment. Furthermore, we describe novel quality-control methodology that has allowed us to select good microarray slides at the prehybridization stage and filter out poor quality data at the stage of posthybridization.

RESULTS AND DISCUSSION

We first started with several functional categories: T cell genes; B cell genes; dendritic cell genes; chemokine and cytokine genes; apoptosis genes; cell cycle genes; cell interaction genes; general hematology and immunology genes; and adhesion genes. We used these keywords to search the Gene Ontology, UniGene, and Swiss-Prot databases, which store the functional annotations of genes and ESTs. This process generated 9 different lists of genes containing the UniGene cluster ID (Hs. No.) as the unique identifier. We decided to use the Hs. No. as the unique identifier because the sequence information for ESTs and known genes is assembled into a nonredundant set of gene-oriented clusters by the UniGene clustering process. A UniGene cluster is a compilation of sequences that represent one unique gene (www.ncbi.nlm.nih.gov/unigene). A verified representative clone in a cluster can be used to amplify the gene of interest for use on a chip. We included one more list of genes (Seattle Transcript list), which came from our collaborator, Gerald Nepom (Benaroya Institute, Seattle, WA). This list contained many monocyte transcripts relating to activation, chemotaxis or presentation, and growth factors involved in stromal cell interactions with T cells. To remove redundancy, we merged the 10 lists into one master list with no duplicate entries. We then updated the Hs. No. with UniGene Build #157, the most current build at the time. The final immunology chip list contained 1903 known genes. There are 192 T cell genes, 12 B cell genes, 402 dendritic cell genes, 353 chemokine and cytokine genes, 182 apoptosis genes, 161 cell cycle genes, 255 cell interaction genes, 388 general hematology/immunology genes, 35 adhesion genes, and 1115 Seattle Transcript genes. There are quite a few genes that belong to more than one functional group.

We acquired 46,656 IMAGE (Integrated Molecular Analysis of Genomes and Their Expression) consortium clones rearrayed and sequence-verified by Research Genetics. The Research Genetics Human cDNA Library consists of clones in bacterial culture, arrayed into 486 plates (96-well). The various Hs. No. for the clones in the clone information spreadsheet were updated with UniGene Build #157. Once we had updated lists, we determined that 1411 of the 1903 genes in the immunology chip list were available in our Research Genetics Human cDNA Library. These 1411 clones are being "cherry-picked" out of the library plates and rearrayed into 384-well plates. The remaining unavailable 492 clones will be ordered from two companies, RZPD (Berlin, Germany) and ATCC (Manassas, VA). Some of the 1903 clones will be sequenced for clone verification. The use of cDNA microarrays begins with construction of the array where hundreds to thousands of cDNA probes are amplified by polymerase chain reaction, purified, and printed onto glass coated slides (typically poly-L-lysine). The printed array subsequently is prepared for hybridization after it is fixed/blocked in a series of steps, commonly termed postprocessing.[2] Finally, the array is then hybridized with Cy3- and Cy5-labeled cDNA targets derived from the two biological samples being compared for differential gene expression. After hybridization, the array is analyzed with a fluorescence scanner, and the relative amount of an mRNA species in the original two samples is defined as a ratio between the two fluorophores at the homologous array element using specially designed software.[2] All of our arrays are printed with positive and negative control elements, including serial dilutions of precisely quantified housekeeping genes (GAPDH and β-actin), which are utilized for laser focusing, for assessment of target labeling, and as a reference for quantifying bound probe of other array elements.[3]

Array technology has drawn criticism because of its lack of reproducibility, which stems from normal biological variation,[4] technical issues in target preparation, and array fabrication. Array fabrication is technically complex and, typically, construction methodologies lack the ability to determine array integrity before hybridization, leaving the array itself a source of uncontrolled experimental variation. Thus, we have developed a novel three-color cDNA array platform where arrays are directly visualized before hybridization.[5] This is accomplished by spotting cDNA probes that are labeled with a third fluorescent dye, which is covalently attached to the oligonucleotide primers used for library amplification. Our system utilizes fluorescein as the third dye, which is compatible with Cy3 and Cy5 target labeling dyes when using confocal laser scanners possessing narrow bandwidths. Comparison of hybridization results between high- and low-quality replicate pairs has revealed a direct and significant relationship between prehybridization fluorescein image quality and posthybridization replicate consistency, illustrating that microarray data quality can be improved through prehybridization slide selection based on quality analysis.[5] Hence, all arrays fabricated in our lab undergo a quality-control analysis using the third dye image and the following putative slide acceptance criteria: mean array element intensity > 5000 RFU/pixel; CV intensity < 10%; mean (signal/signal + noise) ratio > 0.85; and CV of spot size < 20%.[6] On average, more than 80% of slides of a print run meet these criteria, yielding arrays that are able to detect gene expression changes as low as 1.5-fold and generate replicate consistencies typically >0.85. We believe that our novel visualization approach has broad application, improving microarray data reproducibility not only for laboratories using cDNA arrays, but also for those spotting oligonucleotide probes.

As part of our effort to build an in-house LIMS for microarrays, we have developed Matarray, a software package for image processing and data acquisition that provides quantitative quality control for each array element as well as the entire slide,[7] and have built a quantitative data filtering and normalization scheme that has proved to be more efficient than the existing methods.[8] We have extended this work to develop a module that utilizes the fluorescein dye image before hybridization to quality control printed arrays and to incorporate the fluorescein information in data filtering and normalization. Every one of our immunology chips will be certified and quantified by this module after printing.

By designing a gene chip containing known genes in many immunological pathways, we hope to increase the amount of informative gene expression data, which then may be used to unravel these pathways. With our methods of chip design and improved quality control, the gene expression data will also be more reliable. The list of genes on the immunology chip is available from us on request.

ACKNOWLEDGMENTS

J. Waukau, P. Jailwala, X. Wang, and M. J. Hessner contributed equally to this work. We thank Kathryn Tushaus, Nirupma Pati, and Yan Wu for their help in generating some of the initial gene lists for this project. We thank Gerald Nepom for the generous contribution of his gene list to this project. We also thank David D. Eckels, Bart O. Roep, and Sun-Wei Guo for numerous insightful discussions. This work has been supported by a special fund from the Children's Hospital Foundation, Children's Hospital of Wisconsin.

REFERENCES

1. ALIZADEH, A., M. EISEN, R.E. DAVIS et al. 1999. The lymphochip: a specialized cDNA microarray for the genomic-scale analysis of gene expression in normal and malignant lymphocytes. Cold Spring Harb. Symp. Quant. Biol. **64:** 71–78.
2. EISEN, M. & P. BROWN. 1999. DNA arrays for analysis of gene expression. Methods Enzymol. **303:** 179–205.
3. WANG, Y., X. WANG, S-W. GUO et al. 2002. Conditions to ensure competitive hybridization in two-color microarray: a theoretical and experimental analysis. BioTechniques **32:** 1342–1346.
4. PRITCHARD, C.C., L. HSU, J. DELROW et al. 2001. Project normal: defining normal variance in mouse gene expression. Proc. Natl. Acad. Sci. USA **98:** 13266–13271.
5. HESSNER, M.J., X. WANG, K. HULSE et al. 2003. Three-color cDNA microarrays: quantitative assessment through the use of fluorescein-labeled probes. Nucleic Acids Res. **31:** E14.
6. HESSNER, M.J., X. WANG, S. KHAN et al. 2003. Use of a three-color cDNA microarray platform to measure and control support-bound probe for improved data quality and reproducibility. Nucleic Acids Res. **31:** E60.
7. WANG, X., S. GHOSH & S-W. GUO. 2001. Quantitative quality control in microarray image processing and data acquisition. Nucleic Acids Res. **29:** E75–E82.
8. WANG, X., M.J. HESSNER, Y. WU et al. 2003. Quantitative quality control in microarray experiments and the application in data filtering, normalization, and false-positive rate prediction. Bioinformatics **19:** 1341–1347.

Relationship between T and B Cell Responses to Proinsulin in Human Type 1 Diabetes

IVANA DURINOVIC-BELLÓ,[a] NICOLA MAISEL,[a] MICHAEL SCHLOSSER,[b] HUBERT KALBACHER,[c] MARTIN DEEG,[d] THOMAS EIERMANN,[e] WOLFRAM KARGES,[a] AND BERNHARD O. BOEHM[a]

[a]*Department of Internal Medicine I, Division of Endocrinology, University of Ulm, Ulm, Germany*

[b]*Institute of Pathophysiology Karlsburg, University of Greifswald, Greifswald, Germany*

[c]*Medical Scientific Center, University of Tübingen, Tübingen, Germany*

[d]*Section of Transplantation and Immunology, Medical Clinic, University of Tübingen, Tübingen, Germany*

[e]*Institute of Transfusion Medicine, University Hospital Hamburg-Eppendorf, Hamburg, Germany*

ABSTRACT: In type 1 diabetes, humoral and cell-mediated responses to insulin and proinsulin are detectable. Autoantibodies to insulin are associated with impending disease in young individuals and are used as predictive markers to determine disease risk. The aim of this study was to investigate whether different cytokine patterns of cellular reactivity to insulin might serve as additional specific markers of disease maturation and might improve disease prediction in individuals at risk. We correlated T and B cell responses to insulin in subjects with increased genetic risk (HLA-DRB1*04, DQB1*0302) for diabetes with or without islet autoantibodies (Ab+ subjects and controls, respectively) and HLA-matched patients. Peripheral blood mononuclear cells were stimulated with 15 overlapping proinsulin peptides (16-mer), and proinflammatory Th1 (IFNγ) and anti-inflammatory Th2 (IL-4) cytokines were analyzed. We observed a simultaneous increase in IL-4 and IFNγ secretion in early islet autoimmunity of Ab+ subjects, but not in insulin-treated T1D patients. Furthermore, the increase in IL-4 secretion in Ab+ subjects was associated with insulin autoantibody responses. There was no correlation of either IFNγ or IL-4 secretion with insulin antibody responses in patients already treated with exogenous insulin. In conclusion, our findings reveal that quantification of cytokine responses to proinsulin in peripheral blood may prove to be a promising specific marker of diabetes progression and could, in addition to insulin autoantibodies, be used in the prediction of type 1 diabetes.

KEYWORDS: proinsulin; insulin; T cells; autoantibodies; cytokines

Address for correspondence: Dr. Ivana Durinovic-Belló, Department of Internal Medicine I, Division of Endocrinology, University of Ulm, Robert-Koch Strasse 8, 89081 Ulm, Germany. Voice: +49-731-500-24732; fax: +49-731-500-24302.
ivana.durinovic-bello@medizin.uni-ulm.de

INTRODUCTION

Type 1 diabetes (T1D) is considered to be a T cell–mediated autoimmune disease resulting from a disturbed cellular immunoregulation. Insulin and proinsulin are target antigens of β cell destruction. The effects of insulin to prevent T1D has currently been investigated in a large clinical trial.[1] In experimental models of T1D, insulin therapy has been shown to delay diabetes onset, while more recently disease induction was observed after preproinsulin treatment in NOD and RIP-B7.1 mice.[2]

T cells specific for islet β cell proteins also exist in healthy individuals, but are restrained by regulatory mechanisms.[3,4] In T1D, if regulatory T cell responses fail, it has been postulated that autoreactive T helper cells specific for β cell antigens become activated and clonally expand.[5–7] They provide help to B cells that secrete autoantibodies specific for the same autoantigens.[8,9] However, the pathogenesis of T1D is considered to be cell-mediated because T cells can transfer disease in animal models and in human T1D, while autoantibodies do not have pathogenic properties.[10–12]

Insulin and proinsulin autoantibodies develop spontaneously prior to the onset of clinical disease and correlate closely.[13–15] Insulin autoantibodies are also early sensitive markers of the impending disease onset in the young[16] and can precede other islet autoantibodies.[9,17] Moreover, in young subjects, increased T cell proliferation to insulin and proinsulin is associated with an inductive phase of the autoimmune response;[4,18] in contrast, in adult subjects, responses to insulin or proinsulin are generally weak.[3,6,19–21]

The intriguing question of whether Th1 and Th2 autoimmunity in human T1D could be associated with different stages of diabetes development or disease risk has still not been addressed. Autoantibodies and T cells to insulin appear predominantly in younger individuals[17,18,20,22] and more frequently in subjects with high genetic risk of T1D (HLA-DRB1*04).[4,23,24]

The aim of this study was to determine whether T cell cytokine phenotype of *in vivo* primed autoimmune response to proinsulin correlates with different stages of disease progression in individuals with genetic HLA-DRB1*04, DQB1*0302 risk for T1D. In addition, it was analyzed whether specific patterns of cytokine secretion correlate with the level of insulin autoantibodies.

METHODS

Subjects

A total of 35 HLA-DRB1*04, DQB1*0302–positive individuals were analyzed: 12 patients with T1D (median age, 26 years; range, 2–56 years; median duration of insulin treatment, 6 months; range, 1–12 months), 12 autoantibody-positive (Ab+) schoolchildren without family history of T1D from the Karlsburg Type 1 Diabetes Risk Study[25] (median age, 20 years; range, 8–24 years), and 11 healthy control subjects without family history of T1D (median age, 22 years; range, 2–43 years). Out of 12 Ab+ individuals, 9 were classified as "high risk" subjects since they were positive for more than one additional antibody specificity, that is, insulin autoantibodies (IAA), antibodies against glutamic acid decarboxylase (GADA) or islet tyrosine phosphatase (IA-2A), and/or with a high titer of cytoplasmic islet cell antibodies

(ICA > 20 JDF-U).[8,26] Informed consent was obtained from all individuals prior to analysis, and studies were performed in accordance to the Declaration of Helsinki.

HLA Typing

HLA typing was performed using a locus-specific PCR amplification procedure as described elsewhere.[27]

Autoantibody Assays

Autoantibody assays used have been previously described in detail.[25,28] Insulin autoantibodies were determined by the microassay using the protein A/G method with and without the addition of unlabeled insulin. In the Second Diabetes Antibody Standardization Program (DASP-2) proficiency evaluation, this assay achieved a diagnostic sensitivity and specificity of 26% and 99%, respectively, at or above the 99th percentile calculated from 991 (537 m/454 f) healthy schoolchildren (204.6 μU/L). If the 97th percentile is used as threshold, this assay achieved a sensitivity and specificity of 52% and 98%, respectively, in the workshop.

Autoantigens and Peptides

Human proinsulin (Eli Lilly International, Indianapolis, IN) and insulin (Aventis, Frankfurt, Germany) were tested simultaneously with 15 proinsulin peptides (16 amino acids long and 12 amino acids overlapping), which were synthesized according to the primary preproinsulin structure (GenBank accession no. P01308). All antigens and peptides were highly purified and did not contain significant levels of endotoxin as determined by the Limulus lysate assay (<0.06 EU/mL at 10 μg peptide/mL).

Cell Separation and Stimulation Assay

Peripheral blood mononuclear cells (PBMC) were isolated from heparinized blood by Ficoll-paque (Pharmacia, Freiburg, Germany) density centrifugation, aliquoted, and cryopreserved in liquid nitrogen until use as described previously.[29] Microtiter plates were prepared by adding 50 μL of autoantigens (proinsulin and insulin, 10 μg/mL) or peptides (5 μg/mL) per well in triplicates, followed by addition of 150 μL of PBMC (15×10^4/well). On day 5 of incubation, supernatants of replicate cultures were pooled and stored at −80°C for cytokine analysis.

Cytokine Secretion Assay

IFNγ and IL-4 were analyzed according to the manufacturer's instructions using an antigen-capture ELISA from PharMingen (San Diego, CA). Detection limits were 34.2 pg/mL for IFNγ and 19.5 pg/mL for IL-4. Quantification of spontaneous cytokine release was performed by incubating the cells of each individual under the same conditions, but in the absence of antigens. Positive cytokine secretion was defined by subtracting spontaneous cytokine release + 2 SD from experimental values. The amount of secreted cytokines is expressed in pg/mL.

Statistical Analysis

Data were analyzed using the SPSS software package (SPSS GmbH Software, Munich, Germany). Correlation between autoantibody responses and cytokine responses was analyzed by Bravais-Pearson correlation analysis. The nonparametric Mann-Whitney U test was used for unpaired observations, with an appropriate adjustment to the significance level for multiple comparisons.

RESULTS AND DISCUSSION

In the present study, we investigated T and B cell responses to insulin and its precursor, proinsulin. We quantified cytokine responses in the supernatants of PBMC cultures stimulated with 15 overlapping peptides spanning the proinsulin molecule. These cytokine responses were correlated with antibody responses to insulin.

Two groups of subjects with islet autoimmunity, Ab+ subjects and insulin-treated T1D patients with median insulin therapy duration of 6 months, and nondiabetic controls were investigated. All three groups of subjects were strictly selected for the expression of DRB1*04, DQB1*0302 haplotype associated with high risk for T1D. Our aim was to investigate whether cytokine responses, in addition to antibody responses, may prove to be additional specific markers of disease progression in subjects with increased genetic risk for T1D.

In early islet cell autoimmunity of Ab+ subjects, an increase in the magnitude of both investigated cytokines, IL-4 ($p < 0.0001$) and IFNγ ($p < 0.007$), was seen compared to the other two groups, resulting in a Th0 phenotype of cytokine responses (FIG. 1). In Ab+ subjects, T cell responses characterized by increased levels of IL-4 secretion correlated well with increased levels of IAA ($r = 0.8$, $p < 0.01$) (FIG. 2a).

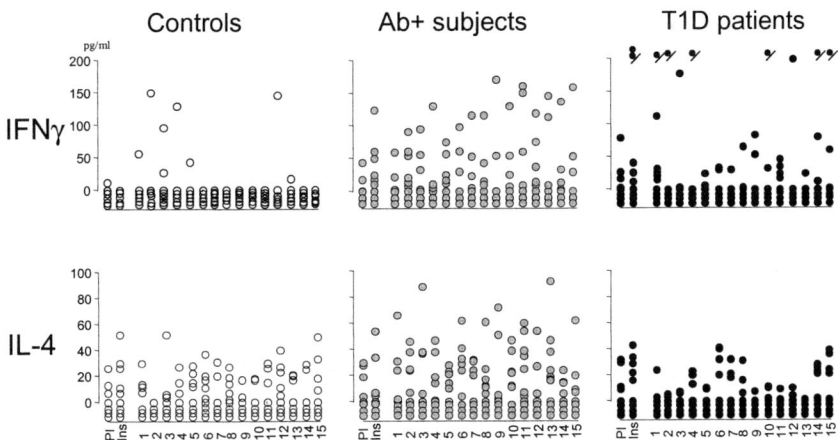

FIGURE 1. *In vitro* IFNγ and IL-4 secretion in response to proinsulin, insulin, and 15 overlapping proinsulin peptides in PBMC of nondiabetic control subjects, Ab+ subjects, and recent-onset T1D patients. PI = proinsulin, Ins = insulin, 1–15 = overlapping proinsulin peptides (16 amino acids long).

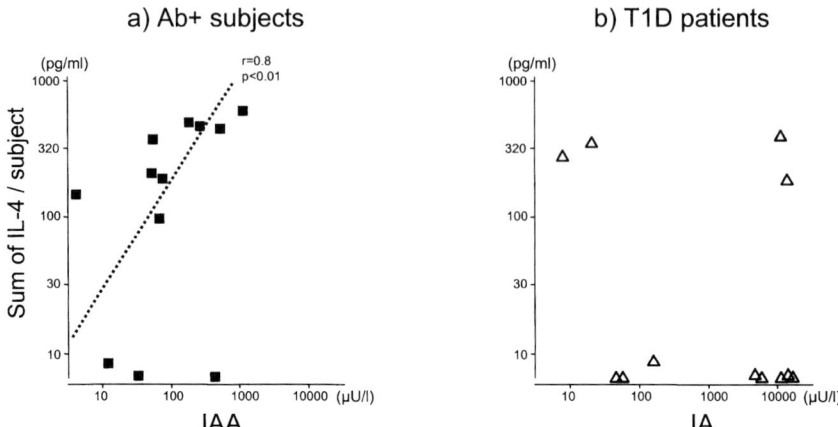

FIGURE 2. Positive correlation of T cell IL-4 secretion to proinsulin peptides with autoantibody response to insulin (IAA) in Ab+ subjects (*black squares and dotted line*) **(a)**. No correlation of IL-4 secretion to proinsulin peptides with antibody response to insulin (IA) in insulin-treated T1D patients (*open triangles*) **(b)**.

IAA develop in subjects at high risk for T1D prior to the onset of clinical disease and exposure to exogenous insulin.[16] In our study, 5 out of 12 Ab+ subjects were positive for IAA; and in 4 out of these 5, the sum of IL-4 responses to proinsulin peptides was higher than 300 pg/mL.

In contrast, in T1D patients (receiving insulin therapy for a median duration of 6 months), no correlation of cytokine responses with insulin antibody (IA) responses was observed (FIG. 2b). IA frequently develop in patients treated with exogenous insulin and reach higher levels in individuals who were IAA-positive before the diagnosis of T1D.[30] Eight out of 12 T1D patients in our study were positive for IA, and only 2 of these 8 had high IL-4 responses. The other patient had IFNγ responses higher than 300 pg/mL.

Different studies have analyzed the relationship between the proliferative T cell versus antibody responses to insulin with conflicting results. An inverse relation of IAA and insulin-reactive T cells was found in the study where recent-onset T1D patients were combined with nondiabetic subjects.[3] No relationship was observed between humoral and cellular responses to insulin in T1D patients, although both T cell responses and autoantibody titers were higher in younger subjects.[20] In our previous study where we analyzed young Ab+ subjects and T1D patients at diagnosis, a weak positive association of antibodies and T cell reactivity to insulin was observed.[31]

Number and level of circulating autoantibodies as indirect markers of the disease activity accompany active autoimmunity in T1D.[26] In this study, we postulated that T cells of subjects with islet autoimmunity (i.e., Ab+ subjects and T1D patients) have been primed *in vivo* during a spontaneous autoimmune response and, therefore, should exhibit a cytokine pattern of activated peripheral memory cells characterized by high IFNγ and IL-4 secretion.[32] By analyzing cytokine secretion patterns and Th1/Th2 differentiation state of these cells, we defined the cytokine specificity of the proinsulin T cell response and correlated their cytokine profile with autoantibody response and with disease progression.

In conclusion, we propose that both autoreactive T cells and autoantibodies to proinsulin simultaneously coexist in T1D and preclinical T1D, and both may play a significant role in the pathogenesis of the disease. Autoantibody responses to insulin are in an early preclinical stage of T1D autoimmunity (Ab+ subjects) associated with Th2 (IL-4) phenotype of cytokine responses. Both in combination may become of increasing value in the prediction and diagnosis of preclinical T1D and in the monitoring of prevention trials.

ACKNOWLEDGMENTS

Wolfram Karges and Bernhard O. Boehm contributed equally to this paper.

This work was supported by grants from the Deutsche Forschungsgemeinschaft, Sonderforschungsbereich, SFB 518 (to I. Durinovic-Belló, W. Karges, and B. O. Boehm); Eli Lilly Foundation International (to I. Durinovic-Belló); Deutsche Diabetes Stiftung, Stiftung "des Zuckerkranke Kind" (to I. Durinovic-Belló); and Deutsche Diabetes Gesellschaft (to I. Durinovic-Belló). We acknowledge H-J. Schreckling, B. Feldmann, and M. Kuhn-Halder for clinical care of the patients.

REFERENCES

1. DIABETES PREVENTION TRIAL–TYPE 1 DIABETES STUDY. 2002. Effects of insulin in relatives of patients with type 1 diabetes mellitus. N. Engl. J. Med. **346:** 1685–1691.
2. KARGES, W., K. PECHHOLD, S. AL-DAHOUK et al. 2002. Induction of autoimmune diabetes through insulin (but not GAD65) DNA vaccination in nonobese diabetic and in RIP-B7.1 mice. Diabetes **51:** 3237–3244.
3. SCHLOOT, N.C., B.O. ROEP, D. WEGMANN et al. 1997. Altered immune response to insulin in newly diagnosed compared to insulin-treated diabetic patients and healthy control subjects. Diabetologia **40:** 564–572.
4. DURINOVIC-BELLÓ, I., B.O. BOEHM & A.G. ZIEGLER. 2002. Predominantly recognized proinsulin T helper cell epitopes in individuals with and without islet cell autoimmunity. J. Autoimmun. **18:** 55–66.
5. ROEP, B.O., A.A. KALLAN, G. DUINKERKEN et al. 1995. T-cell reactivity to beta-cell membrane antigens associated with beta-cell destruction in IDDM. Diabetes **44:** 278–283.
6. DURINOVIC-BELLÓ, I., M. HUMMEL & A.G. ZIEGLER. 1996. Cellular immune response to diverse islet cell antigens in IDDM. Diabetes **45:** 795–800.
7. ENDL, J., H. OTTO, G. JUNG et al. 1997. Identification of naturally processed T cell epitopes from glutamic acid decarboxylase presented in the context of HLA-DR alleles by T lymphocytes of recent onset IDDM patients. J. Clin. Invest. **99:** 2405–2415.
8. VERGE, C.F., R. GIANANI, E. KAWASAKI et al. 1996. Prediction of type I diabetes in first-degree relatives using a combination of insulin, GAD, and ICA512bdc/IA-2 autoantibodies. Diabetes **45:** 926–933.
9. ZIEGLER, A.G., M. HUMMEL, M. SCHENKER & E. BONIFACIO. 1999. Autoantibody appearance and risk for development of childhood diabetes in offspring of parents with type 1 diabetes: the 2-year analysis of the German BABYDIAB Study. Diabetes **48:** 460–468.
10. THIVOLET, C., A. BENDELAC, P. BEDOSSA et al. 1991. CD8+ T cell homing to the pancreas in the nonobese diabetic mouse is CD4+ T cell–dependent. J. Immunol. **146:** 85–88.
11. LAMPETER, E.F., M. HOMBERG, K. QUABECK et al. 1993. Transfer of insulin-dependent diabetes between HLA-identical siblings by bone marrow transplantation. Lancet **341:** 1243–1244.
12. MARTIN, S., D. WOLF-EICHBAUM, G. DUINKERKEN et al. 2001. Development of type 1 diabetes despite severe hereditary B-lymphocyte deficiency. N. Engl. J. Med. **345:** 1036–1040.

13. KUGLIN, B., F.A. GRIES & H. KOLB. 1988. Evidence of IgG autoantibodies against human proinsulin in patients with IDDM before insulin treatment. Diabetes **37:** 130–132.
14. BOHMER, K., H. KEILACKER, B. KUGLIN *et al.* 1991. Proinsulin autoantibodies are more closely associated with type 1 (insulin-dependent) diabetes mellitus than insulin autoantibodies. Diabetologia **34:** 830–834.
15. WILLIAMS, A.J., P.J. BINGLEY, R.E. CHANCE & E.A. GALE. 1999. Insulin autoantibodies: more specific than proinsulin autoantibodies for prediction of type 1 diabetes. J. Autoimmun. **13:** 357–363.
16. BONIFACIO, E., M. SCIRPOLI, K. KREDEL *et al.* 1999. Early autoantibody responses in prediabetes are IgG1 dominated and suggest antigen-specific regulation. J. Immunol. **163:** 525–532.
17. YU, L., D.T. ROBLES, N. ABIRU *et al.* 2000. Early expression of antiinsulin autoantibodies of humans and the NOD mouse: evidence for early determination of subsequent diabetes. Proc. Natl. Acad. Sci. USA **97:** 1701–1706.
18. DURINOVIC-BELLÓ, I. 1998. Autoimmune diabetes: the role of T cells, MHC molecules, and autoantigens. Autoimmunity **27:** 159–177.
19. KELLER, R.J. 1990. Cellular immunity to human insulin in individuals at high risk for the development of type I diabetes mellitus. J. Autoimmun. **3:** 321–327.
20. SARUGERI, E., N. DOZIO, C. BELLONI *et al.* 1998. Autoimmune responses to the beta cell autoantigen, insulin, and the INS VNTR–IDDM2 locus. Clin. Exp. Immunol. **114:** 370–376.
21. ELLIS, T., E. JODOIN, E. OTTENDORFER *et al.* 1999. Cellular immune responses against proinsulin: no evidence for enhanced reactivity in individuals with IDDM. Diabetes **48:** 299–303.
22. NASERKE, H.E., E. BONIFACIO & A.G. ZIEGLER. 1999. Immunoglobulin G insulin autoantibodies in BABYDIAB offspring appear postnatally: sensitive early detection using a protein A/G–based radiobinding assay. J. Clin. Endocrinol. Metab. **84:** 1239–1243.
23. ZIEGLER, R., C.A. ALPER, Z.L. AWDEH *et al.* 1991. Specific association of HLA-DR4 with increased prevalence and level of insulin autoantibodies in first-degree relatives of patients with type I diabetes. Diabetes **40:** 709–714.
24. PUGLIESE, A., T. BUGAWAN, R. MOROMISATO *et al.* 1994. Two subsets of HLA-DQA1 alleles mark phenotypic variation in levels of insulin autoantibodies in first degree relatives at risk for insulin-dependent diabetes. J. Clin. Invest. **93:** 2447–2452.
25. STREBELOW, M., M. SCHLOSSER *et al.* 1999. Karlsburg Type I Diabetes Risk Study of a General Population: frequencies and interactions of the four major type I diabetes–associated autoantibodies studied in 9419 schoolchildren. Diabetologia **42:** 661–670.
26. BINGLEY, P.J., E. BONIFACIO, A.J. WILLIAMS *et al.* 1997. Prediction of IDDM in the general population: strategies based on combinations of autoantibody markers. Diabetes **46:** 1701–1710.
27. ERLICH, H., T. BUGAWAN, A.B. BEGOVICH *et al.* 1991. HLA-DR, DQ, and DP typing using PCR amplification and immobilized probes. Eur. J. Immunogenet. **18:** 33–55.
28. SCHLOSSER, M., M. STREBELOW, R. WASSMUTH *et al.* 2002. The Karlsburg Type 1 Diabetes Risk Study of a Normal Schoolchild Population: association of beta-cell autoantibodies and human leukocyte antigen–DQB1 alleles in antibody-positive individuals. J. Clin. Endocrinol. Metab. **87:** 2254–2261.
29. DURINOVIC-BELLÓ, I., A. STEINLE, A.G. ZIEGLER & D.J. SCHENDEL. 1994. HLA-DQ-restricted, islet-specific T-cell clones of a type I diabetic patient: T-cell receptor sequence similarities to insulitis-inducing T-cells of nonobese diabetic mice. Diabetes **43:** 1318–1325.
30. SUTTON, M., L.J. KLAFF, C.M. ASPLIN *et al.* 1988. Insulin autoantibodies at diagnosis of insulin-dependent diabetes: effect on the antibody response to insulin treatment. Metabolism **37:** 1005–1007.
31. HUMMEL, M., I. DURINOVIC-BELLÓ & A.G. ZIEGLER. 1996. Relation between cellular and humoral immunity to islet cell antigens in type 1 diabetes. J. Autoimmun. **9:** 427–430.
32. SALLUSTO, F., D. LENIG, R. FORSTER *et al.* 1999. Two subsets of memory T lymphocytes with distinct homing potentials and effector functions. Nature **401:** 708–712.

Inheritance of MHC Class II Genes in Lithuanian Families with Type 1 Diabetes

VAIVA SADAUSKAITE-KUEHNE,[a,b] KEN VEYS,[c] JOHNNY LUDVIGSSON,[b] ZILVINAS PADAIGA,[a] AND CARANI B. SANJEEVI[c]

[a]*Laboratory of Pediatric Endocrinology, Kaunas University of Medicine, Kaunas, Lithuania*

[b]*Division of Pediatrics, Department of Health and Environment, Faculty of Health Sciences, Linköping University, Linköping, Sweden*

[c]*Department of Molecular Medicine, Karolinska Institute, Stockholm, Sweden*

ABSTRACT: Type 1 diabetes mellitus (DM) is caused by genetic and environmental factors. Twice as many fathers as mothers of children with type 1 DM have the disease. The reason for the differences remains unclear. We looked at the transmission rates of diabetes-related alleles from parents to children with diabetes. All children with newly diagnosed type 1 DM from August 1, 1996 to August 1, 2000, aged 0 to 15 years, in Lithuania were invited to participate. Blood samples for full genetic analysis were available from 125 families. HLA DQA1, DQB1, and DRB1 typing was done on DNA extracted from peripheral blood, by polymerase chain reaction amplification, manual dot-blotting onto nylon membranes, synthetic sequence-specific oligonucleotide probe 3′-end labeling with ^{32}P-dCTP, and hybridization, followed by stringency washes, autoradiography, and allele calling. Frequency of diabetes risk–related alleles DQB1*0302, DQA1*0201, DR4, and DR3 was less prevalent among Lithuanian than among Swedish children with type 1 DM. Transmission rates of DR4-DQB1*0302-DQA1*0301 and DR3-DQB1*0201-DQA1*0501 haplotypes from parents were higher than expected: χ^2 (TDT) 30.56, $p < 0.0001$, and χ^2 (TDT) 11.26, $p = 0.0008$, respectively. DQB1*0302 and DR4 were significantly more frequently transmitted from both parents, but DR3 was transmitted more frequently only from mothers. Any of these alleles had similar frequencies among female and male offspring. We conclude that, besides DR4-DQB1*0302-DQA1*0301 and DR3-DQB1*0201-DQA1*0501, there are other inherited alleles that determine risk for type 1 DM among children in Lithuania. Fathers might transfer other alleles of disease susceptibility in higher frequency or mothers might provide a protective environment during pregnancy, which results in higher risk to offspring of fathers than mothers to develop diabetes.

KEYWORDS: type 1 diabetes mellitus; MHC; genes; transmission; Lithuania

Address for correspondence: Vaiva Sadauskaite-Kuehne, Division of Pediatrics, Department of Health and Environment, Faculty of Health Sciences, Linköping University, SE-58185 Linköping, Sweden. Voice: +46-13-221335; fax: +46-13-148265.
vaiva.s@takas.lt

INTRODUCTION

Susceptibility for type 1 diabetes mellitus (DM) is genetically determined. Genes in HLA complex, located on chromosome 6p21.3, are considered to contribute most in the pathogenesis of type 1 diabetes.[1] Alleles on the haplotypes DR4-DQB1*0302-DQA1*0301 and DR3-DQB1*0201-DQA1*0501 have the closest association with type 1 DM in white populations.[2] They determine high risk for diabetes development. Another haplotype, closely associated with type 1 DM, is DRB1*15-DQB1*0602-DQA1*0201. When inherited, it dominantly protects against disease development. Penetrance of the disease is low because approximately 60% of the general population carry high-risk diabetes susceptibility alleles DR3 or DR4, yet only approximately 0.3% develop the disease.

Epidemiological studies have shown that the male to female ratios in type 1 DM incidence and prevalence rates are similar in both sexes in childhood and increase significantly after 15 years of age.[3] This is also observed among parents of the children who develop diabetes. The rates of diabetes prevalence are found to be two to three times higher among fathers than among mothers.[4,5] The risk for an offspring from a father with diabetes is accordingly higher than for one from a mother with diabetes.[6] The reasons for these differences remain unclear.

We studied diabetes-associated allele transmission rates from fathers and mothers to diseased children in Lithuania with a low type 1 DM incidence rate.

MATERIALS AND METHODS

Materials

This work is a part of a case-control study, "Diabetes and Environment around the Baltic Sea", which was conducted in southeast Sweden and Lithuania. All newly diagnosed with type 1 DM children from August 1, 1996 to August 1, 2000, aged 0–15 years, in Lithuania were invited to participate in the study. During this time, 286 new cases were registered. Inclusion of new cases is described elsewhere.[4] Blood samples for full genetic analysis were available from 125 families.

Methods

Genomic DNA was extracted from blood leukocytes by the standard phenol-chloroform method. The DNA was dissolved in sterile double distillate water. Typing of HLA-DRB1, DQA1, and DQB1 was done by polymerase chain reaction amplification of the second exon of the genes specific for DRB1, DQA1, and DQB1 primers in the programmable thermal cycler (Perkin Elmer Cetus, Norwalk, CT). Amplified product was manually dot-blotted onto nylon membranes. Synthetic sequence-specific oligonucleotide probes were 3′-end labeled with αP32-dCTP and used for hybridization, followed by stringency washes, autoradiography, and allele calling as previously described.[7]

Statistical Analysis

The distribution of alleles among children and parents was tested using the PedCheck statistical program.[8] Transmission disequilibrium test (TDT) was used to assess the transmission frequencies of alleles and haplotypes from parents to children. Only parents who were heterozygous for the alleles of interest were included in this analysis. The frequency with which the allele/haplotype is transmitted to the offspring is compared with the expected frequency of 50%, which under null hypothesis determines no linkage. Transmission rates, expressed as χ^2 (TDT), were calculated using the Gene Hunter statistical program.[9] To reject the meiotic segregation distortion, we compared transmission frequencies between those with affected children and those with healthy siblings using χ^2.

RESULTS

Of all children with newly diagnosed type 1 DM, 52.9% had DQB1*0302 allele and 53.8% had DQB1*0201 allele. Of the mothers, 27.9% had DQB1*0302 and 49.0% had DQB1*0201 alleles. Of the fathers, 34.6% had DQB1*0302 and 47.1% had DQB1*0201 alleles. DQB1*0302 was found only in combination with DQA1*0301, and DQB1*0201 was found in combinations with DQA1*0501

TABLE 1. Transmission rates of diabetes-related alleles/haplotypes from parents to offspring

Alleles/haplotypes	From fathers				From mothers				From parents			
	To affected child		To healthy siblings		To affected child		To healthy siblings		To affected child		To healthy siblings	
	N (%)	p	N (%)	p	N (%)	p	N (%)	p	N (%)	p	N (%)	p
DQB1												
*0302	29 (83.3)*	0.0001	12 (36.4)	ns	25 (86.2)*	0.0001	13 (44.8)	ns	54 (84.4)*	<0.0001	25 (40.3)	ns
*0201	20 (55.6)†	ns	21 (55.0)	ns	22 (59.5)†	ns	21 (55.3)	ns	42 (56.0)†	0.987	43 (55.1)	ns
DQB1 *0201-DQA1 *0501	16 (66.7)†	ns	10 (50.0)	ns	22 (82.8)**	0.0004	17 (56.7)	ns	40 (75.5)**	0.0002	27 (50.0)	ns
DR4	32 (81.6)*	0.0001	13 (36.1)	ns	25 (89.3)*	0.0001	10 (38.5)	ns	57 (83.8)*	<0.0001	23 (37.1)	0.05
DR3	16 (64.0)†	ns	11 (52.4)	ns	25 (83.3)*	0.0003	16 (53.3)	ns	41 (74.5)*	<0.0001	27 (53.0)	ns

NOTE: The p value is of χ^2 (TDT); *$p < 0.005$; **$p < 0.03$; †not significant (ns) of χ^2 for comparison of allele/haplotype transmission frequencies between affected and healthy children.

(70.2% in children and 62.7% in parents) and DQA1*0201 (29.8% and 37.3%, respectively). Frequency of either allele was not different between mothers and fathers. None of the parents were homozygous for DQB1*0302 allele, whereas 33.3% of fathers and 27.5% of mothers were homozygous for DQB1*0201.

Allele DR4 was found among 53.8% of children with newly diagnosed type 1 DM, and allele DR3 among 38.5% of children. The frequencies of these alleles among parents was as follows: among mothers, 28.8% and 31.7%, respectively; among fathers, 38.5% and 29.8%, respectively. Here, 2.6% of fathers and 3.4% of mothers were homozygous for DR4, whereas 19.4% of fathers and 9.1% of mothers were homozygous for DR3 (differences not significant).

Assuming that transmission of diabetes-related haplotypes would have an expected rate of 50%, haplotype DR4-DQB1*0302-DQA1*0301 was transmitted from the parents more frequently than expected [χ^2 (TDT) 30.56, $p < 0.0001$], as well as DR3-DQB1*0201-DQA1*0501 [χ^2 (TDT) 11.26, $p = 0.0008$].

We then looked at the transmission frequencies of alleles from each parent and found that DQB1*0302 was significantly more frequently transmitted both from the fathers and from the mothers, whereas DQB1*0201 was not (TABLE 1).

DR4 was transmitted significantly more frequently than expected from both mothers and fathers, and DR3 and DQB1*0201-DQA1*0501 from the mothers, whereas for fathers it was not different from the expected rate (TABLE 1).

The transmission frequencies to healthy siblings from either parent or both parents were not different from the expected 50% rate (TABLE 1).

There was no parent carrying DRB1*15 or DQB1*0602 alleles.

DISCUSSION

Frequency of diabetes-related risk alleles among patients with type 1 DM onset below 15 years of age was 10–20% lower in our Lithuanian group of patients with childhood onset of type 1 DM than in another white population,[10] in which the incidence rate of type 1 DM is three to four times higher.[11]

The null hypothesis of distorted segregation causing the differences observed for DQB1*0302, DQB1*0201-DQA1*0501, DR4, and DR3 transmitted from either parent or both parents was rejected by comparison of transmission to nonaffected children, which was not different from the expected rate.[12]

DR4-DQB1*0302-DQA1*0301 and DR3-DQB1*0201-DQA1*0501 were transmitted from the parents more frequently than expected, which was in agreement with the results from another study.[12] Transmission of DR4 and DQB1*0302 was significantly more frequent than expected from both parents. However, DR3 and DQB1*0201-DQA1*0501, which are usually in linkage,[13] were more frequently transmitted only from mothers, but evenly distributed among male and female offspring with type 1 DM (data not shown). Similarly, only DQB1*0302 was transmitted more frequently from the mothers to the offspring with diabetes in Swedish families, but none of these alleles was transmitted more frequently by fathers.[14] Based on their own research and earlier studies, these authors also found that DR3 was transmitted significantly more frequently from mothers to healthy offspring (82%), whereas fathers showed transmission at the expected rate (48%).[14] Thus, although transmitted more frequently from the mothers, DR3 or DQB1*0201 is not sufficient to predispose high risk for developing type 1 DM in childhood. The fathers might transmit some other diabetes-related alleles that were not investigated here and that predispose higher risk for their offspring compared with offspring of the mothers. On the other hand, mothers, even though transferring DR3 and DQB1*0201-DQA1*0501 in higher frequency to the offspring, already during gestation might provide a certain environment for the children that adjusts their immune system and results in lower frequency of clinically expressed disease among their offspring.

Some environmental factors might affect differently the developing male and female immune system, or even after its maturity, resulting in higher prevalence of diabetes among males older than 15 years of age. These environmental factors, which are not determined yet, might also be expressed differently between the countries because nearly a double frequency of the fathers with DM to children with type 1 DM is observed in Sweden, where the incidence rate is high, compared with Lithuania.[4]

In conclusion, the frequency of some other haplotypes besides DR4-DQB1*0302-DQA1*0301 and DR3-DQB1*0201-DQB1*0501 that confer susceptibility to type 1 DM among the Lithuanian childhood population is higher than in other white populations. Parents who carry the above-mentioned haplotypes transmit them to the offspring more frequently than expected. Fathers transmit DR3 and DQB1*0201-DQA1*0501 in expected frequency, but they might transfer some other alleles of disease susceptibility, or mothers might provide a more protective environment during pregnancy, which results in higher risk to offspring of fathers than mothers to develop diabetes.

ACKNOWLEDGMENTS

This project was supported by the Swedish Medical Research Council, the Swedish Diabetes Association, the Swedish Child Diabetes Foundation, and the Novo Nordisk Pharmaceutical Company. We are sincerely grateful to the children and parents for participating in this project.

REFERENCES

1. NOORCHASHM, H. et al. 1997. Immunology of IDDM. Diabetologia **40**(suppl. 3): B50–B57.
2. SANJEEVI, C.B. et al. 1995. Effects of the second HLA-DQ haplotype on the association with childhood insulin-dependent diabetes mellitus. Tissue Antigens **45**: 148–152.
3. NYSTROM, L. et al. 1992. Risk of developing insulin-dependent diabetes mellitus (IDDM) before 35 years of age: indications of climatological determinants for age at onset. Int. J. Epidemiol. **21**: 352–358.
4. SADAUSKAITE-KUEHNE, V. et al. 2002. Severity at onset of childhood type 1 diabetes in countries with high and low incidence. Diabetes Res. Clin. Pract. **55**: 247–254.
5. LORENZEN, T. et al. 1994. Long-term risk of IDDM in first degree relatives of patients with IDDM. Diabetologia **37**: 321–327.
6. WARRAM, J.H. et al. 1984. Differences in risk of insulin dependent diabetes in offspring of diabetic mothers and diabetic fathers. N. Engl. J. Med. **311**: 149–152.
7. SANJEEVI, C.B. et al. 1992. Different genetic backgrounds for malnutrition-related diabetes and type 1 (insulin-dependent) diabetes mellitus in south Indians. Diabetologia **35**: 283–286.

8. O'CONELL, J.R. *et al.* 1999. A program for identification of genotype incompatibility in linkage analysis. Am. J. Hum. Genet. **63:** 259–266.
 9. KRUGLYAK, L. *et al.* 1996. Parametric and nonparametric linkage analysis: a unified multipoint approach. Am. J. Hum. Genet. **58:** 1347–1363.
10. KOCKUM, I. *et al.* 1999. Complex interaction between HLA DR and DQ in conferring risk for childhood type 1 diabetes. Eur. J. Immunogenet. **26:** 361–372.
11. KARVONEN, M. *et al.* 2000. Incidence of childhood type 1 diabetes worldwide: Diabetes Mondiale (DiaMond) Project Group. Diabetes Care **23:** 1516–1526.
12. KAWASAKI, E. *et al.* 1998. Transmission of DQ haplotypes to patients with type 1 diabetes. Diabetes **47:** 1971–1973.
13. KOCKUM, I. *et al.* 1993. HLA-DQ primarily confers protection and HLA-DR susceptibility in type I (insulin-dependent) diabetes studied in population-based affected families and controls. Am. J. Hum. Genet. **53:** 150–167.
14. KOCKUM, I. *et al.* 1994. Inheritance of major histocompatibility complex class II genes in IDDM studied in population-based affected and control families. Diabetologia **37:** 1105–1112.

Ethnic Differences in the Associations between the HLA-DRB1*04 Subtypes and Type 1 Diabetes

AMANDA REWERS,[a] SUNANDA BABU,[a] TIAN BAO WANG,[a]
TEODORICA L. BUGAWAN,[b] KATHY BARRIGA,[c] GEORGE S. EISENBARTH,[a]
AND HENRY A. ERLICH[b]

[a]*Barbara Davis Center for Childhood Diabetes, University of Colorado Health Sciences Center, Denver, Colorado 80262, USA*

[b]*Department of Human Genetics, Roche Molecular Systems, Incorporated, Alameda, California 94501, USA*

[c]*Department of Preventive Medicine and Biometrics, University of Colorado Health Sciences Center, Denver, Colorado 80262, USA*

ABSTRACT: The HLA genotype DRB1*03,DQB1*0201/DRB1*04,DQB1*0302 confers a 25-fold increase in the risk of type 1 diabetes. In persons with this genotype, DRB1*0405, *0402, and *0401 subtypes have been reported to further increase risk, whereas the *0403 and *0406 alleles confer a relative protection. We compared the frequencies of the DRB1*04 alleles in 193 type 1 diabetic patients with the HLA-DRB1*03,DQB1*0201/DRB1*04,DQB1*0302 genotype (140 non-Hispanic white [NHW] and 53 Hispanic) and 205 nondiabetic controls (142 NHW and 63 Hispanic). In addition, 87 NHW first-degree relatives of type 1 diabetes patients were studied: 33 positive and 54 negative for autoantibodies to insulin, GAD65, or IA-2. The HLA-DRB1 was typed using standard PCR SSOP methods. DRB1*0401 (OR, 2.19; 95% CI, 1.36–3.54) in NHW and *0405 (OR, 3.78; 95% CI, 1.43–10.0) in Hispanics were significantly associated with T1DM, whereas DRB1*0403 was protective (OR, 0.19; 95% CI, 0.04–0.89 in NHWs; OR, 0.10; 95% CI, 0.01–0.83 in Hispanics). Associations between the DRB1*04 alleles and prediabetic islet autoimmunity were generally in the same direction as those with diabetes. Among diabetic patients, the mean age of diagnosis appeared to be higher among those with the *0403 and *0407 allele compared with the others. In summary, on the DRB1*03,DQB1*0201/ DRB1*04,DQB1*0302 genotypes, the *0403 allele confers relative protection from type 1 diabetes and development of islet autoantibodies in both Hispanics and NHWs and is associated with older age at diabetes diagnosis. Although the associations between diabetes and *0401 and *0405 appear to differ somewhat between Hispanics and NHWs, overall there is no significant difference between these two ethnic groups.

Address for correspondence: Sunanda Babu, Barbara Davis Center for Childhood Diabetes, University of Colorado Health Sciences Center, B-140, 4200 East 9th Avenue, Denver, CO 80262. Voice: 303-315-7108; fax: 303-315-4892.
sunanda.babu@uchsc.edu

KEYWORDS: alleles; autoimmune; control; development; diabetes; diabetes mellitus; diabetes mellitus, insulin-dependent; disease; epidemiology; families; first-degree relatives; general population; genetics; genotype; HLA-DQB1; HLA-DRB1; IDDM; insulin-dependent; patients; population; protection; risk; type 1

The cause of type 1 diabetes (T1DM) is multifactorial and includes the effects of genes at several loci.[1,2] The *IDDM1* locus, including the HLA-DR and DQ genes, is the only major genetic determinant, accounting for up to 50% of the familiar clustering of the disease.[3,4] Approximately 95% of all T1DM cases have either the DRB1*03,DQB1*0201 or the DRB1*04,DQB1*0302 haplotype. Although only 2% of the general population are DRB1*0301,DQB1*0201/DRB1*04,DQB1*0302 heterozygotes,[5] this genotype is present in 30–40% of T1DM patients[6] and in up to 52% of those who develop diabetes in the first 10 years of life.[7] Interestingly, minor differences within the DRB1*04 alleles modify the risk of diabetes.[6,8–18] Previous reports have shown that, on DQB1*0302 haplotypes, the DRB1*0405 (in Caucasoids, blacks, and Asians), *0402, and *0401 alleles (in Caucasoids) increase the risk, whereas the *0403 (in Caucasoids and Chinese) and *0406 (in Japanese) alleles confer relative protection. Other alleles appear to be neutral. Comparable data for the U.S. population are lacking.

The goal of this study was to (1) determine the population frequencies of the HLA-DRB1*04 alleles in children with diabetes and nondiabetic controls who have the HLA genotype DRB1*03,DQB1*0201/DRB1*04,DQB1*0302; (2) explore the effect of various DRB1*04 alleles on the age of diabetes diagnosis; (3) compare the frequencies of DRB1*04 alleles in nondiabetic relatives of diabetic children to explore if the same alleles are associated with diabetes and the preclinical phase of diabetes marked by the presence of islet autoantibodies; and (4) determine whether the frequencies of the DRB1*04 alleles and the association with diabetes differ between Colorado Hispanic and non-Hispanic white (NHW) children.

METHODS

Study Population

Only persons with the HLA-DRB1*03,DQB1*0201/DRB1*04,DQB1*0302 genotype that live in Colorado were eligible. Diabetic patients were identified from the Barbara Davis Center for Childhood Diabetes in Denver. Nondiabetic controls were children without T1DM among the first-degree relatives followed by the Diabetes Autoimmunity Study in the Young.[5] In addition, 95 nondiabetic first-degree relatives of people with type 1 diabetes were included. Of those, 35 had pre-diabetes (normal blood sugar, but persistent islet autoantibodies present), whereas 60 were negative for islet autoantibodies.

Ethnicity was self-reported (for minors reported by parents) using the U.S. Census classification. Informed consent to genetic typing was obtained from all study participants.

HLA Typing

Samples were first typed for the presence of the HLA-DRB1*03,DQB1*0201/DRB1*04,DQB1*0302 genotype at Roche Molecular Systems, Inc., in Alameda, California, or at the Barbara Davis Center for Childhood Diabetes in Denver. At the Roche Molecular Systems, whole blood (15–25 µL) was used in PCR amplification with 11 biotinylated primers to specifically coamplify the DRB1 and the DQB1 locus.[5] The amplification was conducted in the 9600 Thermal Cycler (Perkin-Elmer). Hybridization and detection were performed by adding the amplified DNA to strips containing 18 immobilized sequence specific oligonucleotide primers (SSOP) for DRB1 and DQB1. Each biotinylated DNA was denatured and hybridized to an individual strip for 30 min at 50°C in 4× SSPE/0.5% SDS. The wash step for 15 min at 50°C in 1× SSPE/0.1% SDS was followed by incubation with streptavidin-HRP and a chromogenic substrate. After color development, the strips were scanned and a simple computer program assigned alleles based on the probe reactivity pattern. At the Barbara Davis Center, DNA samples were typed for the HLA-DQB1 and DQA1 using standard kits (Dynal SSP; Dynal Biotech, Ltd., Merseyside, United Kingdom). For all samples, Dynal Classic SSP DRB1*04 kit (Dynal) was used to determine the DRB1*04 sequence.

Measurement of Autoantibodies

A group of 95 first-degree relatives (87 NHWs) with the HLA-DRB1*03,DQB1*0201/DRB1*04,DQB1*0302 genotype were tested for islet autoantibodies, and 35 (including 33 NHWs) were persistently positive. All measures of autoantibodies in blood were performed in the laboratory of George Eisenbarth of the Barbara Davis Center. We used radioassays for insulin, GAD_{65}, and IA-2 autoantibodies as previously described.[19,20] Persistent islet autoimmunity was defined as presence of at least one autoantibody (IAA, GAA, or IA-2) above the 99th percentile on two or more consecutive visits and at the most recent visit. This definition is highly predictive of type 1 diabetes. As of September 2002, 21 of the 35 islet autoantibody positive and initially nondiabetic relatives who met this definition had converted to diabetes.

Statistical Analysis

All analyses were conducted in SAS version 8.3 (SAS Institute, Cary, NC). Comparisons between frequencies of DRB1*04 subtypes among T1DM patients and control subjects were done by PROC FREQ, using χ^2 test or Fisher's exact test, when appropriate, with the acceptance p level of 0.05 and no correction for multiple comparisons. The univariate odds ratios (OR) and the 95% confidence intervals (CI) were calculated using the PROC LOGISTIC to evaluate potential association between the DRB1*04 alleles and diabetes or prediabetes.

PROC LOGISTIC was also used to formally test if the association between various DRB1*04 subtypes varied by ethnicity. Mean age at diabetes onset by the DRB1*04 allele status was compared using the Kruskal-Wallis test.

TABLE 1. Distribution of DRB1*04 alleles among Colorado T1DM patients and nondiabetic healthy controls with the DRB1*03,DQB1*0201/DRB1*04,DQB1*0302 genotype

DRB1*04 allele	Non-Hispanic whites				Hispanics			
	Diabetic patients ($n = 140$)	Controls ($n = 142$)	p	OR (95% CI)	Diabetic patients ($n = 53$)	Controls ($n = 63$)	p	OR (95% CI)
0401	90 (64%)	64 (45%)	**0.0013**	**2.19 (1.36–3.54)**	7 (13%)	16 (25%)	0.11	0.45 (0.17–1.19)
0402	10 (7%)	12 (9%)	0.83	0.83 (0.35–2.00)	6 (11%)	2 (3%)	0.14	3.89 (0.75–20.1)
0403	2 (1%)	10 (7%)	**0.034**	**0.19 (0.04–0.89)**	1 (2%)	10 (16%)	**0.011**	**0.10 (0.01–0.83)**
0404	35 (25%)	44 (31%)	0.29	0.72 (0.44–1.25)	18 (34%)	15 (24%)	0.30	1.65 (0.73–3.71)
0405	2 (1%)	8 (6%)	0.10	0.24 (0.05–1.16)	17 (32%)	7 (11%)	**0.010**	**3.78 (1.43–10.0)**
0406	–	1 (1%)	–	–	–	1 (2%)	–	–
0407	1 (1%)	2 (1%)	1.00	0.50 (0.05–5.62)	4 (8%)	10 (16%)	0.25	0.43 (0.13–1.47)
Other	–	1 (1%)	–	–	–	2 (3%)	–	–

NOTE: Significant differences (at $\alpha = 0.05$) are denoted by boldface type.

RESULTS

The frequencies of HLA-DRB1*04 subtypes in T1DM cases and controls with the HLA-DRB1*03,DQB1*0201/DRB1*04,DQB1*0302 genotype are shown, by ethnicity, in FIGURE 1. Formal comparisons of these frequencies are summarized in TABLE 1. The DRB1*0403 allele was protective from diabetes both in NHWs (OR, 0.19; 95% CI, 0.04–0.89) and in Hispanics (OR, 0.10; 95% CI, 0.01–0.83). Consistent with previous reports, the *0401 allele conferred increased risk in NHWs (OR, 2.19; 95% CI, 1.36–3.54), but this was not the case in Hispanics (OR, 0.45; 95% CI, 0.17–1.19). On the other hand, DRB1*0405 (OR, 3.78; 95% CI, 1.43–10.0) conferred increased risk in Hispanics, but not in NHWs. The *0404 allele appeared to be neutral in both ethnic groups, concordant with previous findings. The risk associated with other alleles was inconclusive because of low numbers. Overall, there was no evidence for a statistically significant difference between Hispanics and NHWs in the DRB1*04 subtype associations with diabetes ($p > 0.9$).

In addition, 95 NHW nondiabetic first-degree relatives of type 1 diabetes patients were studied. Of those, 87 were NHW and, among these, 33 were persistently positive and 54 negative for islet autoantibodies to insulin, GAD65, or ICA512. The direction and strength of the association between DRB1*04 alleles and either diabetes or prediabetes were remarkably consistent (FIG. 2). This confirms that the

DRB1*04 alleles affect both the early stages of the process, initiation of autoimmunity and its progression to overt diabetes.

Among the NHW diabetic patients, the mean age of diagnosis (FIG. 3) appeared to be higher among those with the *0403 allele (16.7 years) compared with those with the *0401 (10.0 years), *0402 (8.2 years), *0404 (9.8 years), and *0405 (3.8 years). Thus, generally, the more protective the allele, the older the age at diagnosis.

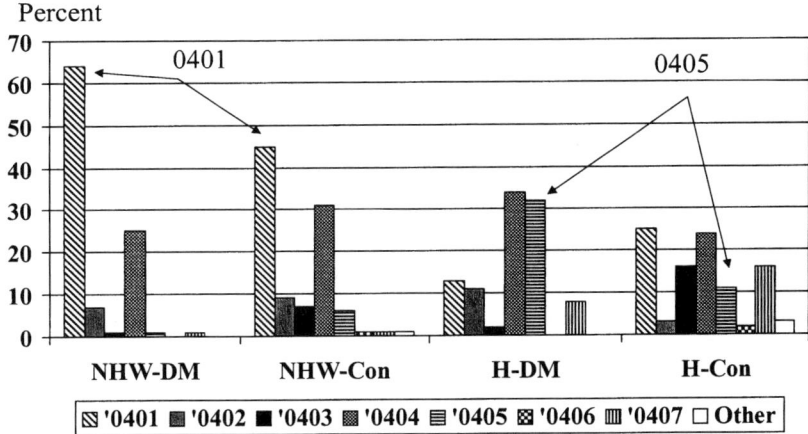

N= controls: 142 NHW and 63H /type 1 DM: 140 NHW and 53 H

FIGURE 1. HLA-DRB1*04 subtypes in T1DM patients and controls with the DR3/4-DQ2/8 genotype (NHW, non-Hispanic white; H, Hispanic).

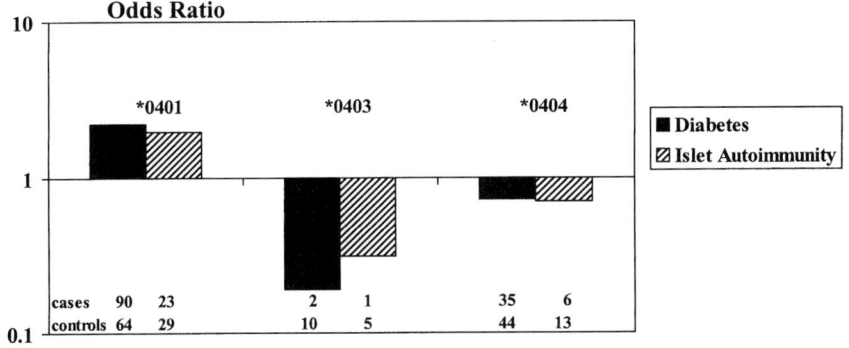

FIGURE 2. Diabetes and islet autoimmunity (persistent insulin, GAD, or IA-2 autoantibodies) are generally associated with the same DRB1*04 alleles.

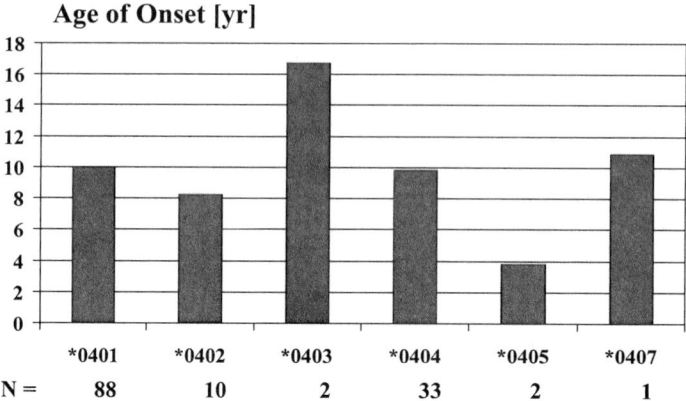

FIGURE 3. Effect of the DQB1*04 allele on the mean age of T1DM onset among children with the HLA-DRB1*03,DQB1*0201/DRB1*04,DQB1*0302 genotype (NHW children, $n = 136$).

DISCUSSION

The DRB1*04 alleles are fairly frequent in the general population (20% of Colorado residents carry at least one DRB1*04 allele) and even more frequent among diabetic children (65% of those carry at least one DRB1*04 allele). We selected individuals with the highest-risk HLA genotype of Hispanic and NHW ethnicity to evaluate previously reported associations between the DRB1*04 subtypes and T1DM. Only 2% in the general population and 30–40% of T1DM patients carry this high-risk DRB1*03,DQB1*0201/DRB1*04,DQB1*0302 genotype.

In NHWs, associations between DRB1*04 alleles and diabetes were similar to those previously reported (*0401 conferred risk, whereas *0403 was protective). The 0402 allele, previously shown to be a high-risk DRB1*04 allele, was unexpectedly not associated with diabetes in this data set. In Hispanics, *0405 allele conferred risk and *0403 was protective. Generally, the same DRB1*04 alleles were associated with development of islet autoimmunity and progression to diabetes. This is most clearly seen in the *0403 allele, which conferred protection to diabetes in both ethnic groups and was associated with an older age at diabetes diagnosis.

This is the first report on the associations between childhood diabetes and the HLA-DRB1*04 alleles in the U.S. population, outside of the multiplex family collection of the Human Biological Data Interchange.[4] In addition, there is a paucity of data on DRB1*04 allele frequencies in Hispanic populations,[21] and our preliminary data for the Hispanic population suggest intriguing similarities and differences compared with NHWs. For instance, the DRB1*0405 allele was a major risk allele in Hispanics (present in 32% of T1DM patients and 11% of controls), whereas it was decreased in frequency in NHWs (both in patients [1%] and controls [6%]; $p < 0.01$). Finally, to our knowledge, this is the first report documenting that the protective

TABLE 2. Prevalence of DRB1*04 alleles in diabetic children and nondiabetic controls with the HLA-DQB1*0201,DQA1*0501,DRB1*03/DQB1*0302,DQA1*0301,DRB1*04 genotype in different populations

		Frequency of specific DR*04 alleles						
		U.S.[4]	Norwegian[13]		Belgian[9]		French[11]	
	T1DM risk	Diabetics ($n = 180$)	Diabetics ($n = 191$)	Controls ($n = 235$)	Diabetics ($n = 174$)	Controls ($n = 73$)	Diabetics ($n = 92$)	Controls ($n = 9$)
0401	Increased	62%	76%	50%	70%	64%	38%	22%
0402	Increased	5%	2%	1%	9%	3%	20%	11%
0403	Lowest	–	1%	3%	–	8%	–	11%
0404	Reduced	30%	19%	44%	11%	14%	21%	56%
0405	Highest	3%	3%	1%	8%	3%	17%	–
0406	Lowest	–	–	–	–	–	–	–
0407	Reduced	–	–	–	–	7%	–	–
0408		–	–	1%	1%	1%	–	–
0410		–	–	–	1%	–	–	–

NOTE: Reported hierarchy of diabetes risk in previous studies: *0405 > *0402 > *0401 > *0404 > *0403 > *0406. The Human Biological Data Interchange data set (U.S.[4]) included diabetic patients only from multiplex families, that is, with more than one affected child.

effect of the *0403 allele extends into the earliest stages of the autoimmune process. Understanding of the structural reasons for this protective effect may yield new clues concerning design of a "diabetes vaccine".

Minor polymorphic substitutions in the peptide-binding groove of class II HLA molecules can lead to drastic variation in peptide-binding selectivity and interactions with specific T cell receptors. Several groups have attempted to develop a model based on characteristics of relevant pockets of HLA-DR and HLA-DQ molecules to explain variability in associations with T1DM.[13,22,23] Undlien et al.[13] presented a plausible hypothesis that the DRB1*0404, 0403, 0406, and perhaps 0407 confer an increasing degree of protection, possibly by binding a common protective peptide.

Note that most studies of the effect of DRB1*04 subtypes have focused on DR4/4 or DR4/X individuals and reported that the DRB1*04 subtype effect was harder to demonstrate in DR3/4 genotypes[21] (TABLE 2). Here, we report that the effect of DRB*04 subtypes can be seen even in the high-risk DR3/4 genotype in two different populations. The previously reported hierarchy of diabetes risk associated with DRB1*04 subtypes, 0405 > 0402 > 0401 > 0404 > 0403 > 0406, generally was confirmed in our study.

This research would have been greatly aided by the inclusion of more Hispanic children as well as other U.S. ethnic groups. U.S. Hispanics are a very heterogeneous group, even within a relatively small state like Colorado. Although ethnicity was defined based on self-reports using the U.S. Census definitions, some degree of misclassification is possible because of variable perception of affiliation with this ethnic group.

In conclusion, the HLA-DRB1*0403 allele confers protection from islet autoimmunity and progression to diabetes. The protective association of the *0403 allele merits further study of the differences in the structure of the peptide-binding domain and deducted structure of peptides that are bound. Hispanics, compared with NHWs with the DRB1*03,DQB1*0201/DRB1*04,DQB1*0302 genotype, appeared to differ only slightly in the associations between different DRB1*04 alleles and diabetes. Further studies of a larger group of Hispanics from Colorado and other areas are needed to validate this observation.

ACKNOWLEDGMENTS

This research was supported by the National Institute of Diabetes and Digestive and Kidney Diseases (Grant Nos. DK-32493, DK-32083, and DK-57516) and the Children's Diabetes Foundation.

REFERENCES

1. TODD, J.A. 1995. Genetic analysis of type 1 diabetes using whole genome approaches. Proc. Natl. Acad. Sci. USA **92:** 8560–8565.
2. COX, N.J. et al. 2001. Seven regions of the genome show evidence of linkage to type 1 diabetes in a consensus analysis of 767 multiplex families. Am. J. Hum. Genet. **69:** 820–830.
3. DAVIES, J.L. et al. 1994. A genome-wide search for human type 1 diabetes susceptibility genes. Nature **371:** 130–136.
4. NOBLE, J.A. et al. 1996. The role of HLA class II genes in insulin-dependent diabetes mellitus: molecular analysis of 180 Caucasian, multiplex families. Am. J. Hum. Genet. **59:** 1134–1148.
5. REWERS, M. et al. 1996. Newborn screening for HLA markers associated with IDDM: Diabetes Autoimmunity Study in the Young (DAISY). Diabetologia **39:** 807–812.
6. RONNINGEN, K.S. et al. 1992. HLA class II associations in insulin-dependent diabetes mellitus among blacks, Caucasoids, and Japanese. In HLA 1991: Proceedings of the 11th International Histocompatibility Workshop and Conference (Yokohama, Japan), pp. 713–722. Oxford University Press. London/New York.
7. VAN DER AUWERA, B. et al. 1995. Genetic susceptibility for insulin-dependent diabetes mellitus in Caucasians revisited: the importance of diabetes registries in disclosing interactions between HLA-DQ– and insulin gene–linked risk—Belgian Diabetes Registry. J. Clin. Endocrinol. Metab. **80:** 2567–2573.
8. ERLICH, H.A. et al. 1990. HLA-DQb sequence polymorphism and genetic susceptibility to IDDM. Diabetes **39:** 96–103.
9. VAN DER AUWERA, B. et al. 1995. DRB1*0403 protects against IDDM in Caucasians with the high-risk heterozygous DQA1*0301-DQB1*0302/DQA1*0501-DQB1*0201 genotype: Belgian Diabetes Registry. Diabetes **44:** 527–530.
10. CUCCA, F. et al. 1995. The distribution of DR4 haplotypes in Sardinia suggests a primary association of type I diabetes with DRB1 and DQB1 loci. Hum. Immunol. **43:** 301–308.
11. HARFOUCH-HAMMOUD, E. et al. 1996. Contribution of DRB1*04 variants to predisposition to or protection from insulin dependent diabetes mellitus is independent of dq. J. Autoimmun. **9:** 411–414.
12. YASUNAGA, S. et al. 1996. Different contribution of HLA-DR and -DQ genes in susceptibility and resistance to insulin-dependent diabetes mellitus (IDDM). Tissue Antigens **47:** 37–48.
13. UNDLIEN, D.E. et al. 1997. HLA-encoded genetic predisposition in IDDM: DR4 subtypes may be associated with different degrees of protection. Diabetes **46:** 143–149.

14. NEJENTSEV, S. et al. 1997. The effect of HLA-B allele on the IDDM risk defined by DRB1*04 subtypes and DQB1*0302. Diabetes **46:** 1888–1892.
15. ROEP, B.O. et al. 1999. HLA-DRB1*0403 is associated with dominant protection against IDDM in the general Dutch population and subjects with high-risk DQA1*0301-DQB1*0302/DQA1*0501-DQB1*0201 genotype. Tissue Antigens **54:** 88–90.
16. QIU, C. et al. 1997. Study on the association of HLA-DR4 with IDDM susceptibility in a Chinese population. Zhongguo Yi Xue Ke Xue Yuan Xue Bao **19:** 54–59.
17. BUGAWAN, T.L. et al. 2002. The association of specific HLA class I and II alleles with type 1 diabetes among Filipinos. Tissue Antigens **59:** 452–469.
18. ABID, K.H. et al. 2002. HLA polymorphism in type 1 diabetes Tunisians. Ann. Genet. **45:** 45–50.
19. YU, L. et al. 2000. Early expression of anti-insulin autoantibodies of humans and the NOD mouse: evidence for early determination of subsequent diabetes. Proc. Natl. Acad. Sci. USA **97:** 1701–1706.
20. YU, L. et al. 2001. Expression of GAD65 or ICA512(IA-2) autoantibodies amongst cytoplasmic ICA positive relatives is associated with eligibility for DPT-1. Diabetes **50:** 1735–1740.
21. ERLICH, H.A. et al. 1993. HLA class II alleles and susceptibility and resistance to insulin dependent diabetes mellitus in Mexican-American families. Nat. Genet. **3:** 358–364.
22. DJOULAH, S. et al. 1999. A new predictive model for insulin-dependent diabetes mellitus susceptibility based on combinations of molecular HLA-DRB1 and HLA-DQB1 pockets. Tissue Antigens **54:** 341–348.
23. SANJEEVI, C.B. et al. 2002. The combination of several polymorphic amino acid residues in the DQα and DQβ chains forms a domain structure pattern and is associated with insulin-dependent diabetes mellitus. Ann. N.Y. Acad. Sci. **958:** 362–375.

MIC-A Genotypes 4/5.1 and 9/9 Are Positively Associated with Type 1 Diabetes Mellitus in Brazilian Population

VALERIA TICA,[a,b] LIENE NIKITINA-ZAKE,[b] EDUARDO DONADI,[c] AND CARANI B. SANJEEVI[b]

[a]*Department of Biochemistry, Faculty of Biology, University of Bucharest, Bucharest, Romania*

[b]*Department of Molecular Medicine, Karolinska Hospital, Stockholm, Sweden*

[c]*Department of Medicine, University of São Paulo, Ribeirão Prêto, SP, Brazil*

ABSTRACT: The aim of our study was to evaluate the frequencies of MIC-A alleles and genotypes in Brazilian patients with type 1 diabetes mellitus (T1DM) and healthy controls. MHC class I chain–related gene-A (MIC-A) has been shown to be associated with susceptibility to T1DM in different populations. We analyzed the DNA samples from 86 patients and 201 healthy controls for MIC-A by PCR amplification, and fragment sizes were determined in an ABI prism DNA sequencer. We found increased frequencies of two genotypes, MIC-A 4/5.1 ($pc = 0.006$; OR, 6.1) and 9/9 ($pc = 0.045$; OR, 5.75), in our patients (mean diagnosis age, 11.70 years; SD, 8.86; mean age, 20.44 years; SD, 12.17) compared with the controls (median age, 26.41 years; SD, 8.87).

KEYWORDS: T1DM; MIC-A; genotypes

INTRODUCTION

Type 1 diabetes mellitus (T1DM) is an autoimmune disorder with a strong genetic component. Located in human major histocompatibility complex (MHC) class I region on the short arm of chromosome 6, between TNF cluster and HLA-B genes, the MIC-A gene is extremely polymorphic.[1] It has a microsatellite in exon 5, encoding the transmembrane (TM) part of the protein. Protein consists of three extracellular domains (α1–3), a transmembrane segment, and a cytoplasmic tail, each coded by a separate exon. Microsatellite polymorphism in the TM region consists of various numbers of GCT repeats. Alleles have been denominated according to the number of repeats (A4, A5, A5.1, A6, and A9). Allele 5.1 has an additional insertion of G (GGCT).[2] The association of MIC-A microsatellite polymorphism with T1DM has been reported by many studies, making this gene one of the candidate genes for susceptibility to T1DM.[3–5] MIC-A molecule is expressed during cell stress (e.g., viral

Address for correspondence: Dr. C. B. Sanjeevi, Department of Molecular Medicine, Karolinska Institute, Karolinska Hospital, CMM, L8:00, S-17176 Stockholm, Sweden. Voice: +46-8-51776254; fax: +46-8-51776179.
sanjeevi.carani@molmed.ki.se

TABLE 1. MIC-A allele and genotype frequencies in Brazilian T1DM and healthy subjects

MIC-A	Controls ($n = 201$)	Patients ($n = 86$)
A4 (179 bp)[a]	39 (19.4%)	26 (30.2%)
A5 (182 bp)	46 (22.9%)	16 (18.6%)
A5.1 (183 bp)	93 (46.3%)	44 (51.2%)
A6 (185 bp)	99 (49.3%)	43 (50.0%)
A9 (194 bp)	75 (37.3%)	29 (33.7%)
4*4	2 (1.0%)	1 (1.2%)
4*5	5 (2.5%)	1 (1.2%)
4*5.1[b]	5 (2.5%)	12 (14.0%)
4*6	15 (7.5%)	7 (8.1%)
4*9	12 (6.0%)	5 (5.8%)
5*5	6 (3.0%)	1 (1.2%)
5*5.1	6 (3.0%)	7 (8.1%)
5*6	15 (7.5%)	5 (5.8%)
5*9	14 (7.0%)	2 (2.3%)
5.1*5.1	20 (10.0%)	4 (4.7%)
5.1*6	34 (16.9%)	12 (14.0%)
5.1*9	28 (13.9%)	9 (10.5%)
6*6	18 (9.0%)	7 (8.1%)
6*9	17 (8.5%)	12 (14.0%)
9*9[c]	4 (2.0%)	9 (10.5%)

[a]MIC-A A4: $p = 0.0639$; OR, 1.8; 95% CI, 1–3.2.
[b]MIC-A 4/5.1: $p = 0.0004$; $pc = 0.006$; OR, 6.1; 95% CI, 2.16–18.6.
[c]MIC-A 9/9: $p = 0.003$; $pc = 0.045$; OR, 5.75; 95% CI, 1.7–19.2.

infection, heat shock) on cells of epithelial origin, gastrointestinal epithelium, keratinocytes, endothelial cells, and monocytes.[1,6,7] MIC-A protein binds to NKG2D receptor on γ/δ T cells, CD8+ α/β T cells, and natural killer (NK) cells and activates them.[8] Unlike MHC class I molecules, it is not associated with β-2-microglobulin.

MATERIALS AND METHODS

Eighty-six patients with diagnosed T1DM and 201 healthy controls from Brazil participated in the study. Informed consent was obtained from all subjects. Genomic DNA was extracted from peripheral blood mononuclear cells using a salting-out procedure.

MIC-A Genotyping

To analyze microsatellite repeat polymorphism in the TM region of the MIC-A gene (exon 5), we used two PCR primers: 5′-CCTTTTTTAGGGAAAGTGC as the forward primer and 5′-CCTTACCATCTCCAGAAACTGC as the reverse primer. The reverse primer was labeled at the 5′-end with the fluorescent reagent HEX or 6-FAM. Microsatellite repeat polymorphism of the MIC-A gene was typed by PCR-based fragment length analysis. The PCR mixture contained 10× PCR buffer, 15 mM $MgCl_2$, 10 mM dNTP, 20 μM primers, and 5 U/mL Taq polymerase. PCR amplification was conducted in a programmable thermal controller. Allele sizes were identified using Perkin-Elmer ABI 373 DNA sequencer and analyzed with Genotyper and Genescan software.

Statistical Analysis

Differences in frequency of the alleles and genotypes between patients and controls were done by a χ^2 test or Fisher's exact probability test when applicable. The p values were corrected (pc) for the number of comparisons made; pc values less than 0.05 were considered as significant.

RESULTS AND DISCUSSION

In this study, the frequencies of alleles A4 (179 bp), A5 (182 bp), A5.1 (183 bp), A6 (185 bp), and A9 (194 bp) were, accordingly, 30.2%, 18.6%, 51.2%, 50.0%, and 33.7% in patients and 19.4%, 22.9%, 46.3%, 49.3%, and 37.3% in control subjects. We looked at the genotypes and found that MIC-A 4/5.1 ($pc = 0.006$; OR, 6.1) and MIC-A 9/9 ($pc = 0.045$; OR, 5.75) were positively associated with the disease in our study material. In our study, we did not find association of MIC-A alleles with the disease. As shown in TABLE 1, allele 4 was nonsignificantly increased in patients (30.2%) compared with controls (19.4%).

This suggests that polymorphism of this gene may be important for development of T1DM, and the MIC-A susceptibility can be different in different populations.

ACKNOWLEDGMENTS

This study was supported by grants from the Swedish Medical Research Council (K2001-16X-12532-04B), Karolinska Institute, Novo Nordisk Fond, Svenska Diabetes Förbundet, Barn Diabetes Fonden, and Åke Wiberg Stiftelse. C. B. Sanjeevi is supported by a Swedish MFR's position (K2001-72P-13149-03C).

REFERENCES

1. BAHRAM, S., M. BRESNAHAN, D.E. GERAGHTY & T. SPIES. 1994. A second lineage of mammalian major histocompatibility complex class I genes. Eur. J. Immunogenet. **26:** 239–241.
2. OTA, M., Y. KATSUYAMA, N. MIZUKI et al. 1997. Trinucleotide repeat polymorphism within exon 5 of the MICA gene (MHC class I chain–related gene A): allele frequency data in the nine population groups Japanese, Northern Han, Hui, Uygur, Kazakhstan, Iranian, Saudi Arabian, Greek, and Italian. Tissue Antigens **49:** 448–454.
3. GAMBELUNGHE, G., M. GHADERI, A. COSENTINO et al. 2000. Association of MHC class I chain–related A (MIC-A) gene polymorphism with type I diabetes. Diabetologia **43:** 507–514.

4. PARK, Y., H. LEE, C.B. SANJEEVI & G.S. EISENBARTH. 2001. MICA polymorphism is associated with type 1 diabetes in the Korean population. Diabetes Care **24:** 33–38.
5. KAWABATA, Y., H. IKEGAMI, Y. KAWAGUCHI *et al.* 2000. Age-related association of MHC class I chain–related gene A (MICA) with type 1 (insulin-dependent) diabetes mellitus. Hum. Immunol. **61:** 624–629.
6. GROH, V., A. STEINLE, S. BAUER & T. SPIES. 1998. Recognition of stress-induced MHC molecules by intestinal epithelial gamma, delta T cells. Science **279:** 1737–1740.
7. ZWIRNER, N.W., K. DOLE & P. STASTNY. 1999. Differential surface expression of MICA by endothelial cells, fibroblasts, keratinocytes, and monocytes. Hum. Immunol. **60:** 323–330.
8. BAUER, S., V. GROH, J. WU *et al.* 1999. Activation of NK cells and T cells by NKG2D, a receptor for stress-inducible MICA. Science **285:** 727–729.

HLA-DRB1 and *MICA* in Autoimmunity

Common Associated Alleles in Autoimmune Disorders

J. RAMÓN BILBAO,[a,b] AINHOA MARTÍN-PAGOLA,[a]
GUIOMAR PÉREZ DE NANCLARES,[a] BEGOÑA CALVO,[a]
JUAN CARLOS VITORIA,[c,d] FEDERICO VÁZQUEZ,[a] AND LUIS CASTAÑO[a,d]

[a]*Endocrinology and Diabetes Research Group, Hospital de Cruces, Barakaldo, Basque Country, Spain*

[b]*Department of Nursing, University of the Basque Country, Bilbao, Basque Country, Spain*

[c]*Pediatric Gastroenterology Unit, Hospital de Cruces, Barakaldo, Basque Country, Spain*

[d]*Department of Pediatrics, University of the Basque Country, Bilbao, Basque Country, Spain*

ABSTRACT: Autoimmune disorders such as type 1 diabetes (T1DM), celiac disease (CD), and Addison's disease (ADD) develop in individuals with genetic susceptibility that are exposed to environmental triggering factors not completely defined. Patients with an autoimmune disease (and their relatives) are at increased risk of developing another disorder, and this might be caused by a common genetic origin of autoimmunity; for example, HLA class II region in 6p21 shows a very strong association with most diseases. The aim of this study was to determine whether shared susceptibility markers extend from the central (DRB1) through the telomeric (*MICA*) HLA region. We analyzed three independent sets of families with one autoimmune disease, T1DM, CD, or ADD, and genotyped them for HLA-DRB1 and for the exon 5 GCT polymorphism of *MICA*. For HLA-DRB1, allele DRB1*0301 was the only one associated with risk for all three diseases; in the case of *MICA*, allele A9 was found to be the common protective allele. Haplotype analysis shows that haplotype A5.1-DRB1*0301 confers risk to autoimmunity. Our results show that there are common risk and protection alleles in both loci, suggesting a core of genetic association with autoimmunity (HLA-DRB1*0301 risk; A9 protection) that could be modulated by other alleles/loci or environmental factors toward one or another disease. Some alleles are part of conserved haplotypes (A5.1-DR3, A5.1-DR2), whereas others seem to have independent effect (A9) and support the idea of two independent loci in this region.

KEYWORDS: type 1 diabetes (T1DM); celiac disease (CD); Addison's disease (ADD); autoimmune disorder; HLA-DRB1; *MICA*; haplotype

---

Address for correspondence: Luis Castaño, M.D., Ph.D., Endocrinology and Diabetes Research Group, Hospital de Cruces, Plaza de Cruces s/n, Barakaldo, E48903 Bizkaia, Spain. Voice: +34-94-600-6376; fax: +34-94-600-6076.
lcastano@hcru.osakidetza.net

Ann. N.Y. Acad. Sci. 1005: 314–318 (2003). © 2003 New York Academy of Sciences.
doi: 10.1196/annals.1288.049

INTRODUCTION

Autoimmune diseases result from a complex interaction between genetic susceptibility and environmental triggering factors that are not completely defined. Patients suffering from an autoimmune disorder such as type 1 diabetes (T1DM), celiac disease (CD), or autoimmune Addison's disease (ADD) are at increased risk of developing another autoimmune disease. For instance, among T1DM patients, approximately 7% also have CD[1] and almost 2% develop adrenal autoantibodies.[2] This increased risk could be caused by genetic susceptibility alleles that are common to different autoimmune disorders. In this sense, several polymorphic loci in the HLA region on chromosome 6p21, including HLA-DRB1 and *MICA*, have been linked to and associated with risk to all three autoimmune diseases.[3-5] It could be that there exists a major determinant for autoimmunity in the HLA region and that environmental factors and/or other genetic loci are responsible for deciding which particular organ will be affected.

The aim of the current study was to determine whether genetic susceptibility markers shared by three different autoimmune diseases (T1DM, CD, and ADD) extend from the central (HLA-DRB1) through the telomeric MHC region (*MICA*).

PATIENTS AND METHODS

We analyzed 70 families with autoimmune T1DM (81 patients [42 males, 39 females; mean age at diagnosis, 14.5 ± 9.9 years] and 239 first-degree relatives), 41 families with CD (42 celiac patients [23 males, 19 females; diagnosed at 3.98 ± 3.94 years] and 85 first-degree relatives), and 29 families with ADD (31 patients with autoantibodies against 21-hydroxylase [11 males, 20 females; diagnosed at 33.8 ± 12.14 years] and 53 first-degree relatives). All studies were performed after informed consent was obtained from the subjects or their parents.

Genomic DNA was extracted by standard procedures. HLA-DRB1 was genotyped by reverse hybridization with immobilized oligonucleotides (Dynal RELI SSO HLA-DRB Test; Dynal Biotech, Bromborough, United Kingdom) and SSP (Dynal Resolve DRB1*03/*11/*13) to resolve DRB1*03/*11/*13 ambiguities. Exon 5 of the *MICA* gene was amplified using fluorescent PCR, and GCT triplet repeat units were determined on an ABI sequencing machine, as previously described.[6] Evaluation of Hardy-Weinberg equilibrium (HWE) in the parental generation of each disease group was done comparing expected and observed genotypes in parents with the exact probability test included in the Web version of the *Genepop* program.[7] For disease association studies, family alleles were classified into *disease* or *nondisease* alleles, according to the affected family-based controls (AFBAC) approach.[8] Allele frequencies were compared in 2×2 tables with either χ^2 or Fisher's exact test, and two-tailed probability values (p) were corrected for multiple testing, according to the number of variants in each locus and to the number of groups analyzed. Relative risk values (RR) and 95% confidence intervals (CI) also were calculated. The presence of allelic association within haplotypes was determined in parental gametes using the Web versions of *Genepop* and *LinkDos* software programs.[7,9]

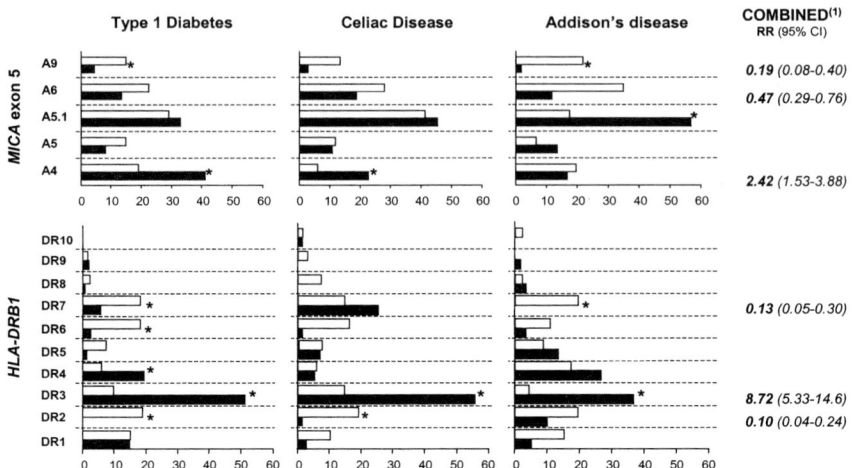

FIGURE 1. Frequency distribution (%) of *MICA* exon 5 and HLA-DRB1 alleles among patients (*black bars*) and AFBAC (*white bars*) in the three disease family sets, and relative risk (RR) values for the combined analysis of all families with autoimmune disease. Asterisks indicate *p* values lower than 0.05 after applying Bonferroni correction for the number of tests (correction factor: 5 for *MICA* and 10 for HLA-DRB1). [1]RR values are shown only for those alleles that showed significant association ($p < 0.05$) after correcting for multiple testing (correction factor: 15 for *MICA* and 30 for HLA-DRB1).

RESULTS AND DISCUSSION

In this study, we have investigated the contribution of genes HLA-DRB1 and *MICA* to the genetic susceptibility to three autoimmune diseases (T1DM, CD, and ADD) in three sets of families with one of each disease. Genotype analysis of both genes identified alleles associated with risk for or protection from disease in all three autoimmune groups (FIG. 1). In the case of HLA-DRB1, allele DRB1*0301 confers the highest risk for all three diseases (RR values of 9.42, 7.34, and 12.74 for T1DM, CD, and ADD, respectively) and is the only allele significantly associated with autoimmunity in the combined analysis. No other disease-associated HLA-DRB1 variant is common to more than one disease. When protective alleles are analyzed, DRB1*1501 is significantly less frequent among T1DM and CD alleles, but this is not so among ADD patients, whereas protection by DRB1*07 is shared only by T1DM and ADD. Combined analysis shows that both DR subtypes confer overall protection from autoimmunity, represented by the three diseases studied in this report.

Regarding the *MICA* exon 5 polymorphism, allele A4 was significantly increased among T1DM and CD alleles, but not so among ADD alleles, where allele A5.1 was found to be the major risk variant, in accordance with previous reports.[5] Although this could indicate that susceptibility alleles might be different between T1DM and CD on one side and ADD on the other side, haplotype analysis shows that, in fact, the A5.1-containing haplotype also includes HLA-DRB1*0301 and that this haplo-

TABLE 1. *MICA*-DRB1 haplotype analysis

	Haplotype	Disease association		Linkage disequilibrium		
		RR (95% CI)	p_c	n	D'	p
T1DM	A5.1-DRB1*0301	3.85 (1.35–13.5)	0.0150	25	−0.0375	ns
	A4-DRB1*0301	6.56 (3.39–25.5)	$<10^{-6}$	48	0.6241	0.0045
	A5.1-DRB1*1501	0.00 (0.00–0.6)	$<10^{-6}$	14	0.6609	0.0430
CD	A5.1-DRB1*0301	4.62 (1.75–13.6)	0.0006	33	0.3533	0.0003
	A4-DRB1*0301	5.70 (1.2–54.9)	$<10^{-6}$	13	0.4067	0.0080
	A6-DRB1*077	5.70 (1.2–54.9)	$<10^{-6}$	14	0.2817	0.0017
ADD	A5.1-DRB1*0301	13.70 (1.9–591.7)	0.0020*	15	0.3810	0.0037

NOTE: For T1DM and CD, only haplotypes significantly associated with disease risk or protection after correction for multiple testing (correction factor: 38) are shown; ns, not significant; *nominal p value.

type is associated with increased risk for all three autoimmune diseases (TABLE 1). Neutrality of A5.1 in both T1DM and CD is, in fact, caused by the presence of a protective A5.1-DRB1*1501 haplotype that is not protective in the case of ADD.

Our study also identified allele A9 as universally protective from autoimmunity, being less frequent among disease alleles in the three groups of families. Moreover, allele A9 does not seem to be in linkage disequilibrium with any HLA-DRB1 allele, suggesting that *MICA* (or another linked gene) has a role in contributing to or modulating genetic susceptibility to autoimmunity. In summary, our results show that different autoimmune diseases share at least some genetic determinants in the MHC region, suggesting that these conditions might have a common major component and that secondary factors, both genetic and environmental, are responsible for driving the autoimmune response against different organs.

ACKNOWLEDGMENTS

J. R. Bilbao is an FIS researcher supported by the Spanish Ministry of Health (Fellowship No. 99/3076). This work was partially funded by Grant Nos. RGDM-G03/212 and RCMN-C03/08 from the Instituto de Salud Carlos III, Madrid, Spain.

REFERENCES

1. VITORIA, J.C. et al. 1998. Association of insulin-dependent diabetes mellitus and celiac disease: a study based on serologic markers. J. Pediatr. Gastroenterol. Nutr. **27:** 47–52.
2. KUKREJA, A. et al. 1999. Autoimmunity and diabetes. J. Clin. Endocrinol. Metab. **84:** 4371–4378.
3. BILBAO, J.R. et al. 2002. HLA-DRB1 and MHC class 1 chain–related A (*MICA*) haplotypes in Basque families with celiac disease. Tissue Antigens **60:** 71–76.
4. GAMBELUNGHE, G. et al. 2000. Association of MHC class I chain–related A (MIC-A) gene polymorphism with type 1 diabetes. Diabetologia **43:** 507–514.

5. GAMBELUNGHE, G. *et al.* 1999. Microsatellite polymorphism of the MHC class I chain–related (MIC-A and MIC-B) genes marks the risk for autoimmune Addison's disease. J. Clin. Endocrinol. Metab. **84:** 3701–3707.
6. BILBAO, J.R. *et al.* 2002. Contribution of *MICA* polymorphism to type 1 diabetes in Basques. Ann. N.Y. Acad. Sci. **958:** 321–324.
7. RAYMOND, M. *et al.* 1995. GENEPOP (version 1.2): population genetics software from exact tests and ecumenicism. J. Hered. **86:** 248–249.
8. THOMSON, G. *et al.* 1995. Mapping disease genes: family-based association studies. Am. J. Hum. Genet. **57:** 487–498.
9. GARNIER-GERE, P. *et al.* 1992. A computer program for testing pairwise linkage disequilibria in subdivided populations. J. Hered. **83:** 239.

5′-Insulin Gene VNTR Polymorphism Is Specific for Type 1 Diabetes

No Association with Celiac or Addison's Disease

GUIOMAR PÉREZ DE NANCLARES,[a] J. RAMÓN BILBAO,[a,b] BEGOÑA CALVO,[a] JUAN CARLOS VITORIA,[c,d] FEDERICO VÁZQUEZ,[a] AND LUIS CASTAÑO[a,d]

[a]*Endocrinology and Diabetes Research Unit, Hospital de Cruces, Barakaldo, Basque Country, Spain*

[b]*Department of Nursing, University of the Basque Country, Bilbao, Basque Country, Spain*

[c]*Pediatric Gastroenterology Unit, Hospital de Cruces, Barakaldo, Basque Country, Spain*

[d]*Department of Pediatrics, University of the Basque Country, Bilbao, Basque Country, Spain*

ABSTRACT: The VNTR region located at the 5′-end of the insulin gene on chromosome 11p15.5 is linked to susceptibility to type 1 diabetes mellitus (T1DM), and class I alleles have been associated with increased risk of disease, whereas class III alleles are considered to be protective. Although a potential effect on the expression level of thymic insulin and a consequent abnormal tolerance have been proposed as an explanation, it is still not clear whether the association is specific for T1DM or whether it is shared by other autoimmune disorders. To investigate the contribution of *INS*-VNTR to the genetic susceptibility to autoimmune disorders, we analyzed 102 autoantibody-positive T1DM patients, 59 patients with celiac disease (CD), and 57 patients with Addison's disease (ADD), as well as 111 unrelated healthy individuals from the general population. When analyzing the results, class I allele frequencies were 85.8% in the T1DM group, 77% among CD patients, 71% in the ADD group, and 76.1% in the general population. Association with increased risk was seen only in the T1DM group ($pc = 0.015$). Risk to T1DM was associated with the class I/class I homozygous genotype (RR, 1.92; 95% CI, 1.03–3.6). In conclusion, *INS*-VNTR does not seem to be involved in the susceptibility to autoimmune diseases other than T1DM and can be considered a diabetes-specific locus.

KEYWORDS: type 1 diabetes mellitus; allele; autoimmune disorder; *INS*-VNTR

INTRODUCTION

The association of type 1 diabetes (T1DM) with other autoimmune diseases such as celiac disease (CD) or Addison's disease (ADD) has been known for some time.

Address for correspondence: Luis Castaño, M.D., Ph.D., Endocrinology and Diabetes Research Group, Hospital de Cruces, Plaza de Cruces s/n, Cruces-Barakaldo E48903, Bizkaia, Basque Country, Spain. Voice: +34-94-600-6376; fax: +34-94-600-6076.
lcastano@hcru.osakidetza.net

In fact, these three disorders share several common genetic characteristics, and evidence has been accumulated to implicate several genes from the HLA class II region on chromosome 6p21.3, which is considered the major genetic contributor to risk of all three diseases. Nevertheless, risk alleles that are also present in the healthy population and several other genes on 6p21 (HLA.DPB1, TAP1, HSP70, *MIC-A*) and elsewhere in the genome (*CTLA-4/CD28* gene region in 2q33) have been associated with these three diseases too, but these findings are not consistent in all populations.[1,2]

INS-VNTR is a polymorphic variable number of tandem repeats located at the 5'-upstream region of the human insulin gene on chromosome 11p15.5. Short VNTR alleles (class I) are positively associated with T1DM, whereas long alleles (class III) are thought to be protective.[3] More recent reports have indicated allele-specific effects on the risk of the disease according to the size or even the sequence of the consensus repeat.[3,4]

The putative role of the *INS*-VNTR in the pathogenesis of T1DM is based on the hypothesis that there is a mechanism for allele-specific tolerance induction in the thymus, which could determine susceptibility to develop autoimmunity against the insulin protein and subsequently risk to develop T1DM. Indeed, class I alleles have been associated with a lower expression level of insulin in the thymus, which could avoid the destruction of insulin-specific autoreactive T cells, whereas class III alleles generate two- to threefold increased transcription levels, which could explain their dominant protective effect.[5,6]

The aim of this study was to determine whether the association of *INS*-VNTR is specific for T1DM or whether it plays a role in the development of other autoimmune diseases.

METHODS

Patients and Controls

We analyzed 102 patients with autoimmune T1DM (45 females, 57 males; mean age at diagnosis, 11.92 ± 7.03 years), 59 CD patients (34 females, 25 males; mean age, 3.16 ± 3.51 years), and a group of 57 patients (39 females, 18 males; mean age, 33.78 ± 12.1 years) with autoimmune ADD (positive for 21-hydroxylase autoantibodies). We also studied 111 unrelated individuals without personal or familiar history of autoimmunity (44 females, 67 males).

INS-VNTR typing was performed as previously described,[7] except that, for allele class assignment, amplification products were loaded onto a 1.5% agarose-TAE gel and run at room temperature and 100-V constant setting. Bands were detected by ethidium bromide staining of the gel.

Statistical Analysis

Evaluation of Hardy-Weinberg equilibrium was conducted comparing expected and observed genotypes with the exact probability test included in the Web version of the *Genepop* program.[8] The χ^2 and Fisher's exact tests were used for statistical comparisons of the case-control study. Only two-tailed p values are reported.

TABLE 1. Distribution of the *INS*-VNTR genotypes in the four populations studied

	T1DM (n = 102)	CD (n = 59)	ADD (n = 57)	CT (n = 111)
Class I/I	74.51%	59.32%	54.39%	60.36%
Class I/II	0%	0%	0%	0.90%
Class I/III	22.55%	35.59%	33.33%	31.53%
Class II/III	0%	0%	1.75%	0%
Class III/III	2.94%	5.08%	10.53%	7.21%

NOTE: T1DM, type 1 diabetes; CD, celiac disease; ADD, Addison's disease; CT, general population.

RESULTS AND DISCUSSION

T1DM, CD, and ADD are three autoimmune disorders that share genetic determinants including several HLA class II gene variants (e.g., HLA-DRB1*03-DQ2 haplotype). More recently, another gene in the class I region, *MIC-A*, has been described as associated with these diseases in an HLA-independent manner, and other non-HLA genes, such as the *CTLA-4/CD28* region, have been implicated in the pathogenesis of these three diseases, although results are somewhat controversial.[1,2] All these results could support some sort of common genetic origin of different autoimmune diseases, with environmental factors (and other genes) responsible for the specificity of the target organ. We analyzed the *INS*-VNTR locus, already known to be involved in the pathogenesis of type 1 diabetes, in 102 T1DM, 59 CD, and 57 ADD patients, as well as 111 control subjects of the same ethnic origin, to resolve whether it plays a general role in the development of autoimmunity or, on the contrary, is specific for T1DM.

INS-VNTR analysis allowed the characterization of class I, II, and III alleles and, among the 329 individuals studied, intermediate-sized class II alleles were shown to be very rare (2 heterozygous individuals). There was a significantly higher prevalence of class I alleles (85.78%) among diabetic patients versus control subjects (76.1%; $p < 0.01$), confirming the association between *INS*-VNTR class I alleles and risk of T1DM. No significant deviation from the healthy population was observed in the CD group (77.1%) or among ADD patients (71.1%). Regarding genotype distribution (TABLE 1), class I/I homozygosity is increased among diabetic patients (74.5% vs. 60.3% in the general population), conferring a relative risk (RR) of 1.92 (95% CI, 1.03–3.6). Again, no differences were observed between ADD or CD patients and the general population.

As in other Caucasoid populations, our study confirms association between class I alleles of the *INS*-VNTR polymorphism and T1DM.[3,9] Because the class I category compiles multiple alleles, some of which have been shown to be associated with protection instead of risk,[9,10] we determined their exact length (FIG. 1) and identified 16 different class I alleles in T1DM individuals (range, 641–858 bp, with allele 814 the most frequent variant [18.14%]), 15 in patients with CD (641–843 bp, alleles 814 and 843 being present in 14.41% of the samples), and 14 variants among ADD patients (655–843 bp, with allele 786 as the major allele, present in 14.91%). We did

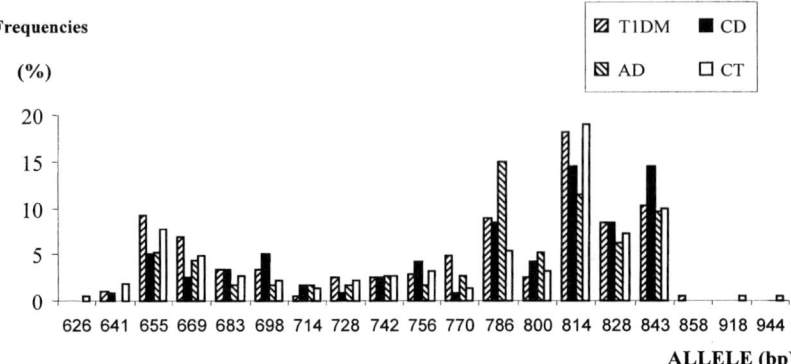

FIGURE 1. Distribution of class I subtypes in the four groups. Frequencies are expressed in percentages. T1DM, type 1 diabetes; CD, celiac disease; AD, Addison's disease; CT, general population.

not observe any allele-specific association with any of the diseases, in contrast with what others have observed for T1DM.[9,10]

On the other hand, no association of this locus with either CD or ADD has been observed, supporting that *INS*-VNTR plays a specific role in the pathogenesis of type 1 diabetes, but not in the susceptibility to autoimmunity in general, as in the case of other genes such as HLA-DRB1-DQB1, *CTLA-4*, and probably *MIC-A*. This specific association is in agreement with the hypothesis of *INS*-VNTR allele–mediated control of tolerance induction toward insulin (and proinsulin) in the thymus.

ACKNOWLEDGMENTS

This work has been partially funded by the Department of Education of the Basque Government (Grant No. BFI98.206 to G. Pérez de Nanclares) and by Grant Nos. RGDM-G03/212 and RCMN-C03/08 from the Instituto de Salud Carlos III, Madrid, Spain. J. R. Bilbao is an FIS Research Scientist supported by the Spanish Ministry of Health (Fellowship No. 99/3076).

REFERENCES

1. DAVIES, J.L. *et al.* 1994. A genome-wide search for human type 1 diabetes susceptibility genes. Nature **371:** 130–136.
2. HOULSTON, R.S. *et al.* 1997. Linkage analysis of candidate regions for celiac disease genes. Hum. Mol. Genet. **6:** 1335–1339.
3. BENNETT, S.T. *et al.* 1995. Susceptibility to human type 1 diabetes at IDDM2 is determined by tandem repeat variation at the insulin gene minisatellite *locus*. Nat. Genet. **9:** 284–292.
4. STEAD, J.D.H. *et al.* 2000. Allele diversity and germline mutation at the insulin minisatellite. Hum. Mol. Genet. **9:** 713–723.

5. PUGLIESE, A. et al. 1997. The insulin gene is transcribed in the human thymus and transcription levels correlated with allelic variation at the INS VNTR-IDDM2 susceptibility *locus* for type 1 diabetes. Nat. Genet. **15:** 293–297.
6. VAFIADIS, P. et al. 1997. Insulin expression in human thymus is modulated by INS VNTR alleles at the IDDM2 *locus*. Nat. Genet. **15:** 289–292.
7. CALVO, B. et al. 2000. Nonisotopic, PCR-based method for 5′ insulin gene VNTR allele class assignment. Biotechniques **29:** 944–948.
8. RAYMOND, M. & F. ROUSSET. 1995. GENEPOP (v1.2): population genetics software for exact test and ecumenicism. J. Hered. **86:** 248–249.
9. URRUTIA, I. et al. 1998. Anomalous behaviour of the 5′ insulin gene polymorphism allele 814: lack of association with type I diabetes in Basques. Diabetologia **41:** 1121–1123.
10. BENNETT, S.T. et al. 1997. Insulin VNTR allele–specific effect in type 1 diabetes depends on identity of untransmitted paternal allele. Nat. Genet. **17:** 350–352.

Nicotinamide Adenine Dinucleotide Phosphate Oxidase (NADPH Oxidase) P22 Phox C242T Gene Polymorphism in Type 1 Diabetes

SEIKO MATSUNAGA,[a] TARO MARUYAMA,[b] SATORU YAMADA,[a] YOSHIKO MOTOHASHI,[a] TOSHIKATSU SHIGIHARA,[a] AKIRA SHIMADA,[a] AND TAKAO SARUTA[a]

[a]*Department of Internal Medicine, Keio University School of Medicine, Tokyo, Japan*
[b]*Department of Internal Medicine, Saitama Social Insurance Hospital, Saitama, Japan*

ABSTRACT: Type 1 diabetes is caused by the immune-mediated destruction of insulin-secreting pancreatic β cells and is thought to be an autoimmune disease resulting from a complex interaction of genetic and environmental factors. In animal models of type 1 diabetes, macrophages and their products, superoxides, have central roles in the β cell destruction, but in humans their roles remain unclear. Nicotinamide adenine dinucleotide phosphate (NADPH) oxidase produces superoxide in macrophages, and its essential component, p22 phox, is a critical enzyme for superoxide production. The C242T polymorphism in the p22 phox coding gene has been reported to be associated with reduced oxidase activity. We therefore investigated whether the p22 phox gene polymorphism affected the susceptibility to and clinical course of type 1 diabetes. We examined 287 Japanese type 1 diabetic patients and 425 unrelated nondiabetic subjects. In addition, we allocated the diabetic patients to the following three groups: (1) acute-onset type 1 diabetes with at least one autoantibody (GADA, IA-2, IAA); (2) acute-onset type 1 diabetes without autoantibodies; and (3) slow-onset type 1 diabetes with autoantibody. We could not find a significant difference in p22 phox genotype and T allele frequency between overall type 1 diabetic patients and control subjects. Regardless of the onset pattern and autoantibody positivity of type 1 diabetes, no difference in p22 phox genotype and T allele frequency was found among the groups. In conclusion, the p22 phox C242T gene polymorphism did not affect the susceptibility to and clinical course of Japanese type 1 diabetes.

KEYWORDS: NADPH oxidase; type 1 diabetes; polymorphism; oxidative stress

INTRODUCTION

Type 1 diabetes is caused by the immune-mediated destruction of insulin-secreting pancreatic β cells and is thought to be an autoimmune disease resulting from a complex interaction of genetic and environmental factors. In animal models of type 1

Address for correspondence: Taro Maruyama, M.D., Ph.D., Department of Internal Medicine, Saitama Social Insurance Hospital, 4-9-3, Kita-urawa, Saitama-shi, Saitama 336-0002, Japan. Voice: +81-48-832-4951; fax: +81-48-833-7527.
n62383@sc.itc.keio.ac.jp

diabetes, macrophages are essential for the initiation of insulitis, and their products, superoxides, destroy the β cells.[1,2] However, the role of macrophages and superoxides in human type 1 diabetes remains unclear.

Nicotinamide adenine dinucleotide phosphate (NADPH) oxidase is the enzyme that produces superoxide in macrophages and has an essential role in innate immunity. In humans, several mutations in the NADPH oxidase genes lead to chronic granulomatous disease and inherited immunodeficiency. The p22 phox is an essential component of NADPH oxidase and is a critical enzyme for superoxide production in phagocytes. The C242T polymorphism in the p22 phox coding gene has been reported to be associated with altered oxidase activity.[3]

The aim of this study was to assess whether the p22 phox gene polymorphism affects the susceptibility to and clinical course of type 1 diabetes.

SUBJECTS AND METHODS

We studied 287 unrelated Japanese patients with type 1 diabetes and 425 unrelated nondiabetic Japanese subjects with no history of autoimmune disease. We allocated the diabetic patients to the following three groups: (1) acute-onset type 1 diabetes with at least one autoantibody (GADA, IA-2, IAA) who met the ADA criteria for type 1 diabetes (group A; $n = 135$), (2) acute-onset type 1 diabetes without autoantibodies (group B; $n = 72$), and (3) slow-onset type 1 diabetes with autoantibody (group C; $n = 80$). We defined "acute-onset" as insulin requirement within 6 months after the onset of diabetes and "slow-onset" as insulin requirement more than 12 months after the onset of diabetes. No control subject was positive for these autoantibodies.

The C242T transition polymorphism in the NADPH oxidase p22 phox gene, exon 6 region, was determined by the TaqMan polymerase chain reaction method.[4] The following primers and probes were included in the reaction: forward primer, 5'-TTC CTC CCT CCC CCA GG-3'; reverse primer, 5'-CCT GGT AAA GGG CCC GAA-3'; T allele–specific probe, 5'-Vic-ACA GAA GTA CAT GAC CG-MGB-3'; and C allele–specific probe, 5'-Fam-AGA AGC ACA TGA CCG-MGB-3'. PCR was performed with an ABI Prism 7700. The frequencies of various alleles were compared among the groups by χ^2 test. The onset age in patients with each phenotype was compared by Mann-Whitney U test. A value of $p < 0.05$ was considered significant.

RESULTS

We could not find a significant difference in p22 phox genotype and T allele frequency between overall type 1 diabetic patients and control subjects (TC + TT genotype frequency 14.6%, T allele frequency 7.8% in diabetic patients; TC + TT genotype frequency 14.6%, T allele frequency 7.8% in control subjects). Regardless of the onset pattern and autoantibody positivity, no difference in p22 phox genotype and T allele frequency was found among the groups (TABLE 1).

TABLE 1. P22 phox genotype and allele frequencies in type 1 diabetic patients analyzed according to clinical classification

	Group A	Group B	Group C	Controls
n	135	72	80	425
Autoantibody	Positive	Negative	Positive	
Onset	Acute	Acute	Slow	
Onset age (years)	32.3 ± 17.0	27.1 ± 15.4	43.5 ± 13.4	
Genotype frequencies				
CC	114 (84.4%)	64 (88.9%)	67 (83.8%)	363 (85.4%)
TC	20 (14.8%)	7 (9.7%)	12 (15.0%)	58 (13.6%)
TT	1 (0.7%)	1 (1.4%)	1 (1.3%)	4 (1.0%)
p	ns	ns	ns	
Allele frequencies				
C	248 (91.9%)	135 (93.8%)	146 (91.3%)	784 (92.2%)
T	22 (8.1%)	9 (6.2%)	14 (8.7%)	66 (7.8%)
p	ns	ns	ns	

NOTE: p versus control subjects; ns, not significant.

DISCUSSION

In animal models of type 1 diabetes, macrophages are essential for the initiation of insulitis, and the depletion of macrophages suppressed the destruction of β cells.[1] At the site of inflammation, superoxide might damage β cells, and administration of superoxide dismutase could protect islet tissue from disease recurrence when transplanted into spontaneously diabetic mice.[2] In human type 1 diabetes, the absolute requirement for macrophages in disease progression remains unclear. However, oxidative stress is reported to be present just before the onset of type 1 diabetes,[5] and polymorphism of the superoxide dismutase gene is thought to affect the susceptibility to type 1 diabetes in humans.[6]

NADPH oxidase is a multicomponent enzyme that mainly consists of p22, gp91, and p47 phox proteins and produces superoxide in macrophages. The p22 phox is an essential component of NADPH oxidase, and the C242T polymorphism in the p22 phox coding gene has been reported to be associated with altered oxidase activity.[3]

Until now, the role of NADPH oxidase in type 1 diabetes has remained unclear. In this report, we could not find a significant difference in p22 phox genotype and T allele frequency between overall type 1 diabetic patients and control subjects. Regardless of the onset pattern and autoantibody positivity, no difference was found among the groups. We concluded that the p22 phox C242T gene polymorphism did not affect the susceptibility to and clinical course of type 1 diabetes.

Recently, however, NADPH oxidase knockout mice were reported to be resistant to the induction of experimental allergic encephalomyelitis, which suggested that superoxide could activate pathogenic T cells in acquired immunity.[7] In addition, lymphocyte migration through endothelial cells was dependent on the expression of

NADPH oxidase in these cells.[8] These results suggest that altered NADPH oxidase activity would affect T cell function. Thus, it may be worth studying antigen-specific T cell function in the patients reported here.

REFERENCES

1. IHM, S.H. & J.W. YOON. 1990. Macrophages essential for development of beta-cell-specific cytotoxic effectors and insulitis in NOD mice. Diabetes **39:** 1273–1278.
2. NOMIKOS, I.N., Y. WANG & K.J. LAFFERTY. 1989. Involvement of O_2 radicals in autoimmune diabetes. Immunol. Cell Biol. **67:** 85–87.
3. GUZIK, T.J., N.E.J. WEST, E. BLACK et al. 2000. Functional effect of the C242T polymorphism in the NAD(P)H oxidase p22phox gene on vascular superoxide production in atherosclerosis. Circulation **102:** 1744–1747.
4. RANADE, K., M.S. CHANG, C.T. TING et al. 2001. High-throughput genotyping with single nucleotide polymorphisms. Genome Res. **11:** 1262–1268.
5. DOMINGUEZ, C., E. RUIZ, M. GUSSINYE et al. 1998. Oxidative stress at onset and in early stages of type 1 diabetes in children and adolescents. Diabetes Care **21:** 1736–1742.
6. POCIOT, F., K. RONNINGEN, R. BERGHOLDT et al. 1994. Genetic susceptibility markers in Danish patients with type 1 (insulin-dependent) diabetes—evidence for polygenicity in man. Autoimmunity **19:** 169–178.
7. VAN DER VEEN, R.C., T.A. DIETLIN, F.M. HOFMAN et al. 2000. Superoxide prevents nitric oxide–mediated suppression of helper T lymphocytes: decreased autoimmune encephalomyelitis in nicotinamide adenine dinucleotide phosphate oxidase knockout mice. J. Immunol. **164:** 5177–5183.
8. MATHENY, H.E., T.L. DEEM & J.M. COOK-MILLS. 2000. Lymphocyte migration through monolayers of endothelial cell lines involves VCAM-1 signaling via endothelial cell NADPH oxidase. J. Immunol. **164:** 6550–6559.

Stromal Cell-Derived Factor-1 Chemokine Gene Polymorphism Is Not Associated with Onset Age of Japanese Type 1 Diabetes

TOSHIKATSU SHIGIHARA,[a] AKIRA SHIMADA,[a] SATORU YAMADA,[a] TARO MARUYAMA,[b] HIROSHI HIROSE,[c] AND TAKAO SARUTA[a]

[a]*Department of Internal Medicine, Keio University School of Medicine, Tokyo, Japan*

[b]*Department of Internal Medicine, Saitama Social Insurance Hospital, Saitama, Japan*

[c]*Institute for Advanced Medical Research, Keio University School of Medicine, Tokyo, Japan*

ABSTRACT: Type 1 diabetes is characterized by cell-mediated autoimmune destruction of pancreatic beta cells. Although the disease shows a strong association with HLA class II alleles, other genes may influence the initiation or the rate of progression of the autoimmune process. Recently, it was reported that a polymorphism of the stromal cell-derived factor-1 (SDF-1) (a kind of chemokine) gene was associated with early onset of type 1 diabetes in Caucasians. Therefore, we examined SDF-1 gene polymorphism in Japanese type 1 diabetes in this study. We examined the SDF-1 gene polymorphism (801G→A) in 298 unrelated Japanese type 1 diabetic patients and 270 healthy subjects by the TaqMan PCR method. Allelic and genotypic frequencies of the SDF-1 A variants were similar in overall type 1 diabetic patients and healthy subjects. We then stratified the patients by their onset pattern (acute vs. slow onset) and islet-associated autoantibody positivity. However, no significant difference was found among each group of type 1 diabetes. Furthermore, unlike the previous report in "Caucasian" type 1 diabetics, the SDF-1 A variant was not associated with early onset of the disease in Japanese type 1 diabetics. The SDF-1 gene polymorphism was not associated with onset age (or onset pattern) of type 1 diabetes in Japanese. Further study is necessary to conclude whether SDF-1 gene polymorphism affects the onset age in type 1 diabetes in general.

KEYWORDS: stromal cell-derived factor-1; gene polymorphism; type 1 diabetes mellitus

INTRODUCTION

Type 1 diabetes is characterized by the destruction of pancreatic beta cells, thereby leading to insulin deficiency, and is mostly considered to be a cell-mediated autoimmune disease.[1] Type 1 diabetes is clinically heterogeneous with regard to the age of onset. Furthermore, although typical cases of type 1 diabetes are abrupt in

Address for correspondence: Toshikatsu Shigihara, M.D., Department of Internal Medicine, Keio University School of Medicine, 35 Shinanomachi, Shinjuku-ku, Tokyo 160-8582, Japan. Voice: +81-3-3353-1211 (ext. 62383); fax: +81-3-5269-3219.

sigihara@sc.itc.keio.ac.jp

onset, some cases are known to have a slow onset.[2] Susceptible genes for type 1 diabetes remain largely unidentified except major histocompatibility complex class II gene (IDDM1) and the insulin gene region (IDDM2). Genetic factors may also influence the rate of disease progression or clinical onset pattern. Some investigators have tried to reveal a genetic difference in the onset age or onset pattern of type 1 diabetes, and we recently reported that the NeuroD/BETA2 gene polymorphism is associated with acute-onset type 1 diabetes.[3]

Recently, the roles of chemokine, which promotes the migration of leukocytes into inflammatory sites and their differentiation or activation, and chemokine receptor in the pathogenesis of autoimmune diseases have been recognized.[4] Stromal cell-derived factor-1 (SDF-1) is one of the CXC chemokines and is a natural ligand for CXCR4, which is also known to be the T-tropic HIV-1 coreceptor. SDF-1 gene polymorphism has been shown to influence the course of HIV infection.[5] SDF-1 is a highly potent chemoattractant for monocytes and naïve T cells.[6] In the role of T cell migration, SDF-1 is also a costimulator of CD4+ T cells.[7] In type 1 diabetes, a recent study revealed that the SDF-1 3′A variant (801G→A in the 3′-untranslated region) was associated with early disease onset in Caucasians.[8] Therefore, in this study, we examined SDF-1 gene polymorphism in Japanese type 1 diabetes to evaluate the role of this gene in the Japanese population.

RESEARCH DESIGN AND METHODS

We studied 298 unrelated Japanese type 1 diabetic patients (mean onset age, 34.3 years) and 270 healthy control subjects. We examined autoantibodies (GADA, anti-insulinoma-associated protein-2 [IA-2], insulin autoantibody [IAA]) and then stratified the patients into the following three groups (group A, B, C). Group A consisted of patients with acute-onset diabetes with autoantibody ($n = 139$; mean onset age, 32.6 years); group B consisted of patients with acute-onset type 1 diabetes without autoantibody who also met the ADA criteria for type 1 diabetes ($n = 74$; mean onset age, 27.1 years); and group C comprised patients with slow-onset type 1 diabetes[2] ($n = 85$; mean onset age, 43.7 years) who met all of the following criteria: (1) originally diagnosed as having type 2 diabetes with no sign of ketosis at diabetes onset; (2) proven autoantibody positivity; (3) insulin treatment started more than 12 months after the diagnosis of diabetes. Insulin treatment was started when ketosis was proven or when at least two diabetologists considered that insulin treatment was necessary for survival.

This study was approved by the institutional review board, and written informed consent was obtained from all subjects.

The 801G→A transition polymorphism in the SDF-1 gene, the 3′-untranslated region, was determined by the TaqMan polymerase chain reaction method (PCR). PCR was carried out with ABI Prism 7700. HLA typing was performed by hybridization protection assay.

RESULTS

First, we compared the SDF-1 3′ genotype and allele frequencies between the overall type 1 diabetes and control groups. Among overall type 1 diabetic patients,

TABLE 1. SDF-1 genotype and allele frequencies in patients with type 1 diabetes analyzed according to clinical classification

	Group A	Group B	Group C	Controls
n	139	74	85	270
Autoantibody	Positive	Negative	Positive	
Onset pattern	Acute onset	Acute onset	Slow onset	
Onset age (years)	32.6 ± 17.1	27.1 ± 15.2	43.7 ± 13.2	
Genotype frequencies				
GG	70 (50.4%)	31 (41.9%)	42 (49.4%)	128 (47.4%)
GA	57 (41.0%)	33 (44.6%)	33 (38.8%)	107 (39.6%)
AA	12 (8.6%)	10 (13.5%)	10 (11.8%)	35 (13.0%)
p (vs. controls)	NS	NS	NS	
Allele frequencies				
G	197 (70.9%)	95 (64.2%)	117 (68.8%)	409 (67.2%)
A	81 (29.1%)	53 (35.8%)	53 (31.2%)	187 (32.8%)
p (vs. controls)	NS	NS	NS	

the SDF-1 3'A allele frequency was 31.4%, with frequencies of 41.3% and 10.7%, respectively, for the SDF-1 3'A heterozygous and homozygous genotypes. There were no significant differences between the overall type 1 diabetes and control groups (32.8%, with 39.6% heterozygous and 13.0% homozygous).

Second, we compared the SDF-1 genotype and allele frequencies between each subgroup of type 1 diabetes, stratified by the disease onset pattern and autoantibody positivity, and the control group, but no significant difference was found (TABLE 1).

Dubois-Laforgue reported that the SDF-1 3'A variant is associated with early-onset type 1 diabetes.[8] Thus, we compared the genotype and allele frequencies of the SDF-1 gene between "typical" type 1 diabetic patients (group A + group B) with onset age below and over 15 years old, but still no significant difference was found.

In the Japanese population, HLA DR4 and DR9 are considered to be major susceptibility genes for type 1 diabetes.[9] Therefore, we examined the HLA types of typical type 1 diabetic subjects ($n = 167$) who participated in this study. However, there was no significant difference regarding genotype and allele frequencies of SDF-1 3'A between HLA DR4- and/or DR9-positive and other phenotype groups.

DISCUSSION AND CONCLUSIONS

In this study, we found no significant difference in SDF-1 genotype and allele frequencies between the overall type 1 diabetes and control groups. Furthermore, the SDF-1 gene polymorphism was not associated with onset pattern or autoantibody positivity in Japanese type 1 diabetes.

It has been reported that the SDF-1 3'A variant is associated with early onset of type 1 diabetes.[8] However, unlike the previous report in "Caucasian" type 1 diabetics, SDF-1 3'A was not associated with early onset of the disease in Japanese type 1 diabetics in this study. There is a possibility that differences in mean onset age and genetic background (Caucasian versus Japanese) could account for the discrepancy between that report and ours. The mean onset age in typical type 1 diabetes in this study was 29.2 years old, which is older than that reported by Dubois-Laforgue.[8] Thus, to reach a conclusion on whether SDF-1 3'A affects the onset age of type 1 diabetes, at least the onset age should be matched.

In conclusion, the SDF-1 gene polymorphism was not associated with onset age (or onset pattern) of type 1 diabetes in Japanese. Further study is necessary to conclude whether the SDF-1 gene polymorphism affects onset age in type 1 diabetes in general.

REFERENCES

1. ATKINSON, M.A. 1994. The pathogenesis of insulin-dependent diabetes mellitus. N. Engl. J. Med. **331:** 1428–1436.
2. KOBAYASHI, T. 1993. Immunogenetic and clinical characterization of slowly progressive IDDM. Diabetes Care **16:** 780–788.
3. YAMADA, S. 2001. NeuroD/BETA2 gene G→A polymorphism may affect onset pattern of type 1 diabetes in Japanese. Diabetes Care **24:** 1438–1441.
4. LUSTER, A.D. 1998. Chemokine: chemotactic cytokines that mediate inflammation. N. Engl. J. Med. **338:** 436–445.
5. WINKLER, C. 1998. Genetic restriction of AIDS pathogenesis by an SDF-1 chemokine gene variant. Science **279:** 389–393.
6. BLEUL, C.C. 1996. A highly efficacious lymphocyte chemoattractant, stromal cell-derived factor 1 (SDF-1). J. Exp. Med. **184:** 1101–1109.
7. NANKI, T. 2000. Cutting edge: stromal cell-derived factor-1 is a costimulator for CD4+ T cell activation. J. Immunol. **165:** 1102–1110.
8. DUBOIS-LAFORGUE, D. 2001. A common stromal cell-derived factor-1 chemokine gene variant is associated with the early onset of type 1 diabetes. Diabetes **50:** 1211–1213.

Mutation Scan of a Type 1 Diabetes Candidate Gene

The Human Interleukin-18 Binding Protein Gene

RÚNA L. NOLSØE,[a] FLEMMING POCIOT,[a] DANIELA NOVICK,[b] MENACHEM RUBINSTEIN,[b] SOO-HYUN KIM,[c] CHARLES A. DINARELLO,[c] AND THOMAS MANDRUP-POULSEN[a,d]

[a]*Steno Diabetes Center, Gentofte, Denmark*

[b]*Department of Molecular Genetics, Weizmann Institute of Science, Rehovot, Israel*

[c]*University of Colorado Health Sciences Center, Denver, Colorado, USA*

[d]*Department of Molecular Medicine, The Rolf Luft Center for Diabetes Research, Karolinska Institute, Stockholm, Sweden*

ABSTRACT: Type 1 (insulin-dependent) diabetes, T1DM, is the result of an immune-mediated destruction of the pancreatic β cells dependent mainly on T helper cells and macrophages. Interleukin-18 (IL-18) is a proinflammatory cytokine produced mainly by macrophages. IL-18 is capable of inducing T lymphocyte synthesis of IFNγ, thereby skewing the T helper response toward a T helper type 1 (Th1) profile. IL-18 binding protein (IL18BP) neutralizes IL-18 and leads to a reduced Th1 response. Polymorphisms in IL18BP may affect the activity of IL-18 and the magnitude of the Th1 response and may play a role in the pathogenesis of T1DM. The aim of the study was therefore to identify polymorphisms in IL18BP and to test these for association with T1DM. We evaluated the human IL18BP gene on chromosome 11q13 as a candidate susceptibility gene for T1DM and scanned the entire IL18BP (promoter, exons 1–6, and 3′UTR) for polymorphisms using single-strand conformational polymorphism analysis and direct sequencing. We identified a total of 11 polymorphisms, all having allele frequencies ranging between 0.05 and 0.10. Four were in the 5′UTR: −257G→T, −78C→T, −65G→A, and −59A→G. Three were in intron 3: IVS3+140A→C, IVS4−147G→T, and IVS4−59G→T. The last four, 38*A→T, 48*T→A, 388*C→G, and 440*_441*insG, were in the 3′UTR of IL18BP. However, none of these were frequent enough to permit association studies in T1DM and we conclude that IL18BP does not contribute to the overall genetic susceptibility to type 1 diabetes.

KEYWORDS: IL-18; IL18BP; T cell; genetics; immune regulation; Th1/Th2 balance; polymorphism

Address for correspondence: Professor Thomas Mandrup-Poulsen, M.D., Ph.D., Steno Diabetes Center, 2 Niels Steensensvej, DK-2820 Gentofte, Denmark. Voice: +45-44-43-91-01; fax: +45-44-43-82-32.
tmpo@steno.dk

INTRODUCTION

Type 1 diabetes is the result of an immune-mediated selective destruction of the pancreatic β cells dependent mainly on T helper 1 (Th1) cells and macrophages. Several genetic as well as environmental factors contribute to disease etiology. The HLA locus on chromosome 6p21.3 (IDDM1) accounts for at least 40% of the familial aggregation of the disease[1,2] and is the major genetic susceptibility component in type 1 diabetes, although genome-wide scans in type 1 diabetes have identified more than 20 candidate susceptibility regions.[3-9]

Interleukin-18 binding protein (IL18BP)[10,11] is a secreted protein that binds and neutralizes interleukin-18 (IL-18). IL18BP is localized in the IDDM4 susceptibility locus on 11q13.[5,6,12,13] IL-18 is a proinflammatory, pleiotropic cytokine closely related to the IL-1 family[14] and is involved in the regulation of innate and acquired immune responses.[15]

IL-18 is produced mainly by activated monocytes/macrophages and is capable of inducing T lymphocyte synthesis of IFNγ in synergy with IL-12, thereby skewing the T helper response toward a Th1 response.[16] Th1 cytokine dominance has repeatedly been implicated in the pathogenesis of type 1 diabetes.[17] IL-18 serum levels are increased in the early subclinical stages of type 1 diabetes in humans.[18]

In the pancreatic islets of nonobese diabetic (NOD) mice, IL-18 mRNA expression was observed early during the spontaneous development of insulitis and subsequent diabetes.[19] IL-18 is also expressed in rodent β cells and is supposed to exacerbate islet inflammation.[20,21] By inducing IFNγ production from infiltrating T cells, IL-18 has no direct action on the pancreatic β cell since this cell type does not express the IL-18 receptor α-chain (IL-1Rrp).[21]

IL18BP binds to IL-18 with high affinity and neutralizes its activity *in vitro* and *in vivo*.[11,22] IL18BP is constitutively expressed in the spleen in healthy individuals and circulates at plasma concentrations of 2.5 ng/mL.[23] IL18BP is induced by IFNγ in various cells, suggesting that it serves as a negative feedback inhibitor of the IL-18-mediated immune response.[24] Several poxviruses encode proteins highly homologous to IL18BP, which can bind to and neutralize human IL-18.[11] IL18BP is a soluble protein consisting of a single immunoglobulin (Ig) domain, which bears little homology to the IL-18 receptor complex, but has limited homology to the decoy IL-1R type II receptor.[11]

There are 4 human isoforms of IL18BP resulting from mRNA splicing. All have a 28-amino-acid signal peptide. Only ILBPa and ILBPc are biologically active and can bind and neutralize IL-18. The mature protein of the predominant form IL18BPa consists of 164 amino acids and is by far the most biologically active. The IL18BPc transcript is longer mainly due to an extended 5′-untranslated region (5′UTR) and the mature protein has 169 amino acids. IL18BPb, a rarer shorter variant of 85 amino acids, and IL18BPd of 135 amino acids lack the complete Ig domain and are biologically inactive. The Ig domain possesses the essential binding requirements for IL-18 and is encoded for by exons 3–5 of the genomic IL18BP sequence (GenBank AC AF110798).[22] The genomic IL18BP sequence comprises 6 exons. The transcription initiator site is at 785 and the translation start site is at 1163 (AF110798).[25]

Since IL-18 has been implicated as an important Th1 cytokine in T1DM, we evaluated IL18BP as a candidate susceptibility gene for type 1 diabetes and scanned the genomic IL18BP sequence (promoter, exons 1–6, introns, and the 3′UTR) for polymorphisms by single-strand conformation polymorphism (SSCP)–heteroduplex analysis and direct sequencing to see if we could identify frequent polymorphisms to be tested for association with type 1 diabetes.

SUBJECTS AND METHODS

Screening for and Identification of Sequence Variants in the Human IL18BP Gene

The screening panel comprised 20 unrelated type 1 diabetes patients and 1 healthy male control of Danish Caucasian ancestry. Approval for the study was obtained from the Ethics Committee of Copenhagen County.

Oligonucleotide sequences for PCR amplification of the entire human IL18BP were designed from the genomic IL18BP sequence (GenBank AC AF110798) to generate 25 overlapping PCR products ranging from 227 to 273 base pairs (bp). PCR amplification of genomic DNA was performed with the primers listed in TABLE 1 and 40 ng DNA. The assay conditions were as follows: primers 1 µM each, dNTPs 50 µM, $MgCl_2$ 1.0–1.5 mM, and Taq DNA polymerase (Gibco) 0.5 U/sample with 1× reaction buffer, all in final concentrations in a reaction volume of 20 µL. PCR cycling conditions were 95°C for 5 min; followed by 35 cycles of 95°C for 30 s, annealing (varying between 59°C and 70°C for different primers) for 30 s, and extension at 72°C for 30 s; followed by a final extension at 72°C for 10 min.

Mutation Screening

The human IL18BP gene was screened for mutations by SSCP-heteroduplex analysis of the 25 overlapping PCR amplicons listed in TABLE 1 using the *Gene Gel Excel12.5/24Kit/GeneGel Clean 15/24 Kit* with the *PhastSystem*™ (Amersham Pharmacia Biotech, Uppsala, Sweden) as described in ref. 26. Samples were run using the *GenePhor Electrophoresis Unit* (Amersham Pharmacia Biotech) at 5°C for the Excel Gels and at 15°C for the Clean Gels containing 1% glycerol, and gels were thereafter stained using the *Plus One*™ *DNA Silver Staining Kit* (Amersham Pharmacia Biotech) on a *Hoefer Automated Gel Stainer* (Pharmacia Biotech, San Francisco, CA). Samples demonstrating mobility shifts or heteroduplex formation, or where sequence variations had been described in GenBank, were directly sequenced by the sequencing facility at *MWGAG BIOTECH* (Ebersberg, Germany). In total, bp 855–1115, 1809–2387, 3016–3621, 4005–4417, and 4612–4854 of IL18BP (AF110798) were sequenced.

RESULTS

We identified a total of 11 novel polymorphisms, listed in TABLE 1, in the genomic sequence (AF110798) of the human IL18BP by SSCP-heteroduplex analysis and direct sequencing. Four of these, g.−257G→T, g.−78C→T, g.−65G→A, and g.−59A→G, were in the 5′UTR region of IL18BP. Three were in intron 3: IVS3+140A→C, IVS4−147G→T, and IVS4−59G→T. The remaining 4, 38*A→T,

TABLE 1. Primers used for SSCP screening and sequencing of IL18BP and identified polymorphisms

Region scanned[a]	Primers (5′–3′)[b]	5′ end[a]	Annealing °C	Amplicon size (bp)	Polymorphism
−1127 → −861	GGTTGGCCGTGA-GAGTTCTA	36	60	267	
	CCCAAGGTCGGC-TACATCT	302			
−911 → −639	GAGAGACAGAGG-GTGTGATGG	252	66	273	
	CCAAGTGTCAGG-ACTTTGGTG	524			
−688 → −419	AAGACCTGGCTG-TGAAGAGG	475	65	270	
	CCCCGACCCTCT-ATTTCACT	744			
−101 → +155	GAGGTGTCACAG-CTGCTCAA	683	66	257	g.−257G→T
	CCAGCTCTCATG-ACCACAAA	939			
−308 → −48	TGGGTCTCAATT-TTGCCTTC	855	66	261	g.−78C→T[b] g.−65G→A[b]
	TGACAACGTCCT-CTTCTCTGG	1115			
−112 → +162	AGAAAAAGCGGG-AGTGGTTT	1051	66	275	g.−59A→G
	TCTGCCCAGGTT-CTTAAAGC	1325			
intron 2 → exon 3	TTCACTCCAAGG-CAAACCAC	1266	70	265	
	GCTGAGGTCTGA-GGAAAGGA	1530			
intron 2 → exon 3	TGGGCTGGAGTT-ACATCCTT	1446	66	258	
	GTCACTTCCAAT-GCTGGACA	1703			
exon 3 → intron 3	TGCCACTGCCTC-AGTTAGAA	1611	66	251	
	GAGAATGGTGCG-TGCTCAG	1861			
intron 3	TTCTGCCCATGT-ACCACCA	1809	67	262	IVS3+140A→C[b]
	ACAGAGGCAGTG-CTGGATG	2070			
intron 3	CAGAGCCTTGGT-TGCAGTG	1968	70	233	

— continued

TABLE 1. Primers used for SSCP screening and sequencing of IL18BP and identified polymorphisms (*Continued*)

Region scanned[a]	Primers (5'–3')[b]	5' end[a]	Annealing °C	Amplicon size (bp)	Polymorphism
	GAGGCCCTAGCC-CTAAACAC	2200			
intron 3 → exon 4	ACGTGAACCAAG-GACCATTC	2149	67	239	IVS4–147G→T[b] IVS4–59G→T[b]
	AGCTCAGCGTTC-CATCTAGG	2387			
intron 3 → exon 5	GCCTGTGTCCCT-AGATGGAA	2359	60	250	
	ACAGCTGCGTAC-CTGTGCT	2608			
exon 5 → intron 5	GAACGTGGGAGC-ACAGGTA	2581	60	255	
	GGAATGCTGGGC-ATTAGTTC	2835			
intron 5 → exon 6	TTCCATATGTGG-GGAGGAAA	2770	62	263	
	TAACCCTGCTGC-TGTGGAC	3032			
exon 6 → 3'UTR	CCACAGCAGCAG-GGTTAAGA	3016	60	232	38*A→T 48*T→A[b]
	GCAGGAGGAGGA-GGCATTAT	3247			
exon 6 → 3'UTR	TTCAAACTCCAT-TCCCACCT	3185	60	238	
	AGCTGTCTGGGA-AAAGCAAG	3422			
3'UTR	TACCTGCATTTC-CCACATGA	3359	59	263	388*C→G[b] 440*_441*insG
	ATCCCTTCCCTG-GAACAGTC	3621			
3'UTR	TCCCCCTTCACT-CTAATGGA	3584	59	259	
	CTTTTTCAAGCG-CCTGTGTT	3842			
3'UTR	GCTGAAGACAAC-ACCTGCTTC	3797	62	228	
	ACTTGATCGGTG-TGGGAAAA	4024			
3'UTR	TTTTCCCACACC-GATCAAGT	4005	59	243	
	AGCACCTGCCAG-AGGATG	4247			

— continued

TABLE 1. Primers used for SSCP screening and sequencing of IL18BP and identified polymorphisms (*Continued*)

Region scanned[a]	Primers (5'–3')[b]	5' end[a]	Annealing °C	Amplicon size (bp)	Polymorphism
3'UTR	AACCCCACTCCT-GAGACACA	4186	62	232	
	TTTGAGGCTGGT-TTTGATGG	4417			
3'UTR	ACCAGCCTCAAA-TCTGGTTG	4406	59	227	
	CTGTCCCTCTCA-GTGCCTTC	4632			
3'UTR	AGAAGGCACTGA-GAGGGACA	4612	62	243	
	GCACAGCCAGCA-ACTGATAA	4854			
3'UTR	GAGCCCCAGGGT-TATCAGTT	4824	60	244	
	AAGGGCAAGGTA-GAGGCACT	5067			

[a]Nomenclature: GenBank AC AF110798 and translation start site (denoted as +1) of IL18BPa in the 1163-bp position. Transcription of IL18BPa starts at the 785-bp position.

[b]Frequency of the rarest allele was 5%; all other polymorphisms had allelic frequencies of 10%.

48*T→A, 388*C→G, and 440*_441*insG, were in the 3'UTR of the gene. The frequency of the polymorphisms ranged from 5% to 10% for the rarest allele, which did not allow testing in our T1DM family material, consisting of 257 families (>1100 individuals) with a sufficient power. We were unable to confirm any of the described single nucleotide polymorphisms (SNPs), submitted to GenBank for IL18BP, by direct sequencing.

DISCUSSION

We have evaluated the human IL18BP, mapping in the IDDM4 locus on chromosome 11q13, as a candidate susceptibility gene for type 1 diabetes by scanning the genomic sequence of IL18BP for polymorphisms with SSCP-heteroduplex analysis and direct sequencing with the intention to test putative frequent polymorphisms for association with type 1 diabetes. We identified 11 novel polymorphisms. However, none of these were frequent enough to allow for testing of association. We could not confirm the presence of any of the SNPs submitted to GenBank, despite direct sequencing of these areas. The likelihood that we could have overlooked polymorphisms in IL18BP is small, also due to the high sensitivity and specificity of SSCP-heteroduplex analysis in our laboratory.[26]

We conclude that the identified polymorphisms in IL18BP do not contribute to the genetic susceptibility to type 1 diabetes. However, there might exist genetically regulated mechanisms that control the translation or posttranslatory modification of the protein.[9]

Finally, genetic susceptibility to T1DM related to the IL-18 system may be conferred by the recently reported functional promoter polymorphism in IL-18 associated with type 1 diabetes.[27,28]

ACKNOWLEDGMENTS

We are grateful for the expert technical assistance of Marja Deckert and Anette Hellgren Adamsen.

This study was supported by the Danish Diabetes Association, the Poul and Erna Sehested-Hansens Foundation, and Novo Nordisk A/S. C. A. Dinarello is a recipient of NIH Grant No. AI-15614.

REFERENCES

1. RISCH, N. 1987. Assessing the role of HLA-linked and unlinked determinants of disease. Am. J. Hum. Genet. **40:** 1–14.
2. NOBLE, J.A., A.M. VALDES, M. COOK et al. 1996. The role of HLA class-II genes in insulin-dependent diabetes-mellitus—molecular analysis of 180 Caucasian, multiplex families. Am. J. Hum. Genet. **59:** 1134–1148.
3. CONCANNON, P., K.J. GOGOLIN-EWENS, D.A. HINDS et al. 1998. A 2nd-generation screen of the human genome for susceptibility to insulin-dependent diabetes-mellitus. Nat. Genet. **19:** 292–296.
4. COX, N.J., B. WAPELHORST, V.A. MORRISON et al. 2001. Seven regions of the genome show evidence of linkage to type 1 diabetes in a consensus analysis of 767 multiplex families. Am. J. Hum. Genet. **69:** 820–830.
5. DAVIES, J.L., Y. KAWAGUCHI, S.T. BENNETT et al. 1994. A genome-wide search for human type-1 diabetes susceptibility genes. Nature **371:** 130–136.
6. HASHIMOTO, L., C. HABITA, J.P. BERESSI et al. 1994. Genetic-mapping of a susceptibility locus for insulin-dependent diabetes-mellitus on chromosome 11q. Nature **371:** 161–164.
7. HOLM, P., C. JULIER, I. KOCKUM et al. 2001. A genomewide scan for type-1 diabetes susceptibility in Scandinavian families: identification of new loci with evidence of interactions. Am. J. Hum. Genet. **69:** 1301–1313.
8. MEIN, C.A., L. ESPOSITO, M.G. DUNN et al. 1998. A search for type-1 diabetes susceptibility genes in families from the United Kingdom. Nat. Genet. **19:** 297–300.
9. POCIOT, F. & M.F. MCDERMOTT. 2002. Genetics of type 1 diabetes mellitus. Genes Immun. **3:** 235–249.
10. AIZAWA, Y., K. AKITA, M. TANIAI et al. 1999. Cloning and expression of interleukin-18 binding protein. FEBS Lett. **445:** 338–342.
11. NOVICK, D., S.H. KIM, G. FANTUZZI et al. 1999. Interleukin-18 binding protein: a novel modulator of the Th1 cytokine response. Immunity **10:** 127–136.
12. ECKENRODE, S., M.P. MARRON, R. NICHOLLS et al. 2000. Fine-mapping of the type 1 diabetes locus (IDDM4) on chromosome 11q and evaluation of two candidate genes (FADD and GALN) by affected sibpair and linkage-disequilibrium analyses. Hum. Genet. **106:** 14–18.
13. NAKAGAWA, Y., Y. KAWAGUCHI, R.C.J. TWELLS et al. 1998. Fine mapping of the diabetes-susceptibility locus, *iddm4*, on chromosome 11q13. Am. J. Hum. Genet. **63:** 547–556.

14. DINARELLO, C.A. 2000. Targeting interleukin 18 with interleukin 18 binding protein. Ann. Rheum. Dis. **59:** 17–20.
15. MCINNES, I.B., J.A. GRACIE, B.P. LEUNG et al. 2000. Interleukin 18: a pleiotropic participant in chronic inflammation. Immunol. Today **21:** 312–315.
16. NEIGHBORS, M., X. XU, F.J. BARRAT et al. 2001. A critical role for interleukin 18 in primary and memory effector responses to Listeria monocytogenes that extends beyond its effects on interferon gamma production. J. Exp. Med. **194:** 343–354.
17. DINARELLO, C.A. 1999. IL-18: a T-H1-inducing, proinflammatory cytokine and new member of the IL-1 family. J. Allergy Clin. Immunol. **103:** 11–24.
18. NICOLETTI, F., I. CONGET, R. DI MARCO et al. 2001. Serum levels of the interferon-gamma-inducing cytokine interleukin-18 are increased in individuals at high risk of developing type I diabetes. Diabetologia **44:** 309–311.
19. ROTHE, H., N.A. JENKINS, N.G. COPELAND et al. 1997. Active stage of autoimmune diabetes is associated with the expression of a novel cytokine, IGIF, which is located near *Idd2*. J. Clin. Invest. **99:** 469–474.
20. FRIGERIO, S., G.A. HOLLANDER & U. ZUMSTEG. 2002. Functional IL-18 is produced by primary pancreatic mouse islets and NIT-1 beta cells and participates in the progression towards destructive insulitis. Horm. Res. **57:** 94–104.
21. HONG, T.P., N.A. ANDERSEN, K. NIELSEN et al. 2000. Interleukin-18 mRNA, but not interleukin-18 receptor mRNA, is constitutively expressed in islet beta-cells and upregulated by interferon-gamma. Eur. Cytokine Netw. **11:** 193–205.
22. KIM, S.H., M. EISENSTEIN, L. REZNIKOV et al. 2000. Structural requirements of six naturally occurring isoforms of the IL-18 binding protein to inhibit IL-18. Proc. Natl. Acad. Sci. USA **97:** 1190–1195.
23. NOVICK, D., B. SCHWARTSBURD, R. PINKUS et al. 2001. A novel IL-18BP ELISA shows elevated serum IL-18BP in sepsis and extensive decrease of free IL-18. Cytokine **14:** 334–342.
24. PAULUKAT, J., M. BOSMANN, M. NOLD et al. 2001. Expression and release of IL-18 binding protein in response to IFN-gamma. J. Immunol. **167:** 7038–7043.
25. HURGIN, V., D. NOVIC & M. RUBINSTEIN. 2002. The promoter of IL-18 binding protein: activation by an IFN-gamma induced complex of IFN regulatory factor-1 and CCAAT/enhancer binding protein beta. Proc. Natl. Acad. Sci. USA **99:** 16957–16962.
26. NOLSØE, R.L., O.P. KRISTIANSEN, K. SANGTHONGPITAG et al. 2000. Complete molecular scanning of the human Fas gene: mutational analysis and linkage studies in families with type I diabetes mellitus. Diabetologia **43:** 800–808.
27. GIEDRAITIS, V., B. HE, W.X. HUANG et al. 2001. Cloning and mutation analysis of the human IL-18 promoter: a possible role of polymorphisms in expression regulation. J. Neuroimmunol. **112:** 146–152.
28. KRETOWSKI, A., K. MIRONCZUK, A. KARPINSKA et al. 2002. Interleukin-18 promoter polymorphisms in type 1 diabetes. Diabetes **51:** 3347–3349.

Caspase 7 Is a Positional Candidate Gene for IDDM 17 in a Bedouin Arab Family

SUNANDA R. BABU, FEI BAO, CHRISTINE M. ROBERTS, ALLISON K. MARTIN, KATHERINE GOWAN, GEORGE S. EISENBARTH, AND PAMELA R. FAIN

Barbara Davis Center for Childhood Diabetes, University of Colorado Health Sciences Center, Denver, Colorado 80262, USA

ABSTRACT: The IDDM 17 locus was mapped to an 8-cM interval at chromosome 10q25.1 based on linkage in a large Bedouin Arab family with 19 affected relatives. Caspase 7 (CASP7), an apoptosis-related cysteine protease, is one of the few known genes in this region. CASP7 is involved in the activation cascade of caspases responsible for apoptosis execution. Only 1 of the 18 SNPs in CASP7 (SNP144692) differed significantly in frequency in the haplotypes found in affected individuals compared to control Bedouin haplotypes. This same SNP showed evidence of association with diabetes in a subset of patients (DR3/DR4*0302) from HBDI families.

KEYWORDS: caspase 7 (CASP7); IDDM 17; Bedouin; locus; gene; chromosome

INTRODUCTION

The IDDM 17 locus was mapped to an 8-cM interval at chromosome 10q25.1 based on linkage in a large Bedouin Arab family with 19 affected relatives.[1] This locus has been confirmed in a large cohort of affected sib-pair families from the United Kingdom and the United States in a subset in which all affected individuals have HLA DR3, but not DR4.[2] We have assembled a set of BACs (bacterial artificial chromosomes) spanning this region, which have been fully sequenced over time in the Human Genome Project, and are looking for candidate genes within this region. Caspase 7 (CASP7), an apoptosis-related cysteine protease, is one of the few known genes in this region. CASP7 is involved in the activation cascade of caspases responsible for apoptosis execution. Overexpression promotes programmed cell death. Other names for this gene are CMH-1, ICE-LAP3, and MCH3. The transcript has 2168 bases; the protein is 303 amino acids long (XM_053352). The enzyme is a heterodimer of 20- and 11-kDa subunits. The 3D structure of caspase has been resolved.[3,4]

Address for correspondence: Sunanda R. Babu, Barbara Davis Center for Childhood Diabetes, University of Colorado Health Sciences Center, 4200 East Ninth Avenue, Denver, CO 80262. Voice: 303-315-6066; fax: 303-315-4892.

sunanda.babu@uchsc.edu

Ann. N.Y. Acad. Sci. 1005: 340–343 (2003). © 2003 New York Academy of Sciences.
doi: 10.1196/annals.1288.054

METHODS

A BAC contig map was assembled and extensive sequence analyses were performed on overlapping BACs surrounding the IDDM 17 locus. The exon-intron structure of CASP7 was identified by comparing the mRNA sequence (XM_053352) to the fully sequenced BAC AL592546. Direct sequencing in Bedouin family members bearing haplotypes found in affected or unaffected members identified several single nucleotide polymorphisms (SNPs). Overlapping amplicons, ~500 bp in length, were sequenced on an ABI 377 Sequencer. SNPs were analyzed for differences in allele frequencies between diabetic and nondiabetic haplotypes, and the transmission disequilibrium test (TDT) was performed in affected offspring of heterozygous parents in the Bedouin family. Fisher's exact tests and χ^2 analyses were the statistical tests; p values less than 0.05 were considered statistically significant.

One significant SNP identified in the Bedouin family (SNP144692) was typed and analyzed in 44 HBDI (Human Biological Data Interchange) families.

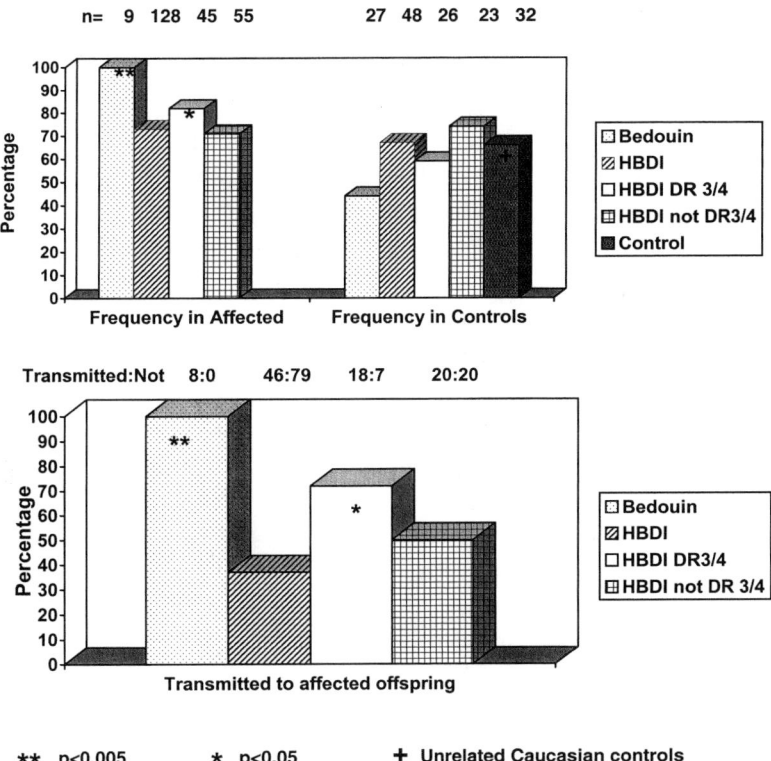

FIGURE 1. Frequency and transmission of "a" variant in caspase SNP144692 in the Bedouin and HBDI haplotypes.

OBSERVATIONS

The "a" allele at a novel SNP (SNP144692 a-c) was found in all 9 Bedouin diabetic haplotypes compared to 15/27 of Bedouin control haplotypes ($p = 0.0046$; FIG. 1). There was no significant difference in the frequency of this allele in the total sample of 44 HBDI families. However, the frequency of the "a" allele was increased significantly among chromosome 10 haplotypes that were transmitted to affected offspring bearing HLA DR3/DR4*0302 compared to haplotypes that were not transmitted to these offspring. In addition, the frequency of transmission from heterozygous parents to HLA DR3/DR4*0302 offspring was also greater than expected (72% vs. 50%; $p = 0.028$; FIG. 1). This SNP is in the 3'-UTR, 353 base pairs (bp) after the stop codon. The 3'-UTR extends for another 1012 bp beyond this SNP.

Seven SNP variations have been reported in CASP7, but only 3 were confirmed in 36 Bedouin and 32 unrelated control Caucasian haplotypes (variations 658, 673, and 1615 in the XM_053352 annotation). Variation 658 (c-g) changes the amino acid

TABLE 1. SNPs identified in the genomic region around CASP7 and frequencies for the less common allele (second base)

BAC no. (AL592546)	SNP[a]	Frequency in Bedouins ($n = 36$ chromosomes)	Frequency in unrelated Caucasians ($n = 32$ chromosomes)	Frequency in 44 HBDI families
142777	a-t	0.257	0.281	
144233 (1615)	c-t	0.194	0.125	
144282	t-c	0.139	0.094	
144692[b]	a-c	0.417	0.469	0.306
144753	a-g	0.333	0.250	
144764	t-c	0.000	0.031	
144890	a +/−	0.028	0.000	
145175 (673)	c-t	0.333	0.281	
145190 (658)	c-g	0.333	0.281	
147732	c-t	0.139	0.187	
149682	c-t	0.472	0.500	
149683	t-c	0.111	0.000	
149893	g-a	0.086	0.118	
150142	a-c	0.371	0.323	
150159	a-g	0.457	0.470	
152555	t-g	0.083	0.176	
153324	g-a	0.306	0.313	
153760	a-g	0.500	0.500	

NOTE: Numbers in parentheses refer to variations designated in XM_053352.
[a]Base change with the second base corresponding to the less common allele.
[b]The more common allele "a" was present in all 9 diabetic Bedouin haplotypes and in 12/27 (44%) control Bedouin haplotypes.

Asp-Glu. Variation 673 is silent and variation 1615 is in the 3′-UTR. The other 4 reported SNPs (variations 202, 586, 1136, and 1145) were not seen in the Bedouin or unrelated Caucasian control samples screened.

In addition, 14 SNPs were identified in the introns, 5′- and 3′-untranslated regions over 12,930 bp of genomic BAC sequence surrounding CASP7 (TABLE 1). The SNPs had similar frequencies in the Bedouin and unrelated Caucasian controls. In this sample size (32–36 chromosomes), there is a 97% chance of identifying a variant with frequency greater than 10%.

CONCLUSIONS

Only 1 of the 18 SNPs in CASP7 (SNP144692) differed significantly in frequency in the haplotypes found in affected individuals compared to control Bedouin haplotypes. This same SNP also showed evidence of association with diabetes in a subset of patients (DR3/DR4*0302) from HBDI families, although these results are in conflict with previous findings of IDDM 17 linkage in HBDI families with HLA DR3 and without DR4.[2] Further analysis of polymorphisms in other populations is needed to confirm the association of this SNP and CASP7 with type 1 diabetes.

Polymorphisms in at least 2 other unknown genes in the region show an association with type 1 diabetes in the Bedouin family.[5]

This extensive SNP map of CASP7 will be useful in analyzing other populations and other autoimmune diseases. Although SNP maps have been generated across the genome, they have to be validated by sequencing in more samples in different populations as many may represent sequencing errors or paralogous sequence variants representing segmental duplications.[6] Only 3 of 7 published SNPs were validated in our study. The published SNPs are a small random sample of the underlying variation; in our study, several more SNPs were discovered by extensive sequencing.

REFERENCES

1. VERGE, C.F. *et al*. 1998. Evidence for oligogenic inheritance of type 1 diabetes in a large Bedouin Arab family. J. Clin. Invest. **102:** 1569–1575.
2. COX, N.J. *et al*. 2001. Seven regions of the genome show evidence of linkage to type 1 diabetes in a consensus analysis of 767 multiplex families. Am. J. Hum. Genet. **69:** 820–830.
3. CHAI, J. *et al*. 2001. Crystal structure of procaspase-7 zymogen: mechanism of activation and substrate binding. Cell **107:** 399–407.
4. RIEDL, S.J. *et al*. 2001. Structural basis for the activation of human caspase-7. Proc. Natl. Acad. Sci. USA **98:** 14790–14795.
5. BAO, F. *et al*. 2002. Characterization of a novel positional candidate gene for IDDM 17 in a Bedouin Arab family. Oral presentation: 155-OR. Am. Diabetes Assoc. San Francisco.
6. ESTIVILL, X. *et al*. 2002. Chromosomal regions containing high-density and ambiguously mapped putative single nucleotide polymorphisms (SNPs) correlate with segmental duplication in the human genome. Hum. Mol. Genet. **11:** 1987–1995.

Interleukin-10 Gene Promoter Region Polymorphisms in Patients with Type 1 Diabetes and Autoimmune Thyroid Disease

AKANE IDE,[a] EIJI KAWASAKI,[b] NORIO ABIRU,[b] FUYAN SUN,[b] TETSUYA FUKUSHIMA,[a] REIKO ISHII,[a] RYOKO TAKAHASHI,[a] HIRONAGA KUWAHARA,[a] NARUHIRO FUJITA,[a] ATSUSHI KITA,[a] MISA IMAIZUMI,[a] KATSUYA OSHIMA,[b] TOSHIRO USA,[a] SHIGEO UOTANI,[a] ERI EJIMA,[a] HIRONORI YAMASAKI,[a] KIYOTO ASHIZAWA,[c] YOSHIHIKO YAMAGUCHI,[a] AND KATSUMI EGUCHI[a]

[a]First Department of Internal Medicine, Graduate School of Biochemical Sciences,
[b]Unit of Metabolism/Diabetes and Clinical Nutrition, and
[c]Department of Radiation Biophysics, Atomic Bomb Disease Institute,
Nagasaki University School of Medicine, Nagasaki, Japan

> ABSTRACT: Type 1 diabetes is a heterogeneous autoimmune disease and is frequently associated with other organ-specific autoimmune diseases, including autoimmune thyroid disease (AITD). Type 1 diabetic patients with AITD are known to show distinct clinical and immunological features from patients without AITD. This study investigated whether interleukin-10 (IL-10) gene promoter region polymorphisms are associated with susceptibility to type 1 diabetes and AITD. The frequency of −1082G/A, −819C/T, and −592C/A polymorphisms was analyzed in 54 type 1 diabetic patients with AITD, 74 type 1 diabetic patients without AITD, 124 nondiabetic patients with AITD, and 107 healthy subjects in a case-control study. No significant differences on the allele and genotype frequencies of three polymorphisms were found not only in type 1 diabetic patients with AITD compared with normal controls, but also between nondiabetic patients with AITD and healthy controls. The distribution of IL-10 gene haplotypes was also similar between both patient groups and normal controls. These results suggest that IL-10 gene promoter region polymorphisms are not associated with genetic susceptibility to type 1 diabetes and AITD.
>
> KEYWORDS: type 1 diabetes; autoimmune thyroid disease (AITD); IL-10; polymorphism; genetics; SNPs

INTRODUCTION

Type 1 diabetes is thought to result from autoimmune destruction of pancreatic β cells. Type 1 diabetes has been known to be frequently associated with other organ-

---

Address for correspondence: Eiji Kawasaki, M.D., Ph.D., Unit of Metabolism/Diabetes and Clinical Nutrition, Nagasaki University School of Medicine, 1-7-1 Sakamoto, Nagasaki 852-8501, Japan. Voice: +81-95-849-7550; fax: +81-95-849-7552.
eijikawa@net.nagasaki-u.ac.jp

specific autoimmune diseases, including autoimmune thyroid disease (AITD), pernicious anemia, and Addison's disease.[1] In Japanese patients with type 1 diabetes, the most common coexisting organ-specific autoimmune disease is AITD.[1] Clinical heterogeneity has been reported between type 1 diabetic patients with and without AITD. Type 1 diabetic patients with AITD were clinically characterized by a late and slow onset of diabetes.[1,2]

A number of studies suggest that cytokines may play a role in the pathogenesis of type 1 diabetes. Interleukin-10 (IL-10) is a pleiotropic T helper type 2 (Th2) cytokine that is usually considered to have a role in the downregulation of cell-mediated and cytotoxic inflammatory responses, thus being a potent anti-inflammatory mediator. It has been suggested that the Th2-induced component of anti–β cell immunity was mediated principally by IL-10.[3,4] In a previous study, we demonstrated that variable production of IL-10 associated with gene polymorphisms might influence the degree of islet β cell destruction.[5] We thus hypothesized that IL-10 gene promoter polymorphisms may participate in the susceptibility to type 1 diabetes with AITD.

SUBJECTS AND METHODS

Subjects used in this study were 128 patients with type 1 diabetes (60 men and 68 women) including 54 patients with AITD and 74 patients without AITD, 124 nondiabetic patients with AITD (19 men and 105 women), and 107 healthy control subjects (48 men and 59 women) after giving informed consent, and protocol was approved by the Institutional Review Board of the Nagasaki University School of Medicine. The diagnoses of type 1 diabetes and AITD were defined by both clinical features and laboratory data.

The 5′-flanking region of the IL-10 gene, spanning from −1351 to +19, was amplified by PCR using genomic DNA isolated from peripheral blood. Allelic polymorphisms in the IL-10 promoter gene at positions −1082 and −819 were analyzed by direct sequencing of the PCR product using an ABI-3100 multicapillary sequencer.

The IL-10 gene polymorphism at position −592 was determined by the PCR-RFLP technique with RsaI restriction enzyme as described previously.[5]

Allele or haplotype frequencies were calculated on patients and control subjects by direct counting. Statistical analysis of the differences between groups was determined by χ^2 test or Fisher's exact probability test. Findings were considered statistically significant at a p value less than 0.05.

RESULTS

TABLE 1 shows the distribution of allele, genotype, and haplotype frequencies in the IL-10 gene promoter polymorphism in type 1 diabetic patients with and without AITD, nondiabetic patients with AITD, and healthy control subjects. The genotype distributions did not differ significantly between patient groups and healthy control subjects. Furthermore, there also was no significant difference in the allele and haplotype frequencies among them.

TABLE 1. Allele, genotype, and haplotype frequencies of IL-10 promoter gene polymorphisms in type 1 diabetic patients with and without AITD, nondiabetic patients with AITD, and healthy controls

Polymorphism	Type 1 diabetes with AITD ($n = 54$)	Type 1 diabetes without AITD ($n = 74$)	Nondiabetic patients with AITD ($n = 124$)	Healthy controls ($n = 107$)
Allele				
Position −1082				
A	104/108 (96)	140/148 (95)	228/248 (92)	200/214 (93)
G	4/108 (4)	8/148 (5)	20/248 (8)	14/214 (7)
Position −819				
T	76/108 (70)	95/148 (64)	168/248 (68)	139/214 (65)
C	32/108 (30)	53/148 (36)	80/248 (32)	75/214 (35)
Position −592				
A	76/108 (70)	95/148 (64)	168/248 (68)	139/214 (65)
C	32/108 (30)	53/148 (36)	80/248 (32)	75/214 (35)
Genotype				
ATA/ATA (low)	26 (48)	29 (39)	52 (42)	42 (39)
ACC/ATA or ACC (intermediate)	24 (45)	37 (50)	55 (44)	51 (47)
GCC/ATA or ACC (intermediate)	4 (7)	8 (11)	17 (14)	14 (13)
GCC/GCC (high)	0 (0)	0 (0)	0 (0)	0 (0)
Haplotype				
ATA (low)	0.70	0.64	0.68	0.65
ACC (intermediate)	0.26	0.31	0.25	0.29
GCC (high)		0.04	0.05	0.07

NOTE: The predicted capacity for IL-10 production for each genotype is indicated in parentheses. Data are n (%).

DISCUSSION

Type 1 diabetes is frequently associated with other organ-specific autoimmune diseases, including AITD, pernicious anemia, and Addison's disease.[1,2] In Japanese patients with type 1 diabetes, the most common coexisting organ-specific autoimmune disease is AITD.[1] We have previously reported that the age at onset of type 1 diabetes in patients with AITD is significantly higher than in patients without AITD, and the prevalence of coma or ketoacidosis at the onset of type 1 diabetes is significantly lower than in patients without AITD.[2] Those results suggested that the degree of islet β cell destruction in type 1 diabetes with AITD is milder than without AITD.

Based on several studies, cytokines were shown to induce and/or exacerbate type 1 diabetes through direct and indirect mechanisms.[6] It is believed that Th1 cytokines promote, whereas Th2 cytokines such as IL-4, -6, and -10 protect from onset and progression of type 1 diabetes.[7,8] However, in some cases, IL-10 accelerated β cell destruction, hence arguing against this exclusive and oversimplistic conclusion.

We previously demonstrated that the IL-10 gene promoter region polymorphisms might influence the degree of islet β cell destruction.[5] In this context, it could be hypothesized that the IL-10 gene polymorphisms affect the susceptibility to type 1 diabetes with AITD.

In the present study, we did not find an association of the IL-10 gene promoter region polymorphisms with type 1 diabetes with or without AITD, as well as with nondiabetic patients with AITD (TABLE 1). Thus, the IL-10 gene polymorphism may not participate in the susceptibility to AITD and type 1 diabetes. These results suggest that clinical heterogeneity in type 1 diabetic patients with AITD is not associated with the IL-10 gene promoter region polymorphisms, and some complicated genetic and/or environmental factors may cause the development of type 1 diabetes with AITD.

ACKNOWLEDGMENTS

We thank Ayako Kaneko for her skillful technical assistance.

REFERENCES

1. KAWASAKI, E. & S. NAGATAKI. 1996. Japanese type 1 diabetic syndrome. Diabetes Metab. Rev. **12:** 175–194.
2. KAWASAKI, E., H. TAKINO et al. 1994. Autoantibodies to glutamic acid decarboxylase in patients with IDDM and autoimmune thyroid disease. Diabetes **43:** 80–86.
3. LEE, M.S., L. WOGENSEN et al. 1994. Pancreatic islet production of murine interleukin-10 does not inhibit immune-mediated tissue destruction. J. Clin. Invest. **93:** 1332–1338.
4. PAKALA, S.V., M.O. KURRER et al. 1997. T helper 2 (Th2) T cells induce acute pancreatitis and diabetes in immune-compromised nonobese diabetic (NOD) mice. J. Exp. Med. **186:** 299–306.
5. IDE, A., E. KAWASAKI et al. 2002. Genetic association between interleukin-10 gene promoter region polymorphisms and type 1 diabetes age-at-onset. Hum. Immunol. **63:** 690–695.
6. FAULKNER-JONES, B.E., M. DEMPSEY-COLLIER et al. 1996. Both Th1 and Th2 cytokine mRNAs are expressed in the NOD mouse pancreas in vivo. Autoimmunity **23:** 99–110.
7. RAPOPORT, M.J., A. JARAMILLO et al. 1993. Interleukin 4 reverses T cell proliferative unresponsiveness and prevents the onset of diabetes in nonobese diabetic mice. J. Exp. Med. **178:** 87–99.
8. PENNLINE, K.J., E. ROQUE-GAFFNEY et al. 1994. Recombinant human IL-10 prevents the onset of diabetes in nonobese diabetic mouse. Clin. Immunol. Immunopathol. **71:** 169–175.

Single Nucleotide Polymorphism Study of IDDM 17 in a Bedouin Arab Family

FEI BAO, SUNANDA R. BABU, CHRISTINE M. ROBERTS, ALLISON K. MARTIN, KATHERINE GOWAN, GEORGE S. EISENBARTH, AND PAMELA R. FAIN

Barbara Davis Center for Childhood Diabetes, University of Colorado Health Sciences Center, Denver, Colorado 80262, USA

ABSTRACT: Type 1 diabetes is an autoimmune disease caused by a combination of genetic and environmental factors. On the basis of a genomic search for linkage in a Bedouin Arab family with 19 members with type 1 diabetes, we previously mapped the IDDM 17 locus to the chromosome 10q25.1 region. The result from a recent genome scan showed suggestive evidence of linkage of IDDM 17 in a subset of Caucasian families in which all affected individuals have DR3, indicating that the IDDM 17 locus might have a measurable effect in Caucasian populations from the United Kingdom and the United States. High-resolution SNP typing provides strong evidence of linkage disequilibrium to the IDDM 17 locus.

KEYWORDS: type 1 diabetes; insulin-dependent diabetes mellitus (IDDM); IDDM 17; single nucleotide polymorphism (SNP)

INTRODUCTION

Type 1 diabetes is an autoimmune disease caused by a combination of genetic and environmental factors. Sequences within or near the major histocompatibility complex (MHC) class II genes (IDDM 1) and the insulin gene (IDDM 2) contribute about 50% to the total familial aggregation of the disease. More than 20 non-MHC loci have been reported to either interact with human leukocyte antigen (HLA) or independently confer genetic susceptibility to type 1 diabetes, but confirmed genes have been identified for few of these putative susceptibility loci.[1–3] The difficulty in defining and confirming non-MHC loci may result from the inadequate sample sizes or, more likely, the genetically heterogeneous nature of the disease. Genetic linkage studies in genetically and environmentally homogeneous populations offer the potential of identifying diabetes susceptibility genes by positional cloning.

On the basis of a genomic search for linkage in a Bedouin Arab family with 19 members with type 1 diabetes, we previously mapped the IDDM 17 locus to the chromosome 10q25.1 region (nonparametric linkage = 4.99, p = 0.00004). In this family, HLA DR3 plus IDDM 17 was associated with a diabetes risk of 40%.[4] The

Address for correspondence: Pamela Fain, M.D., Barbara Davis Center for Childhood Diabetes, University of Colorado Health Sciences Center, 4200 East 9th Avenue, Box B140, Denver, CO 80262. Voice: 303-315-7108; fax: 303-315-4892.
pamela.fain@uchsc.edu

result from a recent genome scan showed suggestive evidence of linkage (LOD score: 2.44) of IDDM 17 in a subset of Caucasian families in which all affected individuals have DR3, indicating that the IDDM 17 locus might have a measurable effect in Caucasian populations from the United Kingdom and the United States.[5] At the IDDM 17 region in the Bedouin family, a high-risk B haplotype was transmitted to 15 affected relatives in 7 different sibships, and a low-risk A haplotype was never transmitted to any affected offspring in 8 opportunities. Recombination events occurring on the B haplotype place the susceptibility locus within an 8-cM candidate region between markers D10S1750 and D10S1773. The strongest evidence for association was apparent with markers D10S592 and D10S554.

STUDY SUBJECTS AND METHODS

Because of recent advances in the Human Genome Project, we were able to construct a contig map with fully sequenced BACs that linked D10S554 and D10S592 in less than 700 kb of genomic DNA. We have examined this candidate region for the presence of known and unknown genes using the Genotator program,[6] which integrates multiple sequence analysis functions. Novel polymorphisms were identified by amplifying multiple regions of about 500 bases in the related BACs and direct sequencing from purified PCR products in 4 Bedouin family members who have the typical diabetic or nondiabetic haplotypes. We have typed these polymorphisms in all 9 diabetic haplotypes transmitted to affected offspring and 27 control haplotypes from the same family that were not transmitted to affected offspring. Single nucleotide polymorphisms (SNPs) were analyzed for differences in allele frequencies between diabetic and nondiabetic haplotypes by applying Fisher's exact test. The transmission disequilibrium test[7] was used to assess the transmission of the high-risk B haplotype allele at each SNP to affected offspring of heterozygous parents.

RESULTS

On the basis of six fully sequenced overlapping BAC clones, the two markers D10S592 and D10S554 showing apparent linkage disequilibrium with the IDDM 17 locus are separated by about 429 kb in the genomic sequence. With 250 amplicons, we generated a sequence of approximately 138 kb covering all the predicted exons identified in the related BAC clones. A total of 205 polymorphisms were identified with an average frequency of 1 in 671 bp genomic DNA. Different types of polymorphisms were found, including SNPs, insertions/deletions, and variable numbers of tandem repeats. Using this ultrahigh-density SNP map, we have determined the fine structure of the haplotypes in the Bedouin family by SNP typing in the candidate region. There are a total of 9 nonidentical haplotypes identified in affected relatives and 27 nonidentical control haplotypes found only in unaffected individuals.

We typed 188 SNPs spanning a region close to 700-kb genomic DNA in the Bedouin family members. Two known genes (CASP7 and ADRB1) and four unknown genes were identified. The hypothetical proteins encoded by the four unknown genes showed homologies to tudor domain containing protein, cutaneous T cell lymphoma associated antigen, von Willebrand factor and epidermal growth factor domains, and

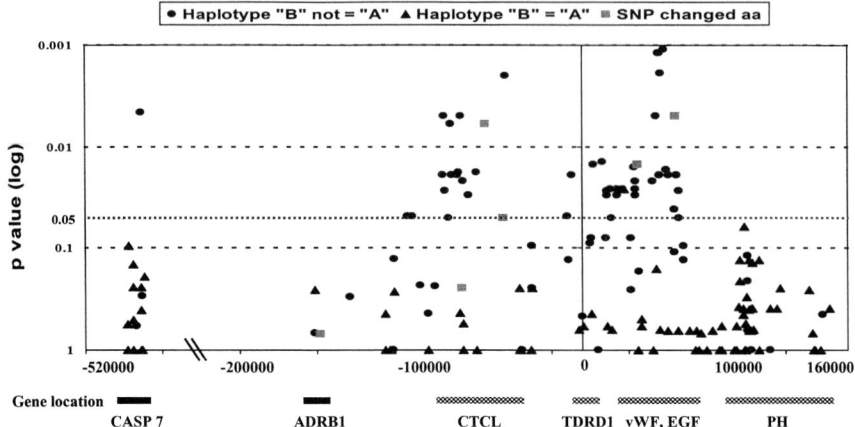

FIGURE 1. The p values shown by the log scale on the y-axis were calculated with Fisher's exact test by comparing each SNP allele frequency on 9 diabetic versus 27 nondiabetic haplotypes. On the x-axis, the sequence position of 188 SNPs and the location of the candidate genes are plotted in a 700-kb genomic region. *Circles* indicate the SNPs for which the allele on the B haplotype was different from that on the A haplotype. *Triangles* indicate the SNPs that had the same allele on both B and A haplotypes. *Squares* show the SNPs that changed amino acids in the proteins encoded by the corresponding genes. CASP7: caspase 7; ADRB1: beta-adrenergic receptor 1; CTCL: unknown gene similar to cutaneous T cell lymphoma associated antigen; TDRD1: unknown gene similar to tudor domain containing protein; vWF, EGF: unknown gene homologous to von Willebrand factor and epidermal growth factor domains; PH: unknown gene similar to the pleckstrin homology domain.

pleckstrin homology domain. Of the 188 polymorphisms, 52 within the exons or introns of four positional candidate genes revealed significantly increased frequencies on the 9 diabetic haplotypes compared to the 27 nondiabetic haplotypes ($p < 0.05$), including 11 polymorphisms with highly significant increased frequencies ($p < 0.01$), as illustrated in FIGURE 1. For all of these polymorphisms, the allele carried by the high-risk B haplotype differed from the allele carried by the low-risk A haplotype. As shown in TABLE 1, 13 SNPs were identified in the exons of the known or predicted genes. Ten of these polymorphisms showed significant evidence of linkage disequilibrium with diabetes, of which 4 resulted in amino acid substitutions in the proteins encoded by these genes. For 29 markers, the allele found on the diabetogenic B haplotype showed 100% transmission to affected offspring out of 16 informative meioses ($p < 0.0001$).

DISCUSSION

High-resolution SNP typing provides strong evidence of linkage disequilibrium to the IDDM 17 locus. Further analysis of polymorphisms is needed to define the boundaries of the region associated with type 1 diabetes. The complete sequence for the entire 8-cM candidate region recently became available, and sequence analysis

TABLE 1. Polymorphisms in exons of the candidate genes

SNP position	Candidate gene	Alleles	Diabetic haplotypes	Nondiabetic haplotypes	p value (DM vs. non-DM)	Amino acid changes
−483493	CASP7	A	9/9	12/27	0.0046**	3′UTR
−167771	ADRB1	G	5/9	16/25	0.7	G-R
−89574	CTCL	A	7/9	7/24	0.019*	3′UTR
−88751	CTCL	insATATT	8/9	8/26	0.007**	3′UTR
−88297	CTCL	A	4/9	2/26	0.027*	3′UTR
−77152	CTCL	GA	1/9	0/27	0.25	E-R
−61896	CTCL	A	7/9	6/26	0.006**	Q-K
−50050	CTCL	C	7/9	9/26	0.05*	T-I
26483	vWF, EGF	A	5/9	4/27	0.026*	5′UTR
26495	vWF, EGF	G	5/9	4/27	0.026*	5′UTR
35641	vWF, EGF	T	7/9	3/26	1	5′UTR
35674	vWF, EGF	A	7/9	7/26	0.015*	A-T
59696	vWF, EGF	G	9/9	12/26	0.005**	E-G

NOTE: CASP7 = caspase 7; ADRB1 = beta-adrenergic receptor 1; CTCL = unknown gene similar to cutaneous T cell lymphoma associated antigen; vWF, EGF = unknown gene homologous to von Willebrand factor and epidermal growth factor domains.

revealed the presence of 49 known and novel genes. The identification of the gene corresponding to IDDM 17 is likely to require continuous study of the patterns of linkage disequilibrium across the region, as well as analyses in other populations, and ultimately functional studies of candidate genes.

REFERENCES

1. DAVIES, J.L. *et al.* 1994. A genome-wide search for human type 1 diabetes susceptibility genes. Nature **371:** 130–136.
2. MEIN, C.A. *et al.* 1998. A search for type 1 diabetes susceptibility genes in families from the United Kingdom. Nat. Genet. **19:** 297–300.
3. CONCANNON, P. *et al.* 1998. A second-generation screen of the human genome for susceptibility to insulin-dependent diabetes mellitus (IDDM). Nat. Genet. **19:** 292–296.
4. VERGE, C.H. *et al.* 1998. Evidence for oligogenic inheritance of type 1 diabetes in a large Bedouin Arab family. J. Clin. Invest. **102:** 1569–1575.
5. COX, N.J. *et al.* 2001. Seven regions of the genome show evidence of linkage to type 1 diabetes in a consensus analysis of 767 multiplex families. Am. J. Hum. Genet. **69:** 820–830.
6. HARRIS, N.L. 1997. Genotator: a workbench for sequence annotation. Genome Res. **7:** 754–762.
7. SPIELMAN, R.S. *et al.* 1993. Transmission test for linkage disequilibrium: the insulin gene region and insulin-dependent diabetes mellitus (IDDM). Am. J. Hum. Genet. **52:** 506–516.

No Evidence for Linkage in Swedish Multiplex T1DM Families to IL12B on Chromosome 5q33–34

PERNILLA HOLM,[a] HOLGER LUTHMAN,[b] AND INGRID KOCKUM[a]

[a]*Department of Molecular Medicine, Karolinska Institutet, Stockholm, Sweden*
[b]*Department of Endocrinology, Lund University, Malmö, Sweden*

ABSTRACT: Type 1 diabetes mellitus (T1DM) is an autoimmune disease in which the β cells in the pancreas are destroyed by the body's own immune system. IL12 plays a role in pathological situations, such as septic shock, tissue damage during inflammation, and organ-specific autoimmune diseases. In NOD mice, administration of IL12 induces T1DM and administration of IL12 antagonists prevents T1DM. Linkage and association of IL12 to T1DM have been reported previously. We are unable to replicate this linkage on chromosome 5q33–34 in 184 Swedish families. Further, we exclude a gene with $\lambda_s > 1.4$ from this region. Together with previously published findings, these data make IL12 an unlikely major susceptibility gene for T1DM.

KEYWORDS: type 1 diabetes mellitus (T1DM); IL12; IL12B; transmission distortion test (TDT); linkage

INTRODUCTION

Destruction of the pancreatic insulin-producing β cells in type 1 diabetes mellitus (T1DM) is a response to an autoimmune reaction induced by cytotoxic T lymphocytes (CTLs) and macrophages. IL12, which is a cytotoxic lymphocyte maturation factor (CLMF) and which is also known as natural killer cell stimulatory factor-2 (NKSF), is produced primarily by antigen-presenting cells and plays an important role in the normal host defense against infections. This proinflammatory cytokine is a heterodimer composed of two disulfide-linked subunits, a smaller 35-kDa subunit (p35) known as IL12A and a larger 40-kDa subunit (p40) known as IL12B. The IL12B gene is located on chromosome 5q33–34 and has previously been linked and associated to T1DM.[1]

IL12 is produced very early during infections or the immune response and leads to the induction of differentiation of T helper type 1 (Th1) cells and the inhibition of the generation of T helper type 2 (Th2) cells. Th1 cells secrete IL2 and interferon-γ and thereby promote cell-mediated immunity. Th1 cells also regulate both T lympho-

---

Address for correspondence: Dr. Ingrid Kockum, Department of Molecular Medicine, Karolinska Institutet, CMM L8:00, Karolinska Hospital, S-171 76 Stockholm, Sweden. Voice: +46-8-517-75713; fax: +46-8-517-76179.
ingrid.kockum@cmm.ki.se

cytes and macrophages that are involved in the autoimmune reaction causing the β cell destruction in T1DM patients. It has been demonstrated previously that daily administration of IL12 in NOD mice induces Th1 cells and accelerates T1DM.[2] In addition, Rothe et al.[3] have shown that administration of IL12 antagonists reduces the T1DM incidence in NOD mice.

METHODS

Three microsatellite markers, D5S2112, D5S412, and D5S1352, were genotyped as described by the European Consortium for IDDM Genome Studies.[4] Linkage analysis was performed using ALLEGRO with equal weight for the families and a linear model. For the exclusion mapping, the GENEHUNTER program was applied using all affected sib-pairs. Furthermore, for the transmission distortion test (TDT) analysis, the pedigree disequilibrium test (PDT) was used, making it possible to correctly use all affected individuals in the families.

RESULTS AND DISCUSSION

When we analyzed the data from chromosome 5 in our whole genome scan, no linkage could be detected in the vicinity of the IL12B gene; however, all the linkage information had not been extracted from this region because the distance between the markers was still quite large.[4] We therefore selected three additional markers,

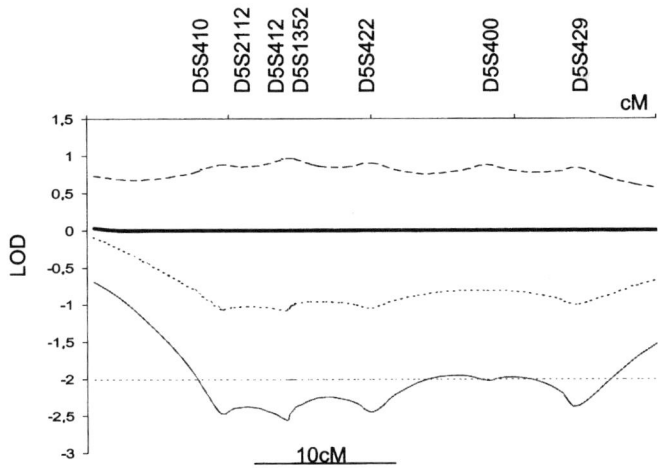

FIGURE 1. LOD values, information content, and exclusion levels for Swedish multiplex T1DM families in the vicinity of the IL12B gene on chromosome 5. *Thick black solid line*: LOD value for Swedish multiplex T1DM families; *thin black dashed line*: information content; *thin black dotted line*: exclusion at $\lambda = 1.2$; *thin gray solid line*: exclusion at $\lambda = 1.4$; *thin gray dotted line*: exclusion level LOD −2.

D5S2112, D5S412, and D5S1352, which were typed in 184 Swedish multiplex families used in the genome scan.[4] As in other recent reports,[5–8] we did not observe any evidence of linkage to T1DM with markers close to the IL12B gene on chromosome 5 (FIG. 1). We are able to exclude a major susceptibility gene from chromosome 5q33–34 because genes with a $\lambda_s > 1.4$ could be excluded from this region (FIG. 1). We also found no association to the markers on 5q33–34 observed using the TDT (data not shown).

Our findings, which do not confirm the involvement of the chromosome 5q33–34 region as a susceptibility region, could be explained by ethnic heterogeneity in the involvement of the IL12B gene as a susceptibility gene. That is, we have investigated Swedish families, whereas the original report was performed using Australian and British families.[1] However, Dahlman et al.,[6] who also failed to show association, reported on an extremely large sample size, 2873 T1DM families derived from the United States, Finland, Romania, Sardinia, and the United Kingdom. Such a large sample size suggests that ethnic heterogeneity is an unlikely explanation. According to McCormack et al.,[8] the most probable explanation for the positive findings in Morahan et al.[1] is the presence of type 1 errors. One possible explanation for our nonexisting linkage is that the disease-causing marker is not in LD with the markers we selected; that is, this explanation may account for why we were unable to detect any association. Furthermore, if the disease-causing allele is a common variant, we may also be unable to detect linkage. However, given the lack of reproduction of linkage and association to IL12B in T1DM families by other investigators,[5–8] the most likely conclusion from their results and ours is that the IL12B gene is not a major susceptibility gene for T1DM.

ACKNOWLEDGMENTS

We thank the Diabetes Incidence Study in Sweden and the Childhood Diabetes Registry for help in the collection of Swedish families. This work was supported by grants from the Juvenile Diabetes Research Foundation International (1-1998-168 and 2-2000-570), the Swedish Scientific Council, Novo Nordisk Fonden, the Swedish Strategic Funds, Svenska Diabetesförbundet, Barndiabetes Fonden, Smedbergs Stiftelse, Sven Järring Fonden, Torsten och Ragnar Söderbergs Stiftelser, Stiftelsen för vetenskapligt arbete inom diabetologin, Magnus Bergvalls Stiftelse, and Borgström & Hedströms forsknings fond.

REFERENCES

1. MORAHAN, G., D. HUANG, S.I. YMER et al. 2001. Linkage disequilibrium of a type 1 diabetes susceptibility locus with a regulatory *IL12B* allele. Nat. Genet. **27**: 218–221.
2. TREMBLEAU, S., G. PENNA, E. BOSI et al. 1995. Interleukin 12 administration induces T helper type 1 cells and accelerates autoimmune diabetes in NOD mice. J. Exp. Med. **181**: 817–821.
3. ROTHE, H., R.M. O'HARA, S. MARTIN & H. KOLB. 1997. Suppression of cyclophosphamide induced diabetes development and pancreatic Th1 reactivity in NOD mice treated with the interleukin (IL)-12 antagonist IL12 (p40)$_2$. Diabetologia **40**: 641–646.
4. EUROPEAN CONSORTIUM FOR IDDM GENOME STUDIES (ECIGS). 2001. A genome-wide scan for type 1 diabetes susceptibility in Scandinavian families: identification of new loci with evidence of interactions. Am. J. Hum. Genet. **69**: 1301–1313.

5. JOHANSSON, S., B.A. LIE, E. THORSBY & D.E. UNDLIEN. 2001. The polymorphism in the 3' untranslated region of IL12B has a negligible effect on the susceptibility to develop type 1 diabetes in Norway. Immunogenetics **53:** 603–605.
6. DAHLMAN, I., I.A. EAVES, R. KOSOY *et al.* 2002. Parameters for reliable results in genetic association studies in common disease. Nat. Genet. **30:** 149–150.
7. NISTICO, L., G. GIORGI, M. GIORDANO *et al.* 2002. IL12B polymorphism and type 1 diabetes in the Italian population: a case-control study. Diabetes **51:** 1649–1650.
8. MCCORMACK, R.M., A.P. MAXWELL, D.J. CARSON *et al.* 2002. The IL12B 3' untranslated region DNA polymorphism is not associated with early-onset type 1 diabetes. Genes Immunity **3:** 433–435.

Frequency of Latent Autoimmune Diabetes in Adults in Asian Patients Diagnosed as Type 2 Diabetes in Birmingham, United Kingdom

VALERIA TICA,[a,b] M. WASIM HANIF,[c] ANNIKA ANDERSSON,[a] G. VALSAMAKIS,[c] A. H. BARNETT,[c] SUDESH KUMAR,[c] AND C. B. SANJEEVI[a]

[a]*Department of Molecular Medicine, Karolinska Institute, Stockholm, Sweden*

[b]*Department of Biochemistry, Faculty of Biology, University of Bucharest, Bucharest, Romania*

[c]*Department of Medicine, University of Birmingham, Birmingham, United Kingdom*

ABSTRACT: The aims of our study were to measure autoantibodies to glutamic acid decarboxylase and autoantibodies to protein tyrosine phosphatase in patients with type 2 diabetes mellitus, patients with impaired glucose tolerance, and healthy controls of Asian origin from Birmingham, United Kingdom. According to our findings, 27% (9/33) of patients initially diagnosed with type 2 diabetes mellitus carry autoantibodies to GAD65.

KEYWORDS: GAD65; IA-2; IGT; LADA

INTRODUCTION

Current classification of diabetes mellitus identifies two forms of type 1 diabetes, the acute-onset form, referred to as classic type 1 diabetes, and the slowly progressive form, referred to as latent autoimmune diabetes in adults (LADA). The LADA patients usually get diagnosed clinically as having type 2 diabetes. Several epidemiological studies have demonstrated that LADA patients represent 10% of those diagnosed with type 2 diabetes.[1] This proportion can vary from population to population. In Asian patients with type 2 diabetes from eastern and southern India, 30% to 40% of the clinical type 2 diabetes patients were positive for either glutamic acid decarboxylase antibodies (GAD65 Abs) or protein tyrosine phosphatase antibodies (IA-2 Abs). One of the reasons cited for this high frequency is the unavailability of the autoantibody assay in several centers. In the absence of this assay, there is an excessive diagnosis of type 2 diabetes, especially in lean type 2 diabetes patients.[2,3]

Both GAD65 and IA-2 are β cell–specific autoantibodies, and their determination is necessary for a correct classification of certain diabetes types, that is, when clinical features are not useful in identifying patients with a form of diabetes that is clinically the same as nonautoimmune type 2 diabetes, but when the presence of

Address for correspondence: Dr. C. B. Sanjeevi, Department of Molecular Medicine, Karolinska Institute, Karolinska Hospital, CMM, L8:00, S-17176 Stockholm, Sweden. Voice: +46-8-5177-6254; fax: +46-8-5177-6179.
sanjeevi.carani@molmed.ki.se

TABLE 1. Frequency of GAD65 and IA-2 Abs in Indian patients with type 2 diabetes, those with IGT, and controls

Autoantibodies	Clinical type 2 diabetes ($n = 33$)	IGT ($n = 50$)	Controls ($n = 98$)
GAD65	9 (27.2%)[a]	6 (12%)[b]	9 (9.18%)
IA-2	1 (3.03%)[c]	0	0

[a]$p = 0.0167$; OR = 3.7; 95% CI = 1.3–4.2.
[b]$p = 0.5779$; OR = 1.3; 95% CI = 0.6–2.3.
[c]$p = 0.4502$; OR = 0.3; 95% CI = 0.05–2.48.

autoantibodies may make the distinction.[4] Autoantibodies to GAD65 can be detected prior to the onset of glucose intolerance. The level of IA-2 Abs in serum from type 2 diabetes patients was reported to be less frequent than GAD65 Abs.[5–7]

In this study, we wanted to test the hypothesis that patients of Asian origin living in the United Kingdom show the same high frequency of autoantibody positivity that is observed in southern and eastern India.

MATERIALS AND METHODS

Patients and Controls

Serum samples were obtained from 33 patients (13 males, 20 females) with type 2 diabetes mellitus and 50 patients (30 males, 20 females) with impaired glucose tolerance (IGT). The group of healthy controls included 98 subjects (61 males, 37 females). Serum samples were collected and stored at –20°C until assayed. Body mass index (BMI) was estimated in all cases and divided into three categories.

Assay

GAD65 Abs were detected by fluoroimmunoassay using a commercial kit (Perkin-Elmer Life Sciences, Finland). The cutoff established from the control group corresponded to 64.5 ng/mL. All samples including positive and negative controls were tested in duplicate.

IA-2 Abs were also detected by fluoroimmunoassay using a commercial kit (Perkin-Elmer Life Sciences, Finland). The cutoff value for solid-phase, IA-2 time-resolved fluoroimmunoassay was established at 1.88 ng/mL.

Statistics

Statistical analysis relied on calculations that used Fisher's exact test. The p values less than 0.05 were considered statistically significant.

RESULTS AND DISCUSSION

In our study, we observed that a BMI value below 25 was recorded in 30% of cases and that BMI values between 25 and 30 (overweight) and above 30 (obese) were recorded in 52.5% and 17% of cases, respectively. The results showed that GAD65 Abs were present in 16.6% of those with a BMI between 25 and 30 and in 7.7% of those with a BMI above 30 in IGT patients.

There was no significant difference in age or BMI between individuals with or without GAD65 or IA-2 Abs.

In the group of patients with type 2 diabetes mellitus, we found that GAD65 Abs were present in 23.8% of those with a BMI between 25 and 30 and in 30% of those with a BMI above 30.

Among the type 2 diabetes mellitus patients, only 1 was positive for IA-2, whereas 9 out of 33 were positive for GAD65. Ninety-eight control subjects were included in this study, of which 9 (9.18%) were positive for GAD65 (TABLE 1).

In our analysis of the serum results, that is, the determination of whether serum was positive for autoantibodies, we carried out calculations for both type 2 diabetes mellitus patients ($p = 0.0167$) and IGT patients ($p = 0.05$). We considered p values less than 0.05 to be statistically significant (TABLE 1).

In conclusion, the frequency of LADA in Asian patients from the United Kingdom is more similar to that observed in European Caucasians than that observed in Asian patients from India. It is interesting to note that the frequency of autoantibodies is raised in IGT patients as well.

ACKNOWLEDGMENTS

This study was supported by grants from the Swedish Medical Research Council (K2001-16X-12532-04B), Karolinska Institute, Novo Nordisk Fond, Eli Lilly (UK), Svenska Diabetes Förbundet, Barn Diabetes Fonden, and Åke Wiberg Stiftelse. C. B. Sanjeevi was supported by a Swedish MFR's position (K2001-72P-13149-03C).

V. Tica and M. W. Hanif contributed equally to this paper.

REFERENCES

1. TUOMI, T., L.C. GROOP, P.Z. ZIMMET et al. 1993. Antibodies to glutamic acid decarboxylase reveal latent autoimmune diabetes mellitus in adults with a non-insulin-dependent onset of disease. Diabetes **42**(2): 359–362.
2. SANJEEVI, C.B., A. KANUNGO, A. SHTAUVERE et al. 1999. Association of HLA class II alleles with different subgroups of diabetes mellitus in eastern India identify different association with IDDM and malnutrition-related diabetes. Tissue Antigens **54**: 83–87.
3. SANJEEVI, C.B., A. KANUNGO, A.K. DAS & V. BALAJI. 1999. Autoimmunity in Indian diabetics. Int. J. Diabet. Dev. Countries **18**: 102–112.
4. LANDIN-OLSSON, M. 2002. Latent autoimmune diabetes in adults. Ann. N.Y. Acad. Sci. **958**: 112–116.
5. MAIOLI, M., G. TONOLO, L. BEKRIS et al. 2002. GAD65 and IA-2 autoantibodies are common in a subset of siblings of Sardinian type 2 diabetes families. Diabetes Res. Clin. Pract. **56**(1): 41–47.
6. ROWLEY, M.J., I.R. MACKAY, Q.Y. CHEN et al. 1992. Antibodies to glutamic acid decarboxylase discriminate major types of diabetes mellitus. Diabetes **41**(4): 548–551.
7. TAKINO, H., H. YAMASAKI, N. ABIRU et al. 2002. Antibodies to GAD in Japanese patients classified as type 2 diabetes at diagnosis: high titre of GAD Ab is a predictive marker for early insulin treatment—report of west Japan (Kyushu, Yamaguchi, Osaka) study for GAD Ab(+) diabetes. Diabet. Med. **19**(9): 730–734.

Two Cases of "Fulminant" Type 1 Diabetes Suggesting Involvement of Autoimmunity

YOSHINORI NAKAGAWA,[a] AKIRA SHIMADA,[a] YOICHI OIKAWA,[a] JUN-ICHIRO IRIE,[a] TOSHIKATSU SHIGIHARA,[a] KAZUHIRO TSUMURA,[a] SHOSAKU NARUMI,[b] AND TAKAO SARUTA[a]

[a]*Department of Internal Medicine, Keio University School of Medicine, Tokyo, Japan*

[b]*Department of Molecular Preventive Medicine, School of Medicine, University of Tokyo, Tokyo, Japan*

ABSTRACT: Recently, a novel subtype of type 1 diabetes, so-called fulminant type 1 diabetes, has been proposed. One of the characteristics of this subtype is the absence of detectable "islet-associated" autoantibody, so it was originally proposed as being "nonautoimmune-mediated"; however, it has not yet been concluded whether autoimmunity is involved. We have previously shown that serum interferon-inducible protein-10 and glutamic acid decarboxylase-reactive $CD4^+$ interferon-γ-producing cells in the peripheral blood are good markers for T cell–mediated autoimmunity in type 1 diabetes. Here, we report two cases of fulminant type 1 diabetes in which these markers were detected and in which the involvement of islet-associated autoimmunity is suggested.

KEYWORDS: fulminant type 1 diabetes mellitus; glutamic acid decarboxylase (GAD); interferon-inducible protein-10 (IP-10)

INTRODUCTION

So-called fulminant type 1 diabetes, which was proposed by Imagawa *et al.*,[1] is characterized by (1) a near-normal HbA1c level regardless of diabetic ketoacidosis, suggesting an extremely acute onset; (2) no detectable islet-associated autoantibodies; (3) elevation of pancreatic exocrine enzyme levels; and (4) infiltration of T cells in exocrine tissue without insulitis on pancreatic biopsy.

This novel subtype was originally proposed as a subtype of type 1B, that is, an idiopathic, "nonautoimmune-mediated" subtype. Because most type 1 diabetes is considered to be mediated by cellular immunity, it is inadequate to conclude that such a subtype is nonautoimmune-mediated on the basis of no detectable islet-associated autoantibodies. However, a system that can directly assess antigen-specific cellular immunity in type 1 diabetes has yet to be established.

We previously reported that the level of serum interferon (IFN)–inducible protein-10 (IP-10), an important chemokine that induces migration of activated

Address for correspondence: Akira Shimada, M.D., Department of Internal Medicine, Keio University School of Medicine, 35 Shinanomachi, Shinjuku-ku, Tokyo 160-8582, Japan. Voice: +81-3-3353-1211 (ext. 62383); fax: +81-3-5269-3219.

asmd@sc.itc.keio.ac.jp

T cells to local lesions, was significantly elevated in type 1 diabetic patients compared with healthy control subjects and type 2 diabetic patients. The number of glutamic acid decarboxylase (GAD)–reactive IFN-γ-producing $CD4^+$ cells, which were measured using an intracellular cytokine staining method, was also elevated in type 1 diabetic patients, and the levels of these two markers were positively correlated with each other.[2] As an important point, elevation of these two markers was also observed in islet-associated autoantibody-negative type 1 diabetic patients.

Thus, the measurement of these markers, serum IP-10 level and GAD-reactive IFN-γ-producing $CD4^+$ cells, is considered useful in assessing whether T cell–mediated autoimmunity is involved. Here, we report two cases of fulminant type 1 diabetes in which these markers were detected and in which the involvement of islet-associated autoimmunity is suggested.

CASE REPORTS

Case 1

A 48-year-old man presented to our hospital with fever (>38.5°C), abdominal discomfort, thirst, polyuria, and weight loss (8 kg reduction in 10 days).[3] On the basis of the presence of diabetic ketoacidosis (blood glucose level of 40.4 mmol/L, urinary ketone bodies, pH 7.28 in blood gas analysis), relatively low HbA1c level (7.3%) at onset, absence of certain antibodies (GAD 65, IA-2, islet cell, and insulin autoantibodies), low level of glucagon-loaded serum C-peptide level (0.4 ng/mL), and low 24-h urinary C-peptide level (<3.0 μg/day), he was diagnosed as having fulminant type 1 diabetes. Moreover, a high level of serum IP-10 (285 pg/mL) was observed, which suggested the involvement of T cell–mediated immunity. Furthermore, although GAD 65 antibody was not detected at the onset of diabetic ketoacidosis, a marked increase was observed one year after the onset (FIG. 1), which indicated that autoimmunity was definitely involved in this case.

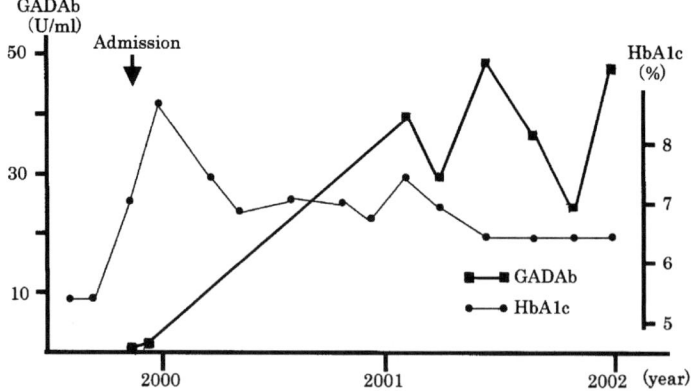

FIGURE 1. Changes in GAD 65 antibody titer in case 1.

Case 2

A 33-year-old man presented to a clinic with abdominal pain, polyuria, and weight loss; in addition, hyperglycemia (23.9 mmol/L) was detected.[4] On the basis of the presence of diabetic ketosis, low HbA1c level (5.8%), negative GAD 65 antibody, negative IA-2 antibody, and elevated pancreatic exocrine enzymes (trypsin 739 ng/mL, elastase-I 567 ng/mL), he was diagnosed as having fulminant type 1 diabetes. In this case, high levels of serum IP-10 (296 pg/mL) and GAD-reactive $CD4^+$ T cells (55 of 50,000 $CD4^+$ cells) were detected. Therefore, we considered that T cell–mediated autoimmunity was involved in this case, although islet-associated autoantibodies were not detected.

CONCLUSIONS

The two cases discussed in this paper suggest the involvement of autoimmunity in fulminant type 1 diabetes. Fulminant type 1 diabetes should not be considered "idiopathic" simply according to the absence of detectable islet-associated autoantibodies, at least at the onset of diabetes. Careful periodic measurement of islet-associated autoantibodies as well as assessment of cellular immunity against islet-associated antigen should be performed for proper classification of type 1 diabetes.

REFERENCES

1. IMAGAWA, A. *et al.* 2000. A novel subtype of type 1 diabetes mellitus characterized by a rapid onset and an absence of diabetes-related antibodies. N. Engl. J. Med. **342:** 301–307.
2. SHIMADA, A. *et al.* 2001. Elevated serum IP-10 levels observed in type 1 diabetes. Diabetes Care **24:** 510–515.
3. SHIMADA, A. *et al.* 2002. A case of fulminant type 1 diabetes with strong evidence of autoimmunity. Diabetes Care **25:** 1482–1483.
4. SHIMADA, A. *et al.* 2002. T-cell-mediated autoimmunity may be involved in fulminant type 1 diabetes. Diabetes Care **25:** 635–636.

Multicenter Prevention Trial of Slowly Progressive Type 1 Diabetes with Small Dose of Insulin (the Tokyo Study)

Preliminary Report

TARO MARUYAMA,[a] AKIRA SHIMADA,[b] AZUMA KANATSUKA,[c]
AKIRA KASUGA,[d] IZUMI TAKEI,[e] JUNICHI YOKOYAMA,[f]
AND TETSURO KOBAYASHI[g]

[a]*Department of Internal Medicine, Saitama Social Insurance Hospital, Saitama, Japan*

[b]*Department of Internal Medicine, Keio University School of Medicine, Tokyo, Japan*

[c]*Department of Internal Medicine, Kasori Hospital, Chiba, Japan*

[d]*Department of Internal Medicine, Tokyo Denryoku Hospital, Tokyo, Japan*

[e]*Department of Laboratory Medicine, Keio University School of Medicine, Tokyo, Japan*

[f]*Third Department of Internal Medicine, Jikeikai University School of Medicine, Tokyo, Japan*

[g]*Third Department of Internal Medicine, Yamanashi University School of Medicine, Yamanashi, Japan*

ABSTRACT: In 1996, we designed a randomized multicenter study to assess the effects of small doses of insulin on beta cell failure in slowly progressive type 1 diabetes (the Tokyo Study). We report here the preliminary results of this study. Glutamic acid decarboxylase 65 antibody (GADA)–positive patients were randomly divided into 2 groups: one group received insulin (Ins group), the other a sulfonylurea (SU group). Fifty-four patients (24 Ins group, 30 SU group) were analyzed at the end of a 4-year period. All patients underwent a 75 g oral-glucose test (O-GTT) every 6–12 months. The insulin-dependent stage was defined based on an integrated value of serum C-peptide levels on O-GTT (ΣCPR; sum of CPR at 0, 30, 60, 90, and 120 min) below 4.0 ng/mL. The ΣCPR in the SU group decreased progressively from 22.0 ± 10.6 to 11.3 ± 7.5 ng/mL over the 48-month period ($p < 0.001$ vs. baseline). The ΣCPR in the Ins group was unchanged. Among the SU group, 30% of subjects (9/30) progressed to IDDM, while 8.3% of Ins group subjects (2/24) progressed to IDDM ($p = 0.087$). With regard to the subjects who had a preserved C-peptide response (ΣCPR $\geq$ 10 ng/mL), the proportion of SU group subjects who progressed to IDDM was significantly higher than that of the Ins group (7/28, 25% vs. 0/21, 0%, $p = 0.015$). Among subjects with a high GADA titer ($\geq$10 U/mL), 9/14 (64.3%) of

Address for correspondence: Taro Maruyama, M.D., Department of Internal Medicine, Saitama Social Insurance Hospital, 4-9-3, Kitaurawa, Urawa-ku, Saitama-shi, Saitama 330-0074, Japan. Voice: +81-48-832-4951; fax: +81-48-825-0322.
taro-m@spn6.speednet.ne.jp

the SU group, but only 2/16 (12.5%) of the Ins group, developed IDDM ($p = 0.0068$). As to those with a high GADA titer and a preserved C-peptide response, SU group subjects progressed to IDDM (7/12, 58.3%) more frequently than Ins group subjects (0/14, 0%) ($p = 0.0012$). In summary, our results suggest that small doses of insulin effectively prevent beta cell failure in slowly progressive type 1 diabetes. We recommend avoiding SU treatment and instead administering insulin to NIDDM patients with high GADA titer.

KEYWORDS: type 1 diabetes; IDDM; NIDDM; GADA; insulin; sulfonylurea

INTRODUCTION

Type 1 diabetes is an autoimmune disease and immunological interventions are thought to be effective for preventing disease development.[1] In animal models of type 1 diabetes, such as the nonobese diabetes (NOD) mouse, the Bio-Breeding/ Worcester (BB/W) rat, and the multiple low-dose streptozotocin-induced diabetic mouse, a large number of successful studies in the prevention of type 1 diabetes have been reported.[2] In these studies, insulin was reported to be effective in animal models.[3–6] Insulin is essential for treating diabetes and physicians can use this drug on diabetic patients safely. Therefore, parenteral insulin therapy is thought to be very convenient, safe, and useful in high-risk subjects with type 1 diabetes. In the United States, a Diabetes Prevention Trial Type 1 (DPT1) was performed for high-risk relatives of type 1 diabetics.[7] On the other hand, patients with type 1 diabetes have preserved endogenous insulin secretion at diagnosis. In slowly progressive type 1 diabetes or latent autoimmune diabetes in adults (LADA) in particular, patients do not require insulin treatment at the onset of diabetes and progress to insulin-dependence within several years.[8,9] A recent preliminary study demonstrated the preventive effect of a small dose of insulin on progressive beta cell dysfunction in islet cell antibody (ICA)–positive patients initially diagnosed as having LADA or slowly progressive type 1 diabetes.[10] To clarify the efficacy of small dose of insulin for progressive beta cell failure in slowly progressive type 1 diabetes, we organized a randomized multicenter prospective trial (the Tokyo Study) over long periods involving a larger patient population in the noninsulin-requiring stage of slowly progressive type 1 diabetes. The Tokyo Study was started in 1996 by seven hospitals in the Tokyo area and has been conducted successfully. We report here the preliminary results of the Tokyo Study.

PURPOSE OF THE TOKYO STUDY

The purposes of the Tokyo Study are as follows: first, to clarify the frequency of glutamic acid decarboxylase 65 antibody (GADA)–positive patients with noninsulin-requiring diabetes mellitus (phenotypically type 2 diabetes, NIDDM in the former classification); second, to clarify the natural course of these GADA-positive patients; and, third, to know the preventive effect of insulin on progressive beta cell failure in these patients.

SUBJECTS

Patients were selected to take part in this study if they fulfilled the following criteria: (1) diagnosis of diabetes according to ADA criteria; (2) not treated with insulin at least 6 months after diagnosis of diabetes; (3) positive GADA (cutoff, 1.5 U/mL) in 2 samples taken within 2 months; (4) disease duration < 10 years (desirable < 5 years); and (5) patients were unrelated. Patients were excluded if they had (1) a history of ketonuria, diabetic ketoacidosis, or marked hyperglycemia requiring insulin, or (2) renal or hepatic dysfunction affecting C-peptide clearance and glucose tolerance.

STUDY PROTOCOL

The study was a randomized, multicenter prospective trial. Patients were randomly assigned to one of two groups. One group received subcutaneous insulin injection after randomization (Ins group) and the other received sulfonylurea if necessary for blood glucose control (SU group). Informed consent was obtained from all patients. The study protocol required good glycemic control at entry and during the study period: fasting plasma glucose (FPG) < 120 mg/dL, HbA1c < 7%, and postprandial hyperglycemia < 200 mg/dL were glycemic goals in both groups. Glibenclamide was used for the SU group patients. At baseline and every 3 months during the follow-up period, levels of FPG, HbA1c, serum creatinine, and urinary microalbumin were checked; and the dosage of insulin or sulfonylurea was adjusted to the above-mentioned target glycemic control levels. Seventy-five g oral-glucose tolerance tests (O-GTT) were performed after overnight fasts annually. When FPG in the SU group patients exceeded over 200 mg/dL and/or HbA1c exceeded 9% despite the maximum dose of glibenclamide (7.5 mg) and strict dietary treatment, the mode of treatment in the SU group patients was changed to insulin. Even after this change in treatment from sulfonylurea to insulin in the SU group, the patients received annual 75 g O-GTT.

END POINTS

The primary outcome measures for the study were serum C-peptide response (CPR) and blood glucose level during 75 g O-GTT. Integrated values of serum C-peptide at 0, 30, 60, 90, and 120 min during O-GTT (ΣCPR) were compared between the insulin and SU groups. The proportion of patients who progressed to an insulin-dependent state was also evaluated in both groups. The insulin-dependent state was defined as ΣCPR below 4 ng/mL.

RESULTS

We screened 3246 patients with type 2 diabetes, phenotypically, not receiving insulin treatment. We analyzed 56 patients at the end of the 4-year period. The baseline characteristics of the analyzed patients are presented in TABLE 1. The two groups were well matched for clinical characteristics in terms of age, sex, duration of diabetes, titer of GADA, BMI, FPG, HbA1c, and ΣCPR.

TABLE 1. Baseline characteristics of the patients in this study

Characteristics	SU group ($n = 30$)	Ins group ($n = 24$)	p
Sex (M/F)	16/14	15/9	NS
Age (years)	50.4 ± 14.1	56.6 ± 13.4	NS
Disease duration	2.4 ± 2.9	2.7 ± 3.8	NS
BMI (kg/m^2)	22.2 ± 4.2	20.0 ± 2.6	NS
HbA1c (%)	7.3 ± 1.8	7.6 ± 1.1	NS
GADA (U/mL)	294 ± 1136	902 ± 3242	NS
ΣCPR (ng/mL)	22.0 ± 10.5	22.1 ± 17.0	NS

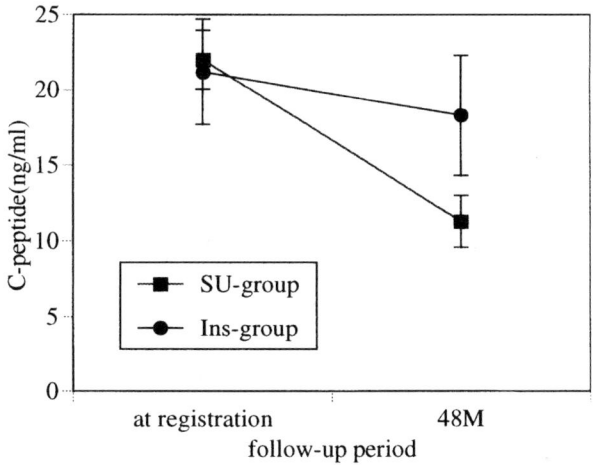

FIGURE 1. Changes in C-peptide response (ΣCPR) during intervention study in the insulin (Ins) group and the sulfonylurea (SU) group.

The ΣCPR value in the SU group decreased progressively from 22.0 ± 10.6 to 11.3 ± 7.5 ng/mL after a 48-month period ($p < 0.001$ vs. baseline). The ΣCPR value in the insulin group was unchanged (FIG. 1).

Among the SU group, 30% of subjects (9/30) progressed to the IDDM stage, while 8.3% in the Ins group (2/24) progressed to this stage ($p = 0.087$) (FIG. 2). With regard to the subjects who had preserved C-peptide responses (ΣCPR ≥ 10 ng/mL), the proportion of SU group subjects progressing to IDDM was significantly higher than that of the Ins group (7/28, 25% vs. 0/21, 0%, $p = 0.015$) (FIG. 3). As to the GADA titer, no subjects with a low GADA titer (<10 U/mL, equivalent to ~200 IU/mL in WHO standard) progressed to IDDM in either group. Among the high GADA titer subjects (≥10 U/mL), 9/14 in the SU group (64.3%), but only 2/16 in the Ins group (12.5%), developed IDDM ($p = 0.0068$) (FIG. 4). Among those with both a high GADA titer (≥10 U/mL) and a preserved C-peptide response (ΣCPR ≥ 10 ng/mL), SU group subjects progressed to IDDM (7/12, 58.3%) more frequently than Ins group subjects (0/14, 0%) ($p = 0.0012$) (FIG. 5).

During follow-up, no adverse reactions, including hypoglycemia, developed in either group.

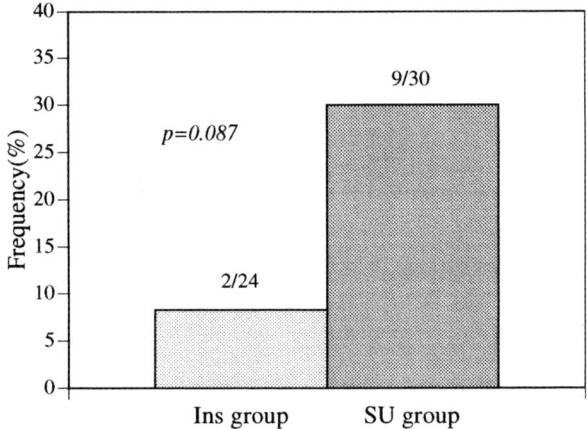

FIGURE 2. Frequency of the patients who progressed to IDDM in the insulin (Ins) group and the sulfonylurea (SU) group.

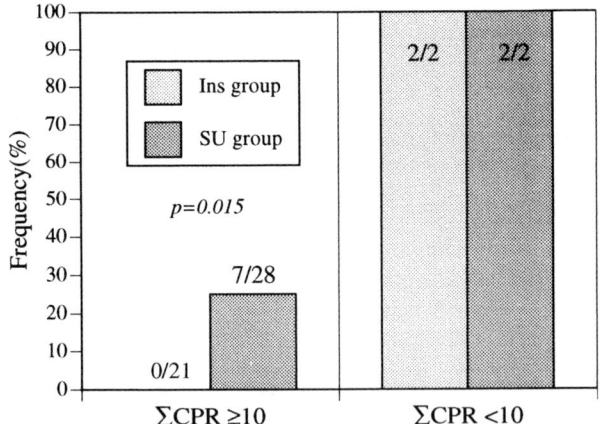

FIGURE 3. Frequency of the patients who progressed to IDDM in the insulin (Ins) group and the sulfonylurea (SU) group with regard to the subjects who had preserved C-peptide response (ΣCPR ≥ 10 ng/mL).

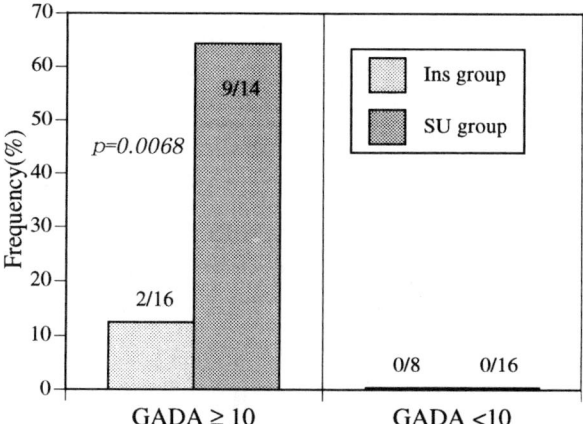

FIGURE 4. Frequency of the patients who progressed to IDDM in the insulin (Ins) group and the sulfonylurea (SU) group concerning GADA titer (GADA ≥ 10 U/mL or <10 U/mL).

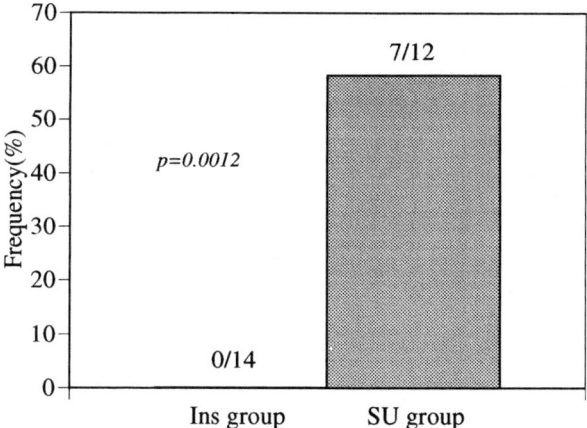

FIGURE 5. Frequency of the patients who progressed to IDDM in the insulin (Ins) group and the sulfonylurea (SU) group among those with both a high GADA titer (≥10 U/mL) and a preserved C-peptide response (ΣCPR ≥ 10 ng/mL).

DISCUSSION

Our data demonstrate that small doses of insulin effectively prevent progressive beta cell failure in slowly progressive type 1 diabetes, specifically in patients with preserved beta cell function and a high GADA titer at the initiation of insulin. Patients who have preserved beta cell function are expected to have good glycemic control for longer periods, and end-stage diabetic complications will be prevented using this insulin treatment. Although the mechanisms of this preventive effect are unclear, several are thought to be possible, including metabolic and immunological mechanisms. First, as insulin is thought to be one of the autoantigens in type 1 diabetes,[11] exogenous insulin may induce immunological tolerance in these patients and suppress the subsequent immunological cascade.[12] Second, suppression of beta cell activity by exogenous insulin will lead to decreased antigen expression on beta cells, with subsequent inactivation of T cell responses to beta cells.[12] Third, exogenous insulin may regulate the IL-4-responsive pathway through the receptor configuration common to IL-4 and insulin. Activation of IL-4 will correct a Th1/Th2 imbalance, which is one of the pathological mechanisms of type 1 diabetes.[13–16] Fourth, insulin is reportedly protective against apoptosis and necrosis of beta cells.[17] Finally, exogenous insulin may prevent beta cell destruction via certain metabolic effects by promoting beta cell rest.[18–21] Although the mechanisms of the preventive effect of insulin are unclear, it seems to be an ideal therapy among immunotherapies because these possible mechanisms do not show systemic immunological adverse effects in patients, unlike systemic immunosuppression or immunomodulation.

Although our data demonstrate preventive effects against progressive pancreatic beta cell failure in patients with slowly progressive type 1 diabetes, parenteral insulin therapy for prediabetic subjects (DPT1 trial) had no preventive effects.[7] We speculate that the difference in results between the two studies is due to differences in some of the pathogenetic mechanisms in typical type 1 diabetes and slowly progressive type 1 diabetes. Infiltrating lymphocytes in pancreatic islets in typical type 1 diabetes are reported to be mainly CD8 T cells.[22,23] In contrast, those in slowly progressive type 1 diabetes are mainly CD4 T cells.[24] The mechanisms of islet beta cell destruction in slowly progressive type 1 diabetes may be similar to those in NOD mice rather than those in typical type 1 diabetes.

In our former study, a major portion of GADA-positive NIDDM patients became insulin-dependent within 5 years, and some took more than 5 years to develop insulin-dependence.[25] Thus, in the protocol of this study, we decided on a follow-up period of 5 years. We plan to follow-up these patients for 5 years at least. However, we conclude that small doses of insulin effectively prevent beta cell failure in slowly progressive type 1 diabetes and we now recommend avoiding sulfonylurea treatment, instead treating NIDDM patients who have a high GADA titer with insulin.

REFERENCES

1. ATKINSON, M.A. & N.K. MACLAREN. 1994. The pathogenesis of insulin-dependent diabetes mellitus. N. Engl. J. Med. **331:** 1428–1436.
2. SHIMADA, A. & G. FATHMAN. 1996. Lessons from animal models: NOD mouse. *In* Prediction and Genetic Counseling in IDDM, pp. 349–368. Wiley. New York.
3. GOTFREDSEN, G.F., K. BUSCHARD & E.K. FRANDSEN. 1985. Reduction of diabetes incidence of BB Wistar rats by early prophylactic insulin treatment of diabetes prone animals. Diabetologia **28:** 933–935.
4. LIKE, A.A., D.L. GUBERSKI & L. BUTLER. 1986. BioBreeding/Worcester (BB/Wor) rats need not be lymphopenic. J. Immunol. **136:** 3254–3258.
5. ATKINSON, M.A., N.K. MACLAREN & R. LUCHETTA. 1990. Insulitis and diabetes in NOD mice reduced by prophylactic insulin therapy. Diabetes **39:** 933–937.
6. ZHANG, Z.J., L. DAVIDSON, G.S. EISENBARTH *et al.* 1991. Suppression of diabetes in nonobese diabetic mice by oral administration of porcine insulin. Proc. Natl. Acad. Sci. USA **88:** 10252–10256.

7. DIABETES PREVENTION TRIAL–TYPE 1 DIABETES STUDY GROUP. 2002. Effects of insulin in relatives of patients with type 1 diabetes mellitus. N. Engl. J. Med. **346:** 4685–4691.
8. KOBAYASHI, T., H. KAJIO, K. TAMEMOT et al. 1993. Immunogenetic and clinical characterization of slowly progressive IDDM. Diabetes Care **16:** 780–788.
9. ZIMMET, P.Z., T. TUOMI, I.R. MACKAY et al. 1994. Latent autoimmune diabetes mellitus in adults (LADA): the role of antibodies to glutamic acid decarboxylase in diagnosis and prediction of insulin dependency. Diabetic Med. **11:** 299–303.
10. KOBAYASHI, T., K. NAKANISHI, T. MURASE et al. 1996. Small dose of subcutaneous insulin as a strategy for preventing slowly progressive β-cell failure in islet cell antibody-positive patients with clinical features of NIDDM. Diabetes **45:** 622–626.
11. EISENBARTH, G.S. 1986. Type 1 diabetes mellitus, a chronic autoimmune disease. N. Engl. J. Med. **314:** 1360–1368.
12. SCHLOOT, N. & G.S. EISENBARTH. 1995. Isohormonal therapy of endocrine autoimmunity [review]. Immunol. Today **16:** 289–294.
13. GLADSTONE, P. & G.T. NEPOM. 1995. The prevention of IDDM: injecting insulin into the cytokine network. Diabetes **44:** 859–862.
14. KEEGAN, A.D., K. NELMS, M. WHITE et al. 1994. An IL-4 receptor region containing an insulin receptor motif is important for IL-4 mediated IRS-1 phosphorylation and cell growth. Cell **76:** 811–820.
15. HANKOCK, W.W., M. POLANSKI, J. AHANG et al. 1995 Suppression of insulitis in non-obese diabetic (NOD) mice by oral insulin administration is associated with selective expression of interleukin-4 and -10, transforming growth factor-β, and prostaglandin-E. Am. J. Pathol. **147:** 1193–1199.
16. FUCHTENBUSCH, M., K. KREDEL, E. BONIFACIO et al. 2000. Exposure to exogenous insulin promotes IgG1 and the T-helper 2–associated IgG4 responses to insulin, but not other islet autoantigens. Diabetes **49:** 918–925.
17. GOTTLIEB, P.A., E.S. HANDLER, M.C. APPEL et al. 1991. Insulin treatment prevents diabetes mellitus, but not thyroiditis in RT6-depleted diabetes resistant BB/Wor rats. Diabetologia **34:** 296–300.
18. BOWMAN, M.A., L. CAMBELL, B.L. DARROW et al. 1996. Immunological and metabolic effects of prophylactic insulin therapy in the NOD-scid/scid adoptive transfer model of IDDM. Diabetes **45:** 205–208.
19. AAEN, K., J. RYGAARD, K. JOSEFSEN et al. 1990. Dependence of antigen expression on functional state of beta-cells. Diabetes **39:** 697–701.
20. BJORK, E., O. KAMPE, A. ANDERSSON et al. 1992. Expression of the 64 kDa/glutamic acid decarboxylase rat islet cell autoantigen is influenced by the rate of insulin secretion. Diabetologia **35:** 490–493.
21. BJORK, E., O. KAMPE, F.A. KARLSSON et al. 1992. Glucose regulation of the autoantigen GAD65 in human pancreatic islets. J. Clin. Endocrinol. Metab. **75:** 1574–1576.
22. ITOH, N., T. HANAFUSA, A. MIYAZAKI et al. 1993. Mononuclear cell infiltration and its relation to the expression of major histocompatibility complex antigens and adhesion molecules in pancreas biopsy specimens from newly diagnosed insulin-dependent diabetes mellitus patients. J. Clin. Invest. **92:** 2313–2322.
23. SOMOZA, N., F. VARGAS, M. MARTI et al. 1992. Immunohistopathological and molecular studies on the pancreas of newly diagnosed type 1 diabetic patients. Diabetologia **35**(suppl.): A41.
24. SHIMADA, A., Y. IMAZU, S. MORINAGA et al. 1999. T-cell insulitis found in anti-GAD65+ diabetes with residual beta-cell function: a case report. Diabetes Care **22:** 615–617.
25. KASUGA, A., T. MARUYAMA, S. NAKAMOTO et al. 1999. High-titer autoantibodies against glutamic acid decarboxylase plus autoantibodies against insulin and IA-2 predict insulin requirement in adult diabetic patients. J. Autoimmun. **12:** 131–135.

Late-Onset Autoimmune Diabetes in Relatives of People with Type 1 Diabetes

SPIROS FOURLANOS,[a] PETER G. COLMAN,[b] AND LEONARD C. HARRISON[a]

[a]*Autoimmunity and Transplantation Division, The Walter and Eliza Hall Institute of Medical Research, Melbourne, Australia*

[b]*Department of Diabetes and Endocrinology, The Royal Melbourne Hospital, Melbourne, Australia*

ABSTRACT: The Melbourne Prediabetes Family Study, a prospective study of first-degree relatives of people with type 1 diabetes (T1D), provided an opportunity to examine late-onset autoimmune diabetes within the context of a family history of T1D. We compared genetic, immunologic, and clinical features in relatives of people with T1D, who developed early- versus late-onset diabetes.

KEYWORDS: type 1 diabetes (T1D); islet autoantibodies; HLA

INTRODUCTION

The establishment of registries for type 1 diabetes (T1D) in the last 20 years has led to increased recognition of late-onset autoimmune diabetes. It is estimated that over 30% of T1D occurs after age 30.[1] In addition, the advent of islet autoantibody screening has enabled detection of β cell autoimmunity in both children and adults. The United Kingdom Prospective Diabetes Study[2] found that 361 of 3672 or 10% of adults with presumed type 2 diabetes had glutamic acid decarboxylase antibody (GAD Ab).

The Melbourne Prediabetes Family Study,[3] a prospective study of first-degree relatives of people with T1D, provided an opportunity for us to examine late-onset autoimmune diabetes within the context of a family history of T1D. We aimed to compare genetic, immunologic, and clinical features in relatives of people with T1D, who developed early- versus late-onset diabetes.

METHODS

One or more islet antibodies were detected in 125 out of 3900 (3.2%) first-degree relatives of T1D probands in the Melbourne Prediabetes Family Study (FIG. 1). Of these, 39 who had GAD Ab at baseline progressed to clinical diabetes. Two-thirds of

Address for correspondence: Spiros Fourlanos, Autoimmunity and Transplantation Division, The Walter and Eliza Hall Institute of Medical Research, The Royal Melbourne Hospital, Parkville VIC 3050, Australia. Voice: +61-(03)-9345-2658; fax: +61-(03)-9342-7970.
 fourlanos@wehi.edu.au

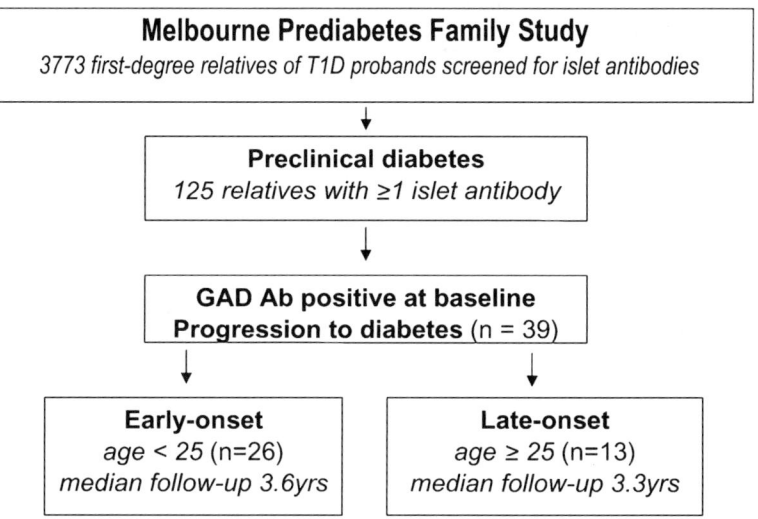

FIGURE 1. The Melbourne Prediabetes Family Study. See text for details.

these progressors ($n = 26$) had early-onset diabetes (age < 25) and one-third ($n = 13$) had late-onset diabetes (age ≥ 25).

Human leukocyte antigen (HLA) A, B, and DR types and islet antibodies in the preclinical phase were analyzed. GAD Ab, tyrosine phosphatase–like insulinoma antigen antibody (IA2 Ab), and insulin autoantibody (IAA) were measured by standardized precipitation assays that have performed optimally in all Immunology of Diabetes Society Combined Antibody Workshops. The cutoffs for the lower limit of detection of antibodies were 5, 3, and 100 units, respectively. GAD IgG Ab subclasses (IgG1, IgG2, IgG3, IgG4) were measured by the binding of ^{35}S-methionine-labeled *in vitro* translated recombinant GAD and precipitation of complexes with 2.5 μg biotinylated mouse monoclonal antihuman subclass antibody coupled to streptavidin-Sepharose beads.[4] Insulin requirement in the first year after diagnosis was assessed.

RESULTS AND DISCUSSION

Relatives with early-onset ($n = 26$) versus late-onset ($n = 13$) diabetes who were GAD Ab+ at baseline were compared for HLA allele distribution, number of different islet antibodies, frequencies of IA2 Ab and IAA, mean concentration of islet antibodies, GAD IgG subclass profile, and insulin requirement in the first year after diagnosis (TABLE 1).

There was no difference in HLA allele distribution between the two groups. The similar HLA allele distribution in early-onset and late-onset subjects may be consistent with the fact that both groups comprised a relatively homogeneous population

TABLE 1. Genetic, immunologic, and clinical features in relatives with early- and late-onset diabetes

	Early-onset (age < 25)	Late-onset (age ≥ 25)	p
Number of subjects (n)	26	13	
Mean age (SD)	12.8 (±9.9)	39.7 (±4.4)	
Sex ratio (m:f)	13:13	7:6	
Mean duration preclinical follow-up	3.2	3.3	
HLA DR distribution			
3,4	46%	41%	
3,3 or 4,4	18%	18%	
3,X or 4,X	36%	41%	
X,X	0%	0%	
Islet Ab number			
1	9	7	
2	8	6	
3	9	0	
Frequency			
IA2 Ab	14	4	0.17
IAA	12	2	0.06
Mean concentration (units ± SEM)			
GAD Ab	38.3 (±4.6)	51 (±6.3)	0.20
IA2 Ab	29.8 (±5.9)	3.0 (±1.0)	0.13
IAA	317 (±55.1)	54 (±12.4)	0.06
GAD IgG subclass (units)			
IgG1	22.2	14.4	0.25
IgG2	1.2	0.7	0.28
IgG3	0.6	0.2	0.99
IgG4	0.2	0.1	0.24
Treatment in first year of diagnosis			
Insulin	26	10	
Diet and oral hypoglycemics	0	3	

of first-degree relatives of people with T1D. Two or more islet antibodies, to GAD, IA2, or insulin, were more common in the early-onset group ($p = 0.05$, chi-square test); no individual in the late-onset group had all three antibodies. The frequency of IAA was lower in the late-onset group (15% vs. 46%, $p = 0.06$, chi-square test), as was the mean concentration of IAA (54 U vs. 317 U, $p = 0.06$, Mann-Whitney test). The frequency of IA2 Ab was also lower in the late-onset group (29% vs. 54%) and there was a trend of lower mean concentration (3.0 U vs. 29.8 U, $p = 0.13$, Mann-Whitney test). GAD IgG Ab subclass profile may be useful for clarifying the nature of the T cell response in T1D.[5] However, the distribution of GAD IgG Ab subclasses was similar between groups, with both groups having a predominant IgG1 response.

Notably, some relatives with late-onset diabetes did not require insulin within the first year of diagnosis.

Thus, we found that one in three first-degree relatives of people with T1D followed to clinical disease had late-onset autoimmune diabetes. The immune profile differed in relatives with late-onset versus early-onset diabetes, those with late-onset being characterized by a lower frequency and concentration of islet antibodies, in particular IAA. This is consistent with other data in older populations with T1D[6,7] and with evidence that the rate of progression to clinical disease is strongly correlated with the frequency and concentration of antibodies in first-degree relatives.

ACKNOWLEDGMENTS

This study was supported by a grant from the Juvenile Diabetes Research Foundation. Spiros Fourlanos is a Postgraduate Research Scholar of the National Health and Medical Research Council of Australia. We thank the staff of the Burnet Clinical Research Unit, The Royal Melbourne Hospital, for collection of blood samples and Shane Gellert, Endocrine Laboratory, The Royal Melbourne Hospital, for technical assistance with islet antibody assays.

REFERENCES

1. LAAKSO, M. & K. PYORALA. 1985. Age of onset and type of diabetes. Diabetes Care **8:** 114–117.
2. TURNER, R., I. STRATTON, V. HORTON et al. 1997. UKPDS 25: autoantibodies to islet-cell cytoplasm and glutamic acid decarboxylase for prediction of insulin requirement in type 2 diabetes: UK Prospective Diabetes Study Group. Lancet **350:** 1288–1293.
3. COLMAN, P.G., P. MCNAIR, H. MARGETTS et al. 1998. The Melbourne Pre-Diabetes Study: prediction of type 1 diabetes mellitus using antibody and metabolic testing. Med. J. Aust. **169:** 81–84.
4. BONIFACIO, E., M. SCIRPOLI, K. KREDEL et al. 1999. Early autoantibody responses in prediabetes are IgG1 dominated and suggest antigen-specific regulation. J. Immunol. **163:** 525–532.
5. COUPER, J.J., L.C. HARRISON, J.J. ALDIS et al. 1998. IgG subclass antibodies to glutamic acid decarboxylase and risk for progression to clinical insulin-dependent diabetes. Hum. Immunol. **59:** 493–499.
6. SABBAH, E., K. SAVOLA, T. EBELING et al. 2000. Genetic, autoimmune, and clinical characteristics of childhood- and adult-onset type 1 diabetes. Diabetes Care **23:** 1326–1332.
7. BINGLEY, P.J. 1996. Interactions of age, islet cell antibodies, insulin autoantibodies, and first-phase insulin response in predicting risk of progression to IDDM in ICA+ relatives: the ICARUS data set—Islet Cell Antibody Register Users Study. Diabetes **45:** 1720–1728.

Insulin Resistance in Latent Autoimmune Diabetes of Adulthood

M. T. BEHME,[a,b] J. DUPRÉ,[a,b,c] S. B. HARRIS,[a] I. M. HRAMIAK,[d] AND J. L. MAHON[a,b,c]

[a]*Lawson Health Research Institute,* [b]*Robarts Research Institute,* [c]*London Health Sciences Centre, and* [d]*St. Joseph's Health Care, University of Western Ontario, London, Ontario, Canada*

> ABSTRACT: Insulin resistance in patients with latent autoimmune diabetes of adulthood (LADA) was determined by homeostasis model assessment (HOMA). LADA was identified by a clinical phenotype of type 2 diabetes with antibodies to GAD65 and/or IA-2/ICA512. All patients were managed with insulin therapy. Insulin resistance in LADA was lower than in antibody-negative type 2 diabetes, higher than in normal humans and in recent-onset type 1 diabetes, and similar to that in long-term type 1 diabetes. Mean values for HOMA varied linearly with mean values for BMI, which accounted for much of the insulin resistance in these forms of diabetes. LADA resembles long-term type 1 diabetes with respect to insulin resistance and BMI, but occurs at an older age.
>
> KEYWORDS: latent autoimmune diabetes of adulthood (LADA); homeostasis model assessment (HOMA); insulin resistance

INTRODUCTION

Latent autoimmune diabetes of adulthood (LADA) is defined as a form of immune-mediated diabetes that occurs in adults and is marked by slowly progressive loss of beta cells.[1] LADA has many of the characteristics of type 1 diabetes, but usually presents clinically as type 2 diabetes and is initially not insulin-requiring. LADA usually progresses to insulin therapy that may be needed earlier than in non-immune-mediated type 2 diabetes, which is usually managed for long periods with oral hypoglycemic agents, exercise, and diet. In Canadian patients with phenotypic type 2 diabetes, conversion to dependence on insulin, within 5 years of diagnosis, occurred in a higher proportion of subjects with LADA than in those without autoimmune diabetes.[2] Insulin resistance occurs commonly in type 2 diabetes, especially with concomitant obesity. In newly diagnosed type 1 diabetes, insulin action may normalize during transient clinical remission, then declines after 1 year, and is inversely proportional to glycemic control and relative body weight.[3] If LADA is a slowly progressive form of type 1 diabetes, insulin resistance in LADA should resemble that in type 1 diabetes. Thus, we compared insulin resistance in insulin-

---

Address for correspondence: Dr. Margaret T. Behme, Siebens-Drake Research Institute, 1400 Western Road, London, Ontario, Canada N6G 2V4. Voice: 519-663-3521; fax: 519-663-3847.
mbehme@uwo.ca

TABLE 1. Insulin resistance estimated by HOMA and characteristics of insulin-treated patients with latent autoimmune diabetes of adulthood (LADA), antibody-negative type 2 diabetes (T2D), type 1 diabetes within 1 year of diagnosis (new T1D), and long-term type 1 diabetes (chronic T1D)

	LADA	T2D	New T1D	Chronic T1D
N	10	8	8	9
M/F	5/5	4/4	4/4	7/2
Age, years	40 ± 5	40 ± 4	29 ± 3^a	23 ± 3^a
BMI, kg/m^2	25.6 ± 1.3	34.2 ± 2.0^a	20.2 ± 3.2^a	24.8 ± 0.7
Diabetes duration, years	1.8 ± 0.5	8.6 ± 2.9^a	0.4 ± 0.1	14 ± 2.7^a
Insulin dose, U/kg/day	0.40 ± 0.08	0.57 ± 0.08	0.35 ± 0.07	0.52 ± 0.04
A1c, %	7.1 ± 0.5	8.0 ± 0.7	5.5 ± 0.2^a	7.1 ± 0.6
Anti-GAD65	10/10 (100%)	0/8 (0%)	7/8 (88%)	6/9 (67%)
Anti-IA-2	4/10 (40%)	0/8 (0%)	6/8 (75%)	6/9 (67%)
HOMA	35.9 ± 7.3^b	78.7 ± 13.2^{a,b}	20.1 ± 2.9^a	38.1 ± 5.3^b

^{a}Differs from LADA, $p < 0.05$.
^{b}Differs from the mean HOMA value of 14.6 ± 2.4 in 10 normal subjects, $p < 0.01$.

treated LADA within 5 years of diagnosis with that in three other insulin-treated groups: recent-onset type 1 diabetes within 1 year of diagnosis, antibody-negative type 2 diabetes, and long-term type 1 diabetes.

METHODS

The characteristics of patients with LADA, type 1 diabetes within 1 year of diagnosis, antibody-negative type 2 diabetes, and long-term type 1 diabetes are shown in TABLE 1. LADA was identified by a clinical type 2 phenotype with antibodies to GAD65 and/or IA-2/ICA512 (IA-2). All subjects received insulin therapy that was initiated without knowledge of antibody status, and they were in good metabolic control. Subjects were ascertained through local endocrine practices and were >20 years of age. Antibodies to GAD65 and IA-2 were determined by radioligand binding with labeled antigen prepared using cDNAs kindly supplied by A. Lernmark and G. Eisenbarth, respectively. Homeostasis model assessment of insulin resistance (HOMA) was calculated as [basal glucose (mmol/L) × basal insulin (pmol/L)]/22.5.[4] Plasma glucose and free immunoreactive insulin levels were determined after overnight fast and ≥10-h withdrawal of exogenous insulin. HOMA values were also determined in 10 normal humans.

RESULTS

Mean values for HOMA varied linearly with mean values for BMI, with $R^2 = 0.98$. Notably, insulin resistance in LADA was much less than in type 2 diabetes. HOMA values indicated that insulin resistance in LADA was similar to that in type 1 diabetes of long duration, but greater than in recent-onset type 1 diabetes and in normal humans (TABLE 1). Mean values for HOMA were not correlated with age, duration of diabetes, insulin dose, or hemoglobin A1c. Patients with LADA were similar in age to the patients with type 2 diabetes, but were significantly older than both groups of patients with type 1 diabetes. Mean values for duration of diabetes were much shorter in LADA and newly diagnosed type 1 diabetes than in the groups with type 2 diabetes and long-term type 1 diabetes. Mean daily doses of insulin did not differ among the groups. Glycemic control indicated by mean hemoglobin A1c values did not differ for LADA, type 2 diabetes, and long-term type 1 diabetes, but mean A1c was lower in recent-onset type 1 diabetes. Due to identification of LADA by the presence of antibodies to GAD65 and/or IA-2, all patients with LADA were antibody-positive, whereas not all with type 1 diabetes were positive. Patients with type 2 diabetes were so defined as antibody-negative.

DISCUSSION

In agreement with reported variations in insulin resistance assessed by euglycemic insulin clamp,[3] HOMA values indicated that insulin resistance was normalized in newly diagnosed type 1 diabetes, but higher than normal in type 1 diabetes of longer duration. The HOMA values also varied in a manner similar to SI assessments of insulin sensitivity ascertained by a modified minimal model of intravenous glucose tolerance tests in normal humans, type 1 diabetes in remission phase, and long-term type 1 diabetes.[5,6] In addition, our mean HOMA values for LADA and long-term type 1 diabetes agree well with the value (32.8 ± 22.7) reported for ICA-positive patients with type 1 diabetes.[7] These results suggest that HOMA provides a valid estimate of insulin resistance in insulin-treated diabetes.

In the patients with insulin-treated antibody-negative type 2 diabetes, obesity may account for much of the insulin resistance in light of the observation that HOMA was correlated with BMI. Duration of diabetes, which was longer in type 2 diabetes than in LADA, may also have influenced insulin resistance, and the very short duration of diabetes characteristic of remission phase type 1 diabetes may be related to lack of insulin resistance in this group. Although insulin resistance estimated by HOMA is most severe in antibody-negative type 2 diabetes, mean values for daily dose of insulin and glycemic control indicated by glycated hemoglobin did not differ from those in LADA and long-term type 1 diabetes. Examination of other factors associated with insulin resistance may clarify further differences between LADA and type 2 diabetes.

CONCLUSIONS

Assuming that estimation of insulin resistance with HOMA is valid in insulin-treated diabetes, lower insulin resistance in LADA than in antibody-negative type 2 diabetes is accounted for by obesity in the latter. LADA resembles type 1 diabetes with respect to insulin resistance and BMI, but occurs at an older age.

ACKNOWLEDGMENTS

This work was supported by a grant from the Canadian Diabetes Association in honor of the late Helen E. Lewis. We thank Anthony M. Jevnikar for consultation, Christine Moogk for technical support, and Janice McCallum for nursing assistance.

REFERENCES

1. POZZILLI, P. & U. DI MARIO. 2001. Autoimmune diabetes not requiring insulin at diagnosis (latent autoimmune diabetes of the adult): definition, characterization, and potential prevention. Diabetes Care **24:** 1460–1467.
2. BEHME, M.T., J.L. MAHON, S.B. HARRIS & I.M. HRAMIAK. 2002. Latent autoimmune diabetes of adulthood in phenotypic type 2 diabetes is associated with conversion to insulin dependence [abstract]. Diabetes **51**(suppl. 2): A283.
3. YKI-JARVINEN, H. & V.A. KOIVISTO. 1986. Natural course of insulin resistance in type 1 diabetes. N. Engl. J. Med. **315:** 224–230.
4. MATTHEWS, D.R., J.P. HOSKER, A.S. RUDENSKI et al. 1985. Homeostasis model assessment: insulin resistance and beta-cell function from fasting plasma glucose and insulin concentrations in man. Diabetologia **28:** 412–419.
5. HRAMIAK, I.M., J. DUPRÉ & D.T. FINEGOOD. 1993. Determinants of clinical remission in recent-onset IDDM. Diabetes Care **16:** 125–132.
6. FINEGOOD, D.T., I.M. HRAMIAK & J. DUPRÉ. 1990. A modified protocol for estimation of insulin sensitivity with the minimal model of glucose kinetics in patients with insulin-dependent diabetes. J. Clin. Endocrinol. Metab. **70:** 1538–1549.
7. GREENBAUM, C.J., D. CUTHBERTSON & J.P. KRISCHER. 2001. Type I diabetes manifested solely by 2-h oral glucose tolerance test criteria. Diabetes **50:** 470–476.

Detection of GAD-Reactive CD4+ Cells in So-Called "Type 1B" Diabetes

AKIRA SHIMADA,[a] KEIICHI KODAMA,[a] JIRO MORIMOTO,[a]
YOICHI OIKAWA,[a] JUNICHIRO IRIE,[a] YOSHINORI NAKAGAWA,[a]
KOICHI MATSUBARA,[b] TARO MARUYAMA,[c] AND TAKAO SARUTA[a]

[a]*Department of Internal Medicine, Keio University School of Medicine, Tokyo, Japan*

[b]*Diagnostic Technology Laboratories, Chugai Pharmaceutical Company, Tokyo, Japan*

[c]*Saitama Social Insurance Hospital, Saitama, Japan*

ABSTRACT: *Objective*—Although the majority of type 1 diabetes is considered to be type 1A, some patients with type 1 diabetes have no islet-associated autoantibody in their serum. This type of type 1 diabetes has usually been diagnosed as type 1B on the basis of islet-associated autoantibody-negativity. In this study, we tried to demonstrate the existence of islet-associated antigen-specific T cells in type 1 diabetes without islet-associated autoantibody. *Research Design and Methods*—Peripheral blood samples were obtained from 110 Japanese diabetic patients, including 15 type 2 diabetic patients. Measurement of islet-associated antigen-specific cytokine response was performed by intracellular cytokine staining for flow cytometry. *Results*—The number of GAD-reactive IFN-γ-producing CD4+ cells in 50,000 CD4+ cells in diabetics with type 1B (113.6 ± 34.6, median 45), type 1A (132.4 ± 33.3, median 25), and LADA (154.4 ± 44.1, median 20) was higher than that in type 2 diabetics (0.3 ± 0.3, median 0) and control subjects (3.8 ± 2.4, median 0). When the normal upper limit of the number of GAD-reactive CD4+ cells was set at the mean + 3SD of values in control subjects, at least half (52.4%) of the so-called "type 1B" patients were positive for GAD-reactive IFN-γ-producing CD4+ cells, a significantly larger proportion than that in type 2 diabetics (0%; $p < 0.001$). *Conclusions*—Assessment of T cell reactivity against islet-associated antigen may contribute to the diagnosis of "autoimmune-related" type 1 diabetes.

KEYWORDS: GAD; T cell; type 1 diabetes; autoimmunity; IFN-γ

INTRODUCTION

Although the majority of type 1 diabetes is considered to be autoimmune, type 1A, some patients with type 1 diabetes meeting the ADA (American Diabetes Association) criteria have no islet-associated autoantibody in their serum.[1,2] However, this type of type 1 diabetes has usually been diagnosed as type 1B (idiopathic type), based on the islet-associated autoantibody-negativity. However, it is obviously necessary to

Address for correspondence: Akira Shimada, M.D., Department of Internal Medicine, Keio University School of Medicine, 35 Shinanomachi, Shinjuku-ku, Tokyo 160-8582, Japan. Voice: +81-3-5363-3797; fax: +81-3-5269-3219.
asmd@sc.itc.keio.ac.jp

assess T cell reactivity against islet-associated antigen in this type of type 1 diabetes to conclude that it really is "idiopathic" because type 1 diabetes with autoimmunity is considered to be a T cell–mediated disease[3] and it is possible that no islet-associated autoantibody is detected in the serum. It has been recognized that detection of an islet-associated antigen-specific response in peripheral blood from human type 1 diabetics is difficult, probably because of the low frequency of such T cells in the periphery. Therefore, we used an intracellular cytokine staining procedure to detect such T cells in this study and tried to demonstrate the existence of islet-associated antigen-specific T cells in type 1 diabetics without islet-associated autoantibody.

METHODS

Patients

Peripheral blood samples were obtained from 110 Japanese diabetic patients, including 15 type 2 diabetic patients (9 males, 6 females; age, 64.3 ± 2.0 years; disease duration, 13.5 ± 1.9 years), recruited from Keio University Hospital and Saitama Social Insurance Hospital, with informed consent from the patients. Serum samples were collected in the morning and frozen at $-80°C$ until assay, and islet-associated autoantibodies (glutamic acid decarboxylase [GAD] and insulinoma-associated protein-2 [IA-2]) were measured as described below. As previously shown,[4] positivity of IA-2 or GAD antibody did not change within 5 years after the onset of diabetes; thus, serum obtained within 5 years after the onset was used in most cases. "Classical" type 1 diabetic patients negative for both of the autoantibodies were designated the type 1B group ($n = 21$; 10 males, 11 females; age, 38.2 ± 2.5 years; disease duration, 5.5 ± 1.5 years), and those positive for either or both (35 out of 38 were GAD antibody-positive and 3 out of 38 were positive for IA-2 antibody only), including patients who had become positive for either of the autoantibodies during the disease course, were designated the type 1A group ($n = 38$; 20 males, 18 females; age, 34.5 ± 2.5 years; disease duration, 5.0 ± 1.0 years) in this study. The diagnoses of type 1B and type 1A diabetes were made based on the ADA criteria for type 1 diabetes: pancreatic β cell destruction as the primary cause of the disorder and a tendency toward ketoacidosis.[1,2] Although there is no specific criterion for C-peptide level to diagnose an "insulin-dependent" state, the serum C-peptide in most cases of classical type 1 diabetes, especially "type 1B" in this study, was below 0.4 ng/mL. The definition of "slow-onset" type 1 diabetes, so-called "latent autoimmune diabetes in adults (LADA)"[5] ($n = 36$; 16 males, 20 females; age, 54.0 ± 2.2 years; disease duration, 8.7 ± 1.4 years), was made based on GAD and/or IA-2 antibody-positivity (35 out of 36 were GAD antibody-positive and 1 out of 36 was positive for IA-2 antibody only) and the requirement for insulin later than 6 months after the diagnosis of diabetes. Blood samples were also obtained from control subjects ($n = 28$; 14 males, 14 females; age, 53.1 ± 3.2 years).

Measurement of Autoantibodies

GAD65 (detection limit < 0.4 U/mL; 100% sensitivity and 100% specificity of the assay in the GAD antibody proficiency test [Immunology of Diabetes Workshop];

Lab ID number 305) and IA-2 (detection limit < 0.75 U/mL; evaluated in the third proficiency IA-2 antibody test organized under the auspices of the Immunology of Diabetes Workshops by The Research Institute for Children, showing 100% validity, 100% consistency, 100% sensitivity, and 100% specificity[6]) antibodies were detected using a previously described radioligand binding assay.[4,6] Briefly, N-terminal-deleted human GAD65 produced in yeast was labeled with ^{125}I. After purification by gel filtration, 50-μL aliquots of labeled material (30,000–40,000 cpm) were incubated at room temperature with 20 μL undiluted test serum. After separation of unbound labeled GAD65 by addition of protein A, specific radioactivity was counted. Regarding IA-2 antibody assay, purified IA-2 preparations were labeled with ^{125}I to a specific activity of 750 kBq per μg of protein using the chloramine T method. After gel filtration on Sephacryl S300 (Pharmacia), the ^{125}I-labeled IA-2 was freeze-dried in 50-kBq aliquots. In the IA-2 antibody immunoprecipitation assay, 20 μL of patient serum was incubated overnight at 4°C with 50-μL aliquots of ^{125}I-labeled IA-2 (30,000–40,000 cpm) reconstituted in assay buffer (50 mmol/L Tris-HCl, pH 8.0, 150 mmol/L NaCl, 10 mL/L Tween 20, 1.0 g/L BSA, 0.5 g/L sodium azide). Then, 50-μL solid-phase protein A (RSR Limited, Cardiff, United Kingdom) was added and incubation continued for 1 h at 4°C. Assay buffer (1 ml) was then added, the contents of the tubes were thoroughly mixed and centrifuged (1500g for 30 min at 4°C), the supernatants aspirated, and the pellets counted in a gamma counter.

Antigen-Specific Stimulation and Intracellular Cytokine Staining for Flow Cytometry

Measurement of islet-associated antigen-specific cytokine response was performed by a blinded researcher as described previously.[7] First, 500 μL heparinized whole blood was placed in 5-mL polystyrene round-bottom tubes (Becton Dickinson, Franklin Lakes, NJ) containing 500 μL RPMI1640 medium (Gibco-BRL, Grand Island, NY) supplemented with 10% heat-inactivated fetal bovine serum (Gibco-BRL), penicillin/streptomycin (Gibco-BRL), and 1 μg anti-CD28 antibody (L293, Becton Dickinson, San Jose, CA), and with (or without) 5 μg/mL recombinant GAD65 produced in yeast (RSR Limited). The endotoxin level of recombinant GAD65 was below 0.1 EU/mL (at an antigen concentration of 10 μg/mL) by the chromogenic assay method.[8]

To confirm that the system was working, the response to PPD (Japan BCG, Tokyo, Japan) was used as a positive control for subjects with a positive tuberculin. PPD responses did not mimic the GAD65 responses. The tubes were incubated at 37°C in a humidified 5% CO_2 atmosphere for a total of 72 h, with the last 4 h including a final concentration of 10 μg/mL Brefeldin A (Sigma). After incubation, 300 μL activated blood was transferred to other tubes (in duplicate). Then, 20 μL CD4-PC5 antibody (Coulter, Marseille, France) was added, and the tubes were incubated at room temperature (RT) for 15 min. Then, 4 mL FACS lysing solution (Becton Dickinson) was added, and the tubes were vortexed gently and incubated at RT for another 10 min. After centrifuging the tubes at 1600 rpm for 5 min, the supernatant was removed and the cells were washed with 0.1% BSA (bovine serum albumin)–PBS. Then, 1.5 mL FACS permeabilizing solution (Becton Dickinson) was added and the tubes were incubated for 10 min at RT in the dark. After washing with 0.1% BSA-PBS twice, 20 μL antibody mixture (IFN-γ-FITC and IL-4-PE [phycoerythrin],

Becton Dickinson) or isotype control mixture (IgG2a-FITC and IgG1-PE, Becton Dickinson) was added, and the tubes were incubated for 30 min at RT in the dark. After washing, the prepared cells were analyzed by EPICS ALTRA (Coulter). Both intra- and interassay variation in this system were <10%, respectively.

HLA Typing

HLA class II antigen (HLA-DR alleles) was examined by the hybridization protection assay, which is an HLA typing method based on hybridization of acridium-ester-labeled DNA probes to amplified DNA, as described previously.[9]

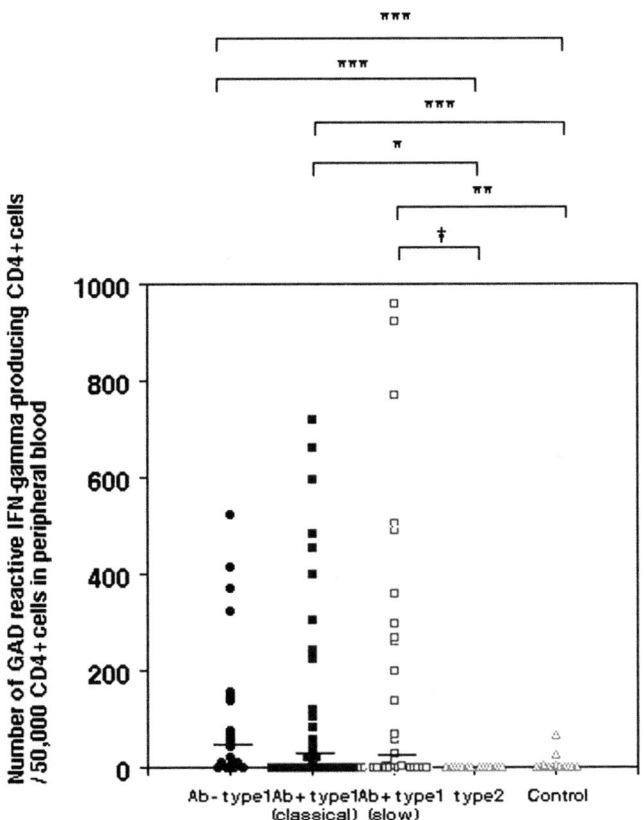

FIGURE 1. Number of GAD-reactive IFN-γ-producing CD4+ cells out of 50,000 CD4+ cells in peripheral blood. Ab− type 1: type 1 diabetes without islet-associated autoantibody; Ab+ type 1 (classical): classical type 1 diabetes with islet-associated autoantibody; Ab+ type 1 (slow): latent autoimmune diabetes in adults; type 2: type 2 diabetes without islet-associated autoantibody; control: control subjects. The bar indicates the median level of each group; ***$p < 0.0001$, **$p = 0.0001$, *$p < 0.001$, †$p < 0.01$.

Statistical Analysis

Results are presented as mean ± SE and median (and interquartile range) in FIGURE 1. Differences in the number of GAD-reactive IFN-γ-producing CD4+ cells between groups were analyzed using the Mann-Whitney U test for nonparametric unpaired observations. The proportion of "GAD-reactive IFN-γ-producing CD4+ cell-positive" patients (level greater than mean + 3SD for control subjects) was compared between the groups using Fisher's exact test.

RESULTS

GAD-Reactive IFN-γ-Producing CD4+ Cells Were Detected in Classical Type 1 Diabetes without Autoantibody

As shown in FIGURE 1, the number of GAD-reactive IFN-γ-producing CD4+ cells in diabetics with type 1B (113.6 ± 34.6, median 45 [interquartile range, 147.5], in 50,000 CD4+ cells), type 1A (132.4 ± 33.3, median 25 [interquartile range, 225], in 50,000 CD4+ cells), and LADA (154.4 ± 44.1, median 20 [interquartile range, 230], in 50,000 CD4+ cells) was significantly higher than that in type 2 diabetics (0.3 ± 0.3, median 0 [interquartile range 0], in 50,000 CD4+ cells) and control subjects (3.8 ± 2.4, median 0 [interquartile range 0], in 50,000 CD4+ cells). There was no significant difference in the number of GAD-reactive IFN-γ-producing CD4+ cells among the type 1B, type 1A, and LADA groups. On the other hand, there was no significant difference in the number of GAD-reactive IFN-γ-producing CD4+ cells between type 2 diabetics and control subjects.

Regarding the proportion of patients possessing HLA DR4 and/or DR9, which are considered to be susceptible alleles in Japanese type 1 diabetes,[9] there was no significant difference among the type 1B, type 1A, and LADA groups (90%, 100%, and 91%, respectively). Of note, however, GAD-reactive IFN-γ-producing CD4+ cells were detected in patients without HLA DR4 and/or DR9 as well.

Regarding age, there was a difference between type 2 diabetics and control subjects, and also there was a difference among the type 1B, type 1A, and LADA groups. However, because there was no significant difference in the number of GAD-reactive IFN-γ-producing CD4+ cells between type 2 diabetics and control subjects and also no significant difference in the number of GAD-reactive IFN-γ-producing CD4+ cells among the type 1B, type 1A, and LADA groups, we assume that age had no effect on the number of GAD-reactive IFN-γ-producing CD4+ cells.

We also assessed the relation between the number of GAD-reactive IFN-γ-producing CD4+ cells and the duration of disease. The number of GAD-reactive IFN-γ-producing CD4+ cells in patients with a shorter disease duration (<3 years) and longer duration (>3 years) was not significantly different in the type 1B, type 1A, and LADA groups, although that in type 1B patients with a shorter duration was higher than that in type 1B patients with a longer duration (162.0 ± 58.0 vs. 69.5 ± 37.4 in 50,000 CD4+ cells).

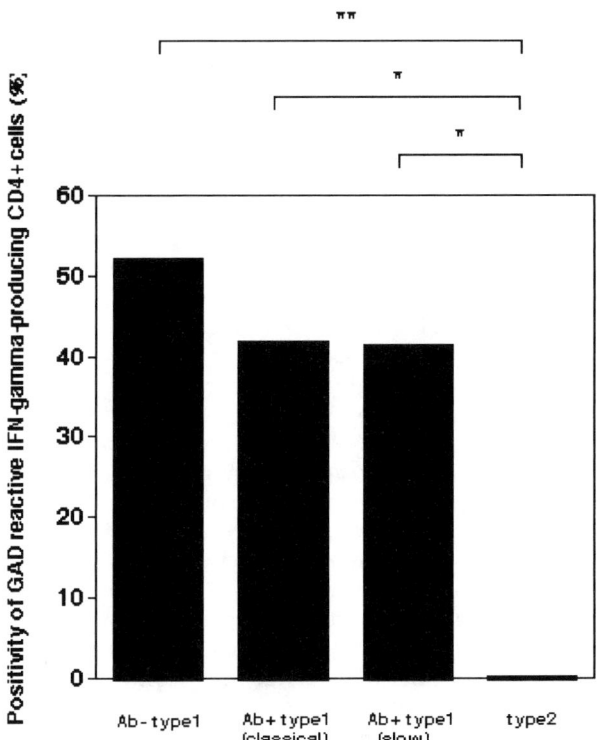

FIGURE 2. Proportion of "GAD-reactive IFN-γ-producing CD4+ cell-positive" patients: Ab– type 1: type 1 diabetes without islet-associated autoantibody; Ab+ type 1 (classical): classical type 1 diabetes with islet-associated autoantibody; Ab+ type 1 (slow): latent autoimmune diabetes in adults; type 2: type 2 diabetes without islet-associated autoantibody; **$p < 0.001$, *$p < 0.01$.

At Least Half of "Type 1B" Patients Had T Cell Reactivity against GAD

As mentioned above, we clearly demonstrated the existence of GAD-reactive T cells in peripheral blood from "type 1B" patients. It is clinically important to assess the proportion of these patients who are positive for GAD-reactive IFN-γ-producing cells. Thus, we set the normal upper limit of the number of GAD-reactive CD4+ cells at the mean + 3SD of values in control subjects (42.6 in 50,000 CD4+ cells) and assessed the "positivity" of GAD-reactive IFN-γ-producing CD4+ cells. Approximately half (52.4%) of "type 1B" patients were positive for GAD-reactive IFN-γ-producing CD4+ cells, whereas none of the type 2 diabetics was positive for GAD-reactive IFN-γ-producing CD4+ cells ($p < 0.001$). Regarding type 1 diabetics with autoantibody, 42.1% of type 1A and 41.7% of LADA patients were considered positive, showing almost the same level as type 1B patients (FIG. 2).

DISCUSSION

Usually, the diagnosis of "idiopathic" (nonautoimmune) type 1 diabetes is made based on the negativity of islet-associated autoantibodies such as GAD and IA-2 antibodies. However, some researchers have reported that negativity of islet-associated autoantibodies in type 1 diabetes does not rule out autoimmunity, based on the fact that the frequency of susceptible HLA types in islet-associated autoantibody-negative type 1 diabetic patients is almost the same as that in islet-associated autoantibody-positive type 1 diabetic patients (C. N. Cornell *et al.*, presented at the ADA meeting, 2000). Therefore, the entity of type 1B diabetes itself has not yet been defined. Of course, most cases of type 1 diabetes are considered a T cell–mediated autoimmune disease; hence, assessment of T cell reactivity against islet-associated antigen is essential. Although attempts have been made to detect the reactivity of T cells against GAD,[10–12] it has been recognized that it is difficult to show a difference in the proliferative responses to GAD between type 1 diabetics and controls.[11,12] In our case also, it was difficult to observe any difference in proliferative responses between type 1 diabetics and controls; thus, we selected an intracellular cytokine staining procedure for use in the present study. The frequency of antigen-specific T cells detected using the ELISPOT assay, etc., in the literature is 1/1000 to 1/10,000 mononuclear cells, whereas the detectable precursor frequency can be 1/1000 to 2/100 CD4+ T cells using this kind of intracellular cytokine staining for FACS according to a report by Waldrop *et al.*[13] The increased sensitivity of the flow cytometric assay is likely to be the result of several factors: (1) the high sensitivity of fluorescence detection by current flow cytometers, (2) the highly efficient capture of cytokine within the cytoplasm of the secretion-inhibited responding cell using Brefeldin A (as compared to only partial capture in ELISPOT-type assays), and (3) the independence of antigen stimulation conditions and the single cell signal detection strategy, allowing these conditions to be set up with optimization of response as the only concern.[13] Moreover, when we compared the numbers of antigen-specific T cells at different time points, at least a 2- to 5-fold increase in responsive cells was detected with culture for an additional 48 h (24 vs. 72 h; data not shown). Furthermore, as described by Waldrop *et al.*,[13] providing exogenous costimulation in the form of an anti-CD28 monoclonal antibody augmented the response in the presence of specific antigen, and the degree of augmentation provided by anti-CD28 was approximately 2-fold. Moreover, augmentation of detectable effector frequencies by anti-CD28 inclusion has been observed for all antigens examined. These results prompted routine inclusion of anti-CD28 in all assays, with control groups having anti-CD28 alone or anti-CD28 added to control antigen preparations.[13] In addition to the issues discussed above, we think that use of whole blood to reduce the background may partly contribute to the better results as compared to the previous reports. In this study, by using an intracellular cytokine staining procedure, we found GAD-reactive T cells in the peripheral blood from islet-associated autoantibody-negative type 1 diabetic patients, and the level was almost the same as that in islet-associated autoantibody-positive type 1 diabetic patients. In addition, at least half of the type 1 diabetic patients without islet-associated autoantibody were found to be positive for GAD-reactive T cells. These data clearly indicate that at least half of the cases of type 1 diabetes without islet-associated autoantibody can be considered as autoimmune type. If we say exactly that islet-associated antibody-negative patients in this study were

"GAD and IA-2 antibody-negative" patients, we therefore cannot perfectly neglect the possibility of inclusion of other antibody such as ICA-positive (and/or IAA-positive) patients. However, according to previous reports, a combination of GAD and IA-2 covers approximately 90% of type 1 diabetic patients; thus, GAD/IA-2 combined assay is considered the first-line screening for type 1 diabetes.[14,15] Of course, we would like to confirm the negativity of ICA (and IAA) in a future study. Recently, it has been reported that insulitis can be observed even in type 1 diabetic patients without islet-associated autoantibodies such as GAD and IA-2 antibody.[16] If possible, we would like to confirm the correlation between pancreatic histology (insulitis) and the number of GAD-reactive IFN-γ-producing CD4+ cells in peripheral blood lymphocytes in a future study as well.

The present study shows data of T cell reactivity against GAD only. We first thought that the IA-2 antigen could not be used as an antigen for the assessment of T cell reactivity in type 1 diabetes because it is produced by *E. coli*, based on the concept that the GAD antigen produced by *E. coli* is not a suitable antigen to assess antigen-specific T cell reactivity in type 1 diabetes. Recently, however, it has been proposed that the IA-2 antigen can be used to assess T cell reactivity in type 1 diabetes even though it is produced by *E. coli*.[17] Therefore, preliminary assessment of IA-2-specific reactivity in type 1 diabetes was also done in some of the patients. However, more detailed assessment and accumulation of data are required to discuss this issue.

Recently, we have found that polymorphisms of the neuroD/BETA2 gene[18] and the vitamin D receptor gene[19] are correlated with the onset pattern of type 1 diabetes. In a future study, combined assessment of the polymorphisms of these genes and islet-associated antigen-specific T cell response may be worthwhile for proper classification of type 1 diabetes. Thus far, immunotherapy for type 1 diabetes has been applied regardless of islet-associated autoantibody-positivity. To select the proper population of type 1 diabetics with autoimmunity, autoantibody measurement may be not enough, and additional assessment to detect the existence of autoimmunity such as islet-associated antigen-specific T cell response may be necessary. Assessment of T cell reactivity against islet-associated antigen may contribute to the diagnosis of "autoimmune-related" type 1 diabetes and the proper selection of patients suitable for immunotherapy.

REFERENCES

1. EXPERT COMMITTEE ON THE DIAGNOSIS AND CLASSIFICATION OF DIABETES MELLITUS. 1999. Report of the Expert Committee on the Diagnosis and Classification of Diabetes Mellitus. Diabetes Care **22**(10): 1755–1757.
2. ALBERTI, K. & P. ZIMMET. 1998. Definition, diagnosis, and classification of diabetes mellitus and its complications. Part 1: Diagnosis and classification of diabetes mellitus provisional report of a WHO consultation. Diabetes Med. **15**(7): 535–536.
3. BACH, J. 1994. Insulin-dependent diabetes mellitus as an autoimmune disease. Endocr. Rev. **15**(4): 516–542.
4. NAKAMOTO, S., A. KASUGA, T. MARUYAMA *et al*. 2000. Age of onset, not type of onset, affects the positivity and evanescence of IA-2 antibody. Diabetes Res. Clin. Pract. **50**(2): 147–152.
5. TUOMI, T., L. GROOP, P. ZIMMET *et al*. 1993. Antibodies to glutamic acid decarboxylase reveal latent autoimmune diabetes mellitus in adults with a non-insulin-dependent onset of disease. Diabetes **42**(2): 359–362.

6. MASUDA, M., M. POWELL, S. CHEN et al. 2000. Autoantibodies to IA-2 in insulin-dependent diabetes mellitus: measurements with a new immunoprecipitation assay. Clin. Chim. Acta **291**(1): 53–66.
7. SHIMADA, A., J. MORIMOTO, K. KODAMA et al. 2001. Elevated serum IP-10 levels observed in type 1 diabetes. Diabetes Care **24**(3): 510–515.
8. YANO, S., Y. HOTTA & S. TAKAHASHI. 1986. Determination of endotoxin in injectable antibiotic preparations by the chromogenic assay method using a Limulus reagent (Tachypleus hemocyte lysate) and a chromogenic substrate. J. Clin. Microbiol. **23**(1): 11–16.
9. MARUYAMA, T., A. SHIMADA, A. KASUGA et al. 1994. Analysis of MHC class II antigens in Japanese IDDM by a novel HLA-typing method, hybridization protection assay. Diabetes Res. Clin. Pract. **23**(2): 77–84.
10. ATKINSON, M.A., D.L. KAUFMAN, L. CAMPBELL et al. 1992. Response of peripheral-blood mononuclear cells to glutamate decarboxylase in insulin-dependent diabetes. Lancet **339**(8791): 458–459.
11. ROEP, B.O., M.A. ATKINSON, P.M. VAN ENDERT et al. 1999. Autoreactive T cell responses in insulin-dependent (type 1) diabetes mellitus: report of the First International Workshop for Standardization of T Cell Assays. J. Autoimmun. **13**(2): 267–282.
12. VIGLIETTA, V., T. ORBAN & D.A. HAFLER. 2002. GAD65-reactive T cells are activated in patients with autoimmune type 1a diabetes. J. Clin. Invest. **109**(7): 895–903.
13. WALDROP, S.L., C.J. PITCHER, D.M. PETERSON et al. 1997. Determination of antigen-specific memory/effector CD4+ T cell frequencies by flow cytometry: evidence for a novel, antigen-specific homeostatic mechanism in HIV-associated immunodeficiency. J. Clin. Invest. **99**(7): 1739–1750.
14. BORG, H., P. FERNLUND & G. SUNDKVIST. 1997. Protein tyrosine phosphatase–like protein IA2-antibodies plus glutamic acid decarboxylase 65 antibodies (GADA) indicate autoimmunity as frequently as islet cell antibodies assay in children with recently diagnosed diabetes mellitus. Clin. Chem. **43**(12): 2358–2363.
15. DITTLER, J., D. SEIDEL, M. SCHENKER & A.G. ZIEGLER. 1998. GADIA2-combi determination as first-line screening for improved prediction of type 1 diabetes in relatives. Diabetes **47**(4): 592–597.
16. IMAGAWA, A., T. HANAFUSA, S. TAMURA et al. 2001. Pancreatic biopsy as a procedure for detecting *in situ* autoimmune phenomena in type 1 diabetes: close correlation between serological markers and histological evidence of cellular autoimmunity. Diabetes **50**(6): 1269–1273.
17. PEAKMAN, M., T. TREE, J. ENDL et al. 2001. Characterization of preparations of GAD65, proinsulin, and the islet tyrosine phosphatase IA-2 for use in detection of autoreactive T-cells in type 1 diabetes: report of phase II of the Second International Immunology of Diabetes Society Workshop for Standardization of T-Cell Assays in Type 1 Diabetes. Diabetes **50**(8): 1749–1754.
18. YAMADA, S., Y. MOTOHASHI, T. YANAGAWA et al. 2001. NeuroD/beta2 gene G→A polymorphism may affect onset pattern of type 1 diabetes in Japanese. Diabetes Care **24**(8): 1438–1441.
19. MOTOHASHI, Y., S. YAMADA, T. YANAGAWA et al. 2003. Vitamin D receptor gene polymorphism affects onset pattern of type 1 diabetes. J. Clin. Endocrinol. Metab. **88**(7): 3137–3140.

Autoantibodies to GAD65 and IA-2 Antibodies Are Increased, but Not Tissue Transglutaminase (TTG-Ab) in Type 2 Diabetes Mellitus (T2DM) Patients from South India

C. B. SANJEEVI,[a] M. BALAJI,[b] V. BALAJI,[b] AND V. SESHIAH[b]

[a]*Department of Molecular Medicine, Karolinska Institute, Karolinska Hospital, Stockholm, Sweden*

[b]*Department of Diabetology, Apollo Hospitals, Chennai, India*

ABSTRACT: The frequency of autoantibody-positve T2DM patients identified as LADA was shown to be high in T2DM patients from Eastern India. In this study, we measured autoantibodies to GAD65, IA-2, and TTG in T2DM patients from Southern India. Our results show that either GAD65 or IA-2 was present in 30% of T2DM patients ($n = 155$) and in 3% of controls for GAD65 and 1% of controls for IA-2 ($n = 105$). TTG-Ab was not increased in T2DM patients compared to controls. Our results suggest that LADA is more frequent in Southern Indians than in European Caucasians, but not as high as in Eastern Indians.

KEYWORDS: T1DM; T2DM; GAD65; IA-2; TTG; LADA

INTRODUCTION

Antibodies to tyrosine phosphatase (IA-2-Ab) and glutamate decarboxylase 65 (GAD65-Ab) are major markers for type 1 diabetes (T1DM) in Caucasians. Detection of these autoantibodies in patients diagnosed with type 2 diabetes (T2DM) would suggest the diagnosis of latent autoimmune diabetes in adults (LADA), also referred to as the slowly progressive form of T1DM. The frequency of autoantibodies to GAD65 or IA-2 antigens was measured in Eastern Indians[1] diagnosed as T2DM. The results suggest that either GAD65 or IA-2 antibodies were present in 90/214 patients (42%) compared to a frequency of 4% for GAD65 and 2% for IA-2 antibodies in 120 healthy controls in Eastern India. This finding suggested that the frequency of autoimmune diabetes in those diagnosed as T2DM was high in India. The reason for this could be attributed to a lack of availability of autoantibody assay, which leads to overdiagnosis of T2DM. The frequency of autoantibody positivity in patients diag-

Address for correspondence: Dr. C. B. Sanjeevi, Department of Molecular Medicine, Karolinska Institute, Karolinska Hospital, CMM, L8:00, S-17176 Stockholm, Sweden. Voice: +46-8-5177-6254; fax: +46-8-5177-6179.
sanjeevi.carani@molmed.ki.se

nosed with T2DM in European populations is not more than 10% to 11% in different populations, including those in the UKPDS study.

Tissue transglutaminase (TTG) is a 85-kDa protein. It is an intracellular enzyme released from cells during wounding. It belongs to a family of calcium-dependent enzymes that catalyze cross-linking of proteins. Gliadin is an excellent substrate for TTG. TTG antibodies (TTG-Ab) are specific for celiac disease.[2] Celiac disease is characterized by small intestinal damage with loss of absorptive villi and hyperplasia of the crypts, typically leading to malabsorption. Celiac disease is precipitated by ingestion of the protein gliadin, a component of wheat gluten, and usually resolves on its withdrawal. About 10% to 20% of the celiac disease patients also have T1DM and both diseases are associated with HLA-DR3-DQ2. The frequency of TTG-Ab in Eastern Indian and Northern Indian patients with T1DM is higher than in healthy controls.[3,4]

The aim of this study was to measure autoantibodies to GAD65, IA-2, and TTG in Southern Indian patients diagnosed as T2DM.

PATIENTS AND METHODS

We studied serum samples from 155 NIDDM patients and 105 healthy controls from Chennai, South India. Samples were transported to Karolinska Hospital in Sweden and stored at −20°C until analysis.

TTG-Ab was evaluated by radioligand binding assay using *in vitro* transcribed/translated recombinant human ^{35}S-TTG. Autoantibodies to GAD65 and IA-2 were also measured by radioligand binding assay using ^{35}S-labeled recombinant human GAD65 and IA-2 in an *in vitro* transcription/translation system.

RESULTS AND DISCUSSION

The results show that TTG-Ab is not increased in patients compared to controls, but GAD65-Ab and IA-2-Ab are significantly increased in NIDDM patients compared to controls from South India. Antibody positivity to either GAD65 or IA-2 in T2DM patients is identified as slow-onset T1DM and, according to the current ADA or WHO classification, they should be redesignated as T1DM. TTG-Ab was compared in autoantibody-positive T2DM patients and healthy controls.

Either GAD65-Ab or IA-2-Ab was present in 30% of patients, suggesting that the prevalence of slow-onset T1DM is high in the South Indian population. Frequency of these autoantibodies was lower in healthy controls (TABLE 1).

TABLE 1. Autoantibody frequencies in T2DM patients from Chennai, India

Autoantibodies	T2DM patients ($n = 155$)	Controls ($n = 105$)
GAD65 Ab+	33 (21%)	3 (3%)
ICA512 Ab+	27 (17%)	1 (1%)
Either GAD65 or IA-2 Ab+	47 (30%)	3 (3%)
TTG Ab+	3 (2%)	3 (3%)

The frequencies of GAD65 and IA-2 antibodies observed in Eastern Indian T2DM patients[1] were higher than in South Indians.

We conclude that TTG-Ab is not associated with T2DM from South India. However, GAD65-Ab and IA-2-Ab are significantly increased in clinically diagnosed T2DM patients. The prevalence of GAD65-Ab is higher than that of IA-2-Ab in South Indians.

ACKNOWLEDGMENTS

This study was supported by grants from the Swedish Medical Research Council (K2001-16X-12532-04B), Karolinska Institute, Novo Nordisk Fond, Svenska Diabetes Förbundet, Barn Diabetes Fonden, and Åke Wiberg Stiftelse. C. B. Sanjeevi is supported by a Swedish MFR's position (K2001-72P-13149-03C).

REFERENCES

1. SANJEEVI, C.B., A. KANUNGO, A. SHTAUVERE et al. 1999. Association of HLA class II alleles with different subgroups of diabetes mellitus in Eastern India identify different association with IDDM and malnutrition-related diabetes. Tissue Antigens **54:** 83–87.
2. DIETERICH, W., T. EHINS, M. BAUER et al. 1997. Identification of tissue transglutaminase as autoantigen of celiac disease. Nat. Med. **3:** 797–801.
3. KANUNGO, A., A. SHTAUVERE-BRAMEUS, K.C. SAMAL & C.B. SANJEEVI. 2002. Autoantibodies to tissue transglutaminase in patients from Eastern India with malnutrition-modulated diabetes mellitus, insulin-dependent diabetes mellitus, and non-insulin-dependent diabetes mellitus. Ann. N.Y. Acad. Sci. **958:** 232–234.
4. TANDON, N., A. SHTAUVERE-BRAMEUS, W.A. HAGOPIAN & C.B. SANJEEVI. 2002. Prevalence of ICA-12 and other autoantibodies in North Indian patients with early-onset diabetes. Ann. N.Y. Acad. Sci. **958:** 214–217.

IA-2 Autoantibodies Are Predominant in Latent Autoimmune Diabetes in Adults Patients from Eastern India

ALOK KANUNGO[a] AND C. B. SANJEEVI[b]

[a]*Cuttack Diabetes Research Foundation, Cuttack, Orissa, India*
[b]*Molecular Immunogenetics Group, Department of Molecular Medicine, Karolinska Hospital, Stockholm, Sweden*

ABSTRACT: Autoimmune diabetes or latent autoimmune diabetes in adults (LADA) among the clinically diagnosed type 2 diabetes patients from Cuttack in Eastern India was studied. GAD65 and IA-2 autoantibodies were measured by radioligand binding assay using recombinant human GAD65 and IA-2. The frequency of GAD65 was not significantly different between patients and controls. However, IA-2 antibodies were predominant in LADA patients and there were two distinct peaks, one in the age group of 20 to 30 years and another in the age group of 50 to 60 years. The data suggest that LADA is more frequent in Eastern Indian T2DM patients and the IA-2 is the predominant autoantibody in this population.

KEYWORDS: T1DM; T2DM; LADA; GAD65; IA-2

INTRODUCTION

Type 1 diabetes mellitus (T1DM) develops due to autoimmune destruction of beta cells. This autoimmune destruction can occur at any age, but occurs predominantly in the younger age group. The World Health Organization (WHO) classifies diabetes mellitus into insulin-dependent diabetes mellitus (IDDM), non-insulin-dependent diabetes mellitus (NIDDM), and malnutrition-related diabetes mellitus (MRDM).[1] This classification of diabetes is based on the clinical criteria and not based on the pathophysiologic disease process. IDDM was also referred to as T1DM, and NIDDM as type 2 diabetes (T2DM). These terminologies are used synonymously in almost all countries. However, the American Diabetes Association (ADA) in their recent classification, proposed in 1997, have used the terminology T1DM and T2DM.[2] After this classification, it has become clear that the terms T1DM and T2DM are used to describe the disease process, thereby giving the understanding that the IDDM and NIDDM are terms used to describe diabetes as clinical categories. In the current ADA classification, clinically described IDDM patients and the autoantibody-positive

---

Address for correspondence: Dr. C. B. Sanjeevi, Molecular Immunogenetics Group, Department of Molecular Medicine, Karolinska Institute, Karolinska Hospital, CMM, L8:00, S-171 76 Stockholm, Sweden. Voice: +46-8-517-76254; fax: +46-8-517-76179.
sanjeevi.carani@molmed.ki.se

NIDDM patients are referred to as T1DM. As there are no markers available for the etiologic diagnosis of T2DM, the diagnosis of the T2DM is determined by exclusion of T1DM.[2,3] According to the published literature, based on the WHO's clinical classification of diabetes, IDDM has a low prevalence in India. Antibodies to glutamic acid decarboxylase isoform 65 (GAD65) and tyrosine phosphatase (IA-2) are the main ones used for the identification of autoimmune diabetes or T1DM.

GAD65Ab-positivity was observed in 70–80% of new-onset T1DM in several populations compared to 1–2% of healthy controls.[5–8] It was found that the prevalence of GAD65Ab was significantly higher among T1DM females than among T1DM males. This gender-dependent difference in occurrence of GAD65Ab seems to be more pronounced in patients less than 12 years old: in that group, GAD65Ab were found in 80% of females and 61% of males.[4] In a study of 312 recent-onset Belgian T1DM patients, the prevalence of GAD65Ab among children less than 9 years old (64%) was found to be lower than that of ICA (86%) or IAA (78%). GAD65Ab are associated with slower rates of disease progression.[9,10] However, while the prevalence of ICA and IAA decreased with increasing age at onset of the disease, the prevalence of GAD65Ab remained unchanged (80% and 78% in age groups of 10–19 years and 20–39 years, respectively). These data indicate that GAD65Ab may have the highest diagnostic sensitivity for T1DM among 20- to 39-year-old patients.

There are very few studies on the prevalence of GAD65 antibodies in Indian T1DM patients. The prevalence of the GAD65Ab in South Indian T1DM patients was 59% in recent-onset T1DM patients (duration < 2 years), but the frequency increased to 69% in patients with duration of 6–10 years. All patients below the age of 5 years were GAD65Ab-positive.[11] This suggests that the T1DM seen in India is not different from that seen in Caucasians. Obese T1DM patients had significantly less GAD65Ab when compared to undernourished and normal-nourished subjects. In Indian T1DM patients from Cuttack, IA-2 was the predominant autoantibody and was present in 43% of patients ($n = 74$), and it was lower in patients with short duration of disease, <4 years (32%), than in patients with long duration, >4 years (60%). This finding is opposite to that found in GAD65Ab, which have levels that are higher in Indian patients with short versus long duration of the disease.[12] However, in T1DM patients from Cuttack, GAD65Ab were lower in frequency than in South Indian patients. In this group, the predominant autoantibody was to ICA512 and not GAD65. However, in European Caucasians, the predominant autoantibody was to GAD65 and not ICA512.

In this study, our aim was to measure the GAD65 and IA-2 autoantibodies in T2DM patients from Cuttack and to identify their frequency in relation to age, treatment, and body mass index (BMI).

SUBJECTS AND METHODS

Patients attending the Diabetes Clinic of the SCB Medical College and Cuttack Diabetes Foundation from Cuttack in Eastern India were studied: T2DM patients ($n = 214$); healthy controls ($n = 120$). Plasma was separated and stored from EDTA blood at $-80°C$ until analysis. *In vitro* transcribed and translated ^{35}S-methionine (Promega, Madison, WI)–labeled recombinant human GAD65 and IA-2 were used to measure autoantibodies to GAD65 and IA-2 by immunoprecipitation assay.

TABLE 1. Autoantibodies versus BMI in NIDDM patients from Cuttack

BMI	GAD65 Ab+ NIDDM (n = 15)	ICA512 Ab+ NIDDM (n = 76)
<18.5	3 (20%)	12 (16%)
Normal	10 (67%)*	54 (71%)*
Obese	2 (13%)	10 (13%)

*$p < 0.001$ vs. the <18.5 and obese groups.

TABLE 2. Autoantibodies versus treatment in NIDDM patients from Cuttack

Treatment	GAD65 Ab+ NIDDM (n = 15)	ICA512 Ab+ NIDDM (n = 76)
Diet	2 (13%)	3 (4%)
OHA	6 (40%)	53 (70%)
Insulin	7 (47%)	20 (26%)

RESULTS AND DISCUSSION

In healthy controls, autoantibody frequency was 4% for GAD65 and 2% for IA-2 antibodies. In T2DM patients from Cuttack, GAD65 antibodies were present in 7% of patients and not significantly different from controls. However, the predominant autoantibody in T2DM patients was IA-2, present in 76/214 (36%) patients. In T2DM patients from Madras, GAD65 antibodies decreased with increasing age.[12] Either GAD65 or IA-2 was present in 90/214 (42%) patients.

GAD65 and IA-2 antibodies were significantly high in normal-weight compared to obese T2DM patients (TABLE 1). Among the GAD65Ab-positive T2DM patients (n = 15), the majority of them were already on insulin (7/15). However, among the IA-2-positive T2DM patients (n = 76), the majority were on oral hypoglycemic agents (53/76; 70%) (TABLE 2).

When all the T2DM patients were divided into different age groups, the maximal IA-2 antibody-positivity was present in the 20–30 age group (30/41; 73%) and in the 50–60 age group (14/23; 60%) (FIG. 1). This finding suggests that LADA is higher in all age groups, but there is a definite peak in the older age group of 50–60 years.

Using clinical criteria for the diagnosis of diabetes, patients who did not present with ketoacidosis and ketonuria were grouped under the category of T2DM, regardless of the age group. With the advent of assays to detect autoantibodies becoming simpler, more and more patients were identified as autoantibody-positive in the T2DM category. This led to the identification of a group called "late-onset autoimmune diabetes in adults or LADA".[13,14] This group of LADA, first described by Paul Zimmet, subsequently turned out to be present in the younger individuals with diabetes in the T2DM category. This category has also been described as latent type 1 diabetes, late-onset type 1 diabetes, type 1 masquerading as type 2 diabetes, antibody-positive NIDDM, and type 1 and 1/2 diabetes. The Japanese found a high frequency of these patients and referred to them as slow-onset T1DM. This category has come to be addressed more appropriately as slowly progressive T1DM. It is believed that the autoimmune beta cell destructive process proceeds slowly in this form of diabetes.

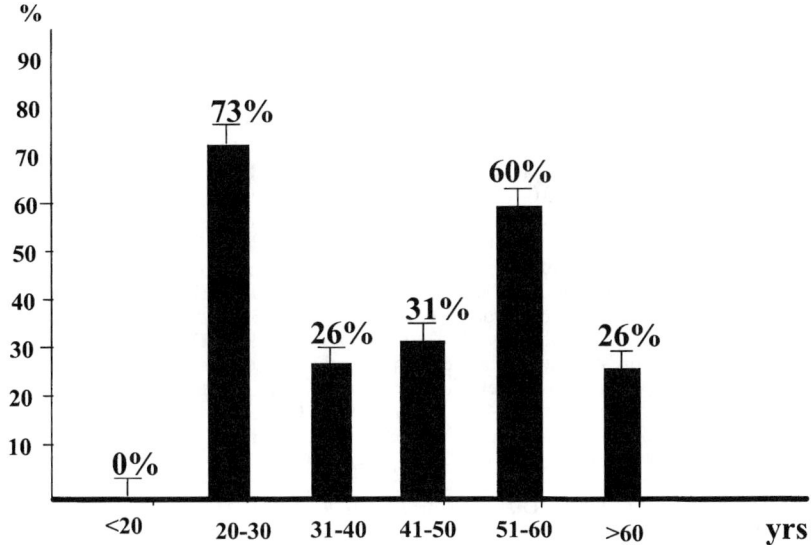

FIGURE 1. Maximal IA-2 antibody-positivity in various age groups of T2DM patients. See text for details.

Several studies have shown that GAD65 and/or IA-2 antibody-positive patients have more rapid decline in C-peptide levels, do not respond adequately to oral drugs, and require early insulin treatment. In a study from Japan, in nonobese and insulin-deficient patients with sulfonylurea failures, 11% were positive for GAD65Ab, suggesting that autoimmune mechanisms may play a role in the secondary failure to sulfonylurea therapy. The GAD65Ab index has also been shown to correlate well with HbA1 in T1DM patients. Patients with low GAD65Ab have better glycemic control and require less insulin. However, the IA-2 index did not correlate with HbA1.[15] Thus, loss of beta cell function in a majority (two-thirds) of individuals with clinical T2DM can be predicted by GAD65Ab and ICA. Early detection of immune markers of beta cell damage creates the potential for immunomodulation to limit such damage.[16]

Insulin treatment has been shown to be the best for the autoimmune variety of diabetes in animal models of autoimmune diabetes and in humans. The action of insulin in an autoimmune situation has been to reduce hyperglycemia, thereby giving beta cell rest and its immunologic effect. A pilot study on the antibody-positive T2DM done in Japanese patients shows the protective effect of small doses of insulin given subcutaneously compared to sulfonylurea-treated patients. Four of the 5 patients in the antibody-positive T2DM group became antibody-negative after follow-up for 30 months and in 0/5 in the sulfonylurea group remained antibody-positive at the end of 30 months.[17]

In conclusion, the frequencies of autoantibody-positive T2DM or LADA patients are high in Cuttack and the predominant autoantibody is that of the IA-2 variety.

REFERENCES

1. WHO STUDY GROUP. 1985. Diabetes mellitus. WHO Technical Report Series 727.
2. ADA. 1997. Classification—The Expert Committee on the Diagnosis and Classification of Diabete Mellitus: report. Diabetes Care **20:** 1183–1197.
3. ALBERTI, K. & P. ZIMMET. 1998. Definition, diagnosis, and classification of diabetes mellitus and its complications. Part 1: Diagnosis and classification of diabetes mellitus—provisional report of a WHO consultation. Diabet. Med. **15:** 539–553.
4. FALORNI, A., E. ÖRTQVIST, B. PERSSON & Å. LERNMARK. 1995. Radioimmunoassays for glutamic acid decarboxylase and GAD65 antibodies using ^{35}S or ^{3}H recombinant human ligands. J. Immunol. Methods **186:** 89–99.
5. HAGOPIAN, W., C. SANJEEVI, I. KOCKUM et al. 1995. Glutamate decarboxylase-, insulin-, and islet cell–antibodies and HLA typing to detect diabetes in a general population-based study of Swedish children. J. Clin. Invest. **95:** 1505–1511.
6. HAGOPIAN, W.A., A.E. KARLSEN, A. GOTTSATER et al. 1993. Quantitative assay using recombinant human islet glutamic acid decarboxylase (GAD-64) shows that 64K autoantibody positivity at onset predicts diabetes type. J. Clin. Invest. **91:** 368–374.
7. PETERSEN, J., K. HEJNAES, A. MOODY et al. 1994. Detection of GAD65 antibodies in diabetes and other autoimmune diseases using a simple radioligand binding assay. Diabetes **43:** 459–465.
8. SANJEEVI, C., A. FALORNI, J. ROBERTSON & Å. LERNMARK. 1996. Glutamic acid decarboxylase in IDDM. Diabet. Nutr. Metab. **9:** 167–182.
9. CHRISTIE, M., S. GENOVESE, D. CASSIDY et al. 1994. Antibodies to islet 37k antigen, but not to GAD, discriminated rapid progression to IDDM in endocrine autoimmunity. Diabetes **43:** 1254–1259.
10. BINGLEY, P., M. CHRISTIE, E. BONIFACIO et al. 1994. Combined analysis of autoantibodies improves prediction of IDDM in islet cell antibodies positive relatives. Diabetes **43:** 1304–1310.
11. SANJEEVI, C., A. SHTAUVERE, A. RAMACHANDRAN et al. 1997. Prevalence of GAD65 autoantibodies in South Indian patients with IDDM and their parents. Diabet. Nutr. Metab. **10:** 60–64.
12. SANJEEVI, C., A. KANUNGO, A. SHTAUVERE et al. 1999. Association of HLA class II alleles with different subgroups of diabetes mellitus in Eastern India identify different associations with IDDM and malnutrition-related diabetes. Tissue Antigens **54:** 83–87.
13. TUOMI, T., L.C. GROOP, P.Z. ZIMMET et al. 1993. Antibodies to glutamic acid decarboxylase reveal latent autoimmune diabetes mellitus in adults with a non-insulin-dependent onset of disease. Diabetes **42:** 359–362.
14. ZIMMET, P., T. TUOMI, L. MACKAY et al. 1994. Latent autoimmune diabetes mellitus in adults (LADA): the role of antibodies to glutamic acid decarboxylase in diagnosis and prediction of insulin dependency. Diabet. Med. **11:** 299–303.
15. HOELDTKE, R., K. BRYNER, G. HORVATH et al. 1997. Antibodies to GAD and glycemic control in recent onset IDDM. Diabetes Care **20:** 1900–1903.
16. NAIK, R. & J. PALMER. 1997. Late-onset type 1 diabetes. Curr. Opin. Endocrinol. Diabetes **4:** 308–315.
17. KOBAYASHI, T., K. NAKANISHI, T. MURASE & K. KOSAKA. 1996. Small doses of subcutaneous insulin as a strategy for preventing slowly progressive beta cell failure in islet antibody positive patients with clinical features of NIDDM. Diabetes **45:** 622–626.

Parents Want to Know if Their Child Is at High Risk of Getting Diabetes

U. GUSTAFSSON STOLT, P-E. LISS, AND J. LUDVIGSSON
FOR THE ABIS STUDY GROUP

Division of Pediatrics, Department of Molecular and Clinical Medicine, Faculty of Health Sciences, Linköping University, Linköping, Sweden

> ABSTRACT: Not least among professionals, voices have been raised against screening research projects, which have been regarded as involving a risk of being unethical as they may disturb, scare, or even harm the included people without giving enough benefit. This problem with large-scale screening should be especially pronounced if increased risk of a serious disease like type 1 diabetes is identified when no effective prevention is available, and even more problematic if children were involved. ABIS (All Babies in Southeast Sweden) is a screening project including 17,000 newborn babies in the general population, followed prospectively to identify children at risk to get diabetes, and to study the influence of environmental factors causing the disease process. Four hundred randomly selected ABIS families received a questionnaire on attitudes and ethical questions regarding the project to be answered anonymously: 293/400 (73.3%) answered; 279/293 (95.3%) stated that they regarded it their right to be informed of results in the study and 278/293 (94.9%) said they really want to know. In fact, 254/293 (86.7%) report wanting to know if their child has increased risk of getting diabetes even if there is no preventive measure available. This clear result supports the view that this type of study may well be ethically justified as long as informed consent can be given based on adequate understanding and voluntariness. The results may have implications for the design of future screening studies.
>
> KEYWORDS: ABIS; children; screening; diabetes; prediction; informed consent; ethics; information

Type 1 diabetes in children is increasing rapidly in most countries.[1–5] This and other facts mean that environmental factors play an important role for this increase in incidence and thus there are several projects ongoing, for example, DIPP, DAISY, BabyDiab, DiPis, and ABIS, to mention a few of the large cohort studies. These studies are using development of autoantibodies (beta cell autoimmunity, BSA) as markers of the disease process, which in some cases lead to manifest type 1 diabetes.

Address for correspondence: Johnny Ludvigsson, Division of Pediatrics, Department of Molecular and Clinical Medicine, Faculty of Health Sciences, Linköping University, SE-58185 Linköping, Sweden. Voice: +46-13-22-13-33; fax: +46-13-14-82-65.
johnny.ludvigsson@lio.se

Such studies seem necessary if we ever shall be able to find the etiology of type 1 diabetes and crucial if we want to prevent the disease.[6–8] However, not least among professionals, voices have been raised against such studies as they are at risk of harming a large population of whom very few ever would have any benefit of the studies. Asking questions and taking biological samples are supposed to scare the population, and identifying high-risk individuals is considered to be unethical if there is no intervention to offer.[9–12]

All Babies in Southeast Sweden (ABIS) includes a general population of children followed from pregnancy and onwards. Out of 21,700 born in the area, 17,055 (78.6%) were included after having given their informed consent. We have earlier reported that an overwhelming majority of these mothers answered that they in fact felt calmer by participating in ABIS and only 1% said they felt more worried.[13]

However, one important question is what to do with results indicating increased risk for the child of getting diabetes. Should the parents be informed even if they do not actively ask for information? Should they be informed even though there is no intervention to offer to reduce the risk?

MATERIALS AND METHODS

The ABIS design involved initially biological samples taken at birth of the child, samples from the mother, and a perinatal questionnaire. Thereafter, during the first year, the children are followed prospectively with a diary, and introductions of new foods, infections, medications, vaccinations, life events, and other environmental factors are registered. At 1 year, new biological samples (e.g., blood) are taken and used for determinations of autoantibodies (GADA, IA-2A) and HLA typing. This procedure is repeated at 2.5 and 5 years. The parents were carefully informed about the study using videotapes, posters, information sheets, and oral information to make it possible for them to give their informed consent to participate. Thus, they were informed that one of the aims of the study is to identify those children with an increased risk of developing type 1 diabetes. However, they were also informed that information about results of such identification markers or determinations would only be given by request.

The ABIS cohort sample comprised all births of a defined geographic area in a 2-year period (October 1997 to October 1999). In 1999, a questionnaire, based on results of explorative interviews of some 20 mothers, was constructed, including questions and visual analogue scales (Likert type scales) covering ethical questions and attitudes. The questionnaire was sent out to 400 randomly selected ABIS families to be answered anonymously. The answer rate was 73.3%, meaning 293 respondents.[14]

RESULTS

Two hundred seventy-eight parents (94.9%) stated that they regard it to be their right to be informed of the results of those investigations made in ABIS indicating that their child could have an increased risk of getting diabetes. In fact, 279 (95.2%) said that they not only regarded it their right to know, but also wanted to be informed. Furthermore, 256 (87.4%) indicated that they want to be informed even if preventive measures were not yet available.[15]

DISCUSSION

Research projects always have to be ethically justified if they are to be performed, and especially when involving children. Even though a research ethics committee makes the initial evaluation, the responsible investigator always has to take the final responsibility and is also the party that has the most complete understanding of the research process.

First of all, the project has to have a quality that makes it plausible that conclusions can be drawn from the results. Then, there are several ethical minimum standards that have to be fulfilled according to the research ethics declarations. Informed consent is one of the most basal ethical requirements in studies or trials involving humans, even though it is not easy to define when somebody is informed enough to give his or her consent freely. For natural reasons, studies in children have special ethical problems as children cannot be expected to fully understand nor to take the autonomous responsibility for serious decisions like participation in research projects.

Screening projects performed in healthy children certainly mean special ethical conflicts. The project may be very scientifically important and of great future value for the health of other children, but may have no therapeutic value for the included individual child. The screening procedure may mean not only pain from blood sampling, but the results of the samples may reveal that the child has an increased risk of getting a serious disease, like type 1 diabetes, some time in the future. This may be a heavy burden to wear for years, especially if there is no effective preventive measure to offer.[16-19] Many physicians and scientists have concluded from this reasoning that the screened subjects or their families should not be informed about results unless these results could lead to a meaningful intervention.

In ABIS, the parents were informed carefully (via videotapes and written and oral information) about the aims of the project. If HLA type or existence of diabetes-related autoantibodies indicates an increased risk of getting diabetes, this information would not be given spontaneously. However, they were told that they have the right to get this information on request according to Swedish law.

So far, very few among all thousands of families have ever asked for information such as results of laboratory determinations. Still, it is clear from the present study of attitudes and ethical questions that an overwhelming majority of Swedish parents, who probably are no different from other educated populations in the world, not only regard it as their right to be informed about results found in the study, but they also do want to know. They want to know if their child has increased risk of developing diabetes, even if there is no preventive measure available.

This clear result supports the view that professionals may have exaggerated their worry for psychological consequences of screening projects, and especially of giving information about results. Such projects like ABIS may certainly be ethically justified as long as informed consent can be given based on adequate information.

Should the conclusion then be that we need to change our primary information, saying that no information about results will be spontaneously sent out, but only if the parents ask for such results? The question is difficult. However, as long as there are parents who do not want to be informed, they must have the right to avoid such knowledge. This means then in ABIS that those who want information have to ask for it.

However, we have also asked all parents in the beginning of the project if they will allow *us* to take the initiative to inform them or, for example, ask for extra blood samples if *we* find that necessary, and those who have said "yes" to that question, the great majority, can be contacted when we, the investigators, find it medically or scientifically justified.

In conclusion, even parents in the general population, having nobody with a certain disease like diabetes in the family, want to be informed about what is found about their children when they are included in screening projects. The way of information and the preparation of how and when to contact parents have to be carefully planned, and our results may have implications for the information design of future studies.[9,15,20–24]

ACKNOWLEDGMENTS

We are extremely thankful to all children and their parents who are participating in ABIS. We are especially grateful to Tommy Svensson, who took part in constructing the questionnaire. We also thank Lennart Nordenfeldt and Bo Pettersson for fruitful discussions. This study, as a part of the ABIS project, was generously supported by the JDRF-Wallenberg Foundations (K98-99D-12813-01A), the Swedish Medical Research Council (MFR; Vetenskapsrådet) (K99-72X-11242-05A), the Swedish Child Diabetes Foundation (Barndiabetesfonden), the Swedish Diabetes Association, Torsten and Ragnar Söderbergs Foundation, and the Novo Nordisk Foundation.

REFERENCES

1. KING, H., R. AUBERT & W. HERMAN. 1998. Global burden of diabetes, 1995–2025: prevalence, numerical estimates, and projections. Diabetes Care **21:** 1414–1431.
2. NARAYAN, K., E. GREGG, A. FAGOT-CAMPAGNA *et al.* 2000. Diabetes—a common, growing, serious, costly, and potentially preventable public health problem. Diabetes Res. Clin. Pract. **50**(suppl. 2): S77–S84.
3. SILINK, M. 2000. Childhood diabetes: a global perspective. Horm. Res. **57**(suppl. 1): 1–5.
4. ZIMMET, P., M. ALBERT & J. SHAW. 2001. Global and societal implications of the diabetes epidemic. Nature **414:** 782–787.
5. KARVONEN, M., M. VIIK-KAJANDER, E. MOLTCHANOVA *et al.* 2000. Incidence of childhood type 1 diabetes worldwide. Diabetes Care **23:** 1516–1526.
6. ATKINSON, M. & G. EISENBARTH. 2001. Type 1 diabetes: new perspectives on disease pathogenesis and treatment. Lancet **358:** 221–229.
7. GRAVES, P. & G. EISENBARTH. 1999. Pathogenesis, prediction, and trials for the prevention of insulin-dependent (type 1) diabetes mellitus. Adv. Drug Delivery Rev. **35:** 143–156.
8. KNIP, M. 1998. Prediction and prevention of type 1 diabetes. Acta Paediatr. Suppl. **425:** 54–62.
9. BURGESS, M. 2003. Beyond consent: ethical and social issues in genetic testing. *In* Contemporary Issues in Bioethics. Sixth edition. Wadsworth/Thomson Learning.
10. BURKE, W., L. PINSKY & N. PRESS. 2001. Categorizing genetic tests to identify their ethical, legal, and social implications. Am. J. Med. Genet. **106**(3): 233–240.
11. ROTH, R. 2001. Psychological and ethical aspects of prevention trials. J. Pediatr. Endocrinol. Metab. **14**(suppl. 1): 669–674.
12. CLARKE, A. 1999. The genetic testing of children. *In* The Ethics of Genetic Screening. Kluwer. Dordrecht.
13. LUDVIGSSON, J., M. LUDVIGSSON & A. SEPA. 2001. Screening for pre-diabetes in the general child population may be reassuring. Pediatr. Diabetes **2:** 170–174.

14. GUSTAFSSON STOLT, U., P-E. LISS, J. LUDVIGSSON & T. SVENSSON. 2002. Attitudes to bioethical issues—a case study of a screening project. Soc. Sci. Med. **54**(9): 1333–1344.
15. GUSTAFSSON STOLT, U., J. LUDVIGSSON, P-E. LISS & T. SVENSSON. 2003. Bioethical theory and clinical practice: results from a research ethics case study of ABIS—a Swedish research screening for pre-diabetes. Med. Health Care Philos. **6:** 45–50.
16. LUDVIGSSON, J. 1993. Ethical aspects on clinical studies of prediabetes. Pediatr. Adolesc. Endocrinol. **23:** 175–179.
17. NORDENFELT, L. 1996. Prevention and ethics in medicine: the case of diabetes prevention. J. Pediatr. Endocrinol. Metab. **9:** 381–386.
18. MICHIE, S. & T.M. MARTEAU. 1996. Predictive genetic testing in children: the need for psychological research. Br. J. Health Psychol. **1:** 3–14.
19. BENNETT JOHNSON, S. 2001. Screening programs to identify children at risk for diabetes mellitus: psychological impact on children and parents. J. Pediatr. Endocrinol. Metab. **14:** 653–659.
20. ATKINSON, M. & G. EISENBARTH. 2001. Type 1 diabetes: new perspectives on disease pathogenesis and treatment. Lancet **358:** 221–229.
21. AVERY, L., D. BORSEY, S. GREENE et al. 1998. British Diabetic Association guidelines on genetic and immune screening for type 1 diabetes mellitus. Diabetes Med. **15**(8): 643.
22. FLANDERS, G., P. GRAVES & M. REWERS. 1999. Prevention of type 1 diabetes from laboratory to public health. Autoimmunity **29**(3): 235–246.
23. BIESECKER, B. & T. MARTEAU. 1999. The future of genetic counselling: an international perspective. Nat. Genet. **22:** 133–137.
24. AMERICAN SOCIETY OF HUMAN GENETICS. 1995. Points to consider: ethical, legal, and psychological implications of genetic testing in children and adolescents. Am. J. Hum. Genet. **57:** 1233–1241.

Population-wide Infant Screening for HLA-Based Type 1 Diabetes Risk via Dried Blood Spots from the Public Health Infrastructure

EMILY WION,[a] MICHAEL BRANTLEY,[a] JEFF STEVENS,[a] SUSAN GALLINGER,[a] HUI PENG,[a] MICHAEL GLASS,[b] AND WILLIAM HAGOPIAN[a,c]

[a]*Pacific Northwest Research Institute, Seattle, Washington, USA*

[b]*Washington State Department of Health, Newborn Screening, Shoreline, Washington, USA*

[c]*Department of Medicine, University of Washington, Seattle, Washington, USA*

ABSTRACT: The frequency of type 1 diabetes mellitus (T1DM)–associated HLA DQ alleles in the U.S. Pacific Northwest is as high as in Scandinavia, which has the highest T1DM incidence in the world. The high regional rate of islet autoimmunity observed among DPT-1 relatives supports this notion. Fortunately, Washington State archives dried blood spots after legislature-mandated newborn screening. The Diabetes Evaluation in Washington (DEW-IT) study aims to show that population-based prospective prediction of T1DM by HLA genotype screening followed by autoantibody surveillance can be performed within the public health infrastructure.

KEYWORDS: type 1 diabetes mellitus (T1DM); blood spots; autoantibody; genetic; prediction; prevention

INTRODUCTION

Although region-specific incidence is unknown, the frequency of type 1 diabetes mellitus (T1DM)–associated HLA DQ alleles in the U.S. Pacific Northwest[1,2] is as high as in Scandinavia, which has the highest T1DM incidence in the world.[3] The high regional rate of islet autoimmunity observed among DPT-1 relatives supports this notion.[4] Fortunately, Washington State (WA) archives dried blood spots (DBS) after legislature-mandated newborn screening. The peer-reviewed Diabetes Evaluation in Washington (DEW-IT) study, sponsored by the U.S. Centers for Disease Control, aims to show that population-based prospective prediction of type 1 diabetes by HLA genotype screening followed by autoantibody surveillance can be performed within the public health infrastructure. (See FIG. 1.)

Address for correspondence: Emily Wion, Pacific Northwest Research Institute, 720 Broadway, Seattle, WA 98122. Voice: 206-568-1460; fax: 206-320-1448.

ewion@pnri.org

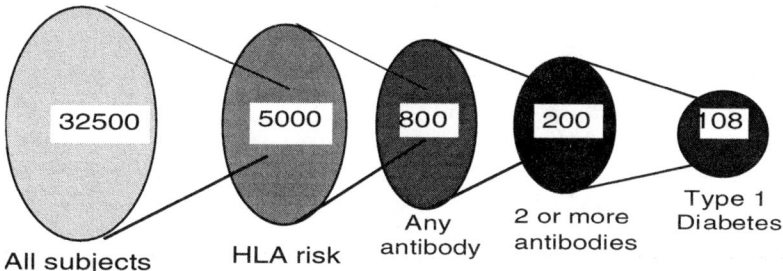

FIGURE 1. Strategy and estimated subject numbers for general population screening and surveillance for childhood T1DM in the DEW-IT study.

METHODOLOGY

For initial regulatory approval, the WA Institutional Review Board required approval of the WA State Medical Association, the WA Chapter of the American Academy of Pediatrics, the Genetic Advisory Committee of the WA DOH, the WA Secretary of Health and Governor's Office, and a study-specific advisory group to review all patient contact material. Because screening results were released to families prior to autoantibody surveillance, HLA and autoantibody tests required certification under the Clinical Laboratories Improvement Act (CLIA).

Public birth record addresses from the DOH were updated using postal records and records from a DOH immunization reminder program. Adopted children and those who had died were not included. A cover letter and brief consent form/questionnaire were mass-mailed in batches to 479,000 WA families inviting enrollment of their young child in the DEW-IT study, coordinated with timed media coverage via eight regional TV stations and three newspapers. Consent forms were signed by parents/guardians and mailed back to the study center. Parents were encouraged to phone with any questions prior to consenting. For consented infants, identity was conveyed to the DOH. Where sufficient reserve sample remained, one 1/8" spot was punched from the DBS record for high-throughput economical genotyping. DBS punches were methanol-fixed prior to multiplex PCR in 96-well microtiter plate format using four primer pairs designed to simultaneously amplify HLA DQA1–exon 2, HLA DQB1–exon 2, the insulin gene promoter, and the CTLA4 gene (exon 1–intron 1). PCR amplicons were 190 to 450 bp in length and were cleaned of leftover PCR reagents and blood products by purification on glass-fiber filters in 96-well microtiter plate format. Products were confirmed by agarose gel electrophoresis prior to microarraying on replicate glass slides for sequence-specific oligonucleotide probe (SSOP) typing, initially for DQA1 and DQB1. Subjects with DQA1-DQB1 haplotypes known to confer TIDM risk, and without haplotypes known to confer dominant protection,[5] were deemed eligible for periodic autoantibody surveillance.

RESULTS

Of the 7.5% of families who returned postage-paid forms, 6.9% (32,547) consented and 0.6% declined. Of these, 47% were girls and 1.2% spoke only Spanish. T1DM was already present in 43 children, verified by phone and confirmatory autoantibody testing. Of 448 total phone calls to the study center, 16 were negative for various reasons. Almost half of these ($n = 7$) were from a parent whose child had died between the time the study obtained birth records and the time the parent received the mailed invitation. Of 62 phone calls to the DOH Newborn Screening Program, only 13 were generally "negative". Two parents asked that their child's blood spot be destroyed (only one completed the necessary paperwork, however). The great majority of phone calls to both locations were quite supportive of the study.

For 2.7% (887) of the subjects, there was insufficient archived blood spot to punch. Families were notified of this by letter. DBS punches were successfully obtained from 97.3% of consented children. PCR amplification for HLA DQA1 and DQB1 typing succeeded in 98.3% of punches. A second punch was requested for all failed tests. Preliminary results suggest the second punch successfully amplifies about 70% of the time, yielding an estimated overall PCR success rate of 99.5%.

Based on initial typing results and a paradigm for assigning HLA risk based on combinations of T1DM-susceptible and T1DM-resistant haplotypes, approximately 17% of children are eligible for the autoantibody surveillance phase of the study. Based on workshops[5] and cross-sectional studies of WA diabetics, the surveillance group should include nearly 75% of new diabetes cases. DR4 subtyping was not part of the initial screening, but will be performed prior to surveillance. Eliminating subjects with the protective allele DRB1*0403 will narrow the surveillance group to about 15% of participants.

Ultimately, effective and safe immunotherapy may be available to prevent progression to clinical T1DM among children developing autoantibodies. However, a current benefit to children taking part in the study is through education of high-risk families to quickly recognize early symptoms and start insulin therapy, to decrease hospitalization, ketoacidosis, cerebral edema, and rarely even death, at onset.[6] The study also helps increase overall knowledge of prediction and prevention of T1DM and will be integrated with studies of T1DM pathogenesis and environmental triggers.

CONCLUSIONS

The DEW-IT study succeeded in general population diabetes recruitment and screening based on the public health infrastructure and high-throughput HLA DQ genotyping via PCR on DBS. The study was well received by parents and the public health community. All recruitment and screening goals were exceeded. Succeeding to the Newborn Screening model will have substantial advantages when intervention therapies preventing clinical T1DM become available and diabetes risk testing becomes standard medical practice.

REFERENCES

1. ROWE, R., N. LEECH, G. NEPOM & D. MCCULLOCH. 1994. High genetic risk for IDDM in the Pacific NW—1st report from the WAn State IDDM prediction study. Diabetes **43:** 87–94.
2. MORI, M., P. BEATTY, M. GRAVES et al. 1997. HLA gene and haplotype frequencies in the North American population: the National Marrow Donor Program Donor Registry. Transplantation **64:** 1017–1027.
3. ONKAMO, P., S. VAANANEN, M. KARVONEN & J. TUOMILEHTO. 1999. Worldwide increase in incidence of type I diabetes—the analysis of the data on published incidence trends. Diabetologia **42:** 1395–1403.
4. COWIE, C., D. CUTHBERTSON, J. KRISCHER et al. 1998. Demographic characteristics of ICA positivity in the DPT-1 trial. Diabetes **47:** A146.
5. CAILLAT-ZUCMAN, S., I. DIILALI-SAIAH, J. TIMSIT et al. 1995. Insulin-dependent diabetes mellitus (IDDM): 12th International Histocompatibility Workshop. *In* HLA: Genetic Diversity of HLA—Functional and Medical Implication. Volume 1. EDK Pub. Paris.
6. EDGE, J., M. HAWKINS, D. WINTER & D. DUNGER. 2001. The risk and outcome of cerebral oedema developing during diabetic ketoacidosis. Arch. Dis. Child. **85:** 16–22.

Vaccinations May Induce Diabetes-Related Autoantibodies in One-Year-Old Children

J. WAHLBERG, J. FREDRIKSSON, O. VAARALA, AND J. LUDVIGSSON FOR THE ABIS STUDY GROUP

Division of Pediatrics, Department of Molecular and Clinical Medicine, Faculty of Health Sciences, Linköping University, Linköping, Sweden

ABSTRACT: Vaccinations have been discussed as one among many environmental candidates contributing to the immune process that later may lead to type 1 diabetes. ABIS (All Babies in Southeast Sweden) is a prospective cohort study following a nonselected birth cohort of general population. In a randomly selected sample collection from 4400 children, GADA and IA-2A have been determined at the age of 1 year. The information on vaccinations was collected from questionnaires answered by the parents and was related to β cell autoantibodies. When studying the induction of autoantibodies using the autoantibody level of 90th percentile as cutoff level, hemophilus influenza B (HIB) vaccination appeared to be a risk factor for IA-2A [OR 5.9 (CI 1.4–24.4; $p = 0.01$)] and for GADA [OR 3.4 (CI 1.1–10.8; $p = 0.04$)] in logistic regression analyses. Furthermore, the titers of IA-2A were significantly higher ($p < 0.01$ in Mann-Whitney test) in those children who had got HIB vaccination. When 99th percentile was used as cutoff to identify the children at risk of type 1 diabetes, BCG vaccination was associated with increased prevalence of IA-2A ($p < 0.01$). We conclude that HIB vaccination may have an unspecific stimulatory polyclonal effect increasing the production of GADA and IA-2A. This might be of importance under circumstances when the β cell–related immune response is activated by other mechanisms.

KEYWORDS: ABIS; children; diabetes; autoantibodies; BCG vaccination; HIB vaccination

The incidence of type 1 diabetes (T1D) in children is increasing rapidly in many countries all over the world.[1] This fact, as well as the remarkable difference in incidence of T1D in children in neighboring countries like Finland and Estonia, with rather similar genetic background in the populations, shows that environmental factors have to play an important role for the development of the disease. Next to Finland, Sweden has the highest incidence of T1D in children in the world and, therefore, environmental factors should be sought for in our country. The age at onset of T1D has decreased in recent years,[2] which strongly suggests that we should look for environmental factors influencing very young children. As manifest diabetes is the end result of a rather long disease process, studies of factors eliciting or influencing

Address for correspondence: Johnny Ludvigsson, Division of Pediatrics, Department of Molecular and Clinical Medicine, Faculty of Health Sciences, Linköping University, SE-58185 Linköping, Sweden. Voice: +46-13-22-13-33; fax: +46-13-14-82-65.
johnny.ludvigsson@lio.se

the very early phase of the autoimmune process have special importance. Diabetes-related autoantibodies such as antibodies against glutamic acid decarboxylase (GADA) and against tyrosine phosphatase (IA-2A) have been shown to be good markers for the disease process sometimes leading to autoimmune diabetes.[3,4] It is thus rational to study how environmental factors influence the development of T1D-associated autoantibodies. The risk for T1D is increased in families with first-degree relatives having T1D; therefore, several studies, such as BabyDiab and DiabFin, have focused on following the first-degree relatives of patients. Another population with increased risk for T1D comprised children with disease-associated HLA risk genotypes, who are studied in other projects, such as the DIPP study and the DAISY project. Our aim is to identify environmental factors associated with β cell auto-immunity by looking at the whole general population, not least those children without high genetic risk, even though they rarely proceed to manifest diabetes. ABIS (All Babies in Southeast Sweden) included 17,055 out of 21,700 newborns (78.6%) in a geographical area with high diabetes incidence. The project was approved by the Research Ethics Committees at the Faculty of Health Sciences, Linköping University, and at the Medical Faculty, Lund University, Sweden.

Among many environmental factors suspected to have a diabetogenic effect, vaccinations have been an interesting candidate.[5] Mumps, hemophilus influenza B (HIB), and pertussis vaccines have been suggested to be associated with the risk of T1D, whereas bacille Calmette-Guérin (BCG) vaccine has been suggested to have a protective effect on the development of T1D.[6] Many other studies have been unable to find any association between vaccinations and increased risk of T1D,[7–13] whereas others obtained results indicating that vaccinations may be a risk factor.[14] However, the information is scarce so far regarding the effect of vaccinations on very early autoimmune response. Thus, it was our aim to elucidate this question.

MATERIALS AND METHODS

Among the ABIS population, a random sample of 4400 1-year-old children was selected. According to the design of the ABIS project, capillary blood samples are taken from the children at the age of 1 year and, at that time point, the parents also answer a questionnaire including questions on vaccinations. As most parents in Sweden follow the recommendations regarding the general vaccination program, it was not expected to find other than exceptional cases not having got vaccinations like tetanus, diphtheria, polio, mumps, rubella, and morbilli. However, BCG vaccination against tuberculosis is not generally recommended, but given mainly to children with parents born or traveling abroad. HIB vaccination and pertussis vaccination have been introduced in recent years. Thus, we can expect to get a group of children without one or the other of those latter three vaccinations before the age of 1 year.

As the marker of diabetes-related autoimmunity, we use GADA and IA-2A, which have been determined by an immune precipitation method using methionine-labeled antigens. The method is described in detail elsewhere[15] and in the DASP (Diabetes Autoantibody Standardization Program) for 2002. Using the autoantibody level of 99th percentile as cutoff for positivity, our methods showed specificity of 96% for GADA and 100% for IA-2A, whereas the sensitivity was 82% for GADA and 54% for IA-2A. Intra-assay coefficient of variation was 5.2% and interassay variation was 13–18%.

The register data in relation to autoantibody data have been analyzed statistically first using univariate analysis (cross-tabulations, Pearson chi-square test, two-sided). Stepwise forward logistic regression was used for factors shown to be significant ($p < 0.05$). Statistics were calculated on a PC using the SPSS 11.0 software.

RESULTS

The 99th percentile cutoff for positivity in our study population corresponds to 40.8 WHO units for IA-2A and 106.6 WHO units for GADA. The 90th percentile cutoff for positivity in our study population corresponds to 32.8 WHO units for IA-2A and 92.3 WHO units for GADA.

Only 1841 out of 4400 answered the question regarding BCG. We found that 5 of 39 who had IA-2A above the 99th percentile had got the BCG vaccination, whereas only 183 of 1828 who had IA-2A levels below the 99th percentile had got BCG vaccination ($p < 0.01$). When the 90th percentile was used as cutoff for detection of β cell autoantibodies, HIB vaccination had an OR of 5.9 (CI 1.4–24.4) ($p = 0.01$) for the induction of IA-2A and of 3.4 (CI 1.1–10.8) ($p = 0.04$) for GADA. Furthermore, the titers of IA-2A were significantly higher ($p < 0.01$ in Mann-Whitney test) in those children who had got HIB vaccination. No other vaccination was related to the prevalence of autoantibodies at the age of 1 year.

DISCUSSION

Autoantibodies to GAD and IA-2 are used as markers for a β cell autoimmune process, which later might lead to T1D. The emergence of autoantibodies is a dynamic process[16] and, so far, there is no consensus as to what age and how often children in the general population should be tested to achieve the best possible prediction value for the clinical T1D. The cutoff for positivity is usually calculated according to the autoantibody level exceeding the 97th to 99th percentile in a normal population. The higher cutoff for positivity improves the specificity of the autoantibody test in population screening. However, one can speculate that children with the highest levels of β cell autoantibodies have already developed a fully maturated immune response against β cell antigens. To study the primary environmental triggers of β cell autoimmunity, lower cutoff levels for positivity may reveal environmental factors that induce the production of β cell autoantibodies. We have therefore based our calculations on two types of cutoff values: the levels above 99th percentile for identifying children at risk of T1D and the levels above 90th percentile to identify children in whom production of autoantibodies has been triggered. Furthermore, it is possible that environmental factors have a more pronounced role in the induction of an abnormal immune response in children without high genetic risk and, thus, we have included the general child population in an area with high incidence of T1D. Vaccinations have been studied as candidate environmental risk factors for T1D mellitus and most studies have found no increased risk of T1D mellitus associated with vaccination.[7–13] Studies of the association of β cell autoimmunity and vaccinations are few and the number of children who have not received the vaccination has been limited in several studies.

BCG vaccine has been suggested to have a protective or delaying effect on T1D in retrospective studies.[17] In animal models, the development of autoimmune diabetes can be prevented by a single injection of BCG vaccine or complete Freund's adjuvant in animal models,[14,18–20] BCG vaccine contains mycobacterium antigens, including heat shock protein 65, an antigen suggested to be autoantigen in T1D mellitus and having a protective immunization effect in the NOD mouse model.[21–23] Interestingly, we found increased risk for development of high levels of IA-2A in relation to BCG vaccination. However, the number of children who received BCG vaccination was relatively small in our study and these children represent a special group of children since BCG vaccination is not included in the general vaccination program in Sweden. It is, however, noteworthy that BCG vaccination is given in all children born in Finland with the highest incidence of T1D mellitus in the world. Although Parent et al. did not find any differences in overall BCG vaccination rates between cases with T1D and their matched control subjects, they found a much lower proportion of cases who developed T1D by the age of 5 years among children who were BCG-vaccinated than in children who were not vaccinated. Our results as well as the findings by Parent et al. suggest that BCG vaccination at birth may increase the risk of β cell autoimmunity and T1D during the first years of life, but does not have a long-lasting effect. Accordingly, the effect of BCG vaccination on the incidence of T1D diagnosed at early age should be evaluated.

In a 10-year follow-up of more than 100,000 Finnish children who participated in a trial of HIB vaccination, no evidence of increased risk for T1D could be found.[24] Others have also been unable to find any association between HIB vaccination and diabetes.[11,25] Our finding indicates that HIB vaccination stimulates the immune system. Such an unspecific stimulation may have a polyclonal effect and thereby increase the production of GADA and IA-2A. We do not dare to draw any conclusion as to risk of getting manifest T1D. However, HIB vaccination might be of importance under special circumstances when the β cell–related immune response is activated by other mechanisms. Our further follow-up of these children will show whether this early stimulation of the immune system, and of production of GADA and IA-2A, has any link to the risk of T1D.

ACKNOWLEDGMENTS

We are very thankful to all children and their parents participating in ABIS, as well as to the health centers where all questionnaires are collected and biological samples taken. We are grateful to Sonja Hellström, Lena Berglert, and Gosia Smolinska, who have been of great help in the autoantibody determinations. This study, as a part of the ABIS project, was generously supported by the JDRF-Wallenberg Foundations (K98-99D-12813-01A), the Swedish Medical Research Council (MFR; Vetenskapsrådet) (K99-72X-11242-05A), the Swedish Child Diabetes Foundation (Barndiabetesfonden), the Swedish Diabetes Association, and the Novo Nordisk Foundation.

REFERENCES

1. KARVONEN, M. et al. 2000. Incidence of childhood type 1 diabetes worldwide: Diabetes Mondiale (DiaMond) Project Group. Diabetes Care **23:** 1516–1526.

2. PUNDZIUTE-LYCKA, A. et al. 2002. Type I diabetes in the 0–34 years group in Sweden. Diabetologia **45:** 783–791.
3. BINGLEY, P.J. et al. 1997. Prediction of IDDM in the general population: strategies based on combinations of autoantibody markers. Diabetes **46:** 1701–1710.
4. SAMUELSSON, U. et al. 2001. Islet autoantibodies in the prediction of diabetes in school children. Diabetes Res. Clin. Pract. **51:** 51–57.
5. LINDBERG, B. et al. 1999. Previous exposure to measles, mumps, and rubella—but not vaccination during adolescence—correlates to the prevalence of pancreatic and thyroid autoantibodies. Pediatrics **104:** E12.
6. LUDVIGSSON, J. et al. 1988. Mumps with laboratory signs of subclinical pancreatitis may cause a disturbed beta-cell function. Diabetes Res. **9:** 193–195.
7. BLOM, L., L. NYSTROM & G. DAHLQUIST. 1991. The Swedish Childhood Diabetes Study: vaccinations and infections as risk determinants for diabetes in childhood. Diabetologia **34:** 176–181.
8. HYOTY, H. et al. 1993. Decline of mumps antibodies in type 1 (insulin-dependent) diabetic children and a plateau in the rising incidence of type 1 diabetes after introduction of the mumps-measles-rubella vaccine in Finland: Childhood Diabetes in Finland Study Group. Diabetologia **36:** 1303–1308.
9. DAHLQUIST, G. & L. GOTHEFORS. 1995. The cumulative incidence of childhood diabetes mellitus in Sweden unaffected by BCG-vaccination. Diabetologia **38:** 873–874.
10. HEIJBEL, H., R.T. CHEN & G. DAHLQUIST. 1997. Cumulative incidence of childhood-onset IDDM is unaffected by pertussis immunization. Diabetes Care **20:** 173–175.
11. GRAVES, P.M. et al. 1999. Lack of association between early childhood immunizations and beta-cell autoimmunity. Diabetes Care **22:** 1694–1697.
12. HUMMEL, M. et al. 2000. No major association of breast-feeding, vaccinations, and childhood viral diseases with early islet autoimmunity in the German BABYDIAB Study. Diabetes Care **23:** 969–974.
13. EURODIAB SUBSTUDY 2 STUDY GROUP. 2000. Infections and vaccinations as risk factors for childhood type I (insulin-dependent) diabetes mellitus: a multicentre case-control investigation. Diabetologia **43:** 47–53.
14. CLASSEN, J.B. 1996. The timing of immunization affects the development of diabetes in rodents. Autoimmunity **24:** 137–145.
15. WAHLBERG, J. et al. 2003. Environmental factors related to the induction of beta-cell autoantibodies in 1-year old healthy children. Submitted.
16. KNIP, M. 1997. Disease-associated autoimmunity and prevention of insulin-dependent diabetes mellitus. Ann. Med. **29:** 447–451.
17. PARENT, M.E. et al. 1997. Bacille Calmette-Guérin vaccination and incidence of IDDM in Montreal, Canada. Diabetes Care **20:** 767–772.
18. HARADA, M., Y. KISHIMOTO & S. MAKINO. 1990. Prevention of overt diabetes and insulitis in NOD mice by a single BCG vaccination. Diabetes Res. Clin. Pract. **8:** 85–89.
19. SADELAIN, M.W. et al. 1990. Prevention of type I diabetes in NOD mice by adjuvant immunotherapy. Diabetes **39:** 583–589.
20. SHEHADEH, N. et al. 1994. Effect of adjuvant therapy on development of diabetes in mouse and man. Lancet **343:** 706–707.
21. ELIAS, D. et al. 1991. Vaccination against autoimmune mouse diabetes with a T-cell epitope of the human 65-kDa heat shock protein. Proc. Natl. Acad. Sci. USA **88:** 3088–3091.
22. BRAS, A. & A.P. AGUAS. 1996. Diabetes-prone NOD mice are resistant to *Mycobacterium avium* and the infection prevents autoimmune disease. Immunology **89:** 20–25.
23. RAZ, I. et al. 2001. Beta-cell function in new-onset type 1 diabetes and immunomodulation with a heat-shock protein peptide (DiaPep277): a randomised, double-blind, phase II trial. Lancet **358:** 1749–1753.
24. KARVONEN, M., Z. CEPAITIS & J. TUOMILEHTO. 1999. Association between type 1 diabetes and haemophilus influenzae type b vaccination: birth cohort study. BMJ **318:** 1169–1172.
25. DESTEFANO, F. et al. 2001. Childhood vaccinations, vaccination timing, and risk of type 1 diabetes mellitus. Pediatrics **108:** E112.

Inhibition of STAT4 Activation by Lisofylline Is Associated with the Protection of Autoimmune Diabetes

ZANDONG YANG, MENG CHEN, LAWRENCE B. FIALKOW, JUSTIN D. ELLETT, RUNPEI WU, AND JERRY L. NADLER

University of Virginia, Charlottesville, Virginia 22908, USA

ABSTRACT: We investigated the signal transduction pathway of IL-12 and showed that lisofylline (LSF) inhibited the signal transducer and activator of transcription factor-4 (STAT4) activation. Interruption of IL-12-mediated STAT4 activation prevented autoimmune diabetes in NOD mice.

KEYWORDS: lisofylline; IL-12; STAT4; NOD mice; autoimmune diabetes

The role of T helper (Th) 1 cells and proinflammatory cytokines in autoimmune diabetes has been recognized.[1] Interleukin-12 (IL-12) is one of cytokines involved in the development of this disease. IL-12 activates Th1 cells and enhances Th1-driven proinflammatory cytokine production.[2,3] Both activated T cells and proinflammatory cytokines cause pancreatic β cell dysfunction and destruction, leading to diabetes.[4] Reduction of IL-12 activity leads to protection of autoimmune diabetes in nonobese diabetic (NOD) mice.[5] In our previous studies, we demonstrated evidence that blockade of IL-12 signaling by a novel anti-inflammatory compound, lisofylline (LSF), could protect NOD mice from autoimmune diabetes,[6] and LSF promoted mitochondrial metabolism in β cells.[7]

In this study, we investigated the signal transduction pathway of IL-12 and showed that LSF inhibited the signal transducer and activator of transcription factor-4 (STAT4) activation. Interruption of IL-12-mediated STAT4 activation prevented autoimmune diabetes in NOD mice.

Seven-week-old female NOD/LtJ mice were purchased from the Jackson Laboratory (Bar Harbor, ME) and received daily ip injections of LSF, 50 mg/kg, for 3 weeks. Normal saline was used as vehicle control. Serum IFN-γ levels were reduced in LSF-treated mice at 1 week after treatment (75 ± 12.1 in saline group vs. 28 ± 4.8 pg/mL in LSF group, $p < 0.05$). IFN-γ mRNA expression was also decreased in LSF-treated

Address for correspondence: Jerry L. Nadler, M.D., Division of Endocrinology and Metabolism, Department of Internal Medicine, University of Virginia, P.O. Box 801405, Charlottesville, VA 22908. Voice: 434-924-9416; fax: 434-924-9730; *or* Zandong Yang, M.D., Division of Endocrinology and Metabolism, Department of Internal Medicine, University of Virginia, P.O. Box 801413, Charlottesville, VA 22908. Voice: 434-924-0229; fax: 434-982-3727.

jln2n@virginia.edu *or* zy4q@virginia.edu

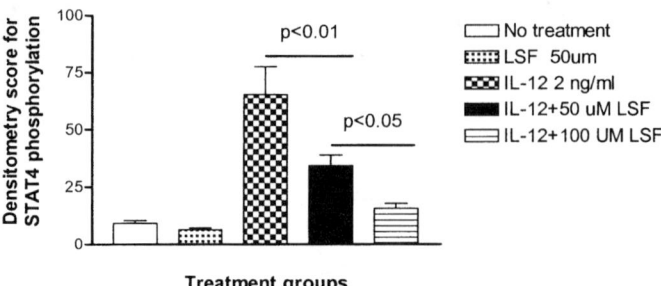

FIGURE 1. STAT4 phosphorylation in NOD splenocytes. Splenocytes were isolated from naive 7-week-old NOD mice and treated with different conditions as indicated for 2 days. Equal amounts of splenocyte protein from each treatment were loaded onto a 10% SDS-PAGE gel. Protein-transferred blots were incubated with an antiphosphorylated STAT4 antibody (H-20, Santa Cruz Biotechnology, Santa Cruz, CA). Radioautographic bands were compared after a densitometry analysis. Statistic analysis was done by ANOVA testing.

NOD pancreata as compared to saline-treated mice. However, we found no effect of LSF on serum levels or pancreatic mRNA expression of IL-12. By 16 weeks after initiation of the treatment, 83% of the mice (10/12) became diabetic in the saline group, whereas only 11% (2/19) were diabetic in the LSF group. LSF prevented cellular infiltration in NOD islets as assessed by pancreatic histology at 3 weeks after withdrawal of treatment. When compared to saline-treated mice, STAT4 activation was remarkably reduced in LSF-treated NOD islets and splenocytes by 5- to 6-fold using quantitative analysis of STAT4 phosphorylation. In contrast, higher levels of STAT4 phosphorylation were correlated with diabetic state in NOD mice. We found that the effect of LSF was dose-dependent in suppressing STAT4 phosphorylation in IL-12-stimulated NOD splenocytes (FIG. 1).

This study extends our research of LSF's mechanism and shows a correlation between LSF-mediated STAT4 inhibition and prevention of diabetes in NOD mice. This evidence supports the notion that LSF interrupts IL-12 signaling[8] and inactivates IL-12 function in T cells and macrophages (Z. Yang et al., unpublished data). Inhibition of STAT4 activation by LSF is associated with reduction of autoimmune diabetes in NOD mice. Further investigations of LSF will allow additional insight in understanding the role of the STAT4 signal pathway in autoimmune diabetes and in developing a therapeutic strategy to prevent autoimmune diabetes in humans.

ACKNOWLEDGMENTS

This study was supported by a center grant from the Juvenile Diabetes Foundation International (JDFI file 1999-805) and a center grant from the National Institutes of Health (P30 DK63609-1, for the islet core grant to Z. Yang and J. L. Nadler). Z. Yang is also supported in part by the Iacocca Foundation and the Manning Foundation.

REFERENCES

1. SCHRANZ, D.B. & A. LERNMARK. 1998. Immunology in diabetes: an update. Diabetes Metab. Rev. **14:** 3–29.
2. TREMBLEAU, S., G. PENNS, E. BOSI et al. 1995. Interleukin 12 administration induces T helper type 1 cells and accelerates autoimmune diabetes in NOD mice. J. Exp. Med. **181:** 817–821.
3. KUKREJA, A. & N.K. MACLAREN. 1999. Autoimmunity and diabetes. J. Clin. Endocrinol. Metab. **84:** 4371–4378.
4. ADORINI, L., J.C. GUERY & S. TREMBLEAU. 1996. Manipulation of the Th1/Th2 cell balance: an approach to treat human autoimmune diabetes? Autoimmunity **23:** 53–68.
5. ROTHE, H., R.M. O'HARA, JR., S. MARTIN & H. KOLB. 1997. Suppression of cyclophosphamide induced diabetes development and pancreatic Th1 reactivity in NOD mice treated with the interleukin (IL)–12 antagonist IL-12 (p40)$_2$. Diabetologia **40:** 641–646.
6. YANG, Z., M. CHEN, R. WU et al. 2002. The anti-inflammatory compound lisofylline prevents type 1 diabetes in non-obese diabetic mice. Diabetologia **45:** 1307–1314.
7. CHEN, M., Z. YANG, R. WU & J.L. NADLER. 2002. Lisofylline, a novel antiinflammatory agent, protects pancreatic β-cells from proinflammatory cytokine damage by promoting mitochondrial metabolism. Endocrinology **143:** 2341–2348.
8. COON, M.E., M. DIEGEL, N. LESHINSKY & S.J. KLAUS. 1998. Selective pharmacologic inhibition of murine and human IL-12-dependent Th1 differentiation and IL-12 signaling. J. Immunol. **163:** 6567–6574.

Reduced Thymic Expression of Islet Antigen Contributes to Loss of Self-Tolerance

C. E. MATHEWS, S. L. PIETROPAOLO, AND M. PIETROPAOLO

Department of Pediatrics, University of Pittsburgh, and Children's Hospital of Pittsburgh, Pittsburgh, Pennsylvania, USA

ABSTRACT: Type 1 diabetes (T1DM) results from a failure of central and peripheral tolerance to islet cell antigens. ICA69 belongs to a group of molecules expressed predominantly in neuroendocrine tissues (including pancreatic islets), which are targets of autoimmune responses in T1DM. These molecules are also expressed in the thymus and peripheral lymphoid organs by dendritic cells. The aim of the present study was to evaluate possible variation in thymic ICA69 expression, comparing diabetes-resistant controls to T1DM-prone NOD mice. Thymic tissue was retrieved from 3- to 6-week-old female B6, NOD-H2^b, and NOD mice. Paraffin-embedded sections were stained with an ICA69-specific antibody in an immunoperoxidase assay. ICA69 staining of thymic sections from B6 and NOD.H2^b showed strong and continual staining, yet the sections from the NOD mice showed significantly reduced staining for ICA69. Corroboration of the reduced level of ICA69 in the thymus of NOD mice has been obtained via analysis for the expression of ICA69 versus other candidate autoantigens (glutamic acid decarboxylase 65, glutamic acid decarboxylase 67, and insulin 2) in the thymus. Real-time PCR analysis, using cDNA generated from the thymus, displayed that the expression of GAD65, GAD67, and INS2 were equivalent when comparing NOD at any age to B6, BALB/cJ, and ALR/LtJ. In marked contrast, the level of ICA69 in the thymus of the NOD mice examined was significantly reduced when compared to the controls. In fact, the real-time PCR analysis strongly suggested that ICA69 was not expressed in the thymus of NOD mice. These findings support the hypothesis that the level of thymic ICA69 expression may be of importance in regulating self-tolerance in T1DM.

KEYWORDS: type 1 diabetes (T1DM); ICA69; NOD; thymus; self-tolerance

INTRODUCTION

A self-tolerant T cell repertoire is contingent on both central and peripheral tolerance.[1–4] Central tolerance is developed in the thymus where positive and negative selection respectively promote or delete nonself or self-reactive thymocytes. Self versus nonself discrimination occurs in the thymic medulla.[2] The medulla is seeded with bone marrow–derived MHC class II$^+$ antigen-presenting cells (APC) such as dendritic cells (DC), which presumably express all self-antigens, including tissue-restricted antigens. Expression and presentation of self-antigens in the context of

---

Address for correspondence: Dr. Clayton E. Mathews, Diabetes Institute, 3460 Fifth Avenue/Rangos Research Center, University of Pittsburgh, Pittsburgh, PA 15213. Voice: 412-692-8574; fax: 412-692-8131.

cem65@pitt.edu

both class I and II MHC in the presence of costimulatory molecules allow for efficient deletion of self-reactive cells.

There is growing evidence that organ-specific molecules are naturally expressed in the thymus and peripheral lymphoid organs. Putative T1DM autoantigens such as the glutamic acid decarboxylases (GAD65 and 67), insulin (INS), and neuroendocrine islet antigen IA-2 (ICA512) are expressed in the thymus[5] and proposed to be presented to developing thymocytes in both diabetes-prone and -resistant mouse strains.[6–9] However, genetic mechanisms controlling the thymic expression of these molecules, such as the insulin VNTR, may influence the development of central tolerance, turning predisposition to autoimmunity. Autoantigens may also utilize alternative core promoters to regulate tissue-specific transcription, such as the case with ICA69.[10] While the thymic expression of some T1DM antigens has been determined, variation in gene expression and age dependency of autoantigen presence in the thymus of NOD mice has not yet been elucidated.

ICA69 is a neuroendocrine protein targeted by autoimmune responses in T1DM in both humans and NOD mice. In this report, we examine the presence of ICA69 and other relevant islet antigens in the thymus of diabetes-prone NOD mice versus control strains. A striking difference was detected in both the expression and presence of this autoantigen, with NOD exhibiting little thymic ICA69 compared to controls. This reduction in the thymic expression of ICA69 may be an important contributor to the loss of self-tolerance in T1DM.

METHODS

Immunohistochemical Staining for ICA69

Seven NOD, 3 C57BL/6, and 6 NOD.B10-$H2^b$ mice (age range: 3–5 weeks) were evaluated for the presence of ICA69 in the thymus. Paraformaldehyde-fixed paraffin-embedded sections were stained with a monoclonal mouse anti-ICA69 IgG1 antibody using a published method.[11] Briefly, paraffin-embedded sections were cut onto Super Frost Plus Slides [Fisher Scientific (Pittsburgh, PA)] and incubated with 30% hydrogen peroxide for 5 min to block endogenous peroxidase activity. Slides were blocked (Super Block [ScyTek Labs (Logan, UT)]) for 5 min and then incubated with the ICA69-specific antibody for 16 h at 4°C. After rinse, a biotinylated secondary antibody (Rat Anti-Mouse Fab[2] [Jackson ImmunoResearch (West Grove, PA)]) was applied for 45 min at room temperature (RT). Then, slides were rinsed and incubated with peroxidase enzyme at RT (Streptavidin/HRP [ScyTek Labs]) and a Chomagen/substrate (AEC, Chomagen/substrate solution [3-amino-9-ethylcarbazole] [ScyTek Labs]) for 10 min for detection.

Real-Time PCR

NOD mice at 2, 4, 6, 8, 10, and 12 weeks of age, as well as ALR/LtJ, BALB/cJ, and C57BL/6J at 8 weeks of age, were examined for thymic expression of the putative T1DM antigens, GAD65, GAD67, INS2, and ICA69. Mice were sacrificed by CO_2 inhalation and the thymus was removed. RNA was isolated using TRIzol Reagent [Life Technologies (Rockville, MD)] and cDNA was generated using the SUPERSCRIPT Choice System [Life Technologies]. Amplification using a primer set specific for glyceraldehyde-3-phosphate dehydrogenase (GAPDH) was also performed. Primer sets, specific for the gene of interest, were validated before use by sequencing of the amplified PCR product to determine specificity. GAD65 and GAD67 primer sets used have been published previously.[5] The primer sequences for GAPDH [GAPDH.F: TCC CAC TCT TCC ACC TTC gA; GAPDH.R: AgT Tgg gAT Agg gCC TCT CTT g], INS2 [INS2.F: AgC AAg CAg gAA gCC TAT CT; INS2.R: TgC CAA ggT CTg AAg gTC AC], and ICA69 [ICA69.F: Agg ggg AgT TCA gCA gAg AgT; ICA69.R: Tgg ATg Agg TgC CgC ggA gTg] were kindly provided by Massimo Trucco. The tests were run using 2 pools of thymus RNA per

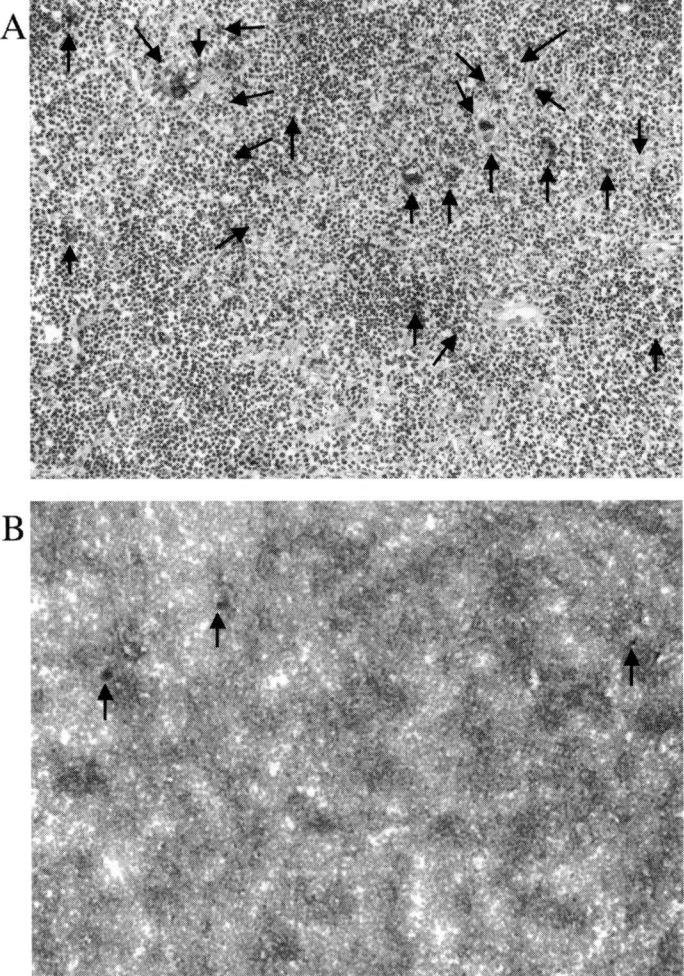

FIGURE 1. Immunohistochemical staining for ICA69 in thymus sections. Higher number of ICA69-positive cells in the thymus from diabetes-resistant C57BL/6 (**A**) as compared to a diabetes-prone NOD (**B**).

group (2 mice per pool). These tests were run on an ABI Prism 7700 using SYBR Green Jump Start Taq Ready Mix (Sigma, St. Louis, MO) for detection as per the manufacturer's protocol. Final reaction contents were 10 mM Tris-HCl (pH 8.3), 50 mM KCl, 3.5 mM $MgCl_2$, 0.2 mM dATP, 0.2 mM dGTP, 0.2 mM dTTP, 0.2 mM dCTP, 13.2 nmol of each primer, 0.625 U Taq DNA polymerase, Jump Start Taq Antibody, SYBR Green I, and template cDNA in a total volume of 50 µL. PCR conditions were a 2-min initial denaturation step at 94°C; followed by 45 cycles of 94°C for 30 s, 55°C for 30 s, and 72°C for 60 s; and then finally a 4°C hold.

RESULTS

T1DM onset in female NOD mice of the Children's Hospital of Pittsburgh Colony begins at approximately 10 weeks of age and reaches a final incidence of 90% by 20 weeks. Male incidence is reduced and delayed compared to females, yet is robust, with initiation at 16 weeks of age and a final incidence reaching 70% by 36 weeks. To determine the presence of ICA69 in the thymus of prediabetic NOD mice, paraffin sections were stained with a monoclonal antibody specific for ICA69.

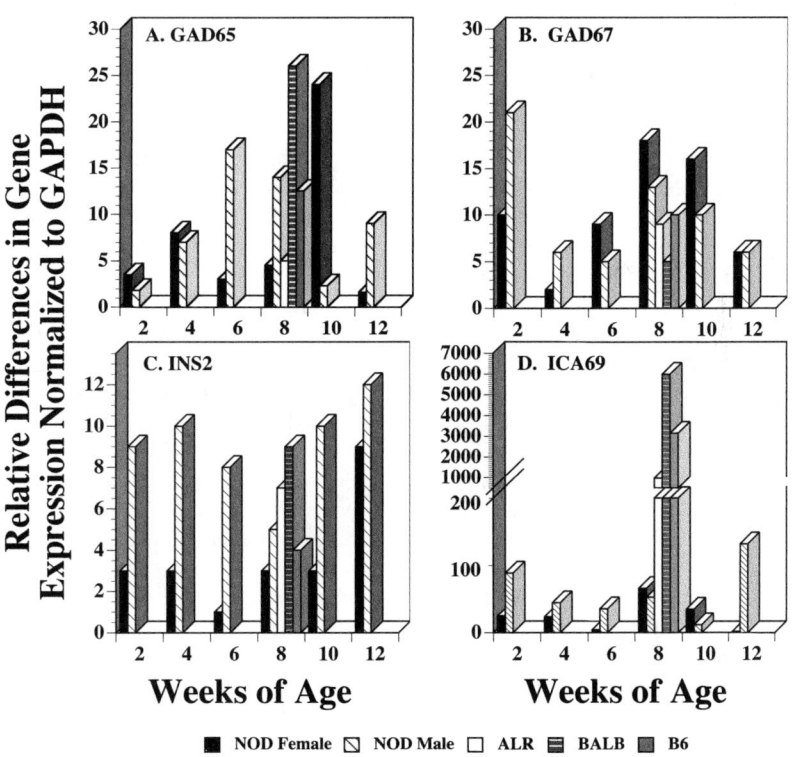

FIGURE 2. Examination of autoantigen expression in mouse thymus by real-time PCR.

Staining of thymic sections of C57BL/6J (FIG. 1A) and prediabetic NOD (FIG. 1B) mice shows a clear reduction in the presence of ICA69 in the thymus of NOD mice.

To assess the gene expression of putative autoantigens in the thymus of prediabetic NOD mice, we compared NOD female and male mice from 2–12 weeks of age to 8-week-old ALR, BALB, and B6 controls by real-time PCR. With the exception of GAPDH, thymic expression of all transcripts was very low. Thymic expression of GAD65 and GAD67 (FIGS. 2A and 2B) was highly variable in intra- and intergroup comparisons and showed no pattern associated with T1DM initiation. In comparison, INS2 expression is significantly lower in NOD females at 2–10 weeks of age compared to NOD males, but at 12 weeks the transcript levels did not differ (FIG. 2C).

Further support for the hypothesis that ICA69 expression is decreased in the thymus of NOD mice of both genders came from the real-time PCR analysis (FIG. 2D). ICA69 expression was detected in the thymus of ALR, BALB, and B6 controls (all 8 weeks of age). Yet, expression of this autoantigen was not detected in any of the thymus samples of NOD mice from 2–12 weeks of age.

DISCUSSION

Immunological tolerance to islet cell autoantigens may be generated and sustained through thymic deletion of islet cell antigen–reactive T cells. A number of pancreatic islet cell autoantigens, such as ICA69, are indeed expressed in the thymus and, under physiological conditions, it is likely that T cells exhibiting high affinity for these antigens may be deleted through the process of negative selection.[7,12,13] In this context, it is intriguing that insulin-requiring diabetes can be prevented in both NOD mice and BioBreeding (BB) rats following intrathymic grafting of syngeneic or allogeneic islets.[14,15] The reduced thymic expression of ICA69 in NOD mice that we describe is also reinforced by preliminary observations indicating that ICA69 transgene expression on thymus and spleen tet1 mice mediates disease protection in NOD mice.[16] Prompted by an interest in understanding how thymic islet cell self-antigen expression relates to autoimmunity, we found that both the number of ICA69-positive cells and the gene expression of ICA69 are reduced in NOD mice compared to diabetes-resistant mice. In addition, INS2 expression was significantly lower in NOD females at 2–10 weeks of age compared to NOD males, but at 12 weeks the transcript levels did not show any difference. With regard to thymic expression of GAD65 and GAD67, there was a high degree of variability in both intra- and intergroup comparisons and there was no pattern associated with T1DM initiation. It remains to be determined, however, whether self-antigen-presenting DCs are fewer in number or less functionally competent in NOD mice. Interestingly, findings from recent literature suggest that DCs can synthesize and express self-antigens. Perhaps the ability to express self-antigens may be an important determinant of their function. There is indeed growing evidence that DCs expressing self-antigens may also have a tolerogenic function. In particular, data from transplantation experiments in transgenic mice provide functional evidence for the tolerogenic properties of these cells.[17] Of note, several reports indicate that DCs can prevent diabetes in NOD mice as well as humans.[18–20]

In sum, our findings reemphasize that ICA69 has a role as an islet autoantigen in NOD mice and that reduced expression of this molecule in the thymus may be important for developing self-tolerance. Studies under way aimed at controlling the degree of ICA69 expression in antigen-presenting cells may reveal that this molecule could induce central and/or peripheral tolerance through deletion of ICA69-reactive T cells, which appear to be involved in the pathogenesis of T1DM.

REFERENCES

1. KISHIMOTO, H. & J. SPRENT. 2000. The thymus and central tolerance. Clin. Immunol. **95:** S3–S7.
2. KISHIMOTO, H. & J. SPRENT. 2000. The thymus and negative selection. Immunol. Res. **21:** 315–323.
3. KISHIMOTO, H. & J. SPRENT. 2001. A defect in central tolerance in NOD mice. Nat. Immunol. **2:** 1025–1031.
4. PUGLIESE, A. 2002. Peripheral antigen-presenting cells and autoimmunity. Endocrinol. Metab. Clin. North Am. **31:** 411–430.
5. PLEAU, J.M., A. ESLING, S. GEUTKENS et al. 2001. Pancreatic hormone and glutamic acid decarboxylase expression in the mouse thymus: a real-time PCR study. Biochem. Biophys. Res. Commun. **283:** 843–848.
6. PIETROPAOLO, M., N. GIANNOUKAKIS & M. TRUCCO. 2002. Cellular environment and freedom of gene expression. Nat. Immunol. **3:** 335 [discussion, p. 336].
7. PUGLIESE, A. et al. 1997. The insulin gene is transcribed in the human thymus and transcription levels correlate with allelic variation at the *INS* VNTR–*IDDM2* susceptibility locus for type 1 diabetes. Nat. Genet. **15:** 293–297.
8. PUGLIESE, A. et al. 2001. Self-antigen-presenting cells expressing diabetes-associated autoantigens exist in both thymus and peripheral lymphoid organs. J. Clin. Invest. **107:** 555–564.
9. PUGLIESE, A. & J. DIEZ. 2002. Lymphoid organs contain diverse cells expressing self-molecules. Nat. Immunol. **3:** 335–336.
10. FRIDAY, R., S. PIETROPAOLO, J. PROFOZICH et al. 2003. Alternative core promoters regulate tissue specific transcription from the autoimmune diabetes-related ICA1 (ICA69) gene locus. J. Biol. Chem. In press.
11. STASSI, G., N. SCHLOOT & M. PIETROPAOLO. 1997. Islet cell autoantigen 69 kDa (ICA69) is preferentially expressed in the human islets of Langerhans than exocrine pancreas. Diabetologia **40:** 120–122.
12. BACH, J.F. & L. CHATENOUD. 2001. Tolerance to islet autoantigens in type 1 diabetes. Annu. Rev. Immunol. **19:** 131–161.
13. PIETROPAOLO, M. & D. LE ROITH. 2001. Pathogenesis of diabetes: our current understanding. Clin. Cornerstone **4:** 1–16.
14. GERLING, I.C., D.V. SERREZE, S.W. CHRISTIANSON & E.H. LEITER. 1992. Intrathymic islet cell transplantation reduces beta-cell autoimmunity and prevents diabetes in NOD/Lt mice. Diabetes **41:** 1672–1676.
15. POSSELT, A.M., C.F. BARKER, A.L. FRIEDMAN & A. NAJI. 1992. Prevention of autoimmune diabetes in the BB rat by intrathymic islet transplantation at birth. Science **256:** 1321–1324.
16. SONG, A., S. WINER, H. TSUI et al. 2003. Deviation of islet autoreactivity to cryptic epitopes protects NOD mice from diabetes. Eur. J. Immunol. **33:** 546–555.
17. SMITH, K., D. OLSON, R. HIROSE & D. HANAHAN. 1997. Pancreatic gene expression in rare cells of thymic medulla: evidence for functional contribution to T cell tolerance. Int. Immunol. **9:** 1355–1365.
18. CLARE-SALZLER, M.J., J. BROOKS, A. CHAI et al. 1992. Prevention of diabetes in nonobese diabetic mice by dendritic cell transfer. J. Clin. Invest. **90:** 741–748.
19. FEILI-HARIRI, M. et al. 1999. Immunotherapy of NOD mice with bone marrow–derived dendritic cells. Diabetes **48:** 2300–2308.
20. PAPACCIO, G., F. NICOLETTI, F.A. PISANTI et al. 2000. Prevention of spontaneous autoimmune diabetes in NOD mice by transferring *in vitro* antigen-pulsed syngeneic dendritic cells. Endocrinology **141:** 1500–1505.

Dietary Microbial Toxins and Type 1 Diabetes

M. A. MYERS,[a] K. D. HETTIARACHCHI,[a] J. P. LUDEMAN,[a] A. J. WILSON,[b] C. R. WILSON,[b] AND P. Z. ZIMMET[c]

[a]*Monash University, Melbourne, Australia*
[b]*University of Tasmania, Hobart, Australia*
[c]*International Diabetes Institute, Melbourne, Australia*

ABSTRACT: Toxins may promote type 1 diabetes by modifying or damaging the β cell causing release of autoantigens. *Streptomyces* is a common soil bacterium that produces many toxic compounds. Some *Streptomyces* can infect vegetables, raising the possibility of dietary exposure to toxins. We aimed to identify toxins that erode cellular proton gradients in extracts of *Streptomyces* and infested vegetables and to establish the effect of low doses of these toxins on pancreatic islets in mice. The vacuolar ATPase inhibitors, bafilomycin and concanamycin, and the ionophore, nigericin, were identified in extracts from 4 of 13 *Streptomyces* isolated from infested potatoes and in potatoes themselves. Injection of bafilomycin A1 into mice impaired glucose tolerance, reduced islet size, and decreased relative β cell mass. Thus, exposure to small quantities of bafilomycin in the diet may contribute to the cause of type 1 diabetes.

KEYWORDS: *Streptomyces*; vacuolar ATPases; diabetes mellitus

INTRODUCTION

Environment contributes approximately 50% of the risk of developing type 1 diabetes. Various environmental agents including viruses, toxins, diet, and microbial exposure in infants have been suggested, but there has been little consistency between studies.[1] We have identified a class of *Streptomyces* toxins as a potential environmental cause of type 1 diabetes. Previously, we have shown that bafilomycin A1, a toxic plecomacrolide antibiotic produced by *Streptomyces* species, has adverse effects on islet β cells in mice.[2] Bafilomycins and the structurally similar concanamycins erode cellular proton gradients through inhibition of the vacuolar ATPase and hence interfere with regulated secretory pathways. In islet β cells, this promotes constitutive release of proinsulin[3] and possibly other incompletely processed secretory granule constituents that may be presented as autoantigens. Some species of *Streptomyces* can infest tuberous vegetables, raising the prospect of dietary exposure to *Streptomyces* toxins including bafilomycin A1. We aimed to identify toxins that can erode cellular proton gradients in cultures of *Streptomyces* isolated from infested vegetables and in infested potatoes and to investigate the effect of low doses of these toxins on pancreatic islets and glucose tolerance in mice.

Address for correspondence: M. A. Myers, Department of Biochemistry and Molecular Biology, Monash University, Melbourne 3800, Australia. Voice: +61-3-9905-1435; fax: +61-3-9905-3726.
mark.myers@med.monash.edu.au

MATERIALS AND METHODS

Detection of Streptomyces Toxins

Cultures of *Streptomyces* species isolated from common scab lesions of potato in Australia, North America, and Europe and peel from potatoes infected with *Streptomyces* were extracted with ethyl acetate or chloroform. Extracts were applied to a C18 column and separated by reverse-phase high performance liquid chromatography (HPLC) using a linear 30–100% acetonitrile gradient followed by an isocratic 100% acetonitrile step. Peaks were detected by absorption at 254 nm. Those fractions with retention times typical of bafilomycins and concanamycins were tested for their ability to ablate intracellular proton gradients by applying 1:20 dilutions of the eluted fractions to COS7 cells in the presence of 2 μg/mL acridine orange. Cells were examined by epifluorescence microscopy for the accumulation of acridine orange into vesicles as an indicator of organelle pH gradients. The molecular mass of compounds with inhibitory activity was determined by electrospray spectrometry.

Effect of vATPase Inhibitors in Mice

The Monash University Animal Ethics Committee approved all animal experiments. BALB/c mice were injected intraperitoneally with 12 ng/g body weight bafilomycin A1. Vacuolar ATPase activity was measured in kidneys (a rich source of vATPase enzyme) from anesthetized treated or control mice. Kidneys were removed and immediately frozen on dry ice and homogenized in 10 mM Tris-Cl, pH 8.0, and 2 mM $MgCl_2$ containing protease inhibitors. Sucrose was added to 0.25 M and the suspension clarified by centrifugation at 700g for 10 min at 4°C. Supernatants were assayed in duplicate for ATPase activity in the presence or absence of 75 nM bafilomycin A1, and inorganic phosphate release was measured by the method of Chan.[4] Results were corrected for background phosphate concentration and ATP autohydrolysis. Protein content was determined using the Bradford reagent (Biorad, Hercules, CA).

Oral glucose tolerance tests were performed on BALB/c mice on days 7 and 21 after bafilomycin A1 injection by anesthetizing the mice with pentobarbitone and delivering 2 mg/g body weight of glucose by gavage. Blood glucose was measured on tail vein blood samples by the glucose oxidase method. Insulin immunostaining and islet size measurement were performed as previously described.[2]

RESULTS AND DISCUSSION

Detection of Streptomyces Toxins

Extracts from cultures of 13 *Streptomyces* species isolated from potato scab lesions were analyzed by HPLC and bioassay. Four of the extracts contained 1 or more molecules that ablated cellular pH gradients. Chromatographic retention times and UV absorbance profiles for many of these were typical of concanamycins and bafilomycins, and mass spectrometry on 2 of the bioactive molecules identified bafilomycin B1 and the toxic ionophore nigericin. Specifically, 2 of the toxin producers were isolates from North America, 1 of which produced predominantly bafilomycin B1 and the other nigericin, while 2 strains isolated from infected potatoes in Australia both produced nigericin along with as yet undetermined members of the plecomacrolide vATPase inhibitor family. The production of more than 1 toxin type by individual *Streptomyces* reflects the existence of more than 20 gene clusters dedicated to secondary metabolite production in the *Streptomyces* genome,[5] and multiple variants of particular toxins reflect either side-chain modifications or biosynthetic intermediates. These results are consistent with previous reports of scab-causative *Streptomyces* producing concanamycins.[6] Applying the same approach to common scab infected potatoes (60% lesion coverage) identified molecules that inhibited acridine orange uptake and exhibited identical retention times and UV absorbance profiles to the bafilomycin variants identified in the culture extract of the Australian isolates. Comparison to standard curves of pure bafilomycin B1 allowed estimation of the quantity of bafilomycins as 240 μg/kg of potato (wet weight). Extrapolating from our data in mice,[2] an equivalent dose to that which causes islet changes in mice (12 ng/g body weight) would be delivered by consumption of 50 g of potato per kg body weight, demonstrating the real possibility of dietary exposure to harmful quantities of bafilomycins and concanamycins.

Effect of vATPase Inhibitors in Mice

The ability of bafilomycin A1 to inhibit vATPase activity *in vivo* was ascertained by measuring bafilomycin A1–sensitive ATPase activity in kidney homogenates (TABLE 1). There was a 50% reduction of bafilomycin A1–sensitive ATPase activity in homogenates of kidneys from mice injected with bafilomycin A1 at either 1 day ($p = 0.03$, Student's *t* test) or 7 days ($p = 0.04$) beforehand. The activity of bafilomycin A1–insensitive ATPases (P-type and F-type ATPases) was not affected, demonstrating specific inhibition of vATPase activity after injection with bafilomycin A1. There were no significant differences in the weight (TABLE 1) or protein contents (data not shown) of the kidneys of control or injected mice.

Glucose tolerance was compared between 6 control mice and 6 bafilomycin A1–treated mice at various times after exposure (FIG. 1). Seven days after injection of bafilomycin A1, glucose tolerance was similar to that of controls; however, 21 days after injection, moderate glucose intolerance was apparent characterized by increased peak blood glucose levels at short time intervals after glucose challenge and a return to normal levels by 120 min. This is consistent with a loss of first-phase insulin release. Islet size was measured on insulin-stained pancreas sections from 4 of the bafilomycin A1–treated mice at day 26 and compared to a group of age-matched

TABLE 1. Bafilomycin A1–sensitive ATP hydrolysis in lysates of kidneys from treated and control mice

	Control	1 day	7 days
Total ATPase activity	5.8 (1.5)	4.4 (0.5)	4.8 (0.8)
Bafilomycin A1–sensitive ATPase activity	1.6 (0.6)	0.80 (0.30)	0.80 (0.30)
Kidney as % of animal weight	0.80 (0.10)	0.90 (0.11)	0.90 (0.15)

NOTE: Terms given in units of ηmol/min/mg protein. Standard deviations given in parentheses.

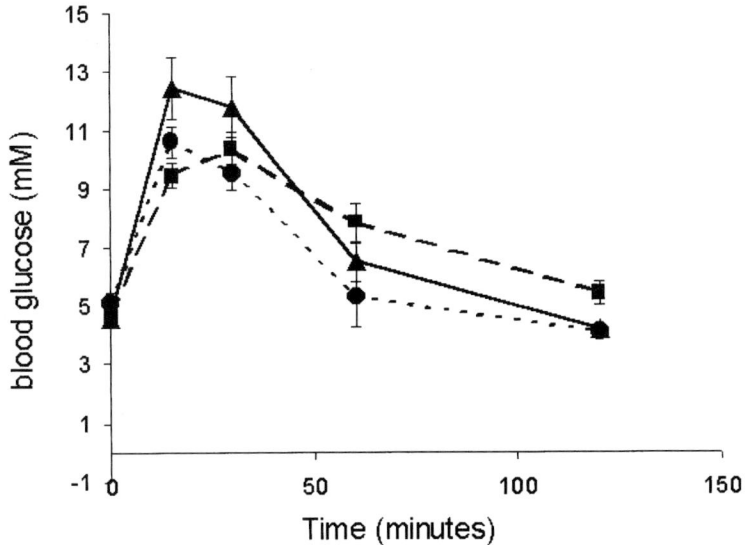

FIGURE 1. Bafilomycin A1 causes glucose intolerance. Blood glucose levels in BALB/c mice were measured over 120 min after an oral glucose challenge for controls (*dashed line with squares*) and mice given bafilomycin A1 at 7 days (*dotted line with circles*) and 21 days (*solid line with triangles*) previously. Controls are derived from 3 measurements at each time point for each of 6 mice. Bafilomycin A1–treated data are derived from 1 measurement at each time point from 6 mice.

controls. The median islet size for the control group was 3204 μm^2 ($n = 223$ islets from 12 mice) versus 1293 μm^2 for the bafilomycin-treated group ($n = 90$ islets from 4 mice, $p = 0.001$, Mann-Whitney U test). The total islet area as a percentage of the total area of pancreas in the histological sections was 0.32% for the control mice and 0.23% for the bafilomycin-treated mice. Impaired glucose tolerance, significantly reduced islet size, and decreased relative β cell mass of mice injected with bafilomycin A1 together indicate either a direct toxic effect of bafilomcyin A1 or an indirect effect on the normal process of islet cell turnover and homeostasis.

CONCLUSIONS

We have demonstrated the presence of vacuolar ATPase inhibitors in potatoes and shown that extremely small quantities of these inhibitors have adverse effects on pancreatic islets in BALB/c mice. *Streptomyces*-derived toxins in the diet have not been considered as causes of disease, and the discovery of their presence in vegetables and effects on glucose tolerance and islet homeostasis suggest a new environmental cause of type 1 diabetes. Dietary bafilomycin A1 and other vATPase inhibitors could contribute to islet autoimmunity through disruption of secretory granule maturation and vesicle turnover and/or other events dependent on acidification of cellular membrane compartments. In the islet β cell, this would lead to the promiscuous release of islet autoantigens that, upon exposure to immune cells in the genetically susceptible individual, could promote islet autoimmunity and the development of type 1 diabetes.

REFERENCES

1. AKERBLOM, H.K. *et al.* 2002. Environmental factors in the etiology of type 1 diabetes. Am. J. Med. Genet. **115:** 18–29.
2. MYERS, M.A. *et al.* 2001. Dietary microbial toxins as a cause of type 1 diabetes: a new meaning for seed and soil. Diabetologia **44:** 1199–1200.
3. KULIAWAT, R. & P. ARVAN. 1994. Distinct molecular mechanisms for protein sorting within immature secretory granules of pancreatic beta-cells. J. Cell Biol. **126:** 77–86.
4. CHAN, K.M. *et al.* 1986. A direct colorimetric assay for Ca2+-stimulated ATPase activity. Anal. Biochem. **157:** 375–380.
5. BENTLEY, S.D. *et al.* 2002. Complete genome sequence of the model actinomycete *Streptomyces coelicolor.* Nature **417:** 141–147.
6. NATSUME, M. *et al.* 1996. Production of phytotoxins, concanamycin A and B by *Streptomyces* spp. causing potato scab. Ann. Phytopathol. Soc. Jpn. **62:** 411–413.

Prevention of Autoimmune Diabetes through Immunostimulation with Q Fever Complement-Fixing Antigen

D. G. SILVA,[a,b] B. CHARLTON,[b] W. COWDEN,[b] AND N. PETROVSKY[a,b]

[a]*Autoimmunity Research Unit, The Canberra Hospital, Canberra, Australia*
[b]*John Curtin School of Medical Research, Canberra, Australia*

ABSTRACT: The most promising strategies for prevention of type 1 diabetes seem to be in the categories of immunomodulation (e.g., nondepleting anti-CD3, Diapep, linomide) and/or immunostimulation (e.g., QFA, BCG). We are currently undertaking a research program directed toward better understanding of immunostimulants to help maximize the likelihood of success of future human clinical trials for diabetes prevention. This program is focused on the key areas of optimization of vaccine dose and route of administration, development of surrogate immune markers, and elucidation of the mechanism of protection. The mechanism whereby QFA protects against diabetes currently is not known. The elucidation of the mechanism should help identify the optimal way in which to administer QFA to provide diabetes protection. It may also assist the development of even more potent immunostimulatory vaccines.

KEYWORDS: QFA; immunostimulation; autoimmune diabetes; type 1 diabetes; vaccine development

INTRODUCTION

Type 1 diabetes results from selective immune-mediated destruction of pancreatic islet β cells. Although predominantly a disease of the young, it may occur at any age, and 5–10% of adult patients with an initial diagnosis of type 2 diabetes have, in fact, a slowly progressive form of type 1 diabetes (latent autoimmune diabetes of adults or LADA).[1] In the absence of clear evidence of an extraneous stimulus, such as an infectious agent or other environmental factor, autoantigens within the β cell are thought to be the target of autoreactive T cells. Multiple strategies including immunosuppression, immunomodulation, cytokine-directed therapies, inhibition of costimulation, free radical scavenging, and antigen-specific tolerance all have been used to develop potential vaccines or immunotherapies for prevention of type 1 diabetes.

Address for correspondence: Nikolai Petrovsky, Autoimmunity Research Unit, The Canberra Hospital, P.O. Box 11, Woden ACT 2606, Australia. Voice: +61-2-6244-3804; fax: +61-2-6260-3372.
nikolai.petrovsky@anu.edu.au

Although immunosuppression with cyclosporine, azathioprine, or cyclophosphamide results in a temporary decrease in insulin requirements in recent-onset type 1 diabetes, such therapies are highly toxic and thus unlikely to be of use in prevention strategies.[2–4] Similarly, immunomodulatory drugs including linomide (quinoline-3-carboxamide), nondepleting anti-CD3 antibodies,[5] or nonhypercalcemic vitamin D analogues (MC1288)[6] all prevent autoimmune diabetes in animal models and are now being tested in early human trials. Cytokines (e.g., IL-4, IL-10, TGF-α) and cytokine antagonists (e.g., anti-TNF, anti-IL-12), although proved to be effective in preventing autoimmune diabetes in animal models, require more understanding of their mechanisms of action and toxicity before being suitable for human intervention studies. The efficacy and toxicity of agents that block cell-cell interaction and costimulation (e.g., anti-VCAM-1,[7] ICAM-1,[8] leukocyte function–associated antigen-1 [LFA-1], and intercellular adhesion molecule-1 [ICAM-1][9]) are yet to be fully addressed, but might again be effective in the prevention of type 1 diabetes. Despite the success of the free radical scavenger, nicotinamide, in animal models, human studies including DENIS and ENDIT failed to show efficacy.[10]

Approaches to develop an antigen-specific tolerance regimen to regulate the autoimmune process also have been taken, including the administration of autoantigens via tolerogenic routes (inhaled, oral, nasal) or antigen modification to make them less immunogenic and more tolerogenic.[11,12] These approaches have not been without problems, primarily through lack of efficacy, but also on safety issues.[13] Human trials on antigen-specific interventions have shown variable results, with the Schwabing Insulin Prophylaxis Pilot Trial suggesting a delay in the onset of diabetes in high-risk relatives treated with systemic insulin.[14] Against this, a trial of oral insulin in subjects with recent-onset diabetes had no effect.[15] Similarly, annual insulin infusions coupled with daily subcutaneous injections (Diabetes Prevention Trial-1) did not prevent or delay the onset of clinical disease.[16] A Phase I study of recombinant human GAD65 recently was completed, and a Phase II study in Sweden using GAD to prevent progression in adult GAD antibody-positive (LADA) patients is understood to be currently under way. Based on these results, although conceptually attractive, antigen-specific tolerance approaches may not live up to their promise, possibly because of an underlying genetic defect in tolerance induction in diabetes-prone individuals.

Failure of antigen-specific tolerance approaches in human autoimmunity trials leaves immunostimulation as the preferred route to avert diabetes development. Immunostimulatory therapies are based on the hypothesis that diabetes-prone individuals have underlying immune system defects that prevent normal tolerance development. Defects in immune function and in antigen-presenting cells (APCs), in particular, are a feature of autoimmune diabetes of humans[17–21] and rodents.[22–26] In support, NOD diabetes is prevented by administration of macrophage activators including OK-432 (a streptococcal-derived preparation),[27] incomplete or complete Freund's adjuvant (CFA),[28–30] and bacillus Calmette-Guérin (BCG).[31] Although the mechanism underlying these protective effects are unknown, a common feature is that the frequency of T cells producing IL-4 is increased and IFN-γ is decreased after BCG or Diapep277, suggesting a Th2 shift.[32] Of these limited interventions, human studies have been performed in recent-onset subjects using BCG and Diapep277.[33] Despite a preliminary study suggesting a benefit of BCG vaccination in recently diagnosed subjects,[34] this has not been supported by subsequent larger studies.[35,36]

Q FEVER ANTIGEN

Q fever is a zoonosis caused by a rickettsia-like organism, *Coxiella burnetii*, which is found in milk, placenta, and excreta of infected animals. Q fever infection induces lifelong immunity. Q fever complement-fixing antigen (QFA) is an inactivated whole-cell derivative of *Coxiella burnetii*. QFA is a potent adjuvant through its ability to activate macrophages. Vaccination with QFA produces a powerful cell-mediated immune response[37–39] and through an adjuvant effect also protects against other unrelated infectious organisms.[40,41] This protection may be related to increased production of TNF and IFN-γ, which are normally associated with cell-mediated immune responses.[40]

Since the 1940s, Australian abattoir workers and laboratory workers handling *C. burnetii* have been given an inactivated QFA-based vaccine called Q-Vax. Although its safety record is good, the vaccine occasionally causes local reactions, particularly in subjects with previous history of Q fever infection. Other minor reactions include fever, headache, local tenderness, erythema, and "flu-like" symptoms.

QFA PROTECTS AGAINST DIABETES IN NOD MICE

Based on the ability of other macrophage stimulants, namely, CFA and BCG, QFA was tested for its ability to protect NOD mice from spontaneous diabetes. Female NOD mice aged 64–69 days were injected with either 200 µL i.p. of QFA Phase I (CSL, Melbourne, Australia; $n = 12$) or 200 µL saline ($n = 13$). At 300 days, 8% of the QFA-treated mice became diabetic, compared with 92% in the saline-treated group. Using lower doses of QFA, we obtained similar results, with 14% and

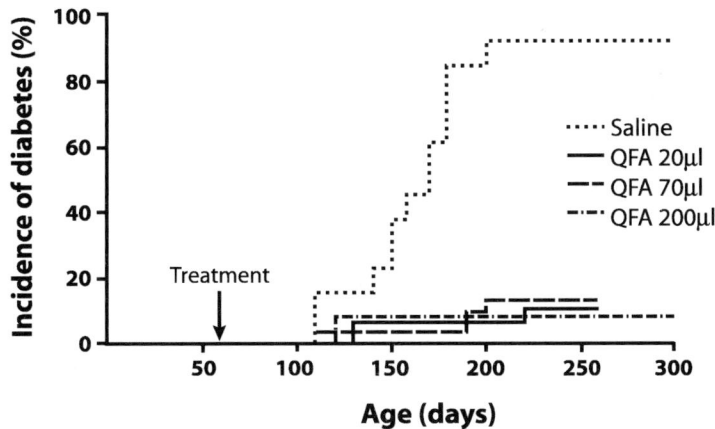

FIGURE 1. Treatment with QFA prevents diabetes in NOD mice. Sixty- to 70-day-old NOD female mice were treated with 20 µL ($n = 28$), 70 µL ($n = 29$), or 200 µL ($n = 12$) of QFA or saline ($n = 13$). At 250 days of age, less than 15% of QFA-treated NOD mice became diabetic. In contrast, by the same age, more than 90% of the saline-treated NOD mice developed diabetes ($p < 0.0001$).

TABLE 1. Effect of QFA on islet histology

Treatment	% Insulin-positive islets	% Collapsed islets
BCG 80 µL	16 (11/69)	84 (58/69)
CFA 50 µL	52 (31/60)	48 (29/60)
QFA 200 µL	87 (105/121)	13 (16/121)
QFA 70 µL	77 (40/52)	23 (12/52)
QFA 20 µL	75 (41/55)	25 (14/55)
Control (age-matched)	73 (22/30)	27 (8/30)

7% of mice developing diabetes at 260 days, when treated with 70 µL ($n = 29$) and 20 µL ($n = 28$) of QFA, respectively (FIG. 1). In the NOD mouse, QFA was more effective than either CFA or BCG in protecting β cells from autoimmune destruction (TABLE 1). QFA treatment resulted in more insulin-positive islets and less "collapsed" islets (staining for glucagon only) compared with BCG or CFA treatment. Islet histology of QFA-treated mice was similar to that in 300-day-old control mice, which represent long-term "survivors" of autoimmune diabetes. These results thus indicate that QFA is more effective than BCG or CFA at preventing frank type 1 diabetes and also subclinical β cell destruction in NOD mice (Silva *et al.*, manuscript in preparation).

HUMAN Q-VAX TRIAL

A multicenter, randomized double-blind, placebo-controlled safety study of a single dose of Q-Vax (CSL) was conducted by the National Health Sciences Center, Canberra, Australia, to test the hypothesis that Q-Vax administration can alter the natural history of type 1 diabetes in recent-onset diabetic subjects. The possibility of Q-Vax inducing the development of antibody-dependent autoimmunity, evidenced by appearance of antinuclear antibodies, positive Coombs' test, and positive thyroid antibodies (antithyroid microsomal peroxidase and antithyroglobulin antibodies), was also examined closely for 24 months after injection.

Patients were enrolled based on the fulfillment of the following inclusion criteria: (1) age ≥ 15 years and <50 years; (2) type 1 diabetes defined as presence of symptoms of hyperglycemia, fasting blood glucose > 7.8 mM or postprandial glucose > 11.1 mM, insulin-requiring in the opinion of the treating physician, ketonuria > trace or body mass index < 30, and either GAD or IA-2 antibody-positive or ICA-positive; (3) duration of type 1 diabetes < 6 weeks since diagnosis; (4) written informed consent by subject; (5) negative skin test and serology for Q fever and absence of prior Q fever infection or previous Q fever vaccination.

Exclusion criteria included (1) known intolerance to Q-Vax, egg yolk protein, or glucagon, (2) participation in another study parallel to or within 4 weeks before study entry, (3) known or suspected to be unable to comply with the study protocol as judged by the investigator, (4) serious concomitant illness, (5) history of disease contraindicating the use of study medication, (6) secondary diabetes, (7) therapy with hypoglycemic agents other than insulin, or hyperglycemic agents, or (8) definitive diagnosis of systemic autoimmune disease or inflammatory arthritis with evidence of current activity or active organ-specific autoimmunity requiring therapy other than replacement.

A total of 44 patients were randomized into either the Q-Vax ($n = 22$) or the placebo ($n = 22$) arm. Patients randomized into the study arm received a single subcutaneous injection of Q-Vax, whereas the placebo arm received saline injection. The majority of the patients were males (70%), with an even distribution of sexes between the groups. Time from diagnosis to vaccination ranged from 10 to 49 days in both groups. Randomized patients were screened for GAD and IA-2 autoantibodies; 39 of 44 patients tested positive for either or both autoantibodies. The primary efficacy parameters included glucagon-stimulated insulin release, insulin dose required to reach target level of glycemic control, and glycosylated hemoglobin. Safety parameters included general clinical observations, biochemistry and hematology evaluation, adverse events, and serum analysis for autoantibodies. Efficacy and safety parameters were measured on day 0 and then at 3, 6, 9, 12, and 24 months. Analysis of safety variables showed no effect of vaccination on biochemistry or hematological parameters, and there was no increment in the levels of antinuclear or thyroid autoantibodies. Statistical analysis of the primary outcomes showed no difference between the treated and placebo groups, and vaccination did not have any significant effect on the levels of C peptide, daily insulin requirements, or levels of glycosylated hemoglobin (unpublished data).

DISCUSSION

The most promising strategies for prevention of type 1 diabetes seem to be in the categories of immunomodulation (e.g., nondepleting anti-CD3, Diapep, linomide) and/or immunostimulation (e.g., QFA, BCG). We are currently undertaking a research program directed toward better understanding of immunostimulants to help maximize the likelihood of success of future human clinical trials for diabetes prevention. This program is focused on the key areas of optimization of vaccine dose and route of administration, development of surrogate immune markers, and elucidation of the mechanism of protection.

A possible reason for the lack of demonstration of efficacy of BCG or QFA (Q-Vax) in human studies is that the doses used were not comparable with and were many times smaller on a weight for weight basis than the protective doses in animal studies. There is currently no available algorithm for translating immunotherapeutic vaccine doses from mice to humans. This is one potential reason for failure of human trials of vaccines validated in small rodent diabetes models. A key question for human trials of a QFA-based immunostimulatory vaccine is the relationship between the maximum tolerated human dose and the dose associated with efficacy. In addition, further research is required on optimizing the dosing regimen and, in particular, the question of whether, in humans, multiple rather than single vaccine doses are required to prevent diabetes progression. It is important that surrogate outcome markers are available to test the efficacy of human diabetes vaccines and also to assist with mouse-human vaccine dose translation. Unfortunately, no surrogate markers currently are validated for use in this context. Development of a surrogate marker of diabetes protection would greatly accelerate all areas of diabetes vaccine development.

The mechanism whereby QFA protects against diabetes currently is not known. The elucidation of the mechanism should help identify the optimal way in which to administer QFA to provide diabetes protection. It may also assist the development of even more potent immunostimulatory vaccines. Although treatment with Q-Vax was relatively free of side effects, the safety/efficacy ratio of a QFA-based protective vaccine potentially could be improved if we were able to identify a subfraction of QFA that mediated the majority of the protective effect.

ACKNOWLEDGMENTS

D. G. Silva is the recipient of a scholarship from the Canberra Hospital Salaried Specialists Private Practice Fund.

REFERENCES

1. ZIMMET, P.Z., T. TUOMI, I.R. MACKAY et al. 1994. Latent autoimmune diabetes mellitus in adults (LADA): the role of antibodies to glutamic acid decarboxylase in diagnosis and prediction of insulin dependency. Diabet. Med. **11:** 299–303.
2. ASSAN, R., G. FEUTREN, M. DEBRAY-SACHS et al. 1985. Metabolic and immunological effects of cyclosporin in recently diagnosed type 1 diabetes mellitus. Lancet **1:** 67–71.
3. STILLER, C.R., J. DUPRE, M. GENT et al. 1984. Effects of cyclosporine immunosuppression in insulin-dependent diabetes mellitus of recent onset. Science **223:** 1362–1367.
4. CAREL, J.C., C. BOITARD, G. EISENBARTH et al. 1996. Cyclosporine delays, but does not prevent clinical onset in glucose intolerant pre-type 1 diabetic children. J. Autoimmunol. **9:** 739–745.
5. CHATENOUD, L., J. PRIMO & J.F. BACH. 1997. CD3 antibody-induced dominant self tolerance in overtly diabetic NOD mice. J. Immunol. **158:** 2947–2954.
6. CASTEELS, K.M., C. MATHIEU, M. WAER et al. 1998. Prevention of type I diabetes in nonobese diabetic mice by late intervention with nonhypercalcemic analogs of 1,25-dihydroxyvitamin D3 in combination with a short induction course of cyclosporin A. Endocrinology **139:** 95–102.
7. JAKUBOWSKI, A., B.N. EHRENFELS, R.B. PEPINSKY & L.C. BURKLY. 1995. Vascular cell adhesion molecule–Ig fusion protein selectively targets activated alpha 4–integrin receptors *in vivo*: inhibition of autoimmune diabetes in an adoptive transfer model in nonobese diabetic mice. J. Immunol. **155:** 938–946.
8. KOMMAJOSYULA, S., S. REDDY, K. NITSCHKE et al. 2001. Leukocytes infiltrating the pancreatic islets of nonobese diabetic mice are transformed into inactive exiles by combinational anti-cell adhesion therapy. J. Leukocyte Biol. **70:** 510–517.
9. MORIYAMA, H., K. YOKONO, K. AMANO et al. 1996. Induction of tolerance in murine autoimmune diabetes by transient blockade of leukocyte function–associated antigen-1/intercellular adhesion molecule-1 pathway. J. Immunol. **157:** 3737–3743.
10. LAMPETER, E.F., A. KLINGHAMMER, W.A. SCHERBAUM et al. 1998. The Deutsche Nicotinamide Intervention Study: an attempt to prevent type 1 diabetes—DENIS Group. Diabetes **47:** 980–984.
11. TIAN, J., M.A. ATKINSON, M. CLARE-SALZLER et al. 1996. Nasal administration of glutamate decarboxylase (GAD65) peptides induces Th2 responses and prevents murine insulin-dependent diabetes. J. Exp. Med. **183:** 1561–1567.
12. POLANSKI, M., N.S. MELICAN, J. ZHANG & H.L. WEINER. 1997. Oral administration of the immunodominant B-chain of insulin reduces diabetes in a co-transfer model of diabetes in the NOD mouse and is associated with a switch from Th1 to Th2 cytokines. J. Autoimmunol. **10:** 339–346.
13. HANNINEN, A. 2000. Prevention of autoimmune type 1 diabetes via mucosal tolerance: is mucosal autoantigen administration as safe and effective as it should be? Scand. J. Immunol. **52:** 217–225.

14. FUCHTENBUSCH, M., W. RABL, B. GRASSL et al. 1998. Delay of type I diabetes in high risk, first degree relatives by parenteral antigen administration: the Schwabing Insulin Prophylaxis Pilot Trial. Diabetologia **41:** 536–541.
15. POZZILLI, P. & M. GISELLA CAVALLO. 2000. Oral insulin and the induction of tolerance in man: reality or fantasy? Diabetes Metab. Res. Rev. **16:** 306–307.
16. YU, L., D.D. CUTHBERTSON, N. MACLAREN et al. 2001. Expression of GAD65 and islet cell antibody (ICA512) autoantibodies among cytoplasmic ICA+ relatives is associated with eligibility for the Diabetes Prevention Trial–Type 1. Diabetes **50:** 1735–1740.
17. CHANDY, K.G., A.M. CHARLES, A. KERSHNAR et al. 1984. Autologous mixed lymphocyte reaction in man: XV. Cellular and molecular basis of deficient autologous mixed lymphocyte response in insulin-dependent diabetes mellitus. J. Clin. Immunol. **4:** 424–428.
18. GUPTA, S., S. FIKRIG & E. ORTI. 1983. Autologous mixed lymphocyte reaction in man: VI. Deficiency of autologous mixed lymphocyte reaction in type I (insulin-dependent) diabetes mellitus. J. Clin. Lab. Immunol. **11:** 59–62.
19. RASANEN, L., H. HYOTY, M. LEHTO et al. 1989. Suppression of autologous mixed leukocyte reaction in type 1 diabetes mellitus by *in vivo*–activated T lymphocytes. Clin. Immunol. Immunopathol. **52:** 406–413.
20. BUSCHARD, K., S. MADSBAD & J. RYGAARD. 1980. Depressed suppressor cell activity in patients with newly diagnosed insulin-dependent diabetes mellitus. Clin. Exp. Immunol. **41:** 25–32.
21. JANSEN, A., M. VAN HAGEN & H.A. DREXHAGE. 1995. Defective maturation and function of antigen-presenting cells in type 1 diabetes. Lancet **345:** 491–492.
22. CRISA, L., J.P. MORDES & A.A. ROSSINI. 1992. Autoimmune diabetes mellitus in the BB rat. Diabetes Metab. Rev. **8:** 4–37.
23. SERREZE, D.V., H.R. GASKINS & E.H. LEITER. 1993. Defects in the differentiation and function of antigen presenting cells in NOD/Lt mice. J. Immunol. **150:** 2534–2543.
24. SERREZE, D.V. & E.H. LEITER. 1988. Defective activation of T suppressor cell function in nonobese diabetic mice: potential relation to cytokine deficiencies. J. Immunol. **140:** 3801–3807.
25. JACOB, C.O., Z. FRONEK, G.D. LEWIS et al. 1990. Heritable major histocompatibility complex class II–associated differences in production of tumor necrosis factor alpha: relevance to genetic predisposition to systemic lupus erythematosus. Proc. Natl. Acad. Sci. USA **87:** 1233–1237.
26. LANGMUIR, P.B., M.M. BRIDGETT, A.L. BOTHWELL & I.N. CRISPE. 1993. Bone marrow abnormalities in the non-obese diabetic mouse. Int. Immunol. **5:** 169–177.
27. TOYOTA, T., J. SATOH, K. OYA et al. 1986. Streptococcal preparation (OK-432) inhibits development of type 1 diabetes in NOD mice. Diabetes **35:** 496–499.
28. MCINERNEY, M.F., S.B. PEK & D.W. THOMAS. 1991. Prevention of insulitis and diabetes onset by treatment with complete Freund's adjuvant in NOD mice. Diabetes **40:** 715–725.
29. SADELAIN, M.W., H.Y. QIN, J. LAUZON & B. SINGH. 1990. Prevention of type I diabetes in NOD mice by adjuvant immunotherapy. Diabetes **39:** 583–589.
30. QIN, H.Y. & B. SINGH. 1997. BCG vaccination prevents insulin-dependent diabetes mellitus (IDDM) in NOD mice after disease acceleration with cyclophosphamide. J. Autoimmun. **10:** 271–278.
31. HARADA, M., Y. KISHIMOTO & S. MAKINO. 1990. Prevention of overt diabetes and insulitis in NOD mice by a single BCG vaccination. Diabet. Res. Clin. Pract. **8:** 85–89.
32. ELIAS, D., A. MEILIN, V. ABLAMUNITS et al. 1997. Hsp60 peptide therapy of NOD mouse diabetes induces a Th2 cytokine burst and downregulates autoimmunity to various beta-cell antigens. Diabetes **46:** 758–764.
33. RAZ, I., D. ELIAS, A. AVRON et al. 2001. Beta-cell function in new-onset type 1 diabetes and immunomodulation with a heat-shock protein peptide (Diapep277): a randomised, double-blind, phase II trial. Lancet **358:** 1749–1753.
34. SHEHADEH, N., F. CALCINARO, B.J. BRADLEY et al. 1994. Effect of adjuvant therapy on development of diabetes in mouse and man. Lancet **343:** 706–707.
35. ALLEN, H.F., G.J. KLINGENSMITH, P. JENSEN et al. 1999. Effect of bacillus Calmette-Guérin vaccination on new-onset type 1 diabetes: a randomized clinical study. Diabetes Care **22:** 1703–1707.

36. ELLIOTT, J.F., K.L. MARLIN & R.M. COUCH. 1998. Effect of bacille Calmette-Guérin vaccination on C-peptide secretion in children newly diagnosed with IDDM. Diabetes Care **21:** 1691–1693.
37. HEGGERS, J.P., L.P. MALLAVIA & D.J. HINRICHS. 1974. The cellular immune response to antigens of *Coxiella burnetii*. Can. J. Microbiol. **20:** 657–662.
38. JERRELLS, T.R., L.P. MALLAVIA & D.J. HINRICHS. 1975. Detection of long-term cellular immunity to *Coxiella burnetii* as assayed by lymphocyte transformation. Infect. Immunol. **11:** 280–286.
39. IZZO, A.A. & B.P. MARMION. 1993. Variation in interferon-gamma responses to *Coxiella burnetii* antigens with lymphocytes from vaccinated or naturally infected subjects. Clin. Exp. Immunol. **94:** 507–515.
40. CLARK, I.A. 1979. Resistance to *Babesia* spp. and *Plasmodium* sp. in mice pretreated with an extract of *Coxiella burnetii*. Infect. Immunol. **24:** 319–325.
41. WAAG, D.M., M. KENDE, T.A. DAMROW *et al.* 1990. Injection of inactivated phase I *Coxiella burnetii* increases non-specific resistance to infection and stimulates lymphokine production in mice. Ann. N.Y. Acad. Sci. **590:** 203–214.

AIRE-1 (Autoimmune Regulator Type 1) as a Regulator of the Thymic Induction of Negative Selection

YONGSOO PARK, YOOMI MOON, AND HEE-YONG CHUNG

Department of Internal Medicine and Microbiology, Hanyang University Hospital, Seoul, Korea

ABSTRACT: The monogenic autoimmune syndrome, APS-1 (autoimmune polyglandular syndrome type 1), is characterized by the loss of self-tolerance to multiple organs. Although mutations in the AIRE (autoimmune regulator) gene are responsible for the APS-1, the function of AIRE is not known. AIRE may determine thymic induction of tolerance to self-antigens in multiple organs. To study the function of AIRE in induction of self-tolerance, an *in vitro* negative selection system was made using 10^6 DO11.10 TCR transgenic thymocytes, 10^5 antigen-presenting cells (APC), and the different constructs of ovalbumin (OVA). In this system, the addition of the immunodominant epitopes of OVA peptide, the antigenic ligand for the DO11.10, made the thymocytes apoptotic and negatively selected. Overexpression of the AIRE gene in APC using retroviral transduction did not cause more thymocytes to become apoptotic. However, the suppression of the expression of AIRE in APC using the dominant-negative gene made the recovery rates of the thymocytes higher than those with the expression of LacZ as a control, and consequently inducing loss of self-tolerance. From these studies, it might be possible to suggest that the AIRE gene might regulate thymic induction of the negative selection process. The target genes for transcriptional regulation by AIRE have been investigated to study the influence of AIRE expression on other proteins in antigen presentation. The expression level of B7.1 was higher in APC expressing the dominant-negative form of AIRE. The target gene regulated by AIRE in transcription will be screened using cDNA microarray.

KEYWORDS: AIRE; negative selection; regulator

INTRODUCTION

Autoimmune diseases are a heterogeneous group of disorders whereby alterations in the immune system may result in a spectrum of diseases that either target specific organs or affect the body systemically. Recent epidemiological studies have described an increased susceptibility of people with one autoimmune disease to other autoimmune diseases. This co-occurrence of autoimmune diseases has been studied

---

Address for correspondence: Yongsoo Park, M.D., Department of Internal Medicine, Hanyang University Hospital, 249-1 Kyomun-dong, Kuri, Kyunggi-do, 471-020 Seoul, Korea. Voice: +82-31-560-2239; fax: +82-31-553-7369.
parkys@hanyang.ac.kr

because the existence of shared pathophysiological mechanisms is hypothesized. Although common susceptibility genes as well as shared environmental triggering factors might contribute to some of its susceptibility, polyclonal immune activation due to the loss of self-tolerance to multiple antigens in various organs might be a better explanation of polyendocrinopathy.[1] Self-antigen expression in the thymus is believed to play a role in the development of immunologic tolerance. Genetically determined variance in the levels of insulin expression in the thymus is associated with differences in susceptibility to type 1 diabetes (T1D).[2] IA-2 expression is differentially regulated in pancreas and thymus.[3] The autosomal recessive form of the co-occurrence of multiple autoimmune syndrome, APS-1 (autoimmune polyglandular syndrome type 1), is characterized by the loss of self-tolerance to multiple organs. Although mutations in the AIRE (autoimmune regulator) gene are responsible for the APS-1, the function of AIRE is not known.[4] AIRE may determine thymic induction of tolerance to self-antigens in multiple organs. Thus, applying the *in vitro* negative selection system, we evaluated the possible role of the AIRE gene in the thymic negative selection process, which led to the induction of self-tolerance, and characterized the target gene for transcriptional regulation by AIRE.

MATERIALS

Unless otherwise stated, all molecular cloning procedures were performed by standard protocols, and reagents were of analytical grade and purchased from Sigma (St. Louis, MO). To study the function of AIRE in induction of self-tolerance of an independent antigen, an *in vitro* thymic negative selection system was established using 10^6 DO11.10 TCR transgenic thymocytes, 10^5 A20 B cell lymphoma lines as APC (antigen-presenting cells), and the different constructs of ovalbumin (OVA). In this system, addition of the immunodominant epitopes of OVA peptide, the antigenic ligand for the DO11.10, made the thymocytes apoptotic and thus negatively selected.[5]

Overexpression of the AIRE gene in APC was induced using retroviral transduction. Suppression of the expression of AIRE in APC was made by using the dominant-negative gene. Three candidate dominant-negative AIRE genes were synthesized and cloned into MFG.ires.puro retroviral vector. Flag tag sequence was attached at the 3′-terminal to visualize the expressed proteins. HEK 293 cells were transduced with the vectors and the expression was detected by Western blot.

To test the influence of the dominant-negative gene on transcriptional activity of AIRE, a modified mammalian two-hybrid system was applied with pFR-Luc (5× GAL4-binding motif with luciferase as a reporter) and pCMV.BD.AIRE (expression vector for GAL4-binding domain and AIRE fusion protein) as basic components.

To explore possible influence on the level of antigen presentation, the surface expression level of B7.1 (CD80), B7.2 (CD86), class II MHC, LFA-1, LFA-3, and ICAM-1 was measured by flow cytometric analysis.

RESULTS

Out of three candidate dominant-negative AIRE genes cloned into MFG.ires.puro retroviral vector, only the constructs including the N-terminal half made the protein.

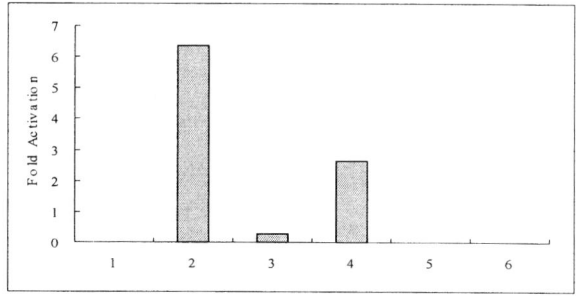

1. p FR-luc
2. p FR-luc + MFG.AIRE.ires.puro + p CMV-BD.AIRE(HA)
3. p FR-luc+ MFG.DN AIRE.ires.puro + p CMV-BD.AIRE(HA)
4. p FR-luc+ p CMV-BD.AIRE(HA)
5. Negative control
6. p FR-luc+ MFG.AIRE.ires.puro

FIGURE 1. The influence of the dominant-negative gene (aa 1–290) on transcriptional activating potential of AIRE. A modified mammalian two-hybrid system was applied with pFR-Luc (5× GAL4-binding motif with luciferase as a reporter) and pCMV.BD.AIRE (expression vector for GAL4-binding domain and AIRE fusion protein) as basic components.

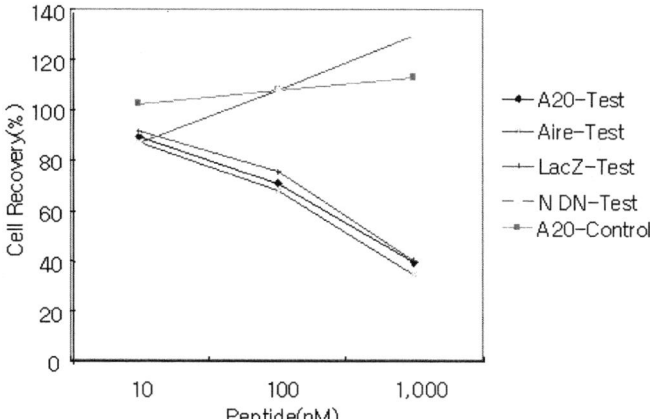

FIGURE 2. The influence of overexpression of the dominant-negative AIRE gene on *in vitro* thymocyte negative selection. An *in vitro* thymic negative selection system was established using 10^6 DO11.10 TCR transgenic thymocytes, 10^5 A20 B cell lymphoma lines as APC, and the different constructs of OVA. In this system, the addition of the immunodominant epitopes of OVA peptide, the antigenic ligand for the DO11.10, made the thymocytes apoptotic and thus negatively selected. "N DN" denotes the APC transduced with the dominant-negative AIRE gene (aa 1–290).

In A20 cells, only the dominant-negative gene of the N-terminal half (aa 1–290) (DN) provided a high level of protein expression and thus used for the suppression of the transcriptional activation of AIRE. The DN AIRE gene was tested for any inhibitory influence on the transcriptional activity over the wild-type AIRE gene, applying a modified mammalian two-hybrid system. There was modest activation of luciferase expression when both plasmids of pFR-Luc and pCMV.BD.AIRE were introduced into HEK 293 cells. When wild-type AIRE was overexpressed at the same time, the luciferase expression was further enhanced. However, overexpression of DN AIRE significantly suppressed the transcriptional activation potential of GAL4-AIRE fusion protein (FIG. 1).

We then made an *in vitro* negative selection system with thymocytes from OVA-specific TCR transgenic mice (DO11.10), with OVA peptide as antigen and A20 cells expressing the different types of AIRE genes as APC. When we measured the recovery rates of the thymocytes after incubating the DO11.10 thymocytes for 24 h in the presence OVA immunodominant peptide and A20 cells, a typical dose-response relationship was found as we increased the concentration of OVA. With this system, we measured thymocyte recovery rates at 1000 nM OVA peptide with A20 cells transduced with different AIRE genes. Overexpression of the AIRE gene did not cause more thymocytes to become apoptotic. However, suppression of the transcriptional activating capability of AIRE by the DN AIRE made the recovery rates of the thymocytes higher than those with the expression of LacZ as a control, indicating the induction of loss of self-tolerance (FIG. 2).

To explore possible influence of the DN AIRE gene expression on the difference in the level of antigen presentation, the surface expression level of B7.1, B7.2, class II MHC, LFA-1, LFA-3, and ICAM-1 was measured by flow cytometric analysis. Only the surface expression level of B7.1 was significantly higher in A20 cells expressing the DN AIRE gene. The expression levels of all other markers were similar between the A20 cells expressing the different types of AIRE.

DISCUSSION

Humans expressing a defective form of the transcription factor AIRE develop multiorgan autoimmune disease. We made an *in vitro* negative selection system and employed DN AIRE gene to influence the transcriptional activating capabilities of AIRE and the thymocyte apoptosis. As we expected, the overexpression of the DN AIRE gene suppressed the transcriptional activation of AIRE, and the APC expressing it was significantly less effective in inducing thymocyte apoptosis. The changes in the level of AIRE expression correlated with the apoptotic markers and, at present, did not seem to influence much on the other proteins in antigen presentation except the level of B7.1. Ultimately, the target gene regulated by AIRE in transcription will be screened (cDNA microarray). Although we have some limitations, these results highlight the importance of thymically imposed "central tolerance" in controlling autoimmunity. Two recent reports that AIRE-deficient mice exhibit autoimmune manifestations are consistent with our proposal, although one study concluded that a problem with peripheral lymphocyte homeostasis was at root[4] and the other concluded that the spectrum of autoimmunity manifested by the AIRE-deficient mice is due to a broad defect in central tolerance induction.[6] The latter report proposed that the AIRE regulates autoimmunity by promoting the ectopic expression of peripheral tissue-restricted antigens in medullary epithelial cells of the thymus. T cell tolerance to self-antigens is considered to reflect a combination of central and peripheral tolerance. Central tolerance leads to deletion of immature T cells in the thymus and is largely responsible for eliminating autoreactive T cells. However, for tissue-specific antigens, the limited representation of these antigens in the thymus is thought to preclude central tolerance. Our cDNA microarray will prove this hypothesis.

Our findings raise several issues. First, we employed an independent antigen, OVA, which is not usually involved in the autoimmune process of the APS-1. From our findings, we might argue that AIRE seems to broadly control central tolerance induction, although the spectrum of autoimmunity resulting from the loss of this transcription factor is quite defined. In both humans with APS-1 and the AIRE-deficient mice, there is disease heterogeneity between individuals and exacerbation with age. There are certain differences between the spectrum of organs targeted in the two cases. This could result from the influence of genetic modifiers. The true molecular mechanism by which AIRE controls thymic induction of self-tolerance should be pursued thoroughly. Second, we applied the A20 cells as an alternative to thymic medullary epithelial cells. We might have evaluated the possible role of the AIRE gene not only in the thymic negative selection process, but also in antigen presentation in general, and characterized the target gene for transcriptional regulation by AIRE-1. We established an *in vitro* negative selection system using thymocytes from DO11+ TcR Tg mice, IA-d-expressing A20 B cell lymphoma lines, and immunogenic OVA peptide. As expected, the influence of DN AIRE overexpression in the APC makes thymocytes less liable to die. However, we should confirm our finding using the thymic epithelial cells as APC.

ACKNOWLEDGMENTS

This work was supported by a grant from the Korea Science and Engineering Foundation (No. R01-2001-00177).

REFERENCES

1. BJORSES, P. *et al.* 1996. Genetic homogeneity of autoimmune polyglandular disease type I. Am. J. Hum. Genet. **59:** 879–886.
2. PUGLIESE, A. *et al.* 1997. The insulin gene is transcribed in the human thymus and transcription levels correlated with allelic variation at the INS VNTR-IDDM2 susceptibility locus for type 1 diabetes. Nat. Genet. **15:** 293–297.
3. PARK, Y. *et al.* 2000. Humoral autoreactivity to an alternatively spliced variant of ICA512/IA-2 in type 1 diabetes. Diabetologia **43:** 1293–1301.
4. RAMSEY, C. *et al.* 2002. AIRE deficient mice develop multiple features of APECED phenotype and show altered immune response. Hum. Mol. Genet. **11:** 397–409.
5. FERRERO, I. *et al.* 1998. Viral superantigen-induced negative selection of TCR transgenic CD4+ CD8+ thymocytes depends on activation, but not proliferation. Blood **91:** 4248–4254.
6. ANDERSON, M.S. *et al.* 2002. Projection of an immunological self-shadow within the thymus by the AIRE protein. Science **298:** 1395–1401.

Association of Interleukin-18 Gene Promoter Polymorphisms in Type 1 Diabetes and Autoimmune Thyroid Disease

AKANE IDE,[a] EIJI KAWASAKI,[b] NORIO ABIRU,[b] FUYAN SUN,[b]
TETSUYA FUKUSHIMA,[a] REIKO ISHII,[a] RYOKO TAKAHASHI,[a]
HIRONAGA KUWAHARA,[a] NARUHIRO FUJITA,[a] ATSUSHI KITA,[a]
MISA IMAIZUMI,[a] KATSUYA OSHIMA,[b] TOSHIRO USA,[a] SHIGEO UOTANI,[a]
ERI EJIMA,[a] HIRONORI YAMASAKI,[a] KIYOTO ASHIZAWA,[c]
YOSHIHIKO YAMAGUCHI,[a] AND KATSUMI EGUCHI[a]

[a]*First Department of Internal Medicine, Graduate School of Biochemical Sciences,*
[b]*Unit of Metabolism/Diabetes and Clinical Nutrition,*
[c]*Department of Radiation Biophysics, Atomic Bomb Disease Institute,*
Nagasaki University School of Medicine, Nagasaki, Japan

ABSTRACT: Type 1 diabetes is a heterogeneous autoimmune disease and is often associated with other organ-specific autoimmune diseases, including autoimmune thyroid disease (AITD). IL-18 is a potent proinflammatory cytokine capable of inducing IFN-γ production that is associated with the development of type 1 diabetes and AITD. The gene for IL-18 is located near *Idd2* and has been reported to be associated with a susceptibility to type 1 diabetes. To test the putative involvement of IL-18 gene polymorphism in predisposition to type 1 diabetes and AITD, we conducted a case-control study in Japanese population. The SNPs at position −607 (C/A) and −137 (G/C) in the promoter region of the IL-18 gene were analyzed by sequence-specific PCR in 74 nondiabetic patients with AITD, 47 type 1 diabetic patients with AITD, and 114 normal controls. There was no significant increase in the genotype and allele frequencies not only in nondiabetic patients with AITD compared with normal controls, but also in type 1 diabetic patients with AITD compared with normal controls. The distribution of IL-18 gene haplotypes was also similar between both patient groups and normal controls. These results suggest that polymorphisms of the IL-18 gene are not associated with a susceptibility to AITD and type 1 diabetes coexistent with AITD in Japanese population.

KEYWORDS: type 1 diabetes; autoimmune thyroid disease (AITD); IL-18; polymorphism; genetics; SNPs

Address for correspondence: Eiji Kawasaki, M.D., Ph.D., Unit of Metabolism/Diabetes and Clinical Nutrition, Nagasaki University School of Medicine, 1-7-1 Sakamoto, Nagasaki 852-8501, Japan. Voice: +81-95-849-7550; fax: +81-95-849-7552.
eijikawa@net.nagasaki-u.ac.jp

INTRODUCTION

Type 1 diabetes is an autoimmune disease characterized by T cell–mediated destruction of pancreatic β cells. A variety of environmental and genetic factors are involved in the development of the disease. Type 1 diabetes is frequently associated with other organ-specific autoimmune diseases and the most common coexisting organ-specific autoimmune disease in Japan is autoimmune thyroid disease (AITD). Previous studies have reported that the clinical and immunogenetic heterogeneity are present between type 1 diabetic patients with and without AITD.[1,2]

The cytokine interleukin-18 (IL-18), a member of the IL-1 superfamily, promotes development of Th1 response by induction of IFN-γ and is associated with the development of type 1 diabetes and AITD.[3] Indeed, it has been reported that the expression of IL-18 mRNA was increased in the pancreas of NOD mice after induction of diabetes by cyclophosphamide, suggesting that IL-18 could be a diabetogenic molecule in these animals.[4] The importance of IL-18 for the occurrence of type 1 diabetes is underscored by the observation that the murine IL-18 gene maps to an interval on chromosome 9 in the vicinity of the diabetes susceptibility gene from the NOD mouse, *Idd2*.[4]

Recently, several polymorphisms in the promoter region of the human IL-18 gene have been identified.[5] In this study, we addressed the question of whether the polymorphisms of the IL-18 gene contribute to the genetic risk for AITD or type 1 diabetes with AITD.

SUBJECTS AND METHODS

We studied 47 Japanese unrelated type 1 diabetic patients with AITD (19 men and 28 women; mean age at onset, 33.0 ± 18.2 years), 74 nondiabetic patients with AITD (14 men and 60 women; mean age, 54.0 ± 13.9 years), and 114 healthy control subjects after giving informed consent, and protocol was approved by the Institutional Review Board of the Nagasaki University School of Medicine. The diagnosis of type 1 diabetes and AITD was defined by both clinical features and laboratory data.

The single nucleotide polymorphisms (SNPs) at position −607 (C/A) and −137 (G/C) in the promoter region of the IL-18 gene were analyzed by sequence-specific PCR method as reported previously.[5] All PCR products were separated in 2% agarose gels stained with ethidium bromide.

Allele or haplotype frequencies were calculated on patients and control subjects by direct counting. Statistical analysis of the differences between groups was determined by χ^2 test or Fisher's exact probability test. Findings were considered to be statistically significant at a p value less than 0.05.

RESULTS

TABLE 1 shows the distribution of allele and genotype frequencies in the IL-18 gene polymorphisms in type 1 diabetic patients coexistent with AITD, nondiabetic patients with AITD, and healthy control subjects. The genotype distributions did not differ significantly between patient groups and healthy control subjects. There were

TABLE 1. Allele and genotype frequencies of IL-18 promoter gene polymorphisms in type 1 diabetic patients with AITD, nondiabetic patients with AITD, and healthy controls

	Type 1 diabetes with AITD ($n = 47$)	AITD ($n = 74$)	Healthy controls ($n = 114$)	P1	P2
Allele frequencies					
Locus −607					
C	41/94 (43.6)	66/148 (44.6)	102/228 (44.7)	0.854	0.978
A	53/94 (56.4)	82/148 (55.4)	126/228 (55.3)		
Locus −137					
G	85/94 (90.4)	131/148 (88.5)	202/228 (88.6)	0.632	0.980
C	9/94 (9.6)	17/148 (11.5)	26/228 (11.4)		
Genotype frequencies					
Locus −607					
CC	6 (12.8)	6 (8.1)	18 (15.8)	0.863	0.094
CA	29 (61.7)	54 (73.0)	66 (57.9)		
AA	12 (25.5)	14 (18.9)	30 (26.3)		
Locus −137					
GG	38 (80.9)	58 (78.4)	90 (78.9)	0.657	0.966
GC	9 (19.1)	15 (20.3)	22 (19.3)		
CC	0 (0)	1 (1.4)	2 (1.8)		
Haplotype frequencies					
Haplotype 1+	41 (87.2)	84 (73.7)	60 (81.1)	0.065	0.242
Haplotype 1−	6 (12.8)	30 (16.3)	14 (18.9)		
Haplotype 2+	9 (19.1)	24 (21.1)	16 (21.6)	0.834	1.000
Haplotype 2−	3 (80.9)	90 (78.9)	58 (78.4)		
Haplotype 3+	28 (59.6)	77 (67.5)	55 (74.3)	0.334	0.321
Haplotype 3−	19 (40.4)	37 (32.5)	19 (25.7)		

NOTE: Haplotypes 1, 2, and 3 indicate −137G/−607C, −137C/−607A, and −137G/−607A, respectively. Data are n (%). "+" or "−" indicates the presence or absence of a particular haplotype. P1, p value between type 1 diabetic patients with AITD vs. healthy controls. P2, p value between AITD vs. healthy controls.

no significant differences in the allele frequencies of −607C and −137G between them either. Furthermore, the frequencies of AITD patients with or without diabetes carrying each haplotype were not significantly different from those in healthy controls.

DISCUSSION

Recently, we and others demonstrated that the IL-18 gene polymorphisms are associated with the susceptibility to type 1 diabetes.[6,7] In this study, we analyzed the

IL-18 promoter gene polymorphisms in nondiabetic patients with AITD and type 1 diabetic patients with AITD. However, we found no differences in the allele, genotype, and haplotype frequencies of the IL-18 gene polymorphisms among type 1 diabetic patients with AITD, nondiabetic patients with AITD, and healthy control subjects.

Kaiser and coworkers reported that serum IL-18 levels were significantly increased in patients with Graves' disease. On the other hand, the serum IL-18 levels in Hashimoto's thyroiditis showed no significant differences compared to those in healthy subjects.[8] This indicates that IL-18 could play a part in the pathogenesis of AITD. In our study, even if we stratified the patients into Graves' disease and Hashimoto's thyroiditis, there were no differences in the allele and genotype frequencies of the IL-18 gene polymorphisms between AITD patients and healthy control subjects.

In conclusion, the results in this study suggest that IL-18 promoter gene polymorphisms are not associated with genetic susceptibility to AITD.

ACKNOWLEDGMENTS

We thank Ayako Kaneko for her skillful technical assistance.

REFERENCES

1. KAWASAKI, E. & S. NAGATAKI. 1996. Japanese type 1 diabetic syndrome. Diabetes Metab. Rev. **12:** 175–194.
2. KAWASAKI, E., H. TAKINO et al. 1994. Autoantibodies to glutamic acid decarboxylase in patients with IDDM and autoimmune thyroid disease. Diabetes **43:** 80–86.
3. NAKANISHI, K., T. YOSHIMOTO et al. 2001. Interleukin-18 is a unique cytokine that stimulates both Th1 and Th2 responses depending on its cytokine milieu. Cytokine Growth Factor Rev. **12:** 53–72.
4. ROTHE, H., N.A. JENKINS et al. 1997. Active stage of autoimmune diabetes is associated with the expression of a novel cytokine, IGIF, which is located near Idd2. J. Clin. Invest. **99:** 469–474.
5. GIEDRAITIS, V., B. HE et al. 2001. Cloning and mutation analysis of the human IL-18 promoter: a possible role of polymorphisms in expression regulation. J. Neuroimmunol. **112:** 146–152.
6. KRETOWSKI, A., K. MIRONCZUK et al. 2002. Interleukin-18 promoter polymorphisms in type 1 diabetes. Diabetes **51:** 3347–3349.
7. IDE, A., E. KAWASAKI et al. 2003. Association between interleukin-18 gene promoter polymorphisms and CTLA-4 gene 49 A/G polymorphism in Japanese patients with type 1 diabetes. J. Autoimmun. In press.
8. KAISER, P., L. ROTHWELL et al. 2000. Increased levels of serum interleukin-18 in Graves' disease. Thyroid **10:** 815–819.

Epitope Analysis of GAD65 Autoantibodies in Japanese Patients with Autoimmune Diabetes

EIJI KAWASAKI,[a] NORIO ABIRU,[a] AKANE IDE,[b] FUYAN SUN,[a]
TETSUYA FUKUSHIMA,[b] RYOKO TAKAHASHI,[b] HIRONAGA KUWAHARA,[b]
NARUHIRO FUJITA,[b] ATSUSHI KITA,[b] KATSUYA OSHIMA,[b] SHIGEO UOTANI,[b]
HIRONORI YAMASAKI,[b] YOSHIHIKO YAMAGUCHI,[b] AND KATSUMI EGUCHI[b]

[a]*Unit of Metabolism/Diabetes and Clinical Nutrition, Nagasaki University School of Medicine, Nagasaki, Japan*

[b]*First Department of Internal Medicine, Graduate School of Biochemical Sciences, Nagasaki University, Nagasaki, Japan*

ABSTRACT: Type 1 diabetes is an organ-specific autoimmune disease characterized by T cell–mediated destruction of pancreatic β cells. In Japanese population, the incidence of type 1 diabetes in children is very low compared to European countries. However, there are more patients with type 1 diabetes in adults, including latent autoimmune diabetes in adults (LADA). The circulating autoantibodies to multiple islet autoantigens including GAD, insulin, and IA-2 are the important immunological features of type 1 diabetes. The prevalences of anti-islet autoantibodies in patients with Japanese type 1 diabetes are 60–70% for GAD autoantibodies, 45–50% for insulin autoantibodies (IAA), and 60–65% for IA-2 autoantibodies at disease onset, which are similar to those reported in Caucasian patients. With combinatorial analysis of these autoantibodies, 90% of patients express at least one of these autoantibodies and are classified as type 1A diabetes. Although the majority of patients with type 1 diabetes are young, lean, and ketosis-prone, there are a number of patients with type 1 diabetes initially diagnosed as having type 2 diabetes at disease onset called LADA. These patients with LADA often progress toward an insulin-deficient state within several years after diagnosis. High levels of GAD autoantibodies have a high predictive value for future insulin deficiency in LADA. Further, epitope analysis of GAD65 autoantibodies may be helpful to predict future insulin dependency in LADA patients. In conclusion, Japanese patients with type 1 diabetes are clinically heterogeneous and the determination of immunological features are helpful to clarify the characteristics of the Japanese type 1 diabetic syndrome.

KEYWORDS: type 1 diabetes; autoantibodies; GAD; LADA; epitope; autoantigen

Address for correspondence: Eiji Kawasaki, M.D., Ph.D., Unit of Metabolism/Diabetes and Clinical Nutrition, Nagasaki University School of Medicine, 1-7-1 Sakamoto, Nagasaki 852-8501, Japan. Voice: +81-95-849-7550; fax: +81-95-849-7552.
eijikawa@net.nagasaki-u.ac.jp

INTRODUCTION

Multiple types of diabetes mellitus have been defined by the recent reports of an American Diabetes Association Expert Committee and a WHO Consultation based on our current understanding of pathogenesis rather than the requirement for insulin therapy.[1,2] Type 1 diabetes is often associated with chronic and progressive autoimmune destruction of islet β cells with a long prodromal phase. This type of type 1 diabetes is classified as "immune-mediated" (type 1A) diabetes. Another type of type 1 diabetes is a disease with no evidence of an autoimmune disorder at disease onset and is classified as "idiopathic" (type 1B) diabetes. On the other hand, type 2 diabetes results from a defect in insulin secretion, almost always with a major contribution from insulin resistance.

Type 1A diabetes is characterized by T cell–mediated destruction of β cells in genetically susceptible individuals[1] and is associated with the presence of autoantibodies to multiple islet cell antigens.[3] During the past decade, there has been a remarkable increase in the number of candidate genes for susceptibility of type 1 diabetes and biochemically defined autoantigens found to be targets of the autoimmune process. In accordance with the view that development of type 1 diabetes involves heterogeneous mechanisms, different clinical courses of β cell destruction have been reported in Japanese population. The most prevalent clinical classification of type 1 diabetes is abrupt-onset with severe clinical symptoms with ketoacidosis. The peak age of onset of type 1 diabetes in Japan is 10–12 years old, in accordance with the age-related distribution in the Caucasian population. Another subtype of type 1 diabetes in the Japanese population is a slow-onset form of diabetes having NIDDM at onset. Slow-onset patients with type 1 diabetes are also referred to as "latent autoimmune diabetes in adults (LADA)" or "slowly progressing IDDM".[4–6] LADA is a special subgroup of autoimmune diabetes, which could represent a late manifestation of type 1 diabetes.[4] The autoimmune destructive process is much slower, making it sometimes difficult to distinguish clinically between type 1 and type 2 diabetes. The development of clinical symptoms is often insidious, without features typical of type 1 diabetes such as severe polydipsia, polyuria, weight reduction, or ketoacidosis. Such patients who have a slowly evolving form of type 1 diabetes retain insulin secretion in their initial stage and are often diagnosed as having type 2 diabetes based on clinical features.[7] Recently, several studies have suggested that GAD autoantibodies might be useful as a predictive marker for the development of insulin-deficiency in type 2 diabetes in Caucasians and in Japanese as well.[4,8–10] The United Kingdom Prospective Diabetes Study (UKPDS) reported that, among patients with type 2 diabetes, the frequency of GAD autoantibodies was from 34% of those aged 25–35 at diagnosis to 7% of those aged 55–65. Of the patients with both ICA and GAD autoantibodies, 94% required insulin therapy versus only 14% without either autoantibody. These insulin-requiring type 2 diabetics with GAD autoantibodies may be classified as SPIDDM or LADA.[9] Takeda and coworkers have recently reported that GAD autoantibody-positive noninsulin-deficient patients differ from GAD autoantibody-positive patients with insulin deficiency with respect to clinical characteristics, humoral autoimmunity to other organ-specific autoimmunity, and HLA class II genes in Japanese population.

AUTOANTIBODIES TO MULTIPLE ISLET AUTOANTIGENS IN JAPANESE TYPE 1 DIABETES

A large number of biochemically defined autoantigens including insulin, GAD65, and ICA512/IA-2 have been found to be targets of the autoimmune process that precedes type 1 diabetes onset.[11] Expression of multiple autoantibodies confers a high risk for progression to type 1 diabetes.[12] We determined the distribution of autoantibodies to ICA512/IA-2, GAD, and insulin in Japanese type 1 diabetes patients. Of 73 new-onset patients, the prevalence was 71% for GAD autoantibodies, 48% for insulin autoantibodies (IAA), 62% for ICA512/IA-2 autoantibodies, and 62% for islet cell antibodies (ICA). Eighty-nine percent of patients with recent onset of type 1 diabetes expressed one or more of three autoantibodies. Of note, 8 out of 73 patients (11%) with type 1 diabetes were negative for all of these anti-islet autoantibodies and classified as having type 1B (idiopathic) diabetes (FIG. 1).[13] Furthermore, with comparison of diagnostic sensitivity for type 1 diabetes for the combined analysis of biochemically defined islet autoantibodies versus ICA measured by immunohistochemistry, the sensitivity for the diagnosis of type 1 diabetes was markedly increased when the test for GAD autoantibodies was used in addition to the tests for other islet autoantibodies. Thus, the test for GAD autoantibodies in addition to ICA512/IA-2 autoantibodies or IAA increased positivity to 86% and 79%, respectively. As expected, at equal specificity, the combined evaluation of autoantibodies to ICA512/IA-2, GAD, and insulin was more sensitive (89%) compared to ICA testing for diagnosis of type 1 diabetes.[13]

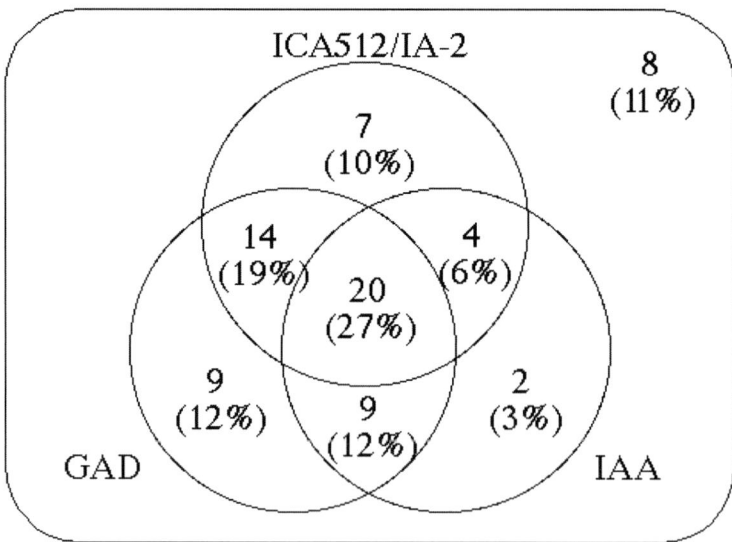

FIGURE 1. Combinatorial autoantibody analysis in Japanese new-onset patients with type 1 diabetes. Modified from ref. 13.

TABLE 1. Anti-islet autoantibodies in unselected patients with type 2 diabetes

Autoantibodies	Overall ($n = 648$)	Diet and/or OHA ($n = 357$)	Insulin-treated ($n = 291$)
GAD65	31 (4.8)	7 (2.0)	24 (8.2)**
ICA512/IA-2	7 (1.1)	1 (0.3)	6 (2.1)*
Insulin	101 (15.6)	12 (3.4)	89 (30.6)***
GAD65 or ICA512/IA-2	33 (5.1)	8 (2.2)	25 (8.6)**

NOTE: Data are n (%). OHA, oral hypoglycemic agent. *$p < 0.05$, **$p < 0.0005$, ***$p < 0.0001$ vs. diet and/or OHA group.

AUTOANTIBODIES TO MULTIPLE ISLET AUTOANTIGENS IN JAPANESE TYPE 2 DIABETES

Autoantibodies to GAD65, ICA512/IA-2, and insulin were evaluated in 648 unselected patients with type 2 diabetes. As illustrated in TABLE 1, the overall prevalence of autoantibodies to GAD65, ICA512/IA-2, and insulin was 4.8%, 1.1%, and 15.6%, respectively. The patients were stratified into two groups according to their current treatment of diabetes: diet and/or OHA ($n = 357$) and insulin-treated ($n = 291$). The frequency of GAD65 autoantibodies was significantly higher in insulin-treated patients compared to the noninsulin-treated group ($p < 0.0005$), as previously reported.[14] Furthermore, the frequency of ICA512/IA-2 autoantibodies in insulin-treated patients was also significantly higher than that in noninsulin-treated patients ($p < 0.05$, Fisher's exact test). These results suggest that not only GAD65 autoantibodies, but also ICA512/IA-2 autoantibodies may be a predictive marker for progression to insulin dependency in LADA patients. Of note, IAA were detected in 3.4% of noninsulin-treated patients, which was more frequent compared to GAD65 autoantibodies. With combinatorial analysis of autoantibodies to GAD65 and ICA512/IA-2, 25 of 291 patients (8.6%) with insulin treatment were positive for either of the autoantibodies.

It is very well known that type 1 diabetes is often associated with other organ-specific autoimmune diseases, including autoimmune thyroid disease (AITD), autoimmune atrophic gastritis, pernicious anemia, and Addison's disease. Furthermore, type 1 diabetic patients without clinical manifestations of organ-specific autoimmune disease have a markedly increased incidence of autoantibodies against other organs or tissues in their sera. Among these autoimmune diseases, the most common coexisting organ-specific autoimmune disease in Japanese patients with type 1 diabetes is AITD.[15,16] FIGURE 2 illustrates the frequency of antithyroid autoantibodies in type 2 diabetic patients with and without GAD autoantibodies. The prevalence of antithyroid autoantibodies in patients with GAD autoantibodies is 40–60%, which is significantly higher than that in GAD autoantibody-negative patients. These results indicate that immunological features of type 2 diabetes with GAD autoantibodies (LADA) are similar to those in classical type 1 diabetes in children.

In 1996, we commenced a longitudinal nationwide study of LADA by 14 centers across western Japan. A total of 2658 Japanese type 2 diabetic patients treated with diet and/or OHA were evaluated for GAD autoantibodies and assessed prospectively

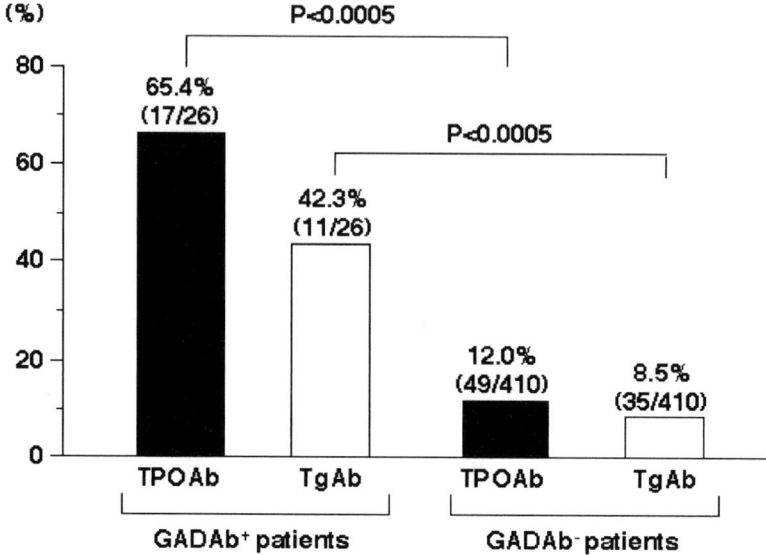

FIGURE 2. Frequency of antithyroid autoantibodies in type 2 diabetic patients with and without GAD autoantibodies. TPOAb: thyroid peroxidase autoantibodies; TgAb: thyroglobulin autoantibodies.

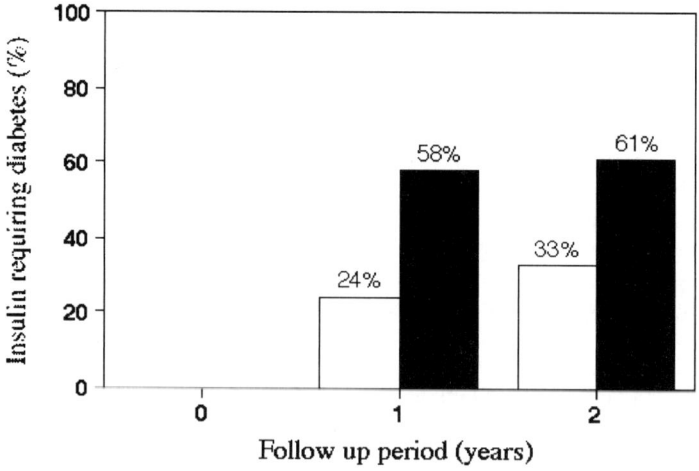

FIGURE 3. Relationship between levels of GAD autoantibodies and the progression to insulin-requiring diabetes in LADA patients. *Open bars*: GAD autoantibodies < 20 units/mL. *Solid bars*: GAD autoantibodies ≥ 20 units/mL. Adapted from ref. 17.

whether the presence of GAD autoantibodies could predict the requirement of future insulin treatment. The overall prevalence of GAD autoantibodies among patients with noninsulin-requiring diabetes was 2.0%, and 2.8% of the patients with disease duration of <5 years and 0.9% with a longer duration of diabetes. The patients with higher levels of GAD autoantibodies (≥20 units/mL) more often progressed to insulin dependency than the lower titer group (<20 units/mL) during the follow-up period.[17] As illustrated in FIGURE 3, the proportion of LADA patients who progressed to insulin-requiring diabetes was 61% in patients with higher levels of GAD autoantibodies compared to 33% in those with GAD autoantibodies at <20 units/mL.

ESTIMATION OF RISK FOR FUTURE INSULIN REQUIREMENT IN LADA

Although the high titer of GAD autoantibodies is a predictive marker of insulin dependency in LADA patients, there is a certain number of patients with high titer of GAD autoantibodies who do not progress to insulin dependency for many years. We estimated the predictive value of GAD autoantibody-positivity for future insulin requirement by Bayes' theorem. In our cross-sectional study on the clinical evaluation of noninsulin-dependent diabetic patients with GAD autoantibodies,[8] 38 of 583 diabetic patients (6.5%) initially diagnosed as having type 2 diabetes at onset subsequently progressed to insulin deficiency. Furthermore, the sensitivity of GAD autoantibodies in new-onset patients with type 1 diabetes is 70% in Japanese population. On the other hand, the specificity of GAD autoantibodies in diabetic patients with noninsulin-deficient state was 97.6%. Using these specificity figures for calculation of the positive predictive value, around two-thirds of diabetic patients initially diagnosed as having type 2 diabetes positive for GAD autoantibodies progress toward insulin deficiency (positive predictive value of 67.1%).

EPITOPE ANALYSIS OF GAD65 AUTOANTIBODIES IN AUTOIMMUNE DIABETES

FIGURE 4 shows a schematic representation of the chimeric molecules used in this study. Chimeric molecules were generated by substitution of regions of human GAD65 with homologous regions of GAD67, an isoform of GAD that is not a major autoantigen in type 1 diabetes. To evaluate the immunoreactivity to the amino-terminal region of GAD65, we used the cDNA coding for a chimeric molecule containing the amino-terminal region of GAD65 (aa 1–245) in fusion with the central/carboxy-terminal regions of GAD67 (aa 253–594), designated 65/67/67. This chimeric molecule and the cDNA of a $GAD67_{1-253}/GAD65_{245-585}$ (67/65/65) were constructed by taking advantage of the single NarI site of GAD65 and GAD67 cDNA and of the ApaI site in the pGEM-T vector.

The cDNA of a $GAD67_{1-451}/GAD65_{443-585}$ (67/67/65) chimera was constructed first by primer extension of a fragment coding for $GAD67_{1-451}$ in pGEM-T vector using an SP6 primer and a primer containing an StuI recognition sequence immediately downstream of the stop codon. Then, by taking advantage of the single StuI site in GAD65 and of the ApaI site in the vector, the ApaI/StuI-cut-amplified $GAD67_{1-451}$

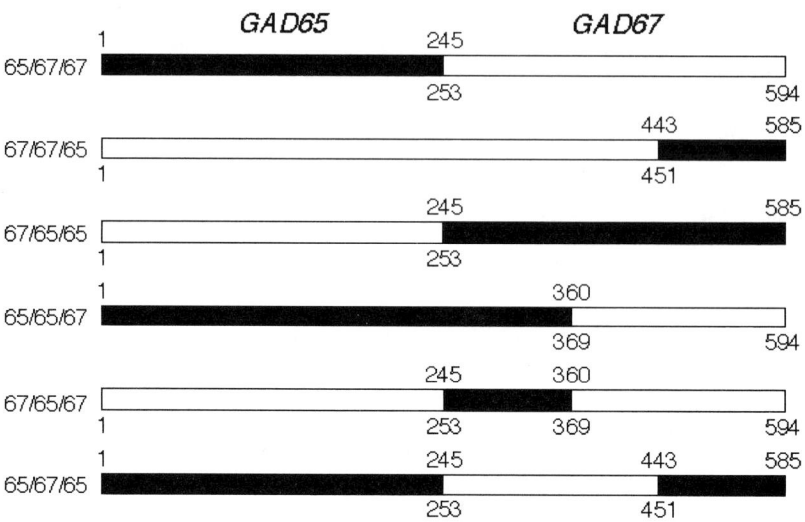

FIGURE 4. Schematic representation of the chimeric molecules used in this study. Numbers are amino acid positions in human GAD65 or GAD67 cloned from a human islet cDNA library.[19,20]

DNA fragment was cloned into the *Apa*I/*Stu*I-cut GAD65 cDNA in pGEM-T vector. This molecule detects antibodies reactive with the carboxy-terminal epitope of GAD65.

The cDNA of a $GAD65_{1-360}/GAD67_{369-594}$ (65/65/67) chimera was constructed first by primer extension of a fragment coding for $GAD67_{369-594}$ in pGEM-T vector using a T7 primer and a primer containing a *Bgl*II recognition sequence immediately upstream of the GAD67 coding sequence. Then, by taking advantage of the single *Bgl*II site in GAD65 and of the *Apa*I site in the vector, the *Apa*I/*Bgl*II-cut-amplified $GAD67_{369-594}$ DNA fragment was cloned into the *Apa*I/*Bgl*II-cut GAD65 cDNA in pGEM-T vector. The cDNA of a $GAD67_{1-253}/GAD65_{245-360}/GAD67_{369-594}$ (67/65/67) chimera was constructed by taking advantage of a single *Nar*I site in the $GAD65_{1-360}/GAD67_{369-594}$ (65/65/67) chimera. Furthermore, the cDNA of a $GAD65_{1-245}/GAD67_{253-451}/GAD65_{443-585}$ (65/67/65) chimera was constructed by taking advantage of a single *Bgl*II site in the $GAD65_{1-360}/GAD67_{369-594}$ (65/65/67) chimera.

The full-length GAD65, GAD67, and chimeric constructs were transcribed and translated *in vitro* in the presence of ^{35}S-methionine (Amersham International, Amersham, Bucks, United Kingdom; >1000 Ci/mmol) using the TNT-coupled rabbit reticulocyte lysate system (Promega) with SP6 RNA polymerase.

Serum reactivity to a series of GAD constructs were determined by radioligand binding assays in a 96-well assay format as described previously with some modifications.[18] In brief, *in vitro* translated ^{35}S-protein (20,000 cpm of TCA precipitable protein) was incubated with human sera in duplicate at a 1:25 dilution overnight at 4°C, and the antibody-bounded and free antigen were separated by Protein A–

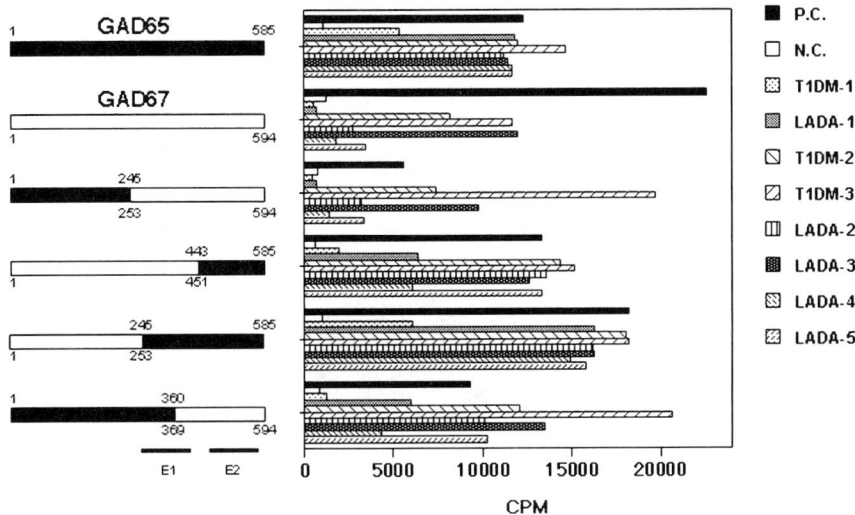

FIGURE 5. Immunoprecipitation (cpm) of human GAD65, human GAD67, and GAD65/GAD67 chimeric molecules with sera from patients with autoimmune diabetes. P.C., positive control serum; N.C., negative control serum; T1DM, typical type 1 diabetes; LADA, latent autoimmune diabetes in adults. The reactivity to each GAD65/GAD67 chimeric molecule was analyzed with competition by recombinant GAD67.

Sepharose 4FF (Pharmacia, Freiburg, Germany). Then, radioactivity was determined with a 96-well microplate scintillation counter (MLC-2001, ALOKA Co., Tokyo, Japan). Because sera double-positive for autoantibodies to GAD65 and GAD67 recognized all of these chimeric molecules, the serum reactivity to chimeric molecules was analyzed by competition assay using recombinant GAD67. For competition studies of autoantibody binding to chimeric GAD65/GAD67 molecules, sera were preincubated with the bacterially produced and purified recombinant GAD67 to absorb the reactivity to GAD67 epitopes followed by the addition of *in vitro* translated ^{35}S-labeled protein.

FIGURE 5 illustrates the representative reactivity to full-length GAD65, GAD67, and chimeric GAD65/GAD67 molecules in sera from autoimmune diabetes. With competition by recombinant GAD67 protein, two major epitopes recognized by GAD65-specific autoantibodies were found, designated epitope 1 (E1, aa 245–360) and epitope 2 (E2, aa 443–585), in sera from patients with type 1 diabetes and LADA. Now, the nationwide prospective study is under way to identify the GAD65 autoantibody epitope(s) for prediction of insulin dependency in LADA patients.

CONCLUSIONS

It is now possible to predict the ongoing β cell destruction using combined measurement of autoantibodies to multiple islet autoantigens. A remarkable number of new agents for immunotherapy are being introduced into clinical practice for autoimmune diseases. If a safe and effective therapy is identified, we should consider the use of agents for high-risk individuals to prevent development of type 1 diabetes as well as for the patients with type 1 diabetes in adults who are often diagnosed as having type 2 diabetes to preserve residual β cell function.

REFERENCES

1. AMERICAN DIABETES ASSOCIATION. 1997. Report of the Expert Committee on the Diagnosis and Classification of Diabetes Mellitus. Diabetes Care **20:** 1183–1197.
2. ABIRU, N. & G.S. EISENBARTH. 2000. Multiple genes/multiple autoantigens role in type 1 diabetes. Clin. Rev. Allergy Immunol. **18:** 27–40.
3. KAWASAKI, E. & G.S. EISENBARTH. 1996. Multiple autoantigens in the prediction and pathogenesis of type I diabetes. Diabet. Nutr. Metab. **9:** 188–198.
4. ZIMMET, P.Z. et al. 1994. Latent autoimmune diabetes mellitus in adults (LADA): the role of antibodies to glutamic acid decarboxylase in diagnosis and prediction of insulin dependency. Diabet. Med. **11:** 299–303.
5. KOBAYASHI, T. et al. 1993. Immunogenetics and clinical characterization of slowly progressive IDDM. Diabetes Care **16:** 780–788.
6. URAKAMI, T. et al. 1989. Type I (insulin-dependent) diabetes in Japanese children is not a uniform disease. Diabetologia **32:** 312–315.
7. KAWASAKI, E., Y. YAMAGUCHI & S. NAGATAKI. 1999. Insulitis in an autoimmune-mediated patient originally classified as having type 2 diabetes. Diabetes Care **22:** 541–542.
8. ABIRU, N. et al. 1996. Clinical evaluation of non-insulin-dependent diabetes mellitus patients with autoantibodies to glutamic acid decarboxylase. J. Autoimmun. **9:** 683–688.
9. TURNER, R. et al. 1997. UKPDS 25: autoantibodies to islet-cell cytoplasm and glutamic acid decarboxylase for prediction of insulin requirement in type 2 diabetes—UK Prospective Diabetes Study Group. Lancet **350:** 1288–1293.
10. TUOMI, T. et al. 1999. Clinical and genetic characteristics of type 2 diabetes with and without GAD antibodies. Diabetes **48:** 150–157.
11. LESLIE, R.D., M.A. ATKINSON & A.L. NOTKINS. 1999. Autoantigens IA-2 and GAD in type 1 (insulin-dependent) diabetes. Diabetologia **42:** 3–14.
12. VERGE, C.F. et al. 1996. Prediction of type I diabetes in first-degree relatives using a combination of insulin, GAD, and ICA512bdc/IA-2 autoantibodies. Diabetes **45:** 926–933.
13. SERA, Y. et al. 1999. Autoantibodies to multiple islet autoantigens in patients with abrupt onset type 1 diabetes and diabetes diagnosed with urinary glucose screening. J. Autoimmun. **13:** 257–265.
14. NAGATAKI, S., N. ABIRU & E. KAWASAKI. 1995. Type 1 Diabetes in Non-Insulin-Dependent Diabetes Mellitus in Japan. Elsevier Science. Amsterdam/New York.
15. MIMURA, G. et al. 1990. Immunogenetics of early-onset insulin-dependent diabetes mellitus among the Japanese—HLA, Gm, BF, GLO, and organ-specific autoantibodies: the J.D.S. Study. Diabetes Res. Clin. Pract. **8:** 253–262.
16. KAWASAKI, E. & S. NAGATAKI. 1996. Japanese type 1 diabetic syndrome. Diabetes Metab. Rev. **12:** 175–194.
17. TAKINO, H. et al. 2002. Antibodies to GAD in Japanese patients classified as type 2 diabetes at diagnosis: high titer of GAD Ab is a predictive marker for early insulin treatment—report of West Japan (Kyushu, Yamaguchi, Osaka) Study for GAD Ab(+) diabetes. Diabet. Med. **19:** 730–734.
18. KAWASAKI, E. et al. 2001. Association between IA-2 autoantibody epitope specificities and age of onset in Japanese patients with autoimmune diabetes. J. Autoimmun. **17:** 323–331.
19. KAWASAKI, E. et al. 1993. Cloning and expression of large isoform of glutamic acid decarboxylase from human pancreatic islet. Biochem. Biophys. Res. Commun. **192:** 1353–1359.
20. YANO, M. et al. 1995. Autoantibodies against glutamic acid decarboxylase 65 in Japanese patients with insulin-dependent diabetes mellitus (IDDM). J. Autoimmun. **8:** 83–96.

Index of Contributors

Abiru, N., 205–210, 218–221, 344–347, 436–439, 440–448
Ahn, Y., 242–249
Ali, C., 157–160
Anderson, J.A., 237–241
Andersson, A., 356–358
Ashizawa, K., 344–347, 436–439
Atkinson, M., 1–12, 237–241

Babu, S., 205–210, 301–309, 340–343, 348–351
Balaji, M., 387–389
Balaji, V., 387–389
Bao, F., 205–210, 340–343, 348–351
Barnett, A.H., 356–358
Barriga, K., 301–309
Bathjat, K., 184–186
Bedian, V., 259–264, 265–268
Behme, M.T., 226–229, 374–377
Bilbao, J.R., 314–318, 319–323
Boehm, B.O., 288–294
Bonifacio, E., 1–12
Bradley, B., 43–54
Bradley, J., 192–195
Branisteanu, D.D., 215–217
Brantley, M., 400–403
Brezner, K., 222–225
Bugawan, T.L., 301–309
Burkhardt, B.R., 237–241

Calvo, B., 314–318, 319–323
Cardozo, A.K., 55–74
Castaño, L., 314–318, 319–323
Charlton, B., 161–165, 423–430
Chen, M., 409–411
Chung, H.-Y., 242–249, 431–435
Clare-Salzler, M.J., 184–186, 222–225
Colman, P.G., 370–373
Cowden, W., 161–165, 423–430
Crawford, J.M., 237–241

Dai, R., 233–236
Darville, M., 55–74
de Nanclares, G.P., 314–318, 319–323

Decallonne, B., 176–177, 215–217
Deeg, M., 288–294
Demeterco, C., 138–147
Dinarello, C.A., 332–339
Donadi, E., 310–313
Donoso-Mantke, O., 170–175
Dupré, J., 374–377
Durinovic-Belló, I., 288–294

Eguchi, K., 218–221, 344–347, 436–439, 440–448
Eiermann, T., 288–294
Eisenbarth, G.S., xiii, 1–12, 109–118, 187–191, 205–210, 218–221, 301–309, 340–343, 348–351
Eizirik, D.L., 55–74
Ejima, E., 344–347, 436–439
El-Kabbani, O., 250–252
Ellett, J.D., 409–411
Ellis, T.M., 237–241
Erlich, H.A., 301–309

Fadok, V., 43–54
Fain, P.R., 340–343, 348–351
Fälth-Magnusson, K., 269–274
Fenalti, G., 250–252
Fialkow, L.B., 409–411
Finco-Kent, D., 259–264, 265–268
Flores, S., 43–54
Flotte, T.R., 237–241
Foley, J., 259–264, 265–268
Fourlanos, S., 370–373
Fredriksson, J., 404–408
Fujisawa, T., 196–204
Fujita, N., 344–347, 436–439, 440–448
Fukushima, T., 344–347, 436–439, 440–448

Gallinger, S., 400–403
Gelderblom, H.R., 170–175
Gerling, I.C., 157–160
Geron, I., 138–147
Ghosh, S., 279–283, 284–287
Glass, M., 400–403

Glimcher, L.H., 187–191
Goodnow, C., 178–183
Goudy, K.S., 237–241
Gowan, K., 340–343, 348–351
Gray, R., 250–252
Greiner, D.L., 148–156

Hagopian, W., 400–403
Hanif, M.W., 356–358
Hao, E., 138–147
Harris, S.B., 374–377
Harrison, L.C., 370–373
Haskins, K., 43–54
Hayakawa, T., 218–221
Hessner, M.J., 279–283, 284–287
Hettiarachchi, K.D., 418–422
Hirose, H., 328–331
Holm, P., 352–355
Holmberg, H., 269–274
Hörnfeldt, B., 170–175
Hramiak, I.M., 374–377
Hyöty, H., 13–22

Ide, A., 344–347, 436–439, 440–448
Ikegami, H., 196–204
Imaizumi, M., 344–347, 436–439
Irie, J., 211–214, 230–232, 359–361, 378–386
Ishii, R., 344–347, 436–439
Itkin-Ansari, P., 138–147

Jailwala, P., 284–287
Juedes, A.E., 128–137

Kalbacher, H., 288–294
Kanatsuka, A., 362–369
Kanungo, A., 390–394
Karges, W., 288–294
Kasuga, A., 362–369
Kawabata, T., 259–264, 265–268
Kawasaki, E., 218–221, 344–347, 436–439, 440–448
Kench, J., 43–54
Khoo, H.-J., 279–283, 284–287
Kilberg, M.S., 237–241
Kim, D., 253–258
Kim, S.-H., 332–339

Kita, A., 344–347, 436–439, 440–448
Kobayashi, T., 362–369
Kockum, I., 352–355
Kodama, K., 211–214, 378–386
Krasner, A., 259–264, 265–268
Kumar, S., 356–358
Kutlu, B., 55–74
Kuwahara, H., 344–347, 436–439, 440–448
Kwok, W.W., 82–87

Lenchik, N., 157–160
Lernmark, Å., 170–175
Lesage, S., 178–183
Levine, F., 138–147
Li, Y., 184–186, 222–225
Ling, X., 43–54
Liss, P-E., 395–399
Litherland, S., 222–225
Liu, E., 187–191, 205–210, 218–221
Loiler, S.A., 237–241
Ludeman, J.P., 418–422
Ludvigsson, J., 269–274, 275–278, 295–300, 395–399, 404–408
Luthman, H., 352–355

Mahon, J.L., 226–229, 374–377
Maisel, N., 288–294
Makino, S., 196–204
Mandrup-Poulsen, T., 32–42, 332–339
Markees, T.G., 148–156
Martin, A.K., 340–343, 348–351
Martín-Pagola, A., 314–318
Maruyama, T., 230–232, 324–327, 328–331, 362–369, 378–386
Mataverde, P., 233–236
Mathews, C.E., 412–417
Mathieu, C., 176–177, 215–217
Matsubara, K., 378–386
Matsunaga, S., 324–327
McDevitt, H., 75–81
Melanitou, E., 187–191, 205–210
Miao, D., 187–191, 205–210, 218–221
Mizuguchi, H., 218–221
Moon, Y., 431–435
Mordes, J.P., 148–156
Morimoto, J., 211–214, 378–386
Moriyama, H., 205–210
Morrone, A., 259–264

INDEX OF CONTRIBUTORS

Motohashi, Y., 230–232, 324–327
Moxness, M., 259–264, 265–268
Myers, M.A., 250–252, 418–422

Nadler, J.L., 409–411
Nagayama, Y., 218–221
Nakagawa, Y., 230–232, 359–361, 378–386
Narumi, S., 359–361
Nepom, G.T., 82–87
Niedrig, M., 170–175
Nikitina-Zake, L., 310–313
Niklasson, B., 170–175
Nolsøe, R.L., 332–339
Novick, D., 332–339
Nyholm, E., 170–175

Oberste, S., 23–31
Ogihara, T., 196–204
Oikawa, Y., 211–214, 230–232, 359–361, 378–386
Oshima, K., 218–221, 344–347, 436–439, 440–448
Overbergh, L., 215–217

Padaiga, Z., 295–300
Pallansch, M.A., 23–31
Park, C.-K., 242–249
Park, H., 242–249, 253–258
Park, Y., 242–249, 253–258, 431–435
Paronen, J., 205–210
Pati, N., 279–283
Pearson, T., 148–156
Peng, H., 400–403
Peng, R., 184–186, 222–225
Peterson, L.B., 148–156
Petrovsky, N., 161–165, 178–183, 423–430
Pierce, M.A., 148–156
Pietropaolo, M., 412–417
Pietropaolo, S.L., 412–417
Pociot, F., 332–339
Powers, K., 43–54
Pugazhenthi, S., 43–54

Rasschaert, J., 55–74
Reddy, S., 166–169, 192–195
Reijonen, H., 82–87

Reusch, J., 43–54
Rewers, A., 301–309
Rjasanowski, I., 98–108
Roberts, C.M., 340–343, 348–351
Ross, J.M., 166–169, 192–195
Rossini, A.A., 148–156
Rowley, M.J., 250–252
Rubinstein, M., 332–339

Sadauskaite-Kuehne, V., 295–300
Salminen, K., 13–22
Sanjeevi, C.B., xiii, 295–300, 310–313, 356–358, 387–389, 390–394
Santamaria, P., 88–97
Saruta, T., 211–214, 230–232, 324–327, 328–331, 359–361, 378–386
Scealy, M., 250–252
Schlosser, M., 98–108, 288–294
Serreze, D.V., 148–156
Seshiah, V., 387–389
Shigihara, T., 324–327, 328–331, 359–361
Shimada, A., 211–214, 230–232, 324–327, 328–331, 359–361, 362–369, 378–386
Shultz, L.D., 148–156
Sikora, K., 205–210
Silva, D., 161–165, 178–183, 423–430
Singh, B., 226–229
Skundric, D.S., 233–236
Socha, L., 161–165, 178–183
Stene, M., 259–264, 265–268
Stevens, J., 400–403
Stolt, U.G., 395–399
Strebelow, M., 98–108
Summers, K.L., 226–229
Sun, F., 218–221, 344–347, 436–439, 440–448
Suzuki, R., 211–214

Takahashi, R., 344–347, 436–439, 440–448
Takei, I., 362–369
Tauriainen, S., 13–22
Thomas, J., 1–12
Tica, V., 310–313, 356–358
Tong, J.C., 250–252
Tsumura, K., 359–361
Tyrberg, B., 138–147

Uotani, S., 344–347, 436–439, 440–448
Usa, T., 344–347, 436–439

Vaarala, O., 269–274, 404–408
Valsamakis, G., 356–358
Vázquez, F., 314–318, 319–323
Veys, K., 295–300
Vitoria, J.C., 314–318, 319–323
von Herrath, M.G., 128–137

Wahlberg, J., 404–408
Wang, T.B., 301–309
Wang, X., 279–283, 284–287
Wang, Y., 284–287
Wasserfall, C., 1–12
Wassmuth, R., 98–108
Waukau, J., 284–287
Wicker, L.S., 148–156

Wilson, A.J., 418–422
Wilson, C.R., 418–422
Wion, E., 400–403
Wu, R., 409–411
Wucherpfennig, K.W., 119–127

Yamada, S., 211–214, 230–232, 324–327, 328–331
Yamaguchi, Y., 344–347, 436–439, 440–448
Yamasaki, H., 218–221, 344–347, 436–439, 440–448
Yang, Z., 409–411
Yokoyama, J., 362–369
Yoo, E., 253–258
Yu, L., 1–12, 187–191

Ziegler, M., 98–108
Zimmet, P.Z., 418–422